Juliet Nichols, MD.

CLINICAL
NEUROLOGY
for
PSYCHIATRISTS

FOURTH EDITION

CLINICAL NEUROLOGY for PSYCHIATRISTS

DAVID MYLAND KAUFMAN, M.D.

Department of Neurology
Montefiore Medical Center
Albert Einstein College of Medicine
Bronx, New York

Juliet Nichols, M.D.

W.B. SAUNDERS COMPANY

A Division of Harcourt Brace & Company

Philadelphia, London, Toronto, Montreal, Sydney, Tokyo

W. B. SAUNDERS COMPANY
A Division of Harcourt Brace & Company

The Curtis Center
Independence Square West
Philadelphia, PA 19106

Library of Congress Cataloging-in-Publication Data

Kaufman, David Myland.
    Clinical neurology for psychiatrists / David Myland Kaufman. — 4th ed.
        p.   cm.
    Includes bibliographal references and index.
    ISBN 0-7216-5829-6
    1. Nervous system—Diseases.   2. Neurology.   3. Psychiatrists. I. Title.
    [DNLM: 1. Nervous System Diseases—psychology. WL 140 K21c 1995]
    RC346.K38   1995
    616.8—dc20
    DNLM/DLC   94-46917

CLINICAL NEUROLOGY FOR PSYCHIATRISTS   ISBN   0–7216–5829–6

Printed in the United States of America.

Last digit is the print number: 9   8   7   6   5   4

*This is dedicated
to the ones I love—*
MY FAMILY:
my wife of 25 years, Rita, and
our three children,
Rachel, Jennifer, and Sarah

ACKNOWLEDGMENTS

For this edition, Ms. Abigail Geman and Drs. Marc Klafter, David Steiner, and Steven Wolf have provided helpfully critical editorial advice. Artists Ms. Meryl Ranzer, Mr. Barry Morden, and Ms. Ann Mannato captured the sense of neurology in their wonderful illustrations.

My students, housestaff, and colleagues at Montefiore Medical Center/Albert Einstein College of Medicine have provided valuable contributions and reviews of each chapter, question and answer sets, and course that gave rise to this book, "Clinical Neurology for Psychiatrists."

My thanks also to Berta Steiner and her staff at Bermedica Production, Ltd. for so capably producing this edition.

NOTES ABOUT REFERENCES

Most chapters provide specific references from the neurologic and general medical literature. Some standard, well-written textbooks contain appropriate information about many topics:

Adams RD, Victor M: Principles of Neurology (5th ed.). New York, McGraw-Hill, Inc., 1993.

Barclay L (Ed.): Clinical Geriatric Neurology. Lea & Febiger, Philadelphia, 1993.

Fenichel GM: Clinical Pediatric Neurology: A Signs and Symptoms Approach (2 ed.). Philadelphia, W. B. Saunders, 1993.

Fitzgerald MJT: Neuroanatomy: Basic and Clinical. Philadelphia, Baillière Tindal, 1992.

Goldstein PJ, Stern (Eds.): Neurological Disorders of Pregnancy, (2nd ed.). Mount Kisco, NY, Futura Publishing, 1992.

Heilman KM, Valenstein E: Clinical Neuropsychology, (3rd ed.). New York, Oxford University Press, 1993.

Kaufman DM, Solomon G, Pfeffer C (Eds.): Child and Adolescent Neurology for Psychiatrists. Baltimore, Williams & Wilkins, 1992.

Joynt RJ (Ed.): Clinical Neurology. Philadelphia, J.B. Lippincott Co., 1994.

Rowland L (Ed.): Merritt's Textbook of Neurology (8 ed.). Philadelphia, Lea & Febiger, 1989.

Swaiman KF: Pediatric Neurology: Principles and Practice (2nd ed.). St. Louis, The C.V. Mosby Co., 1994.

PREFACE

I have written *Clinical Neurology for Psychiatrists*, from my perspective as a neurologist at a major teaching hospital, as a collegial, straight-forward guide. In a format combining traditional neuroanatomic correlations with symptom-oriented discussions, the book should help the reader learn about neurologic illnesses that are common, illustrate a principle, and cause or mimic psychiatric symptoms. Having evolved from the course by the same name that I founded in 1971, the book should also help prepare readers for specialty examinations, particularly the one given by the American Board of Psychiatry and Neurology.

The first half of the book reviews classical anatomic neurology and describes how a physician might approach patients with a suspected neurologic disorder, identify central or peripheral nervous system disease, and correlate physical signs. The second half discusses clinical areas. For each area, chapters describe the relevant history and neurologic findings, easily performed office and bedside examinations, appropriate laboratory tests, differential diagnosis, and, where appropriate, suggestions for management.

One feature of this book is its visual approach. Each chapter includes abundant illustrations because they help explain neuroanatomy, reinforce or personify clinical descriptions, best describe several uncommon but important disorders, and serve as the basis for question-based learning. Moreover, despite the availability of highly sophisticated procedures, the diagnosis of entire categories of neurologic illnesses, such as gait abnormalities, psychogenic neurologic deficits, neurocutaneous disorders, and facial dyskinesias, relies almost entirely on observation or "diagnosis by inspection." In fact, many highly sophisticated procedures – computed tomography (CT), magnetic resonance imaging (MRI), and electroencephalography (EEG) – are visual records, which are also reproduced.

Many chapters are supplemented with outlines of the relevant history; reproductions of standard tests, such as the Blessed Mental Status Test, Mini-mental Status Test, hand-held visual acuity card, and Abnormal Involuntary Movement Scale (AIMS); and references to recent articles, reviews, and classic studies. Appendices contain information that pertain to virtually every chapter: Patient and Family Support Groups (Appendix 1), Expenses for Tests and Common Treatments (Appendix 2), Chromosome and Mitochondria Abnormalities, which are cross-referenced with the illnesses they produce (Appendix 3). Readers are expected to consult these lists without constant prompting.

Another feature of the book is its question-based learning. Most chapters and two review sections are followed by short-answer, essay, or illustrated questions. They are an integral part of this book's teaching, not just preparation for examinations. Question-based learning reflects current medical school teaching where questions following case presentations draw students into an interactive educational process.

The first three editions of *Clinical Neurology for Psychiatrists* have enjoyed considerable success in the United States, Canada, and abroad. The book has been translated into Japanese and Italian. For the fourth edition, which has been rewritten five years after the previous edition, I have included advances in etiology, diagnosis, and treatment that have occurred in virtually all subjects; added still more illustrations; and, while keeping the book to a manageable size, introduced or greatly expanded the following topics:

- Muscle diseases and molecular genetics, including mitochondria muscle disorders.
- Neurotransmitters and their NMDA receptors.
- Head trauma: the post-concussive syndrome and whiplash injuries.
- Sleep disorders and the new American Sleep Disorder Association classification.
- Pediatric neurology: myelomeningocele and other neural tube defects, Rett and fragile X syndromes, and dopa-responsive dystonia.
- Illnesses where major advances have taken place: Parkinson's, Huntington's, and Alzheimer's diseases.
- Recently described diseases: post-polio syndrome, AIDS dementia, Lyme disease, and chronic fatigue syndrome.
- New diagnostic tests: visual analogue scales for pain, SPECT, and thermography.
- New treatments for headaches, epilepsy, dementia, impotence, pain, mental aberrations in Parkinson's disease, and focal dystonias.

DAVID MYLAND KAUFMAN, M.D.

CONTENTS

Physician-Readers, Please Note:

Clinical Neurology for Psychiatrists discusses current, effective, and relatively safe medications, testing, procedures, and other aspects of medical care. However, these discussions are not recommendations and are not intended to apply to individual patients. The physician must be responsible for indications, dosage, contraindications, precautions, side effects, and alternatives, including doing nothing. Some aspects of medical care are widely and successfully used for particular purposes not approved by the Food and Drug Administration (FDA) or other review panel. In regard to these unorthodox treatments, as well as conventional ones, this book is merely reporting on neurologists' use of various medicines, diagnostic techniques, and other aspects of their practice.

DAVID MYLAND KAUFMAN, M.D.

CLASSICAL ANATOMIC NEUROLOGY

1 First Encounter with a Patient: Examination and Formulation

Despite the ready availability of sophisticated tests, the neurologic examination remains the fundamental aspect of the specialty. Beloved by neurologists, their examination provides a vivid portrayal of function and illness. When neurologists say they have seen a case of a particular illness, they mean that they have really *seen* it.

Although patients' histories often suggest certain neurologic illnesses, psychiatrists should be familiar with the neurologic examination. Even if they themselves will not actually be examining patients, psychiatrists should appreciate certain neurologic signs and be able to assess a neurologist's conclusion.

Physicians should examine patients systematically. They should test interesting areas in detail during a sequential evaluation of the nervous system's major components. Undeviating adherence to routine is vital to avoid omission, duplication, and ultimately confusion. Despite obvious dysfunction of one part of the nervous system, all areas are evaluated. A physician can complete an initial or screening neurologic examination in about 20 minutes and return to perform special testing of particular areas, such as the mental status.

EXAMINATION

Physicians should note the patient's age, sex, and handedness, and then review the chief complaint, present illness, past medical history, family history, and social history. They should include standard questions about the primary symptom, associated symptoms, and possible etiologic factors. If a patient cannot relate the history, the physician might interrupt the process to look for language, memory, or other cognitive deficits. Many chapters in Section II of this book contain outlines of standard questions related to common symptoms.

After obtaining the history, physicians should anticipate the patient's neurologic deficits and be prepared to look for disease primarily of the central nervous system (CNS) or the peripheral nervous system (PNS). At this point, without yielding to rigid preconceptions, the physician should have developed some feeling for the problem at hand.

Then physicians should look for the site of involvement, i.e., "localize the lesion." "Localization" is a hallowed goal of the examination and is useful in most cases. However, it is partly an art, is often supplanted by imaging, and is inapplicable to several important neurologic illnesses.

The examination, which overall remains invaluable to diagnosis, consists of a functional neuroanatomy demonstration: mental status, cranial nerves, motor system, reflexes, sensation, and cerebellar system (Table 1–1). This format should be followed during every examination. Until it is memorized, a copy should be taken to the patient's bedside to serve both as a reminder and a place to record neurologic findings.

The examination usually starts with an assessment of the mental status because it is the most important neurologic function, and impairments may preclude an accurate assessment of other neurologic functions. The examiner should consider specific intellectual deficits, such as language impairment (see Aphasia, Chapter 8), as well as general intellectual decline (see Dementia, Chapter 7). Tests of cranial nerves may reveal malfunctions of nerves either individually or in groups, such as the *ocular motility nerves* (III, IV, and VI) and the *cerebellopontine angle nerves* (V, VII, and VIII; see Chapter 4).

The examination of the motor system is usually performed more to detect the pattern than the severity of weakness. Whether weakness is mild to moderate (*paresis*) or complete (*plegia*), the pattern indicates its origin. Three common important patterns are easy to recognize. If the lower face, arm, and leg on one side of the body are paretic, the pattern is called *hemiparesis* and indicates damage to the contralateral cerebral hemisphere or brainstem. Both legs being weak, *paraparesis*, indicates spinal cord damage. Paresis of the distal portion of all the limbs indicates PNS rather than CNS damage.

TABLE 1–1.   NEUROLOGIC EXAMINATION

Mental status
  Cooperation
  Orientation
  Language
  Memory for immediate, recent, and past events
  Higher intellectual functions: arithmetic, similarities/differences
Cranial nerves
  I Smell
  II Visual acuity, visual fields, optic fundi
  III, IV, VI Pupils' size and reactivity, extraocular motion
  V Corneal reflex and facial sensation
  VII Strength of upper and lower facial muscles, taste
  VIII Hearing
  IX–XI Articulation, palate movement, gag reflex
  XII Tongue movement
Motor system
  Limb strength
  Spasticity, flaccidity, or fasciculations
  Abnormal movements, e.g., tremor, chorea
Reflexes
  Deep tendon reflexes (DTRs)
    Biceps, triceps, brachioradialis, quadriceps, Achilles
  Pathologic reflexes
    Extensor plantar response (Babinski sign), frontal release
Sensation
  Position, vibration, stereognosis
  Pain
Cerebellar system
  Finger-nose, heel-shin, and rapid alternating movements
  Gait

Eliciting two categories of reflexes assists in determining whether paresis or another neurologic disorder originates in the CNS or PNS. *Deep tendon reflexes (DTRs)* are normally present with uniform reactivity in all limbs, but neurologic injury often alters their activity or symmetry. In general, with CNS injury that includes corticospinal tract damage, DTRs are hyperactive, whereas with PNS injury, DTRs are hypoactive.

In contrast to DTRs, *pathologic reflexes* are not normally elicitable beyond infancy. If found, they are a sign of CNS damage. The most widely recognized pathologic reflex is the infamous *Babinski sign*. Judging from current medical conversations, the terminology regarding this sign must be clarified. After plantar stimulation, the great toe normally moves downward, i.e., it has a flexor response. With brain or spinal cord damage, plantar stimulation typically causes the great toe to move upward, i.e., to have an extensor response: The reflex extensor movement is the Babinski sign (see Fig. 19–3). This sign and others may be "present" or "elicited," but they are never "positive" or "negative." In the same way, a traffic stop sign may be present or absent, but never positive or negative.

Frontal release signs, which are other pathologic reflexes, reflect frontal lobe injury. They are helpful in indicating an "organic" basis for a change in personality. Also, to a limited degree, they are associated with intellectual impairment (see Chapter 7).

The examination of the sensory system is long and tedious. Moreover, unlike abnormal DTRs and Babinski signs, which are reproducible, objective, and virtually impossible to mimic, the sensory examination relies almost entirely on the patient's report. Its subjective nature has led to the practice of disregarding the sensory examination if it varies from the rest of the evaluation. Under most circumstances the best approach is to test the major sensory modalities in a clear anatomic order and tentatively accept the patient's report.

Depending on the nature of the suspected disorder, the physician may test sensation of position, vibration, and stereognosis (appreciation of an object's form by touching it)—all of which are carried in the posterior columns of the spinal cord. Pain (pinprick) sensation, which is carried in the lateral columns, should be tested carefully with a nonpenetrating, disposable instrument.

Cerebellar function is evaluated by observing the patient for intention tremor and incoordination during several standard maneuvers that include the *finger-nose test* and rapid repetition of *alternating movement test* (see Chapter 2). The patient's gait is observed for incoordination (*ataxia*); for noncerebellar disorders, including hemiparesis, involuntary movements, and apraxia (see Table 2–4); and even for orthopedic conditions. Keep in mind that gait impairment is not merely a neurologic or orthopedic sign, but is a dangerous condition that leads to fatal falls or permanent incapacity for numerous elderly people each year.

FORMULATION

The classic *formulation* is an appraisal of the four aspects of the examination: symptoms, signs, localization, and differential diagnosis. The clinician might also have to support a conclusion that neurologic disease is present or, equally important, absent. For this step, psychogenic signs must be separated, if only tentatively, from neurologic ones. Evidence must be demonstrable for a psychogenic or neurologic etiology while acknowledging that neither is a diagnosis of exclusion. As if to confuse the situation, patients often have thought or mood disorders and grossly exaggerated deficits resulting from an underlying neurologic illness (see Chapter 3). Although somewhat ritualistic, a succinct and cogent formulation remains the basis of neurologic problem solving.

Localization of neurologic lesions requires the clinician to determine at least whether the illness affects the CNS, PNS, or muscle system (see Chapters 2 through 6). Precise localization of lesions within them is possible and generally expected. The physician must also establish whether the nervous system is affected diffusely or in a discrete area. The site and extent of neurologic damage will indicate certain diseases. A readily apparent example is that cerebrovascular accidents (strokes) and tumors generally involve a discrete area of the brain, but Alzheimer's disease causes widespread, symmetric changes.

Finally, the differential diagnosis is the disease or diseases—up to three—most consistent with the patient's symptoms and signs. When specific diseases cannot be suggested, major categories, such as "structural lesions," should be offered.

A typical formulation might be as follows: "Mr. Jones, a 56-year-old man, has had left-sided headaches for 2 months and a generalized seizure on the day before admission. He is lethargic. He has papilledema, a right hemiparesis with hyperactive DTRs, and a Babinski sign. The lesion seems to be in the left cerebral hemisphere. Most likely, he has a tumor, but a stroke is possible." This formulation recounts the symptoms, offers an abbreviated relevant medical history, and details the salient physical findings. It tacitly assumes that neurologic disease is present because of the obvious, objective physical findings. The localization is based on the history of seizures and the right-sided hemiparesis and abnormal reflexes. The differential diagnosis is based on the high probability of these conditions being caused by a discrete cerebral lesion.

To review, the physician should present a formulation that answers *The Four Questions of Neurology*:

- What are the *symptoms* of *neurologic* disease?
- What are the *signs* of *neurologic* disease?
- *Where* is the lesion?
- *What* is the lesion?

2 Central Nervous System Disorders

Lesions in the two components of the central nervous system (CNS)—the brain and the spinal cord—typically cause paresis, sensory loss, and visual deficits (Table 2–1). In addition, lesions in the cerebral hemispheres (the cerebrum) cause neuropsychologic impariments. Symptoms and signs of CNS disorders must be contrasted to those resulting from peripheral nervous system (PNS) and psychogenic disorders. Neurologists tend to rely on their physical rather than verbal evaluations and thereby honor an updated Confucian proverb, "One Babinski sign is worth a thousand words."

SIGNS OF CEREBRAL HEMISPHERE LESIONS

Of the various signs of cerebral hemisphere injury, the most prominent is usually *contralateral hemiparesis* (Table 2–2): weakness of the lower face, trunk, arm, and leg opposite to the side of the lesion. It results from damage to the *corticospinal tract*, which is also called the *pyramidal tract* (Fig. 2–1). During the corticospinal tract's entire path from the cerebral cortex to the anterior horn cells of the spinal cord, it is considered the *upper motor neuron (UMN)* (Fig. 2–2). The anterior horn cells are the beginning of the *lower motor neuron (LMN)*.

The division of the motor system into upper and lower motor neurons is a basic tenet of clinical neurology. Cerebral lesions that damage the corticospinal tract are characterized by *signs of UMN injury* (Figs. 2–3 to 2–5):

- Paresis with muscle spasticity
- Hyperactive deep tendon reflexes (DTRs)
- Babinski signs

In contrast, peripheral nerve lesions, including anterior horn cell or motor neuron diseases, are associated with *signs of LMN injury*:

- Paresis with muscle flaccidity and atrophy
- Hypoactive DTRs
- No Babinski signs

Cerebral lesions are not the only cause of hemiparesis. Because the corticospinal tract has such a long course (see Fig. 2–1), hemiparesis and other signs of UMN damage may originate from lesions in the brainstem and spinal cord, as well as the cerebrum. Signs pointing to injury in various regions of the CNS can indicate the origin of hemiparesis.

TABLE 2-1.   SIGNS OF COMMON CNS LESIONS

Cerebral hemisphere[a]
   Hemiparesis with hyperactive DTRs, spasticity, and Babinski sign
   Hemisensory loss
   Homonymous hemianopsia
   Partial seizures
   Aphasia, hemi-inattention, and dementia
   Pseudobulbar palsy
Basal ganglia[a]
   Movement disorders: parkinsonism, athetosis, chorea, and hemiballismus
Brainstem
   Cranial nerve palsy with contralateral hemiparesis
   Internuclear ophthalmoplegia (MLF syndrome)
   Nystagmus
   Bulbar palsy
Cerebellum
   Tremor on intention
   Impaired rapid alternating movements (dysdiadochokinesia)
   Ataxic gait
   Scanning speech
Spinal cord
   Paraparesis or quadriparesis
   Sensory loss up to a "level"
   Bladder, bowel, sexual dysfunction

[a]Signs contralateral to lesions.

Another indication of a cerebral lesion is loss of certain sensory modalities over one half of the body, i.e., *hemisensory loss* (Fig. 2–6). A patient with a cerebral lesion characteristically loses contralateral position sensation, two-point discrimination, and the ability to identify objects by touch (stereognosis). Loss of those modalities is often called a "cortical sensory loss."

Pain sensation, a "primary" sense, is perceived in the thalamus. Since the thalamus is the uppermost portion of the brainstem, pain sensation is retained with cerebral lesions. For example, patients with cerebral infarctions may be unable to identify a painful area, but will still feel the intensity and discomfort of pain. Also, patients in intractable pain do not obtain relief when they undergo experimental surgical resection of the cerebral cortex. The other aspect of the thalamus' role in sensing pain is seen when patients with thalamic

TABLE 2-2.   SIGNS OF COMMON CEREBRAL LESIONS

Either hemisphere[a]
   Hemiparesis with hyperactive DTRs and Babinski sign
   Hemisensory loss
   Homonymous hemianopsia
   Partial seizures: simple, complex, or secondarily generalized
Nondominant hemisphere
   Hemi-inattention
   Anosognosia
   Constructional apraxia
Dominant hemisphere
   Aphasias
   Gerstmann's syndrome
   Alexia without agraphia
Both hemispheres
   Dementia
   Pseudobulbar palsy

[a]Signs contralateral to lesions.

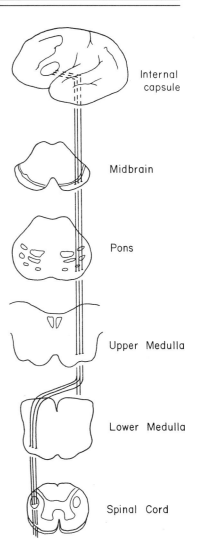

FIGURE 2-1.

The corticospinal tract originates in the cerebral cortex, passes through the internal capsule, and descends into the brainstem. It crosses in the pyramids, which are located in the medulla, to descend in the spinal cord as the *lateral corticospinal tract*. It terminates by synapsing onto the *anterior horn cells* of the spinal cord, which give rise to peripheral nerves. The corticospinal tract is called the *pyramidal* tract because it crosses in the pyramids. A complementary tract, which originates in the basal ganglia, is called the *extrapyramidal* tract.

infarctions develop spontaneous, disconcerting, burning pains over the contralateral body, i.e., thalamic pain (see Chapter 14).

Visual loss of the same half-field in each eye, *homonymous hemianopsia* (Fig. 2–7), is a characteristic sign of a contralateral cerebral lesion. Other equally characteristic visual losses are associated with lesions involving the eye, optic nerve, or optic tract (see Chapters 4 and 12). Of course, brainstem, cerebellar, or spinal cord lesions do not lead to visual field loss.

Another prominent sign of a cerebral hemisphere lesion is the development of *partial seizures* (see Chapter 10). Although the origin of primary generalized seizures has not been established, partial seizures that are elementary, complex, or secondarily generalized are clearly the result of cerebral lesions. In fact, about 90 per cent of partial complex seizures originate in the temporal lobe.

Although hemiparesis, hemisensory loss, homonymous hemianopsia, and partial seizures may result from lesions of either cerebral hemisphere, several neuropsychologic deficits are referable specifically to either the dominant or nondominant hemisphere. Since approximately 95 per cent of people are right-handed, unless the physician knows otherwise the left hemisphere should be

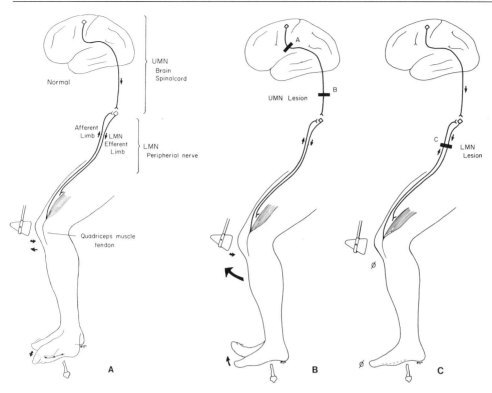

FIGURE 2-2.

A, Normally, when the quadriceps tendon is struck with the percussion hammer, a deep tendon reflex (DTR) is elicited. Also, when the sole of the foot is stroked to elicit a plantar reflex, the big toe bends downward (flexes). *B,* When brain or spinal cord lesions involve the corticospinal tract and cause UMN damage, the DTR is hyperactive and the plantar reflex is extensor, i.e., a Babinski sign is present. *C,* When peripheral nerve injury causes LMN damage, the DTR is hypoactive and the plantar reflex is absent.

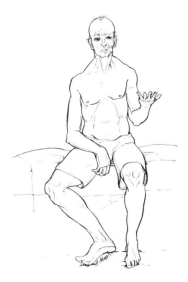

FIGURE 2-3.

This patient with severe right hemiparesis typically has weakness of the right lower face, the arm, and the leg. The right-sided facial weakness causes the widened palpebral fissure and flat nasolabial fold; however, the forehead muscles are normal (see Chapter 4 regarding this discrepancy). The right arm is limp, and the elbow, wrist, and fingers are flexed. The right hemiparesis also causes the right leg to be externally rotated and the hip and knee to be flexed.

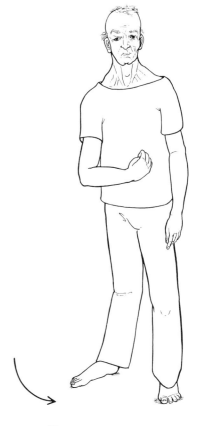

FIGURE 2-4.

When the patient arises, his weakened arm retains its flexed posture. His right leg remains externally rotated, but he can walk by swinging it in a circular path. This is an effective maneuver that results in *circumduction* or a *hemiparetic gait*.

assumed to be dominant. Lesions of the dominant hemisphere usually cause *aphasia*, which is language impairment (see Chapter 8). Moreover, with these lesions, a right hemiparesis typically accompanies aphasia because the language centers are adjacent to the cortical areas controlling voluntary movement (the corticospinal tract; see Fig. 8−1).

Disorders of the nondominant hemisphere usually cause subtle and transient neuropsychologic abnormalities. When the nondominant parietal lobe is

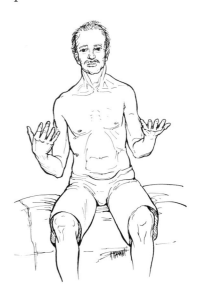

FIGURE 2-5.

Mild hemiparesis may not be obvious. To exaggerate a subtle hemiparesis, the physician has asked this patient to close his eyes and extend both arms with his palms held upright, as though he were holding a water glass on his outstretched hand. After a minute, the weakened arm slowly sinks (drifts), and the palm turns inward (pronates). The imaginary water glass would spill inward, falling off the right palm. This arm's drift and pronation represents a *forme fruste* of the posture seen with severe paresis (Fig. 2-3).

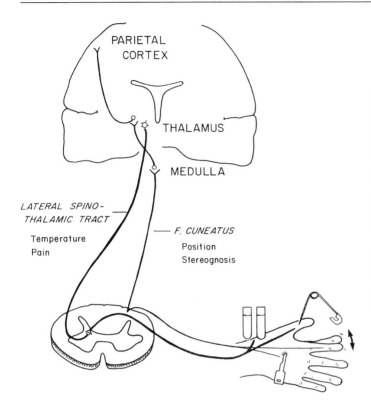

FIGURE 2-6.

Pain and temperature sensation are carried to the spinal cord where, after a synapse, these sensations cross and ascend in the *contralateral lateral spinothalamic tract*. For practical purposes, pain tracts terminate in the thalamus. Position sense (tested by movement of the distal finger joint) and stereognosis (tested by tactile identification of common objects) are carried in the *ipsilateral fasciculus cuneatus* and *f. gracilis*, which together constitute the *posterior columns* (Fig. 2-14). These tracts cross, synapse in the thalamus, and terminate in the cortex of the contralateral parietal lobe. (When testing pain, examiners should not use a pin.)

injured, patients typically have *hemi-inattention*, a constellation of disorders in which patients neglect left-sided visual perceptions and touching and experience hemiparesis (see Chapter 8). Patients may not even acknowledge their (left) hemiparesis—a condition known as *anosognosia*. Patients with *constructional apraxia*, another manifestation of nondominant lesions, cannot arrange match-sticks into certain patterns nor copy simple forms (Fig. 2–8).

All signs discussed so far are referable to one cerebral hemisphere. Bilateral cerebral hemisphere damage produces *pseudobulbar palsy*. This condition, best known for its emotional lability, results from damage to the *corticobulbar tract*. This is the UMN tract, which is a counterpart of the corticospinal tract, that innervates the brainstem motor nuclei (see Chapter 4).

Dementia also indicates that both cerebral hemispheres are damaged. It is usually caused by Alzheimer's disease, multiple infarctions, alcohol-related damage, or other *diffuse* structural or metabolic injuries (see Chapter 7). Since the CNS damage is usually extensive, dementia is associated with bilateral hyperactive DTRs, Babinski signs, and frontal lobe release reflexes, although not necessarily with hemiparesis or other lateralized findings. Whenever possible, a diagnosis of dementia or other neurologically based mental aberration should be buttressed by a description of physical abnormalities.

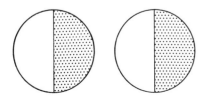

FIGURE 2-7.

In homonymous hemianopsia, the same half of the visual field is lost in each eye. In this case, a right homonymous hemianopsia is attributable to damage to the left cerebral hemisphere.

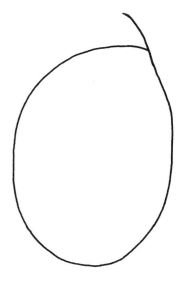

FIGURE 2-8.

With constructional apraxia from a right parietal lobe infarction, a 68-year-old woman was hardly able to complete a circle (*top figure*). She could not draw a square on request (*second highest figure*) or even copy one (*third highest figure*). She spontaneously tried to draw a circle and began to retrace it (*bottom figure*). Her constructional apraxia is seen in the rotation of the forms, perseveration of certain lines, and the incompleteness of the second and lowest figures. Also, the figures tend toward the right-hand side of the page, which indicates that she is ignoring or has neglect of the left-hand side of the page.

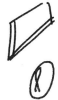

In general, in large urban acute care hospitals, the five conditions most likely to cause discrete unilateral or bilateral cerebral lesions are cerebral infarctions and other cerebrovascular accidents ("strokes"), primary or metastatic brain tumors, trauma, complications of acquired immune deficiency syndrome (AIDS), and multiple sclerosis (MS). Partial complex seizures, which are an important exception, are usually the result of sclerosis, cryptic vascular malformations, or small tumors. (A broader listing is offered in Table 2–3, and detailed discussions of strokes, tumors, seizures, and MS are presented in Section 2.)

SIGNS OF BASAL GANGLIA LESIONS

To complement the corticospinal or pyramidal tract, the *extrapyramidal* tract originates in the basal ganglia and modulates motor tone and activity. Unlike the corticospinal tract, its efferent fibers play upon the corticospinal

TABLE 2-3.   COMMON CONDITIONS THAT DAMAGE THE CNS

Genetic
  Down's syndrome
  Wilson's disease
  Huntington's chorea
Congenital ("cerebral palsy," mental retardation, or both)
  Cerebral anoxia, kernicterus (jaundice), prematurity
  Congenital malformations[a]
  Neurocutaneous disorders[a]
Toxic
  Hepatic or renal failure
  Medications
  Illicit drugs, especially cocaine
  Alcohol (and malnutrition)
Infectious
  Bacterial: abscess[a] or meningitis
  Viral: encephalitis or meningitis
  Acquired immune deficiency syndrome (AIDS) and its complications
Inflammatory[a]
  Multiple sclerosis
  Systemic lupus erythematosus (SLE)
Traumatic[a]
Neoplastic (tumors)[a]
  Primary: glioblastoma, astrocytoma, meningioma
  Metastatic: lung, breast, melanoma
Vascular ("strokes")
  Infarction[a]
  Embolus[a]
  Hemorrhage[a]
  Anoxia from cardiopulmonary arrest
Degenerative (etiology unknown)
  Alzheimer's disease
  Creutzfeldt-Jakob disease
  Amyotrophic lateral sclerosis (ALS)

[a]Discrete cerebral damage.

tract, cerebral cortex, and other CNS structures. They do not act on the spinal cord or LMNs. The major components of the extrapyramidal tract are the caudate nucleus, the globus pallidus, the putamen, the substantia nigra, and the subthalamic nucleus (corpus of Luysii; see Fig. 18–1).

Basal ganglia injury often causes dramatic, *involuntary movement disorders* (see Chapter 18):

- *Parkinsonism* is the combination of resting tremor, rigidity, bradykinesia (slowness of movement) or akinesia (absence of movement), and postural abnormalities. Minor features include festinating gait (Table 2–4) and

TABLE 2-4.   GAIT ABNORMALITIES

Gait	Associated Illness	Figure
Apraxia	Normal pressure hydrocephalus	7-7
Astasia-abasia	Hysteria	3-2
Ataxia	Cerebellar damage	2-13
Festinating	Parkinson's disease	18-9
Marche à petits pas		
Hemiparetic	Cerebrovascular accidents	2-4
Circumduction		
Spastic hemiparesis		13-2
Steppage	Tabes dorsalis (CNS syphilis)	2-18
	Peripheral neuropathies	

micrographia. Parkinsonism is associated with damage to the substantia nigra from degeneration (Parkinson's disease), antipsychotic medications, or toxins.

- *Athetosis* is the slow, continuous, writhing movement of the fingers, hands, face, and throat. It is usually caused by kernicterus or other perinatal brain injury.

- *Chorea* is intermittent jerking of limbs and trunk. The infamous hereditary condition, *Huntington's* disease, is associated with caudate nucleus atrophy.

- *Hemiballismus* is the intermittent flinging of the arm and leg on one side of the body. It is associated with small infarctions of the contralateral subthalamic nucleus.

In general, when damage is restricted to the extrapyramidal tract, as in many cases of hemiballismus and athetosis, patients have no paresis, DTR abnormalities, or Babinski signs—signs of corticospinal (pyramidal) tract damage. More important, in many of these cases, patients have no intellectual abnormality. On the other hand, several illnesses that damage the cerebral cortex as well as the basal ganglia are characterized by a notorious association with dementia and involuntary movement disorders. The most noteworthy are Huntington's disease, Wilson's disease, and advanced Parkinson's disease (see Table 18–4).

Unlike illnesses that affect the cerebrum, most basal ganglia diseases are slowly progressive, cause bilateral damage, and result from biochemical abnormalities, rather than discrete structural lesions. When there is unilateral basal ganglia damage, the signs are found contralateral to the lesion. One example is hemiballismus, which results from infarction of the contralateral subthalamic nucleus. Another is unilateral parkinsonism ("hemiparkinsonism"), which results from degeneration of the contralateral substantia nigra.

SIGNS OF BRAINSTEM LESIONS

The brainstem contains the cranial nerve nuclei, the corticospinal tracts and other "long tracts" that travel between the cerebral hemispheres and the limbs, and several self-contained systems (Fig. 2–9). Massive brainstem injuries, such as extensive infarctions or barbiturate overdoses, cause coma, but otherwise brainstem injuries do not impair mentation. Also, few illnesses simultaneously damage the brainstem and the cerebrum.

Combinations of cranial nerve and long tract signs indicate the presence and location of a brainstem lesion. The localization should be supported by the absence of visual field cuts, neuropsychologic impairments, and other signs of cerebral injury. For example, brainstem injuries cause *diplopia* (double vision) because of cranial nerve impairment, but visual acuity and visual fields remain normal because the visual pathways, which pass from the optic chiasm to the cerebral hemispheres, do not travel within the brainstem (see Fig. 4–1). Similarly, a right hemiparesis associated with a left third cranial nerve palsy indicates that the lesion is in the brainstem and that aphasia will not be present.

Several syndromes are important because each illustrates critical anatomic relationships, such as the location of the different cranial nerve nuclei or the course of the corticospinal tract, but none of them involves neuropsychologic abnormalities. Although each syndrome has an eponym, for practical purposes

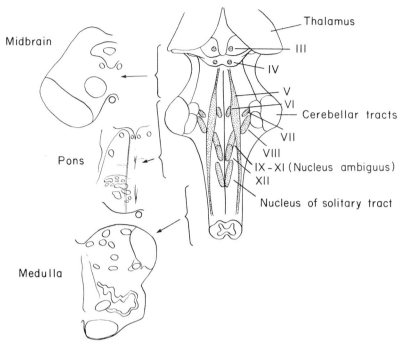

FIGURE 2-9.

In cross-section (*Left*) and overview (*Right*), the midbrain contains the nuclei of cranial nerves III and IV; the pons, nuclei V through VIII; and the medulla, nuclei IX through XII. The brainstem also contains the long tracts that pass from the cerebellum and cerebrum to the spinal cord. In addition, several other tracts, including the medial longitudinal fasciculus, some cerebellar tracts, and the reticular activating system, are contained and act solely within the brainstem.

it is only necessary to identify them as the result of a lesion in the brainstem or, possibly, in one of the *three divisions of the brainstem: midbrain, pons, or medulla*. Most cases are caused by infarctions in small branches of the basilar or vertebral arteries.

In the midbrain, where the oculomotor (third cranial) nerve passes through the descending corticospinal tract, both pathways can be damaged by a single small infarction. Patients with oculomotor nerve paralysis and contralateral hemiparesis typically have a midbrain lesion ipsilateral to the paretic eye (see Fig. 4–8).

Patients with abducens (sixth cranial) nerve paralysis and contralateral hemiparesis likewise have a pons lesion that is ipsilateral to the paretic eye (see Fig. 4–10).

Lateral medullary infarctions create a classic but complex picture. Patients have paralysis of the ipsilateral palate because of damage to cranial nerves IX through XI; ipsilateral facial hypalgesia because of damage to cranial nerve V, with contralateral anesthesia of the body *(alternating hypalgesia)* because of ascending spinothalamic tract damage; and ipsilateral ataxia because of ipsilateral cerebellar dysfunction. Fortunately, it is not necessary to recall all the features of this syndrome: Physicians only need to realize that those cranial nerve palsies and the alternating hypalgesia are characteristic of a lower brainstem lesion (Fig. 2–10 A and B).

Although these particular brainstem syndromes are distinctive, the most frequently observed sign of brainstem dysfunction, which is nonspecific, is

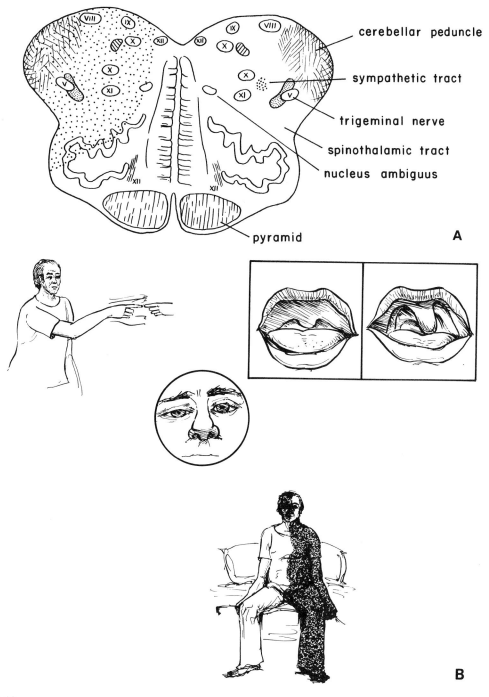

FIGURE 2-10.

A, Whenever the posterior inferior cerebellar artery (PICA) is occluded, the lateral portion of the medulla suffers infarction. This infarction damages important structures: the cerebellar peduncle, the nucleus of the trigeminal nerve, the spinothalamic tract, the nucleus ambiguus (motor nuclei of cranial nerves IX to XI), and poorly delineated sympathetic fibers. Medial structures that escape damage are the corticospinal tract, hypoglossal nerve, and medial longitudinal fasciculus. The stippled area represents the lateral medulla, which would be infarcted when the right PICA or its parent artery, the vertebral artery, is occluded. *B*, This patient, who suffered an infarction of the right lateral medulla, has a right-sided Wallenberg syndrome. He has a right-sided Horner's syndrome (ptosis and miosis) because of damage to the sympathetic fibers (also see Fig. 12-15B). He has right-sided ataxia because of damage to the ipsilateral cerebellar tracts. He has an alternating hypalgesia: diminished pain sensation on the *right* side of his face, accompanied by loss of pain sensation on the *left* trunk and extremities. Finally, he has hoarseness and paresis of the right soft palate because of damage to the right nucleus ambiguus: On voluntary phonation or in response to the gag reflex, the palate deviates upward toward his left because the right side of the palate is weak.

nystagmus (repetitive jerk-like eye movements). Resulting from any injury of the brainstem's large vestibular nuclei, nystagmus is usually a manifestation of one of the following disorders: MS; intoxications with alcohol, phenytoin (Dilantin), or barbiturates; Wernicke-Korsakoff syndrome; ischemia of the vertebrobasilar artery system; or merely viral labyrinthitis. It may also be associated with *internuclear ophthalmoplegia*, a disorder of ocular motility in which the brainstem's medial longitudinal fasciculus (MLF) is damaged by MS or an infarction (see Chapters 4 and 15).

SIGNS OF CEREBELLAR LESIONS

The cerebellum is composed of two hemispheres and a central portion, the *vermis*. Each hemisphere controls motor coordination of the ipsilateral limbs, and the vermis controls coordination of "midline structures," which are the head, neck, and trunk. The control of coordination of the limbs on the *same side of the body* gives the cerebellum a unique quality captured by the aphorism, "Everything in the brain, except for the cerebellum, is backwards." Another unique feature of the cerebellum is that when one hemisphere is damaged, the other will eventually be able to perform almost all the functions for both. Thus, although loss of one cerebellar hemisphere will cause incapacitating ipsilateral incoordination, the disability improves as the remaining hemisphere compensates almost in full.

Cerebellar lesions cause ipsilateral incoordination, but they do not cause paresis or significant reflex abnormality. Moreover, since the cerebellum is isolated from the cerebral hemispheres, even its total destruction does not cause intellectual abnormalities. A good example is the normal intellect of children who have undergone resection of a cerebellar hemisphere for removal of a cerebellar astrocytoma (see Chapter 19).

The characteristic sign of a cerebellar lesion is *intention tremor*, which is elicited during the finger-nose test (Fig. 2–11) and heel-shin test (Fig. 2–12). It is present when the patient moves willfully, but absent when the patient rests. In contrast, Parkinson's disease causes a *resting tremor* that is present when the patient is sitting quietly and is reduced or abolished during movements (see Chapter 18).

Another sign of a cerebellar lesion is an impaired ability to perform rapid alternating movements, *dysdiadochokinesia*. When asked to slap the palm and then the back of the hand rapidly and alternately on his or her own knee, for example, a patient with dysdiadochokinesia will use uneven force, move irregularly, and lose the alternating pattern.

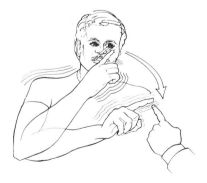

FIGURE 2-11.

This young man, who has a MS plaque in the right cerebellar hemisphere, has an *intention tremor*. During repetitive *finger-nose* movements, as his finger approaches his own nose and then the examiner's finger, it develops a coarse and irregular path. The irregular rhythm is called *dysmetria*.

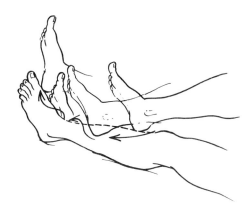

FIGURE 2-12.

In the *heel-shin test*, the patient with the right-sided cerebellar lesion in Figure 2-11 displays limb *ataxia* or *tremor on intention* as his right heel wobbles when he moves it along the crest of his left shin.

Damage to either the entire cerebellum or the vermis alone causes incoordination of the trunk, i.e., *truncal ataxia*. It forces patients to place their feet widely apart when standing and produces a lurching, unsteady, and wide-based pattern of walking known as an *ataxic gait* (Table 2–4 and Fig. 2–13). This gait abnormality is dramatically apparent in the staggering and reeling of people who are drunk.

With extensive cerebellar damage, voice production is impaired by poor modulation, irregular cadence, inability to separate adjacent sounds, and prolonged pauses between syllables. In a form of *dysarthria* called *scanning speech*, patients tend to speak as though reading a poem. Dysarthria—from cerebellar injury, bulbar and pseudobulbar palsy, and other CNS conditions—should be distinguishable from aphasia (see Chapter 8). (The nomenclature of dysdiadochokinesia, dysarthria, and dysmetria suggests that cerebellar disease

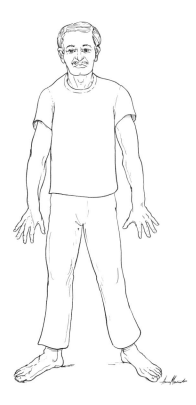

FIGURE 2-13.

This man is a chronic alcoholic who suffers from diffuse cerebellar degeneration. He has a typical *ataxic gait*: broad-based, unsteady, and uncoordinated. He stands with his feet pointed outward to widen and thus steady his stance.

gives rise to the "dys" words.) Finally, a subtle sign of cerebellar disease is that muscle tone is hypotonic and DTRs are pendular.

The illnesses that are responsible for most *cerebral* lesions—strokes, tumors, trauma, AIDS, and MS—also cause most *cerebellar* lesions. In a virtually unique situation, alcoholism or taking certain medications, such as phenytoin (Dilantin), leads to damage to the vermis. In the infamous Wernicke-Korsakoff syndrome, poor nutrition, which is usually but not necessarily related to alcoholism, leads to cognitive impairment, which is characterized by memory loss (amnesia), as well as ataxia and nystagmus. Any patient even suspected of having Wernicke-Korsakoff syndrome should immediately receive thiamine 50 mg intravenously to prevent serious brain injury.

SIGNS OF SPINAL CORD LESIONS

At the spinal cord's center is a broad H-shaped, gray matter structure composed largely of neurons that transmit nerve impulses in a horizontal plane. White matter, composed of myelinated tracts conveying information in a vertical direction, surrounds the gray matter (Fig. 2–14). Curiously, the spinal cord's arrangement—gray matter on the inside with white outside—is the opposite of that of the cerebrum.

The major descending pathway is the *lateral corticospinal tract*.

The major ascending pathways, which are virtually all sensory, include the following:

- *posterior columns*, which carry position and vibration sensations to the thalamus
- *lateral spinothalamic tracts*, which carry temperature and pain sensations to the thalamus
- *anterior spinothalamic tracts*, which carry light touch sensations to the thalamus
- *spinocerebellar tracts*, which carry joint position and movement sensations to the cerebellum

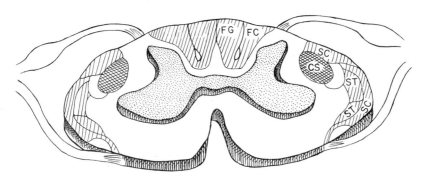

FIGURE 2-14.

In this drawing of the spinal cord, the centrally located gray matter is stippled. The surrounding white matter contains myelin-coated tracts that ascend and descend within the spinal cord. Clinically important ascending tracts are the spinocerebellar tracts (SC), the lateral spinothalamic tract (ST), and the posterior columns [fasciculus cuneatus (FC), from the upper limbs, and fasciculus gracilis (FG), from the lower limbs]. The most important descending tract is the lateral corticospinal tract (CS).

A spinal cord lesion will interrupt both the descending motor and ascending sensory myelinated tracts. Since most signs of spinal cord injury are due to interruption of the myelinated tracts, it is often called "myelopathy." On a microscopic level, spinal cord lesions cause the breakup of distal or "downstream" myelin.

A cervical spinal cord injury causes the loss of motor function and sensation below the neck. The arms and legs will be paralyzed (*quadriparesis*). After 1 to 2 weeks, spasticity, hyperactive DTRs, and Babinski signs will develop. Also, limb and trunk sensations will be interrupted, and bladder fullness and genital stimulation will not be appreciated. Similarly, a midthoracic spinal cord injury will lead to leg paralysis (*paraparesis*), reflex changes, and sensory loss of the legs and trunk below the nipples (Fig. 2–15). As a general rule, all spinal cord injuries disrupt sexual function (see Chapter 16).

Even with devastating spinal cord injury, however, cerebral function is preserved. In an admittedly tragic example, patients with a penetrating gunshot wound of the cervical spinal cord, although quadriplegic, retain intellectual, visual, and verbal facilities. Patients surviving spinal cord injuries are often beset with depression, which is more closely related to isolation than to physical impairment, and an have increased rate of suicide.

Of the various spinal cord lesions, the most instructive of neuroanatomy is the *Brown-Séquard syndrome*. This is a classic disturbance that results from an injury that transects the lateral half of the spinal cord (Fig. 2–16). It is characterized by unilateral corticospinal tract damage that causes paralysis of the ipsilateral limb(s) and by lateral spinothalamic tract damage that causes pain loss (*hypalgesia*) in the contralateral limb(s). Simply put, one leg is weak and the other is numb.

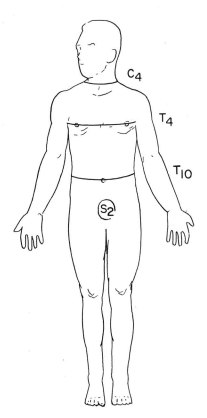

FIGURE 2-15.

In a patient with a spinal cord injury, the "level" of hypalgesia will indicate the site of the damage: C4 injuries cause hypalgesia below the neck; T4 injuries, hypalgesia below the nipples; T10 injuries, hypalgesia below the umbilicus.

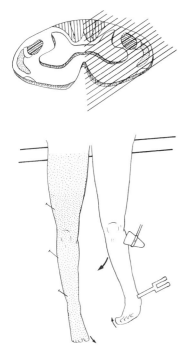

FIGURE 2-16.

In this case of hemitransection of the spinal cord (Brown-Séquard syndrome), the left side of the thoracic spinal cord has been transected, as by a knife wound. Injury to the left lateral corticospinal tract results in the combination of left-sided leg paresis, hyperactive DTRs, and a Babinski sign; injury to the left posterior column results in impairment of left leg vibration and position sense. Most striking, injury to the left spinothalamic tract causes loss of temperature and pain sensation in the right leg. The loss of pain sensation contralateral to the paresis is the readily identifiable hallmark of the Brown-Séquard syndrome.

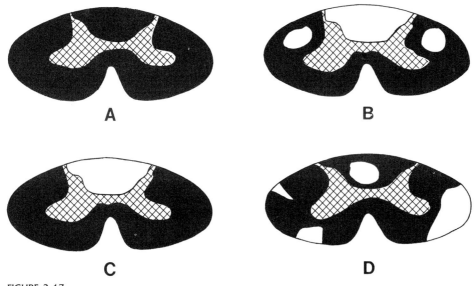

FIGURE 2-17.

A, A standard spinal cord histologic preparation stains normal myelin (white matter) black and leaves the central H-shaped column gray. B, In combined system disease (vitamin B$_{12}$ deficiency), damage to the posterior column and corticospinal tracts causes their demyelination and lack of stain. C, In tabes dorsalis (syphilis), damage to the posterior column leaves them unstained. D, MS, however, leads to asymmetric, irregular, demyelinated plaques.

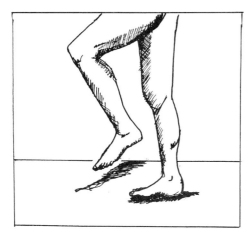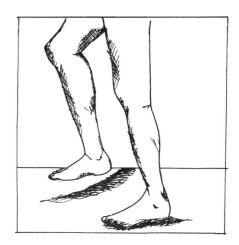

FIGURE 2-18.

The steppage gait consists of each knee being excessively raised when walking to compensate for a loss of position sense. This maneuver elevates the feet to ensure that they will clear the ground, stairs, and other obstacles. It is a classic sign of posterior column spinal cord damage from tabes dorsalis; however, peripheral neuropathies more commonly impair position sense and cause this gait impairment.

Capitalizing on the well-known position and function of the pain-carrying lateral spinothalamic tract, neurosurgeons can sometimes alleviate severe, unilateral pain with a relatively simple procedure, *cordotomy*. By severing the lateral spinothalamic tract contralateral to the painful side, neurosurgeons can produce considerable analgesia.

The cervical region of the spinal cord is particularly susceptible to common, nonpentrating trauma because in most accidents, hyperextension of the neck crushes the cervical vertebrae. Approximately 50 per cent of civilian spinal cord injuries result from motor vehicle accidents; 20 per cent from falls; 15 per cent from gunshot wounds and other violence; and 15 per cent from sports injuries, mostly diving accidents. The other dangerous sports are football, skiing, surfing, trampoline work, and horseback riding. Also, hangings fracture the cervical spine, which crushes the cervical spinal cord and cuts off the air supply. Survivors are likely to be quadriplegic as well as brain damaged.

MS, which is the most common disabling illness in North America and Northern Europe, typically causes myelopathy alone or in combination with cerebellar, optic nerve, or brainstem damage (see Chapter 15). Lung, breast, and other tumors that spread to the vertebral bodies often compress the spinal cord.

People who develop paraplegia or quadriplegia, usually as the result of an injury, have a high rate of divorce and suicide. Several patients with quadriplegia have requested withdrawal of life support not only immediately after the injury, when their plans may be attributed to depression, but also several years later when they are clear-headed and not overtly depressed.

With several illnesses, only specific tracts of the spinal cord may be affected (Fig. 2–17). The posterior columns seem to be particularly vulnerable. For example, in tabes dorsalis (syphilis), combined system disease (B_{12} deficiency), and the familial spinocerebellar degenerations, such as Friedreich's ataxia, the posterior columns are damaged alone or in combination with other tracts. In these conditions, impairment of the posterior columns leads to the loss of position sense that prohibits affected people from standing erect with their eyes closed (*Romberg's sign*), as well as to a *steppage gait* (Fig. 2–18).

Another example of specific tract injury is demyelination above a spinal cord transection. After a thoracic spinal cord gunshot wound, for example, the cervical region's corticospinal tract and *f. cuneatus* will be normal, but the *f. gracilis* and portions of the lateral spinothalamic tract, which would have ascended from the legs, are demyelinated.

Most importantly, myelopathy is associated with dementia because of concomitant cerebral damage in several illnesses. Examples of this association are tabes dorsalis, combined system disease, and AIDS. Unless the disease is advanced, patients with MS usually have no mental impairment; however, in advanced cases, when plaques are disseminated throughout the CNS, patients have myelopathy, dementia, and other neurologic signs (see Chapter 15).

3 Psychogenic Neurologic Deficits

Classic studies of hysteria, conversion reactions, and related conditions that were associated with neurologic deficits included patients who had only rudimentary physical examinations and minimal, if any, laboratory testing. Studies that re-evaluated the same patients after many years found that as many as 20 per cent eventually had specific neurologic conditions, such as movement disorders, multiple sclerosis (MS), or seizures, that probably had been responsible for the original symptoms. In addition, some patients had been suffering from systemic illnesses, such as anemia or congestive heart failure, that could have at least contributed to their symptoms. Another interesting aspect of those studies is that many illnesses assumed to be psychogenic in the first two thirds of the twentieth century are now acknowledged to be neurologic, such as Tourette's syndrome, writer's cramp and other focal dystonia, migraines, and trigeminal neuralgia.

Today, psychogenic neurologic deficits are rarely misdiagnosed. Routine evaluations include powerful, sophisticated testing, such as computed tomography (CT), magnetic resonance imaging (MRI), and closed circuit television (CCTV) monitoring. Physicians can also avoid overdiagnosing psychiatric disturbances by applying specific, relatively strict diagnostic criteria.

THE NEUROLOGISTS' ROLE

Nevertheless, even in the face of flagrant psychogenic signs, neurologists have a burden in confirming the absence of neurologic disease. They generally test for most neurologic conditions that could explain the symptoms and particularly for those that are serious or life threatening. In addition, although the course of the illness proves to be the best test, neurologists tend to request extensive testing at the onset of symptoms to obtain objective evidence of disease or its absence.

Neurologists typically disregard specific psychiatric diagnoses, such as conversion reactions, factitious disorders, somatoform disorders, and malingering, and merge them all into the category of psychogenic disturbance. In addition, neurologists often consider gross exaggeration of a neurologic deficit, *embellishment*, to be a psychogenic disturbance. Within the context of this potential oversimplification, they routinely and reliably diagnose psychogenic seizures (see Chapter 10), diplopia and other visual problems (see Chapter 12), and tremors and other movement disorders (see Chapter 18). Also, neurologists are keenly aware of the psychogenic aspects of pain (see Chapter 14), sexual function (see Chapter 16), and post-traumatic headaches and whiplash injuries (see Chapter 22).

In dealing with patients who have psychogenic disturbances, neurologists usually offer reassurances, strong suggestions that the deficits will resolve by a certain date, and a referral for psychiatric consultation. Sometimes they offer patients "face-saving" exits by prescribing placebos or nonspecific treatment, such as physical therapy. However, physicians should avoid ordering invasive diagnostic procedures, surgery, and medications, especially those that are habit forming or otherwise dangerous.

Patients often have mixtures of neurologic and psychogenic deficits, disproportionately great post-traumatic disabilities, and minor neurologic illnesses that preoccupy them. As long as serious, progressive physical illness has been excluded, physicians can consider some symptoms to be chronic illnesses. For example, low back injury or surgical incision pain can be treated as a "pain syndrome" with empiric combinations of antidepressant medications, analgesics, and psychotherapy, without expecting either to cure the pain or determine its exact cause (see Chapter 14).

PSYCHOGENIC SIGNS

When a deficit violates the *Laws of Neuroanatomy*, a physician should suspect a psychogenic origin. For example, if temperature sensation is preserved, but pain perception is "lost," the deficit is *non-anatomic* and therefore likely to be psychogenic. Likewise, tunnel vision is a classic psychogenic disturbance (see Fig. 12–8).

Another guideline is that, if a deficit changes, it is likely to be psychogenic. For example, someone with psychogenic paralysis might either walk when unaware of being observed or walk despite seeming to have paraplegia while in bed. Another noted example occurs when someone with a psychogenic seizure momentarily "awakens" and stops convulsive activity, but resumes it when assured of being observed. The psychogenic nature of a deficit can be confirmed if it is reversed during an interview under hypnosis.

Motor Signs

One indication of psychogenic weakness is that it is not in an anatomic distribution, such as loss of vision in one eye, hearing in one ear, and strength in the arm and leg—all on the same side of the body. Other indications are the absence of functional impairment despite claims of profound weakness, and limb movements with a slow, tremulous, and easily fatigued quality.

Intermittent paresis is evident in a "give-way" effort, in which the patient has a brief (several second) exertion before returning to an apparent paretic position. Intermittent paresis is also demonstrable using the *face-hand test*, in which the patient momentarily exerts sufficient strength to deflect a falling hand from hitting the face (Fig. 3–1).

An indication of unilateral psychogenic leg weakness is the infamous *Hoover's sign* (Fig. 3–2). Normally, when someone attempts to raise a genuinely paretic leg, the other leg presses down. The examiner can feel the downward force at the patient's normal heel and can use the straightened leg, as a lever, to raise the entire leg and lower body. In contrast, Hoover's sign consists of the patient unconsciously pressing down with a "paretic" leg when at-

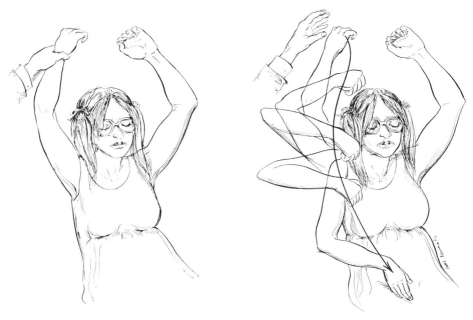

FIGURE 3-1.

In the face-hand test, a young woman with psychogenic right hemiparesis inadvertently demonstrates her preserved strength by deflecting her falling "paretic" arm from striking her face as it is dropped by the examiner.

tempting to raise the unaffected leg and failing to press down with the unaffected leg when attempting to raise the "paretic" leg.

A similar test involves adduction of the legs. Normally, when asked to adduct their legs, people squeeze both knees together. Someone with psychogenic weakness who is asked to adduct both legs against resistance might unconsciously adduct the "paretic" leg or fail to adduct the normal leg.

Gait Impairment

Many psychogenic gait impairments closely mimic neurologic disturbances, such as tremors in the legs, ataxia, or weakness of one or both legs. However, a readily identifiable, characteristic psychogenic gait impairment is *astasia-abasia*. This disorder consists of patients staggering, balancing momentarily, and appearing to be in great danger of falling, but never actually falling, as they grab hold of railings, furniture, and even the examiner (Fig. 3–3).

Another blatant psychogenic gait impairment occurs when patients drag a "weak" leg as though it were a totally lifeless object apart from their body. Patients with true hemiparesis, in contrast, swing their leg outward with a circular motion, i.e., they "circumduct" their leg or have a "hemiparetic" gait (see Fig. 2–4).

Sensory Deficits

Although the sensory examination is the least reliable portion of the neurologic examination, several sensory abnormalities reasonably predict a psychogenic basis. Loss of sensation to pinprick that stops abruptly at the middle

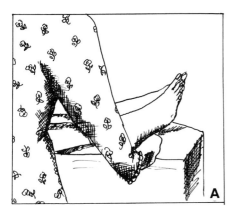
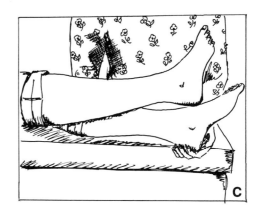
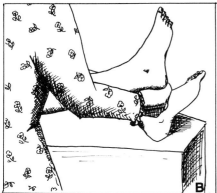
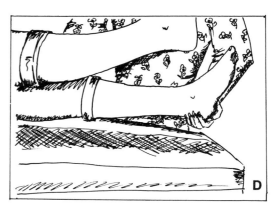

FIGURE 3-2.

Hoover's sign is demonstrated in a 23-year-old man who has a psychogenic left hemiparesis. *A*, The physician asks him to raise his left leg as she holds her hand under his right heel. *B*, Revealing his lack of effort, he exerts so little down force with his right leg that she easily raises it. *C*, When she asks him to raise his right leg while cupping his left heel, he reveals his intact strength as he unconsciously forces down his left, "paretic" leg—the Hoover sign. *D*, In an extreme example, he forces down the left leg with enough force to allow the physician to use his left leg as a lever to raise his lower torso.

of the face and body is the classic *splitting the midline*. (Neurologists now use pins cautiously, if at all, to avoid blood-borne-infections. Testing for pain is performed with nonpenetrating, disposable instruments, such as cotton sticks.) This finding suggests a psychogenic loss because the sensory nerve fibers of the skin normally spread across the midline (Fig. 3–4). Likewise, since vibrations naturally spread across bony structures, loss of vibration sensation over half the forehead, jaw, sternum, or spine is consistent with a psychogenic disturbance.

A similar abnormality is loss of sensation of the entire face, but not the scalp. This pattern is inconsistent with the anatomic distribution of the trigeminal nerve, which innervates the scalp anterior to the vertex and the face, but not the angle of the jaw (see Fig. 4–11).

A psychogenic sensory loss, as already mentioned, can be a discrepancy between pain and temperature sensations, which are normally carried together by the peripheral nerves and then the lateral spinothalamic tracts. (Discrepancy between pain and *position* sensations in the fingers, in contrast, is indica-

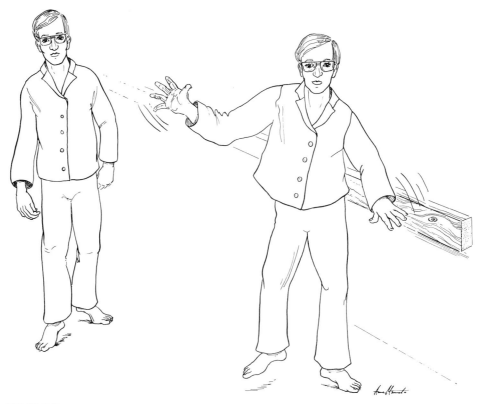

FIGURE 3-3.

A young man demonstrates astasia-abasia by seeming to fall when walking, but catching himself by balancing carefully. He even staggers the width of the room in order to grasp the rail. When possible, he grasps physicians and pulls them toward himself and then drags them toward the ground. While dramatizing his purported impairment, he actually displays good strength, balance, and coordination through a series of acrobatics.

tive of syringomyelia: In this condition the central fibers of the spinal cord, which carry pain sensation, are ripped apart by the expanding central canal.) A maneuver designed to expose a psychogenic sensory loss in the limbs is testing for sensory loss when the arms are twisted, placed out of sight behind the patient's back, or seen in a mirror.

Finally, because sensory loss impairs function, patients with genuine sensory loss in the feet or hands cannot perform many tasks if their eyes are closed. In contrast to this expectation, patients with psychogenic sensory loss, with their eyes closed, can still generally button their shirt, walk short distances, and stand with their feet together and their eyes closed. People with a true sensory loss in both feet who keep their eyes closed when standing erect tend to fall, i.e., they have a *Romberg sign*. Similarly, people with injury of the posterior columns of their spinal cord, usually from tabes dorsalis, MS, or vitamin B_{12} deficiency, have a Romberg sign (see Chapter 2).

Special Senses

Blindness, tunnel vision, and diplopia are commonly diagnosed as psychogenic disturbances when they violate the Laws of Neuroanatomy. Psychogenic and neurologic visual disorders may be readily separated (see Chapter 12.)

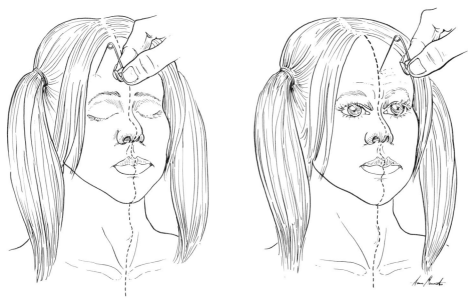

FIGURE 3-4.

A young woman with psychogenic right hemisensory loss appears not to feel a pinprick until the pin reaches the midline of her forehead, face, neck, or sternum, i.e., she splits the midline. When the pin is moved across the midline, she appears to feel a sharp stick. (The pin in this sketch is used for teaching purposes only.)

A patient with psychogenic deafness usually responds to unexpected noises or words. Unilateral hearing loss in the ear ipsilateral to a hemiparesis is highly suggestive of a psychogenic etiology because extensive auditory tract synapses in the pons ensure that some tracts reach the upper brainstem and cerebrum despite CNS lesions (see Fig. 4–15). If doubts about hearing loss remain, audiometry, brainstem auditory evoked responses, and other technical procedures can performed.

Patients can genuinely lose their sense of smell (suffer from anosmia) from a head injury (see Chapter 22) or age; however, they can usually perceive noxious volatile substances, such as ammonia or alcohol, because these chemicals irritate the nasal mucosa endings of the trigeminal nerve, rather than the olfactory nerve. This distinction is unknown to individuals with psychogenic anosmia who typically claim not to be able to smell any substance.

Miscellaneous Conditions

A distinct but common psychogenic disturbance, the *hyperventilation syndrome*, occurs in people with underlying anxiety or panic attacks. It leads to lightheadedness and paresthesias around their mouth, fingers, and toes, and, in severe cases, to *carpopedal spasm* (Fig. 3–5). Although the disorder seems distinctive, physicians should be cautious before diagnosing it because partial complex seizures and transient ischemic attacks (TIAs) produce similar symptoms.

In this disorder, hyperventilation first causes a fall in carbon dioxide tension that leads to respiratory alkalosis. The rise in blood pH from the alkalosis produces hypocalcemia, which produces the tetany of muscles and paresthe-

FIGURE 3-5.

Carpopedal spasm, which is the characteristic neurologic manifestation of hyperventilation, consists of flexion of the wrist and proximal thumb and finger joints. Also, although the thumb and fingers remain extended, they are drawn together and tend to overlap.

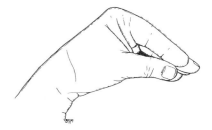

sias. Sometimes, to demonstrate to the patient that the symptoms are from hyperventilation, physicians attempt to re-create them by having a patient hyperventilate. This procedure may induce excessive giddiness or irrationality. If so, the physician should abort it by having the patient continually rebreathe expired air from a paper bag cupped around the mouth.

POTENTIAL PITFALLS

The neurologic examination of a patient suspected of having a psychogenic deficit should be sensitive. It can be undertaken in conjunction with a psychiatric evaluation, need not follow the conventional format, and can be completed in two or more sessions. The evaluation should not be threatening or embarrassing to the patient. An inept evaluation may obscure the diagnosis, harden the patient's resolve, or precipitate a catastrophic reaction.

Moreover, the guidelines are fallible. Patients may display psychogenic signs because of pain, fatigue, desire to please the examiner, or to exaggerate a neurologic deficit. Changes in affect and many other psychiatric guidelines to psychogenic deficits are unreliable. In particular, one famous psychiatric guideline, *la belle indifférence*, is found in hemi-inattention, Anton's syndrome, frontal lobe injury, and other neurologic problems.

Although the neurologic examination itself seems rational and reliable, it contains many potentially misleading findings. Probably because of anxiety, many patients with psychogenic paresis have deep tendon reflexes that are briskly reactive and plantar reflexes that appear to be extensor—as they would with cerebral or spinal cord damage. Another problem is that a right hemiparesis unaccompanied by aphasia or right homonymous hemianopsia might be interpreted as a psychogenic sign, but that combination might be found if patients were left-handed or if a stroke were small and located in the internal capsule, deep cerebrum, or upper brainstem, i.e., a "pure motor stroke."

Neurologists tend to misdiagnose several types of disorders as psychogenic when they are unique or bizarre or when their severity is greater than expected. This error may simply reflect an individual neurologist's lack of experience. Neurologists also misdiagnose disorders as psychogenic when a patient has no accompanying objective physical abnormalities. This determination might be faulty in illnesses where objective signs are often transient or subtle, such as in MS, partial complex seizures, and small strokes. With an incomplete history, neurologists may not appreciate transient neurologic conditions, such as transient hemiparesis induced by migraines, postical paresis, or TIAs and transient mental status aberrations induced by alcohol, medications, seizures, or other conditions (see Table 9–4).

Another potential pitfall is dismissing an entire case because a patient is grossly exaggerating a deficit. Patients may be seeking attention for a problem by overstating or overreacting to it. Also, a neurologic disorder may be triggering fear or overwhelming anxiety.

Possibly the single most common error is failure to recognize MS because its early signs may be evanescent, exclusively sensory, or so disparate as to appear to violate *several* Laws of Neuroanatomy. The correct diagnosis can now usually be made early and reliably with MRIs, visual evoked response testing, and cerebrospinal fluid analysis (see Chapter 15). On the other hand, trivial sensory or motor symptoms that are accompanied by normal variations in these highly technical tests are likely to lead to some false-positive diagnoses of MS.

Neurologists are also prone to err in diagnosing involuntary movement disorders as being psychogenic. These disorders, in fact, have some stigmata of psychogenic illness (see Chapter 2): They can be bizarre, associated with mental abnormalities, precipitated or exacerbated by anxiety, or apparently relieved by tricks, such as when a dystonic gait can be alleviated by walking backward. Also, involuntary movements will usually be reduced or even abolished during an interview under an hypnotic. Since laboratory tests are not available for many disorders—chorea, tics, tremors, and focal and generalized dystonia—the diagnosis rests on the neurologist's clinical evaluation. As a general rule, movement disorders should always first be considered neurologic (see Chapter 18).

Epileptic and psychogenic seizures are often misdiagnosed in both directions (Chapter 10). In general, psychogenic seizures are clonic and unaccompanied by incontinence, tongue biting, or loss of body tone (Fig. 3–6). Immediately afterward, patients regain awareness and have no retrograde amnesia. However, numerous exceptions exist. Frontal lobe seizures and mixtures of epileptic and psychogenic seizures notoriously mimic psychogenic seizures. CCTV correlations between convulsions and EEG changes have become the most reliable diagnostic test.

Individuals with emotional and thought disorders have often been misdiagnosed in the past as having psychogenic disturbances; however, the mental changes have been found in many cases to result from frontal lobe meningiomas and other frontal lobe tumors. The error has arisen because patients with these tumors often have had no overt intellectual or physical abnormalities. With the ready availability of the CT and MRI, physicians now rarely overlook any structural lesion.

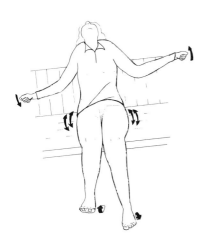

FIGURE 3-6.

This young woman, who is screaming during an entire 30-second episode, is having a psychogenic seizure. Its non-neurologic nature is revealed in several typical features. In addition to verbalizing throughout the episode rather than only at its onset (as in an epileptic cry), she maintains her body tone, which is required to keep her sitting upright; has alternating flailing limb movements, rather than organized bilateral clonic jerks; and has subtle but suggestive pelvic thrusting. After psychogenic seizures, patients are fully alert, oriented, and able to recall events preceding and possibly during the episode, rather than being lethargic, dull, and amnestic.

In general, neurologists rely on physical findings, CTs, and MRIs. They tend to invoke a Confucian attitude of "One Babinski sign is worth a thousand words."

REFERENCES

Baker GA, Hanley JR, Jackson HF, et al: Detecting the faking of amnesia: Performance differences between simulators and patients with memory impairments. J Clin Exp Neuropsychol *15*: 668–684, 1993

Baker JHE, Silver JR: Hysterical paraplegia. J Neurol Neurosurg Psychiatry *50*: 375–382, 1987

Caplan LR, Nadelson T: Multiple sclerosis and hysteria: Lessons learned from their association. JAMA *243*: 2418–2421, 1980

Fishbain DA, Goldberg M: The misdiagnosis of conversion disorder in a psychiatric emergency service. Gen Hosp Psychiatry *13*: 177–181, 1991

Glatt SL, Kennedy D, Barter R, et al: Conversion hysteria: A study of prognosis with long-term follow-up. Neurology *41* (Suppl 1): 120, 1991

Hurst LC: What was wrong with Anna O? J Roy Soc Med *75*: 129–131, 1982

Keane JR: Hysterical gait disorders. Neurology *39*: 586–589, 1989

Lazare A: Conversion symptoms. N Engl J Med *305*: 745–748, 1981

Maloney MJ: Diagnosing hysterical conversion reactions in children. J Pediatr *97*: 1016–1020, 1980

Matas M: Psychogenic voice disorders. Can J Psychiatry *36*: 363–365, 1991

Reich P, Gottfried LA: Factitious disorders in a teaching hospital. Ann Intern Med *99*: 240–247, 1983

Richtsmeier AJ: Pitfalls in diagnosis of unexplained symptoms. Psychosomatics *25*: 253–255, 1984

Saint-Hilaire MH, Saint-Hilaire JM, Granger, L: Jumping Frenchmen of Maine. Neurology *36*: 1269–1271, 1986

Wolf M, Birger M, Ben Shoshan J, et al: Conversion deafness. Ann Otol Rhinol Laryngol *102*: 349–352, 1993

4 Cranial Nerve Impairments

The evaluation of cranial nerve impairment is complex. Individually, in pairs, or in groups, the cranial nerves are vulnerable to numerous conditions. Moreover, when a nerve seems to be impaired, the problem might not be damage to the cranial nerve itself, but rather an underlying cerebral injury or psychogenic disturbance. Following custom, this chapter uses the 12 cranial nerves' Roman numeral designations that can be recalled using the old mnemonic, "On old Olympus' towering top, a Finn and German viewed some hops."

I	Olfactory	VII	Facial
II	Optic	VIII	Acoustic
III	Oculomotor	IX	Glossopharyngeal
IV	Trochlear	X	Vagus
V	Trigeminal	XI	Spinal accessory
VI	Abducens	XII	Hypoglossal

THE OLFACTORY NERVE (FIRST CRANIAL NERVE)

Olfactory nerves transmit the sensation of smell to the brain. From sensory receptors within each nasal cavity, branches of the pair of olfactory nerves pass upward through the multiple holes in the cribriform plate of the skull to several areas of the brain. They terminate mostly in the undersurface of the frontal cortex, which is the home of the olfactory sensory areas, and more deeply in the hypothalamus and amygdala, the cornerstones of the limbic system (see Fig. 16–5). The bringing of olfactory sensation into the limbic system accounts for the influence of smell on psychosexual behavior.

When both olfactory nerves are impaired, patients, who are then said to have *anosmia*, cannot perceive smells or appreciate the aroma of food. Sometimes anosmia has life-threatening consequences, as when people cannot smell escaping gas. More commonly, food without a perceptible aroma is virtually tasteless. People with anosmia, to whom food is completely bland, tend to have a decreased appetite.

To test the olfactory nerve, the patient is asked to identify certain substances by smelling through one nostril while the other is compressed. Testing must be done with readily identifiable and odoriferous but innocuous substances, such as coffee. A set of "scratch 'n sniff" odors has been manufactured for detailed testing. Volatile and irritative substances, such as ammonia and alcohol, are not suitable because they may trigger intranasal trigeminal nerve receptors and bypass a (possibly damaged) olfactory nerve.

Unilateral anosmia may result from tumors adjacent to the olfactory nerve, such as olfactory groove meningiomas (see Fig. 20–5). In the classic Foster-Kennedy syndrome, anosmia is associated with optic atrophy when these tumors also compress the nearby optic nerve. If the tumors grow into the frontal lobe, anosmia is accompanied by personality changes, dementia, seizures, or hemiparesis. However, head trauma is the most common cause of anosmia. In addition to direct nasal injuries, frontal head trauma tends to shear the delicate olfactory nerve fibers as they pass through the cribriform plate (see Head Trauma, Chapter 22).

Anosmia may of course be psychogenic. Patients with psychogenic anosmia are apparently unable to "smell" either irritative or innocuous substances. This complete sensory loss would be possible only if both trigeminal and both olfactory nerves were obliterated. However, most individuals have a genetically based anosmia to one of several hundred perceptible smells.

Olfactory hallucinations may be a manifestation of partial complex seizures that originate in the medial-inferior surface of the temporal lobe, the *uncus*. Formerly called "uncinate fits," these seizures consist of episodes lasting only several seconds in which ill-defined but often sweet smells are superimposed on a background of impaired consciousness and behavioral aberrations (see Chapter 10). Of course, olfactory hallucinations can be purely psychogenic. In contrast to those of uncinate seizures, psychogenic "odors" are almost always foul smelling, continual, and not associated with impaired consciousness.

Although these neurologic and psychogenic disturbances may be tantalizing, most disturbances of smell are mundane. In older people, normal age-related neuronal degeneration causes anosmia: more than 50 per cent of individuals older than 65 years and 75 per cent of those older than 80 years have an impaired sense of smell. Anosmia is also found in anyone with nasal congestion. In addition, since the olfactory nerve can be sheared off as it passes through the cribriform plate, even minor head trauma from almost any direction can cause anosmia. Abnormal smells most often originate in head and neck infections, such as sinusitis, bronchitis, and pyorrhea.

THE OPTIC NERVE (SECOND CRANIAL NERVE)

The optic nerves and their tracts convey visual information from the eye to the cerebral cortex and light intensity status from the eye to the brainstem. The optic nerves, unlike other cranial nerves, are actual myelin-coated projections of the brain, which makes them part of the central nervous system (CNS). They are susceptible to CNS illnesses, particularly childhood-onset metabolic storage diseases, migraines (Chapter 9), and multiple sclerosis-induced optic neuritis (see Chapter 15). Compared to other cranial injuries, visual impairments are the ones most often associated with mental impairments.

The optic *nerves'* receptors are in the retinas. At the optic chiasm, their nasal fibers cross while the temporal fibers continue uncrossed (Fig. 4–1). Temporal fibers of one eye join nasal fibers of the other to form the optic *tracts*. The tracts pass through the temporal and parietal lobes to terminate in the calcarine cortex of the occipital lobe. Thus, each occipital lobe receives visual information from the contralateral visual field.

In their other function, the optic nerves and tracts form the afferent limb of the *light reflex* by sending small branches containing information about light intensity status to the midbrain. After a synapse, the oculomotor nerves (the

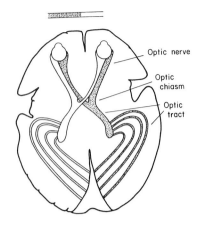

FIGURE 4–1

The optic nerves extend from the retinas to the optic chiasm where they divide to form the optic tracts. The primary effect of this system is that the impulses from each visual field are brought to the cortex of the contralateral occipital lobe.

third cranial nerves) form the efferent limb. The light reflex adjusts pupil size to the brightness of light that strikes the retina: It constricts the pupils in response to increased light. A similar mechanism, the *accommodation reflex,* constricts the pupils when gaze is moved from a distant to a close object.

Routine testing of the optic nerve includes examination of (1) visual acuity (see Fig. 12–2), (2) visual fields (Fig. 4–2), and (3) the ocular fundi (Fig. 4–3). Since the visual system is important, complex, and subject to numerous ocular, neurologic, iatrogenic, and psychogenic disturbances, those visual dis-

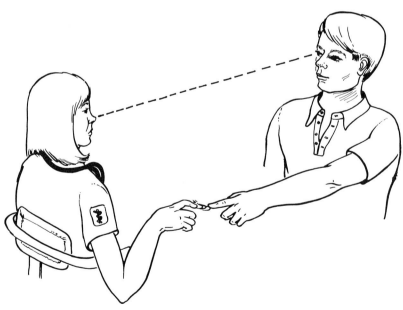

FIGURE 4–2

In testing visual fields by the confrontation method, this physician wiggles her index finger as the patient points to it without deviating his eyes from her nose. Each eye must be tested individually, and the four quadrants of each eye's visual field must be tested. (Only in this way will the examiner detect a bitemporal quadrantanopia, which is a characteristic of pituitary adenomas.) Young children and others unable to comply with this testing method may be examined in a more superficial but still meaningful manner: The physician assesses their response to an attention-catching object introduced to each visual field. If a dollar bill, toy, or glass of water fails to capture the patient's attention, visual field deficit(s) may be present.

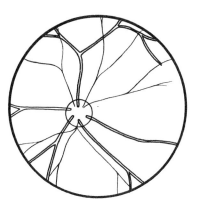

FIGURE 4-3

The normal optic fundus or disk is yellow, flat, and clearly demarcated from the surrounding red retina. The retinal veins, as everywhere else in the body, are larger than their corresponding arteries. The retinal veins can normally be seen to pulsate except with increased intracranial pressure.

turbances particularly relevant to a psychiatrist's practice are given an entire chapter (see Chapter 12).

THE OCULOMOTOR, TROCHLEAR, AND ABDUCENS NERVES (THIRD, FOURTH, AND SIXTH CRANIAL NERVES)

The oculomotor, trochlear, and abducens nerves are considered as a group because they move the eyes in unison to provide normal *conjugate gaze*. The oculomotor nerves (third cranial nerves) originate in the midbrain (Fig. 4-4) and eventually supply the pupil constrictor, eyelid, and adductor and elevator muscles of each eye (medial rectus, inferior oblique, inferior rectus, and superior rectus). Oculomotor nerve impairment, which is a frequently occurring situation, leads to an obvious constellation: a dilated pupil, ptosis, and outward deviation (abduction) of the eye (Fig. 4-5).

The trochlear nerves (fourth cranial nerves) also originate in the midbrain. They supply only the superior oblique muscle, which is responsible for depression of the eye when it is adducted (turned inward). Since this maneuver is difficult to detect and the nerve is rarely injured, only specialists are responsible for recognizing trochlear nerve impairment.

The abducens nerves (sixth cranial nerves), unlike the third and fourth cranial nerves, originate in the pons (Fig. 4-6). They too have only a single function—abduction—for which they innervate only a single muscle, the lat-

MIDBRAIN

FIGURE 4-4

The oculomotor nerves (third cranial nerves) arise from nuclei in the dorsal portion of the midbrain. Each descends through the red nucleus, which carries cerebellar outflow fibers to the contralateral limbs. Then they also pass through the cerebral peduncle, which carries the corticospinal tract that is destined to innervate the contralateral limbs.

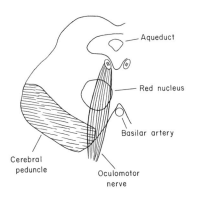

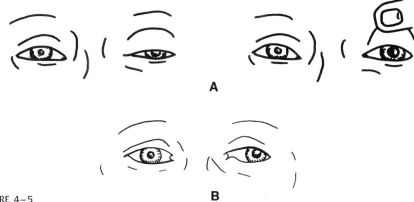

A

B

FIGURE 4–5

A, The patient with paresis of the left oculomotor nerve has ptosis and lateral deviation of the left eye, which has a dilated and unreactive pupil. *B,* In a milder case, close inspection reveals subtle ptosis, lateral deviation of the eye, and dilation of the pupil. In both cases, patients have diplopia that increases when adducting the left eye because looking to the right requires increased reliance on the paretic left medial rectus muscle (also see Fig. 12–13).

eral rectus. Abducens nerve impairment, which is relatively common, causes inturning (adduction) of the eye, but no ptosis or pupil changes (Fig. 4–7). In summary, the lateral rectus muscle is innervated by the sixth cranial nerve, the superior oblique by the fourth, and all the rest by the third. A mnemonic captures this relationship: LR_6SO_4

PONS

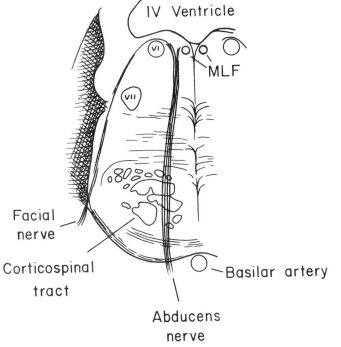

FIGURE 4–6

The abducens nerves (sixth cranial nerves) arise from nuclei located in the dorsal portion of the pons. These nuclei are adjacent to the medial longitudinal fasciculus (MLF; see Fig. 15–3). As the abducens nerves descend, they pass medial to the facial nerves and then penetrate the corticospinal tract.

FIGURE 4-7

The patient with paresis of the left abducens nerve has medial deviation of the left eye. There will be diplopia on looking ahead and toward the left, but not when looking to the right (see Fig. 12-14).

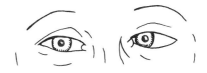

In terms of conjugate ocular motility, the oculomotor nerve on one side is complementary to the abducens nerve on the other. For example, when looking to the left, the left sixth nerve and right third nerve innervates their respective muscles to produce conjugate leftward eye movement. Complementary innervation is essential for conjugate gaze. If both third nerves were to innervate their muscles, the eyes would look toward the nose, and if both sixth nerves were innervated, they would look toward opposite walls.

Dysconjugate gaze results in diplopia (double vision). Diplopia is most often explainable by a lesion in the oculomotor nerve on one side or the abducens nerve on the other. For example, if a patient has diplopia when looking to the left, then either the left abducens nerve or the right oculomotor nerve is paretic. Diplopia on right gaze, of course, suggests a paresis of either the right abducens nerve or left oculomotor nerve. Although elaborate diagnostic tests may be performed, the presence or absence of other signs of oculomotor nerve palsy (a dilated pupil and ptosis) usually indicates whether that nerve is responsible.

The ocular cranial nerves may be damaged by lesions in the brainstem, in the nerves' course from the brainstem to the ocular muscles, or in their neuromuscular junctions, but not in the cerebral hemispheres (the cerebrum). Cerebral lesions spare these and other cranial nerves, and conjugate gaze is preserved. Thus, patients with advanced Alzheimer's disease and those who have sustained cerebral anoxia have devastating cerebral lesions but normal ocular motility. These patients typically exist in a persistent vegetative state while retaining full, conjugate eye movements.

Brainstem lesions, which routinely damage cranial nerves, produce combinations of injuries of the ocular nerves and the adjacent corticospinal (pyramidal) tract. That tract carries motor function to the contralateral limbs, or occasionally the red nucleus, which carries cerebellar outflow to the contralateral limbs. These lesions cause diplopia and contralateral hemiparesis or ataxia. Almost all cases result from brainstem infarctions caused by occlusion of a small branch of the basilar artery (see Chapter 11).

Despite generating complex neurologic deficits, brainstem lesions generally do not impair the mental status. However, some well-known exceptions exist. Wernicke's encephalopathy, one exception, consists of memory impairments (amnesia) accompanied by nystagmus and signs of damage to the oculomotor and abducens nerves (see Chapter 7). Another exception is transtentorial herniation, in which a cerebral mass lesion, such as a subdural hematoma, squeezes the temporal lobe through the tentorial notch. In this situation, the mass compresses the oculomotor nerve and brainstem to cause coma and a dilated pupil (see Fig. 19-3).

With a right-sided midbrain infarction—a typical brainstem lesion—a patient would have a right oculomotor nerve palsy, which would cause right ptosis, a dilated pupil, and diplopia, accompanied by left hemiparesis (Fig. 4-8). With a slightly different right-sided midbrain infarction, a patient might have right oculomotor nerve palsy and left tremor (Fig. 4-9). A right-sided

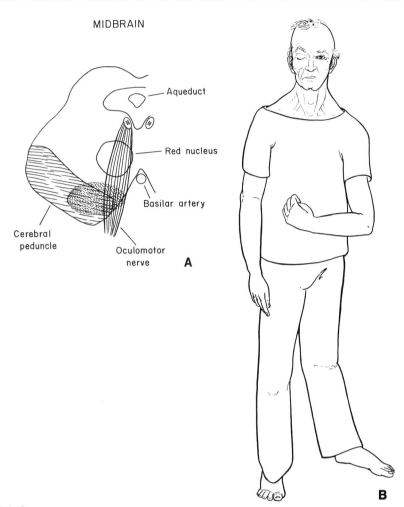

MIDBRAIN

Aqueduct

Red nucleus

Basilar artery

Cerebral
peduncle

Oculomotor
nerve   **A**

B

FIGURE 4–8

A, A right midbrain infarction damages the oculomotor nerve that supplies the ipsilateral eye and the adjacent cerebral peduncle, which contains the corticospinal tract that subsequently crosses in the medulla, ultimately supplying the contralateral arm and leg. *B,* The patient has right-sided ptosis from the right oculomotor nerve palsy and left hemiparesis from the corticospinal tract injury. Also note that the ptosis elicits a compensatory, unconscious elevation of the eyebrow to uncover the eye. (Similar eyebrow elevations can be seen in other conditions that cause ptosis, including cluster headache, myasthenia gravis, and lateral medullary syndrome.)

pontine lesion translates into a right abducens nerve paresis and left hemiparesis (Fig. 4–10). Notably, in each of these brainstem injuries, the mental status is normal because the cerebrum is unscathed.

Another common site of brainstem injury that affects the ocular nerves is the *medial longitudinal fasciculus (MLF)*. This structure is the heavily myelinated, midline tract that links the nuclei of the oculomotor and abducens nerves (see Figs. 4–10 and 15–3). Its interruption produces the *MLF syndrome*, which is often called *internuclear ophthalmoplegia (INO)*. This syndrome, which is characteristic of multiple sclerosis, consists of nystagmus of the abducting eye and failure of the adducting eye to cross the midline (see Fig. 15–4).

Lesions occur more frequently in the long paths of the oculomotor or abducens nerves, between the brainstem and the ocular muscles than in the

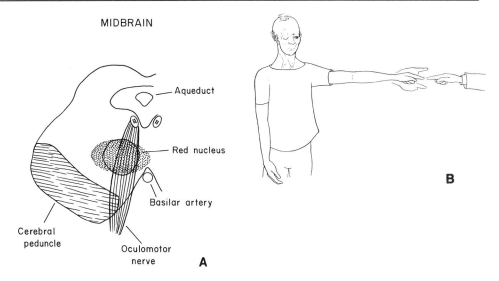

MIDBRAIN

Aqueduct

Red nucleus

Basilar artery

Cerebral peduncle

Oculomotor nerve

A

B

FIGURE 4–9

A, A right midbrain infarction damages the oculomotor nerve and the *red nucleus,* which conveys left cerebellar hemisphere outflow to the left arm and leg by a "double-cross." *B,* This patient has right ptosis from the oculomotor nerve palsy and left arm ataxia from the damage to the cerebellar outflow tract.

brainstem. Moreover, these lesions produce simple, readily identifiable clinical pictures. *Diabetic infarction,* the most frequently occurring lesion of the oculomotor nerves, produces a sharp headache and paresis of the affected muscles that lasts several months. Although otherwise typical, diabetic oculomotor nerve infarctions characteristically spare the pupil, i.e., the pupil remains normal in size but as usual, the eye is abducted and ptosis is present.

The oculomotor nerve, just as it exits from the midbrain, may also be injured by ruptured aneurysms of the posterior communicating artery. In this case, oculomotor nerve palsy—which would be the least of the patient's problems—is one component of a subarachnoid hemorrhage that usually renders patients prostrate with a severe headache. Similarly, children occasionally have migraine headaches that cause temporary oculomotor nerve paresis (see Ophthalmoplegic Migraine, Chapter 9). In contrast, in the motor neuron diseases amyotrophic lateral sclerosis (ALS) and poliomyelitis, the oculomotor and abducens nerves are normal despite destruction of large numbers of motor neurons. Patients may have full and conjugate eye movements despite being unable to breathe, lift their limbs, or move their head.

Even disorders of the neuromuscular junction produce oculomotor or abducens nerve paresis. In myasthenia gravis (see Fig. 6–3) and botulism, for example, impairment of acetylcholine transmission leads to combinations of ocular and other cranial nerve paresis (see Fig. 6–1). These deficits may be perplexing to physicians because the muscle weakness is subtle and variable in severity and pattern. These disorders are always important, especially in their extremes: Respiratory impairment may ensue in severe cases, and mild cases may be overlooked or misdiagnosed as psychogenic.

In a related issue, people with congenital dysconjugate or "crossed" eyes, *strabismus,* do not have double vision. Their brain suppresses one of the images. If uncorrected in childhood, strabismus leads to blindness of the deviated eye, *amblyopia.*

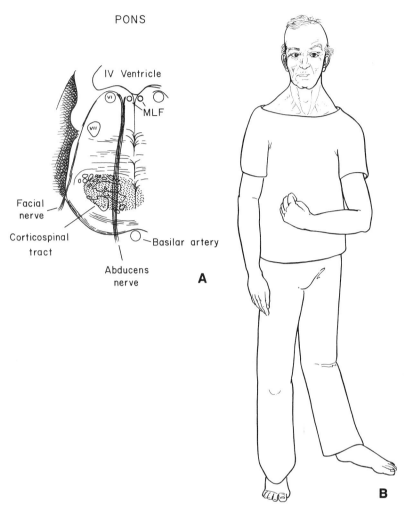

PONS

IV Ventricle

MLF

Facial nerve

Corticospinal tract

Basilar artery

Abducens nerve

A

B

FIGURE 4–10

A, A right pontine infarction damages the abducens nerve, which supplies the ipsilateral eye, and the adjacent corticospinal tract, which supplies the contralateral limbs. (This situation is analogous to midbrain infarctions; see Fig. 4–8.) *B,* The patient has inward turning of the right eye from paresis of the right abducens nerve, and left hemiparesis from right corticospinal tract damage.

As for psychogenic disturbances, people can usually feign ocular muscle weakness only by staring inward, as if looking at the tip of their nose. Children often do this playfully; however, adults with their eyes in such a position are easily recognized as displaying voluntary, bizarre activity. Another psychogenic disturbance, relatively common in health care workers, is surreptitiously instilling eye drops that dilate the pupil to mimic ophthalmologic or neurologic disorders.

THE TRIGEMINAL NERVE (FIFTH CRANIAL NERVE)

The trigeminal nerves' main jobs are to convey sensation from the face and to innervate the large, powerful muscles that protrude and close the jaw. Since these muscles' main function is to chew, they are often called the "muscles of mastication." The motor nucleus of the nerve is situated in the pons, but its sensory nucleus extends from the midbrain through the medulla (see Fig. 2–9). The nerves leave the brainstem at the side of the pons to become one of the three cranial nerves passing through the cerebellopontine angle: V, VII, and VIII.

Examination of the trigeminal nerve begins by testing sensation in its three sensory divisions (Fig. 4–11). The examiner touches the side of the patient's forehead, cheek, and jaw. Areas of reduced sensation, *hypalgesia*, should conform to anatomic outlines.

Assessing the *corneal reflex* is useful, especially in examining patients whose sensory loss does not conform to neurologic expectations. The corneal reflex is a "superficial reflex" that is basically independent of upper motor neuron (UMN) status. This reflex begins with stimulation of the cornea by a wisp of cotton or a breath of air that triggers the trigeminal nerve, which forms the afferent limb. A brainstem synapse stimulus innervates both facial (seventh cranial) nerves, the efferent limb, which innervate both sets of orbicularis oculi muscles. If the cotton tip is first applied to the right cornea and neither eye blinks, and then to the left cornea and both eyes blink, the explanation is that the right trigeminal nerve (the afferent limb) is impaired. If cotton on the right cornea fails to provide a right eye blink, but succeeds in provoking a left eye blink, the explanation is that the right facial nerve (the efferent limb) is impaired.

Testing jaw muscle strength is done by asking the patient to clench and then protrude the jaw. The *jaw jerk reflex*, which is similar to a deep tendon reflex, consists of a prompt but not overly forceful closing after a tap (Fig. 4–12). A hyperactive response indicates an UMN (corticobulbar tract) lesion, and a hypoactive response indicates a lower motor neuron (LMN) or cranial nerve lesion. The physician should test the jaw jerk in patients with dysarthria, dysphagia, and emotional lability—mostly to assess the likelihood of pseudobulbar palsy (see below).

Injury of a trigeminal nerve causes facial hypalgesia, afferent corneal reflex impairment, jaw jerk hypoactivity, and deviation of the jaw toward the side of the lesion. Such deficits may be caused by nasopharyngeal tumors, gunshot wounds, and tumors of the cerebellopontine angle, such as acoustic neuromas.

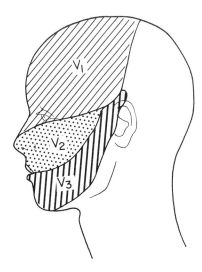

FIGURE 4–11

The three divisions of the trigeminal nerve convey sensory innervation of the face. The first division (V_1) supplies the forehead, the cornea, and the scalp up to the vertex; the second (V_2) supplies the malar area; and the third (V_3) supplies the lower jaw except for the angle. These distributions have more than academic importance. They may be mapped by *Herpes zoster* infections ("shingles"), trigeminal neuralgia (see Chapter 9), and facial angioma in the Sturge-Weber syndrome (see Fig. 13–7), but not be respected in psychogenic facial sensory loss.

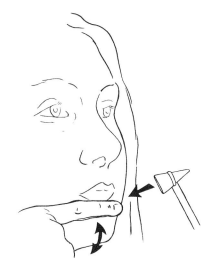

FIGURE 4–12

Tapping the normal, open, relaxed jaw will move it slightly downward. The jaw jerk reflex is the soft rebound. Abnormalities are mostly a matter of rapidity and strength. In a hypoactive reflex, as found in bulbar palsy and other LMN injuries, there is little or no rebound. In a hyperactive reflex, as in pseudobulbar palsy and other UMN (corticobulbar tract) lesions, there is a quick and forceful rebound.

In the opposite situation, *trigeminal neuralgia* (tic douloureux) results from trigeminal nerve irritation by an aberrant vessel or other lesion in the cerebellopontine angle. Instead of having hypalgesia, patients with trigeminal neuralgia have bursts of lancinating face pain in the distribution of the third or other division of the nerve (see Chapter 9). Another common trigeminal nerve problem is *Herpes zoster* infection, which causes a rash followed by an excruciating pain (*postherpetic neuralgia*) in one division of the nerve (see Chapter 14).

Finally, a psychogenic sensory loss involving the face will usually encompass the entire face or be included in a sensory loss of one half the body. In almost all cases, the following three non-anatomic features will be present: (1) The sensory loss will not involve the scalp (although the portion anterior to the vertex is supplied by the trigeminal nerve); (2) the corneal reflex will remain intact; and (3) when only one half the face is affected, sensation will be lost sharply rather than gradually at the midline, i.e., the midline will be split (see Fig. 3–4).

THE FACIAL NERVE (SEVENTH CRANIAL NERVE)

The facial nerves' major functions are to convey taste sensation and to innervate the facial muscles. While the trigeminal nerves supply the muscles of mastication, the facial nerves supply the "muscles of facial expression." Their motor and sensory nuclei are in the pons and the nerves exit through the side of the brainstem with the other cerebellopontine angle nerves.

In a unique and potentially confusing arrangement in neuroanatomy, cerebral impulses innervate both the contralateral and ipsilateral facial nerve motor nuclei. The facial nerves supply the ipsilateral temporalis, orbicularis oculi, and orbicularis oris muscles—the muscles responsible for a person's frown, raised eyebrows, wink, smile, and grimace. Because of their crossed and uncrossed supply, the upper facial muscles are ultimately innervated by both cerebral hemispheres, whereas the lower ones are innervated only by the contralateral cerebral hemisphere (Fig. 4–13).

Taste sensation is more straightforward. The facial nerve conveys impulses from taste receptors of the anterior two thirds of the tongue, and the glosso-

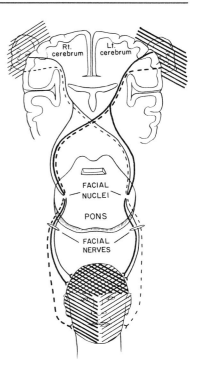

FIGURE 4–13

In a unique arrangement, corticobulbar tracts originating in the ipsilateral as well as in the contralateral
cerebral hemisphere supply each facial nerve nucleus.
Each facial nerve supplies the ipsilateral muscles of
facial expression. Since the upper half of the face receives cortical innervation from both hemispheres, cerebral injuries lead to paresis only of the lower half of
the contralateral face. In contrast, facial nerve injuries
lead to paresis of both the upper and lower half of the
ipsilateral side of the face.

pharyngeal nerve (the ninth cranial nerve) conveys those from the posterior
third. Also, despite the extraordinary variety of foods, taste sensation is surprisingly limited. Taste receptors detect only four fundamental sensations: bit-
ter, sweet, sour, and salty. Food actually derives most of its flavor from its
aroma, which is detected by the olfactory nerve. Moreover, the olfactory nerve,
not the facial nerve, has extensive connections with the frontal lobe cortex and
limbic system.

Routine facial nerve testing involves examining the strength of the facial
muscles and, at certain times, assessing taste. An examiner observes the patient's face, first at rest and then during a succession of maneuvers that employ
various facial muscles: looking upward, closing the eyes, and smiling. When
weakness is detected, the examiner should try to ascertain if it involves both
the upper and lower, or only the lower, facial muscles. Upper and lower paresis suggests a lesion of the facial nerve itself. In this case, taste is also likely
to be impaired. Of course, with unilateral or even bilateral facial nerve injuries,
patients have no mental changes. In contrast, paresis of only the lower facial
muscles suggests a lesion of the contralateral cerebral hemisphere that may be
associated with ipsilateral hemiparesis and mental changes. With weakness of
the right lower face, aphasia may be present. In these cases, taste sensation
will be preserved.

To test taste, the examiner applies either a dilute salt or sugar solution to
the anterior portion of each side of the tongue, which must remain protruded
to prevent the solution from spreading. A patient will normally be able to
identify the fundamental taste sensations, but not those "tastes" that depend
on aroma, such as onion and garlic.

Facial nerve damage results in paresis of the ipsilateral upper and lower
face muscles with or without loss of taste sensation. Of the various facial nerve
injuries, _Bell's palsy, an_ idiopathic inflammatory condition, is probably the
most frequently encountered illness (Fig. 4–14). Lyme disease (see Chapters 5

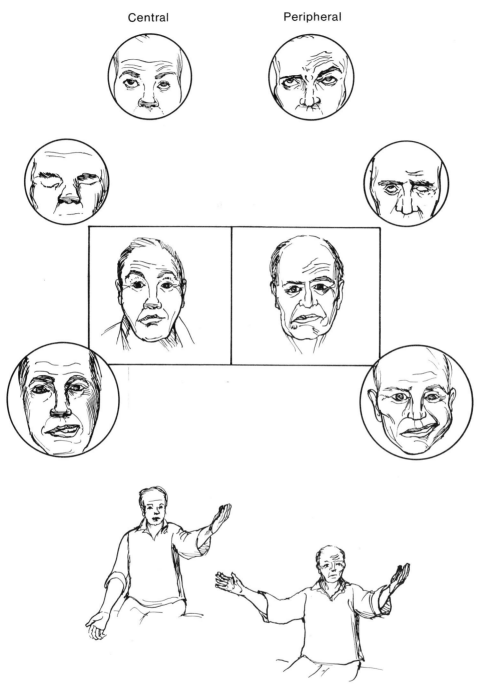

FIGURE 4–14

The patient on the left has weakness of his right lower face from thrombosis of the left middle cerebral artery. He might be said to have a "central" (CNS) paralysis. The patient on the right has right-sided weakness of both the upper and lower face from a right facial nerve injury (Bell's palsy). He might be said to have a "peripheral" (cranial nerve) paralysis.

In the *center, boxed sketches*, the man with the central palsy, on the left, has flattening of the right nasolabial fold and sagging of the mouth downward to the right. This pattern of weakness indicates paresis of only the lower facial muscles. The man with the peripheral palsy on the right, however, has right-sided loss of the normal forehead furrows, in addition to flattening of the nasolabial fold. This pattern of weakness indicates paresis of the upper as well as the lower facial muscles. *Legend continued on opposite page* and 7), a relatively common infectious illness in several regions of the United States, can mimic Bell's palsy. Destructive injuries include lacerations and cerebellopontine angle tumors.

Lesions that stimulate the nerve have the opposite effect. As in trigeminal neuralgia, aberrant vessels in the cerebellopontine angle irritate the facial nerve. Intermittent facial nerve stimulation produces involuntary contractions of the muscles on one side of the face. This condition, *hemifacial spasm* (see Chapter 18), is the facial nerve's counterpart of trigeminal neuralgia.

Patients with psychologic aberrations cannot mimic unilateral facial paresis. People who refuse to be examined, particularly children, might forcefully close their eyelids and mouth. The willful nature of this maneuver is evident when the examiner finds resistance on opening the eyelids and jaw, and sees, when the eyelids are pried open, that the eyeballs retrovert (Bell's phenomena).

THE ACOUSTIC NERVE (EIGHTH CRANIAL NERVE)

Each acoustic nerve is actually composed of two divisions with separate courses and functions: hearing and balance. The *cochlear nerve*, one of the two nerves, transmits auditory impulses from the middle and inner ear mechanisms to the superior temporal gyri of both cerebral hemispheres (Fig. 4–15). This bilateral cortical representation of sound explains the fact that damage to the acoustic nerve or ear itself may cause deafness in that ear, but unilateral lesions of the brainstem or cerebral hemisphere—CNS damage—will not cause hearing impairment. Cerebral lesions that spare hearing occur in patients whose extensive cerebrovascular accidents or tumors cause aphasia without impairing their (nonspecific) response to sounds. Although Alzheimer's disease patients often have hearing loss, that impairment results from age-related nerve and inner ear changes.

During the routine examination, hearing is tested initially by the examiner whispering into each of the patient's ears while covering the other. Acoustic nerve injury may result from medications, such as aspirin or streptomycin, by skull fractures severing the nerve, or by cerebellopontine angle tumors, particularly acoustic neuromas associated with neurofibromatosis. Congenital deafness, as well as mental retardation, commonly results from *in utero* rubella infections or kernicterus (see Chapter 13).

In the *circled sketches at the top,* the patients have been asked to look upward—a maneuver that would exaggerate upper facial weakness. The man with central weakness has normal upward movement of the eyebrows and furrowing of the forehead. The man with peripheral weakness has no eyebrow or forehead movement, and the forehead skin remains flat.

In the *circled sketches second from the top,* the men have been asked to close their eyes—a maneuver that also would exaggerate upper facial weakness. The man with the central weakness has widening of the palpebral fissure, but he is able to close his eyelids and cover the eyeball. The man with the peripheral weakness is unable to close the affected eyelids, although his genuine effort is apparent by the retroversion of the eyeball (Bell's phenomenon).

In the *lowest circled sketches,* the men have been asked to smile—a maneuver that would exaggerate lower facial weakness. Both men have strength only of the left side of the mouth, and thus it deviates to the left. If tested, the man with Bell's palsy would have loss of taste on the anterior two thirds of his tongue on the affected side.

The *bottom sketches* show the response when both men are asked to elevate their arms. The man with the central facial weakness also has paresis of the adjacent arm, but the man with the peripheral weakness has no arm paresis.

In summary, the man on the left with the left middle cerebral artery occlusion has paresis of his right lower face and arm. The man on the right with right Bell's palsy has paresis of his right upper and lower face and loss of taste.

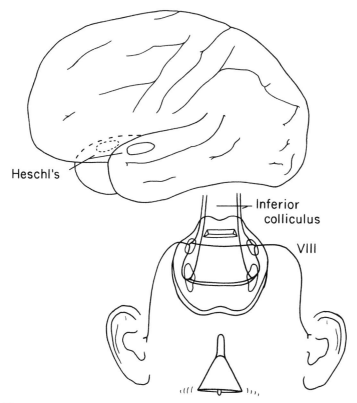

Heschl's

Inferior
colliculus

VIII

FIGURE 4–15

The cochlear division of the acoustic nerve synapses extensively in the pons. Crossed and uncrossed fibers pass upward through the brainstem to terminate in the auditory (Heschl's area) cortex of both temporal lobes. In the dominant hemisphere, Heschl's area is adjacent to Wernicke's language area (see Fig. 8–1).

On the other hand, when patients seem to mimic deafness, the examiner may attempt to startle them with a loud sound or may watch for an *auditory-ocular reflex* (seeing if they look involuntarily toward a noise). Factitious hearing loss may be confirmed by testing brainstem auditory evoked responses (BAERs; see Chapter 15).

About 25 per cent of people older than 65 years have hearing impairments from degeneration of the acoustic nerve or the middle or inner ear structures. Not only might hearing impairment contribute to inattention and feelings of isolation, but also when visual and hearing impairments are superimposed on a marginal cognitive capacity, sensory deprivation may precipitate hallucinations and other mental aberrations. In helping the elderly, physicians should dispense hearing aids readily and even on a trial basis.

Another common problem among the elderly is a persistent ringing or whistling sound, *tinnitus*. Although it may be caused by medications that damage the inner ear, tinnitus is most often caused by ischemia from atherosclerotic cerebrovascular disease. An audible heartbeat, while often the result of heightened sensitivity, may also be a manifestation of atherosclerosis because a rigid arterial tree transmits undampened cardiac contractions all the way to the small vessels of the inner ear.

Auditory evaluations are necessary in patients suspected of having a psychogenic hearing impairment; children with autism, cerebral palsy, mental retardation, speech impediments, and poor school performance; and most older adults.

The other division, the *vestibular nerve*, transmits impulses from the labyrinth governing equilibrium, orientation, and change in position. The most characteristic symptom of vestibular nerve damage is *vertigo*, a sensation that one is spinning within the environment or that the environment is itself spinning. Unfortunately patients casually say "dizziness" when they mean lightheadedness, anxiety, weakness, or unsteadiness, rather than vertigo. The most common cause of vertigo is vestibular injury, such as viral infections of the inner ear, *labyrinthitis*, or ischemia.

Ménière's disease, which deserves special attention, is a relatively common, chronic vestibular disorder of unknown etiology that causes attacks of unequivocal vertigo, unilateral tinnitus, and nystagmus. Developing in women more often than in men, it also leads to progressive hearing loss. Although most attacks of Ménière's disease are obvious, they may be indistinguishable from basilar artery transient ischemic attacks (TIAs), basilar artery migraines, and mild hyperventilation.

THE GLOSSOPHARYNGEAL, VAGUS, SPINAL AND ACCESSORY NERVES (NINTH THROUGH ELEVENTH CRANIAL NERVES)

A group of *bulbar* cranial nerves (IX through XII) arise from nuclei in the brainstem caudal to the ocular (III, IV, and VI) and the cerebellopontine (V, VII, and VIII) cranial nerves. The bulb is technically equivalent to the medulla; however, from a clinical viewpoint, the bulb includes the pons, as well as the medulla. In addition to containing the nuclei and initial portions of cranial nerves IX through XII, the bulb contains the descending corticospinal tracts, ascending sensory tracts, and sympathetic nervous system tracts. The cranial nerves innervate the muscles of the soft palate, pharynx, larynx, and tongue. They implement speaking and swallowing. The lateral medullary infarction, the most common brainstem stroke, has already illustrated the bulbar cranial nerves' relationship to certain CNS tracts and signs of their injury (Wallenberg syndrome, see Fig. 2–10).

Even though the bulbar cranial nerves originate in the lower end of the brainstem, which is nowhere near the brain's cognitive centers, and their functions are simple and mechanical, they are involved in several neurologic illnesses that have psychiatric aspects. Their impairment often leads to *bulbar palsy*, that is most notable in comparison to the infamous pseudobulbar palsy that appears to induce overwhelming emotional changes (see below). Likewise, the *locked-in syndrome*, which is important itself, may be contrasted to the persistent vegetative state (see Chapter 11), in which cognitive function is obliterated but vegetative functions—respiration, sleeping, and swallowing—persist. Finally, bulbar nerve overactivity leads to certain bizarre disorders, such as spasmodic dysphonia and spasmodic torticollis, that until recently have been considered psychogenic and untreatable (see Chapter 18).

Bulbar Palsy

Bulbar cranial nerve injury within the brainstem or along the course of the nerves leads to bulbar palsy. This commonly occurring disorder is characterized by *dysarthria* (speech impairment), *dysphagia* (difficulty in swallowing), and a hypoactive jaw and gag reflexes (Table 4–1).

To assess bulbar nerve function, the examiner should listen to the patient's spontaneous speech during the casual conversation and while eliciting the history. The patient should be asked to repeat syllables that require lingual ("la"), labial ("pa"), and guttural ("ga") speech mechanisms. Most bulbar palsy patients speak with a thick, nasal intonation. Some are mute. Even if a patient's speech is not strikingly abnormal during casual conversation, repetition of the guttural consonant, "ga...ga...ga....," will usually evoke typically thickened, nasal sounds, uttered "gna...gna...gna...." Also, when saying "ah," a patient with bulbar palsy will have little or no palate elevation because of paresis.

Patients with cerebellar dysfunction will have irregularities in the rhythm of speech that are akin to ataxia. The speech of those patients with spasmodic dysphonia has an intermittent, strained quality that often has a superimposed tremor (see Chapter 18).

In contrast to patients with aphasia, those with bulbar palsy, despite marked dysarthria, express full meaning when speaking and have normal verbal comprehension. Moreover, bulbar palsy patients can express themselves in writing. For example, a patient with bulbar palsy might be unable to repeat the phrase, "Please, pick up your hand," but would be able to comprehend and comply with the request. Patients with aphasia, in contrast, typically would be unable to repeat, comprehend, or execute the request (see Aphasia, Chapter 8).

Impaired palatal and pharyngeal movement in bulbar palsy causes dysphagia. Food tends to lodge in the trachea or go into the nasopharyngeal cavity; liquids tend to be regurgitated through the nose. Impairment of palate sensation or movement also leads to the characteristic loss of the gag reflex (Fig. 4–16). Finally, extensive bulbar damage will injure the medullary respiratory center or the nerves that innervate respiratory muscles. In particular, the bulbar form of poliomyelitis ("polio") forced its childhood victims into "iron lungs" to support their respirations. Today, many patients with Guillain-Barré syndrome, myasthenia gravis, and similar conditions must undergo tracheostomy and temporary respirator support.

Depending on its cause, bulbar palsy is associated with still other physical findings. When the jaw muscles are involved, the jaw jerk reflex will be depressed (Fig. 4–12). If the corticospinal tract is also damaged by a brainstem lesion, patients may have hyperactive deep tendon reflexes (DTRs) and Babinski signs. However, as in other conditions with brainstem damage, bulbar palsy is not associated with mental aberrations.

TABLE 4–1. Comparison of Bulbar and Pseudobulbar Palsy

	Bulbar	Pseudobulbar
Dysarthria	Yes	Yes
Dysphagia	Yes	Yes
Movement of palate		
Voluntary	No	No
Reflex	No	Yes
Jaw jerk	Hypoactive	Hyperactive
Emotional lability	No	Yes
Intellectual impairment	No	Yes

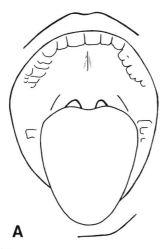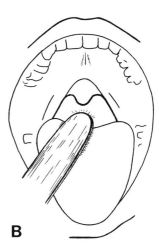

A   B

FIGURE 4-16

A, The soft palate normally forms an arch from which the uvula seems to hang. *B,* When the pharynx is stimulated, the gag reflex elicits pharyngeal muscle contraction; the soft palate rises with the uvula remaining in the midline. With bulbar nerve injury (bulbar palsy)—LMN injury —the palate has little, no, or an asymmetric movement. With corticobulbar tract injury (pseudobulbar palsy)—UMN injury—the reaction is brisk and forceful and often causes retching, coughing, or crying.

Conditions that commonly cause bulbar palsy by damaging the nerves within the brainstem are ALS, poliomyelitis, and infarctions, such as the lateral medullary infarction. Diseases that damage the cranial nerves after they have emerged from the brainstem are the Guillain-Barré syndrome, chronic meningitis, and tumors that grow along the base of the skull or within the adjacent meninges. Myasthenia gravis and botulism cause bulbar palsy by impairing neuromuscular junction transmission (Chapter 6). Most important, none of these conditions *directly* changes the mental status.

Pseudobulbar Palsy

When dysarthria and dysphagia result from frontal lobe damage, the condition is termed pseudobulbar palsy. Better known than bulbar palsy, pseudobulbar palsy is typically associated with dementia, aphasia, and unprovoked emotions (emotional lability) that overshadow physical changes.

Pseudobulbar patients' dysarthria is characterized by variable rhythm and intensity and is often said to have an "explosive" cadence. For example, when asked to repeat the consonant "ga," patients might blurt out "GA.. GA... GA.. ga... ga... ga." Their dysphagia often results in inadequate nutrition and aspiration. Although these complications might be circumvented by surgical placement of gastrotomy tubes, installing these mechanical devices has created almost as much controversy as the use of respirators in artificially prolonging life.

From an admittedly narrow neurologic perspective, an important distinguishing characteristic of pseudobulbar palsy is hyperactivity of reflexes because of damage to the UMN corticobulbar tracts (Fig. 4–17): Thus, it is sometimes called "suprabulbar" palsy. As in bulbar palsy, pseudobulbar patients have little or no palatal or pharyngeal movement in response to voluntary effort, as when attempting to say "ah." However, when the gag reflex is tested,

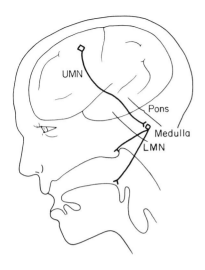

FIGURE 4–17

Damage to the bulbar cranial nerves (bulbar palsy) abolishes the jaw jerk and gag reflexes, which is a characteristic of LMN injury (see Fig. 2–2C). Although mental changes may be the most conspicuous feature of pseudobulbar palsy, corticobulbar tract damage leads to hyperactive reflexes, which is a characteristic of UMN injury (see Fig. 2–2B).

pseudobulbar palsy patients have brisk elevation of the palate and contraction of the pharynx, often overreacting with coughing, crying, and retching (Fig. 4–16). Likewise, the jaw jerk reflex, depressed in bulbar palsy, is hyperactive in pseudobulbar palsy because of UMN corticobulbar tract damage. Also in pseudobulbar palsy, damage to the frontal lobes is so common that it almost always leads to signs of bilateral corticospinal tract damage, such as hyperactive DTRs and Babinski signs. Frontal lobe damage also leads to corticobulbar tract damage that makes the face sag and impairs expression (Fig. 4–18).

The most notorious feature of pseudobulbar palsy is emotional lability, which is a tendency to cry or, less often, laugh in response to minimal provocation, with fluctuations between euphoria and depression. Patients, certainly not as expressive as the crying and laughing would suggest, often describe themselves as being awash with emotions. Amitriptyline, given in relatively low doses (e.g., 75 mg or less daily), may suppress the unwarranted, *pathologic laughing* and *crying* apart from its antidepressant effect.

Although pseudobulbar palsy has become the commonly accepted explanation for unwarranted emotional states in people with brain damage, tearfulness should not always be ascribed to brain damage. A great deal of true sadness can be expected with neurologic illness.

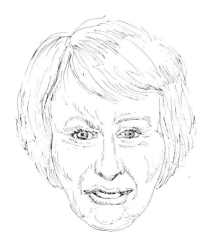

FIGURE 4–18

Patients with pseudobulbar palsy, such as this woman who has suffered multiple cerebral infarctions, often sit with a slack jaw, furrowed forehead, and vacant stare.

Pseudobulbar palsy is associated with dementia as well as with emotional lability because extensive cerebral damage usually underlies pseudobulbar palsy (see Chapter 7). Likewise, when the left cerebral hemisphere is heavily damaged, pseudobulbar palsy may be associated with aphasia, usually of the nonfluent variety (see Chapter 8). This association, seen in reverse, might account for aphasic patients crying at minimal provocation, even in frustration at naming objects. In any case, pseudobulbar palsy patients should be carefully evaluated for dementia and aphasia.

Damage to both frontal lobes or, more often, the entire cerebrum by any of a wide variety of degenerative, structural, or metabolic disturbances causes pseudobulbar palsy. The most common causes are Alzheimer's disease, multiple cerebral infarctions, head trauma, and multiple sclerosis. Congenital cerebral damage (i.e., cerebral palsy), causes pseudobulbar palsy along with bilateral spasticity and choreoathetotic movement disorders. Finally, since ALS causes both UMN and LMN damage, it leads to a mixture of bulbar and pseudobulbar palsy; however, since ALS is exclusively a motor neuron disorder, it is not associated with either dementia or aphasia (see Chapter 5).

THE HYPOGLOSSAL NERVE (TWELFTH CRANIAL NERVE)

The hypoglossal nerves originate from paired nuclei near the midline of the medulla and descend through the base of the medulla. They pass through the base of the skull and travel through the neck to innervate the tongue muscles. Each nerve innervates the ipsilateral tongue muscles. These muscles move the tongue within the mouth, protrude it when people eat and speak, and push it contralaterally. Since the pressure on each side is balanced, the tongue protrudes in the midline.

If one hypoglossal nerve was injured, that side of the tongue would become weak and, with time, atrophic. When protruded, the tongue would deviate toward the weakened side (Fig. 4–19), which illustrates the adage, "the tongue points toward the side of the lesion." If both nerves were injured, as in bulbar palsy, the tongue would become immobile. Patients with ALS have tongue fasciculations, as well as atrophy (see Fig. 5–4).

The most frequently occurring conditions in which one hypoglossal nerve is damaged are lower brainstem infarctions, penetrating neck wounds, and

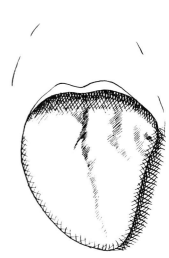

FIGURE 4–19

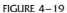

With (left) hypoglossal nerve damage, the tongue deviates toward the weaker side, and its affected (left) side undergoes atrophy.

nasopharyngeal tumors. Guillain-Barré syndrome, myasthenia gravis, and ALS usually injure both hypoglossal and other bulbar cranial nerves.

QUESTIONS and ANSWERS: CHAPTERS 1 to 4

1. A 68-year-old man has the sudden, painless onset of paresis of the right upper and lower face, inability to abduct the right eye, and paresis of the left arm and leg. Where is the lesion and what structures are involved?

> *answer:* The damaged structures include the right-sided abducens (VI) and facial (VII) nerves and the corticospinal tract destined to supply the left limbs. Only a relatively small lesion of the pons' right side could damage all these structures. A large brainstem lesion would cause coma and quadriparesis. Small infarctions are the most common cause of small brainstem lesions. (If the lesion pictured in Figure 4–10 extended more laterally, it would create these deficits.)

2. What deficits would be produced with occlusion of the left internal carotid artery?

> *answer:* Occlusion of the left internal carotid artery can destroy the left hemisphere, which would cause right-sided hemiparesis, hemisensory loss, homonymous hemianopsia, and global aphasia. Circulation through three sets of anastomoses, however, may provide collateral blood supply. These anastomotic channels are the Circle of Willis, which is completely patent in only 20 per cent of individuals; meningeal connections to cerebral vessels; and retrograde flow in the ophthalmic artery.

3. What symptoms and signs will a patient have with sudden occlusion of the right internal carotid artery?

> *answer:* As in the previous case, patients may have contralateral hemiparesis, hemisensory loss, and homonymous hemianopsia, but not aphasia. Since patients with these deficits frequently have hemi-inattention, they may not describe their hemiparesis because they also have anosognosia.

4. A 20-year-old man has the subacute onset of complete loss of vision in the right eye, incoordination of the left hand, and moderate spastic paraparesis. Where is the localization?

> *answer:* The patient probably has lesions in the right optic nerve, left cerebellum, and thoracic spinal cord. Disseminated lesions are typically found in multiple sclerosis.

5. A 20-year-old woman complains of right eye "blindness," right hemiparesis, and right hemisensory loss. Pupil and deep tendon reflexes are normal. She does not press down with her left leg while attempting to lift her right leg. Where is the lesion?

> *answer:* The symptoms cannot be explained by a single lesion, cannot be confirmed by objective signs, and lack the usual accompanying symptom of right hemiparesis, aphasia. If she had had a left cerebral lesion, the visual impairment would have been a right homonymous hemianopsia. Moreover, she fails to exert maximum effort with one leg while "trying" to lift the other against resistance (Hoover's sign). Neurologic disease may not be present. Rather, she might have a psychogenic disturbance, such as a conversion reaction.

6. What frequently occurring diseases are characterized by involuntary movement disorders associated with dementia?

> *answer:* Dementia is part of Wilson's disease, Huntington's disease, and Creutzfeldt-Jakob disease, but not necessarily part of Parkinson's disease (in its early stages), Sydenham's chorea, or choreoathetotic cerebral palsy.

7. What physical abnormalities are frequently found with Alzheimer's disease?

> *answer:* Frontal release signs and corticospinal tract abnormalities (hyperactive DTRs and Babinski signs) may be found in patients with Alzheimer's disease.

However, usually in the early and middle stages of the illness, physical deficits are subtle and do not impair function. These Alzheimer's disease patients typically talk, walk, or wander without needing assistance. In contrast, patients with multi-infarct dementia often have corticobulbar signs (dysarthria, hyperactive gag reflex, briskly reactive jaw jerk—pseudobulbar palsy), as well as pronounced corticonspinal tract signs. These patients typically have hemiparesis and other impediments that impair their mobility, communication, and self-sufficiency.

8. A 45-year-old previously healthy woman had the sudden onset of jargon speech, uncontrollable crying, and agitated behavior, for which she was admitted with a diagnosis of schizophrenia. The physical examination revealed only a right Babinski sign and an equivocal right hemiparesis. Which common neurologic condition frequently mimics her psychiatric disturbance?

> ***answer:*** Schizophrenia almost never begins with a "word salad." The patient probably developed a fluent aphasia and subtle corticospinal tract signs from a left temporoparietal lesion. The sudden onset of fluent aphasia, which often precipitates a catastrophic reaction, is attributable to a small cerebral embolus.

9. An elderly man has left ptosis and a dilated and unreactive left pupil with external deviation of the left eye; a right hemiparesis; and right-sided hyperactive DTRs and Babinski sign. He does not have either aphasia or hemianopsia. Where is (are) the lesion(s)?

> ***answer:*** Since the patient has only a left oculomotor nerve palsy and right hemiparesis, the lesion is in the left midbrain. He does not have a language or visual field deficit because the lesion is in the brainstem, nowhere near the cerebrum.

10. Where is the lesion that causes a left superior homonymous quadrantanopia?

> ***answer:*** This visual field loss is usually found with destruction of the right temporal or inferior occipital lobe, which would be caused by a brain tumor or occlusion of the posterior cerebral artery. Alternatively, an optic tract lesion may occasionally be responsible.

11. A 60-year-old man has seizures that begin with clonic activity of the left hand that spreads to the left arm, then face, and then leg. Subsequently, he has transient paresis of the left arm. Where is the lesion?

> ***answer:*** The lesion is located in the right lateral cerebral cortex. It gives rise to focal motor seizures that undergo a Jacksonian march. After the seizure, he has postictal (Todd's) paresis. Todd's paresis lasts less than 24 hours.

12. A 50-year old woman complains of many years of gait impairment and right-sided decreased hearing. The right corneal reflex is absent. The entire right side of her face is weak. Auditory acuity is diminished on the right. There are left-sided hyperactive DTRs with a Babinski sign and right-sided difficulty with rapid alternating movements. What structures are involved? Where is (are) the lesion(s)?

> ***answer:*** The right-sided corneal reflex loss, facial weakness, and hearing impairment all indicate damage to the trigeminal, facial, and acoustic cranial nerves, respectively. These nerves (V, VII, VIII) emerge together from the brainstem at the cerebellopontine angle. The right-sided dysdiadochokinesia reflects right-sided cerebellar damage. The left-sided DTR abnormalities are caused by compression of the pons. Common cerebellopontine lesions are acoustic neuromas and meningiomas, which are often manifestations of neurofibromatosis.

13. A 60-year-old man developed interscapular back pain, paraparesis with hyperreflexia, loss of sensation below the umbilicus, and incontinence. Where is the lesion?

> ***answer:*** The lesion is in the thoracic spinal cord at the T10 level.

14. After a minor motor vehicle accident, a young man complains of visual loss, paralysis of his legs, and loss of sensation to pin and position below the waist; however, sensation of warm versus cold is intact. He can see only 2 m² at every distance. He is unable to raise his legs or walk. He has brisk DTRs, but his plantar responses are flexor. Where is the lesion?

> *answer:* Many features of the examination indicate that the basis of his symptoms and signs is not neurologic, i.e., there is no lesion. A psychogenic origin is suggested by the following: (1) the constant area (2 m²) of visual loss at all distances—tunnel vision—is contrary to the optics of vision, in which a greater area of vision is encompassed at greater distances from the eye; (2) the sensory loss to pain (pin) is inconsistent with preservation of temperature sensation because pain and temperature sensory systems are contained in the same pathway; and (3) despite his apparent paraparesis, the normal plantar response indicates that both the upper and lower motor neurons are intact. His DTRs are typically brisk because of anxiety.

15. A 50-year-old man with mild dementia has absent reflexes, loss of position and vibration sensation, and ataxia. What nonstructural diseases must be considered?

> *answer:* Conditions that cause dementia and dysfunction of the posterior columns of the spinal cord and the cerebellar system are combined system disease (pernicious anemia), tabes dorsalis, some spinocerebellar degenerations, and heavy metal intoxication. The posterior columns seem to be especially vulnerable to environmental toxins and are frequently involved in hereditary illnesses.

16. A 55-year-old woman, thought to have depression, is then found to have right optic atrophy and papilledema on the left. Where is the lesion?

> *answer:* She has the classic Foster-Kennedy syndrome. Probably a right frontal lobe tumor compresses the underlying optic nerve, causing optic atrophy and raising intracranial pressure, causing papilledema of the other optic nerve.

17. A middle-aged man complains of impotence. He has been in excellent health except for hypertension. He has orthostatic hypotension and lightheadedness, but the neurologic examination is otherwise normal. What neurologic conditions may be contributing?

> *answer:* Impotence, as well as orthostatic hypotension, may be the result of autonomic nervous system dysfunction. In this patient, antihypertensive medications may be responsible.

18. A 60-year-old man with right upper lobe pulmonary carcinoma has the rapid development of lumbar spine pain, weak and areflexic legs, loss of sensation below the knees, and urinary and fecal incontinence. Where is the lesion?

> *answer:* The development of paraparesis and incontinence in cancer patients naturally triggers a search for metastatic spinal cord compression. However, in this case, the lumbar spine pain and absent DTRs suggest that the lesion is in the cauda equina. This structure is composed of lumbosacral nerve roots, is part of the peripheral nervous system, and is located in the canal of the lumbar spine.

19. Subsequently, the man in Question 18 develops a flaccid, areflexic paresis of the right arm and a right Horner's syndrome. Where is the lesion?

> *answer:* His problem is now a lesion of the right C4-6 nerve roots and the thoracic sympathetic chain. He has a Pancoast's tumor. He must have a chest x-ray or CT.

20. A 60-year-old man complained of left leg stiffness. Examination reveals that he has a spastic paraparesis, DTR hyperreflexia in all extremities, and bilateral extensor plantar response. He has fasciculations in the left leg, both arms, and tongue. The left arm muscles are atrophied. However, all sensation, bladder and bowel function, and ocular movements are intact. What process is developing?

> *answer:* The patient has signs of corticospinal tract (upper motor neuron) disease in all limbs: generalized hyperreflexia, stiffness (spasticity) in the legs, and Babinski signs. In addition, he has signs of anterior horn cell (lower motor neuron) injury: fasciculations and atrophy. Mentation, sensation, sphincter function,

and ocular motility are uninvolved. He has the motor neuron disease amyotrophic lateral sclerosis (ALS).

21.   A 21-year-old woman has the mildly painful loss of vision in the left eye; a mild left hemiparesis with hyperactive DTRs and a Babinski sign; and right-sided ataxia. She had a similar episode 5 years before. Where is the lesion?

> *answer:*   Several areas of the CNS are involved: the left optic nerve, the right corticospinal tract, and the right cerebellar hemisphere. Moreover, this is the second episode. Since she has lesions that are disseminated in space and time, she probably has multiple sclerosis. Although a single lesion in the midbrain might produce similar corticospinal tract and cerebellar signs, it would not affect vision. Testing that might support a diagnosis of multiple sclerosis would include an MRI, visual and brainstem auditory evoked responses, and a lumbar puncture (LP) for oligoclonal bands.

22.   A 40-year-old man has interscapular spine pain, paraparesis with hyperactive DTRs, bilateral Babinski signs, and a complete sensory loss below his nipples. What would be the localization, differential diagnosis, and preliminary approach?

> *answer:*   The lesion clearly affects the spinal cord at the T4 level. Common causes include benign and malignant mass lesions (a herniated thoracic intervertebral disk or an epidural metastatic tumor), infections (abscess or tuberculoma), and inflammations (transverse myelitis or multiple sclerosis). HIV infection itself does not produce such a discrete lesion; however, complications of AIDS, such as lymphoma, toxoplasmosis, and tuberculosis might create a mass lesion that would compress the spinal cord. An MRI of the thoracic spine or myelography is routinely performed to rule out mass lesions compressing the spinal cord.

23.   Lesions of either hemisphere can cause contralateral hemiparesis, hemisensory loss, and hemianopsia. Which neuropsychologic deficits are specifically referable to lesions of the dominant or nondominant hemisphere?

> *answer:*   Aphasias and Gerstmann's syndrome are usually referable to dominant hemisphere lesions. Hemi-inattention, anosognosia, somatotopagnosia, and constructional apraxia are usually referable to nondominant hemisphere lesions. Bilateral or diffuse cerebral disease leads to perseverations, dementia, and pseudobulbar palsy.

24.   An elderly man has vertigo, nausea, and vomiting. He has a right Horner's syndrome, loss of the right corneal reflex, and dysarthria because of paresis of the palate. What are the other features of this common eponymic syndrome? Which way does the palate deviate?

> *answer:*   The patient has a right-sided lateral medullary (Wallenberg's) syndrome. This syndrome includes crossed (right-facial and left-truncal) hypalgesia and right-sided ataxia. The palate deviates to the left because of right-sided palatal muscle weakness. Even though the lateral medullary syndrome is the most common brainstem infarction, psychiatrists are not asked to see patients with this disorder. Since the cerebrum is spared, patients do not have emotional or cognitive impairments or other signs of cerebral damage, such as visual field cuts or seizures.

25.   A 54-year-old woman complains of having experienced several episodes of shaking of her left leg that begins in the foot. There is a hyperactive left knee and ankle DTR and a left Babinski sign. What sensory abnormalities might be detected?

> *answer:*   The lesion causing focal motor seizures and paresis of the left leg must involve the medial surface of the right frontal lobe. In that location, which is adjacent to the falx, i.e., "parafalcine," the lesion would be in a position to damage the upper motor neuron fibers destined to supply the contralateral leg. Since the lesion that causes seizures is superficial, it might only cause loss of cortical sensations, such as stereognosis and two-point discrimination. Pain and temperature sensations would be preserved because they are perceived in the thalamus.

Common causes would be a parasagittal meningioma, glioblastoma, or a scar from an anterior cerebral artery infarction.

26. Where is the primary damage in Wilson's disease, Huntington's chorea, and choreiform cerebral palsy?

answer: These diseases, like Parkinson's disease, damage the basal ganglia, which are the foundation of the extrapyramidal motor system. Basal ganglia dysfunction causes tremor, chorea, athetosis, rigidity, and bradykinesia. In contrast, corticospinal tract dysfunction causes spasticity, DTR hyperreflexia, clonus, and Babinski signs.

27. What are the frontal lobe release reflexes? Are they pathologic?

answer: The frontal release reflexes involve the face (snout, suck, and rooting reflex), jaw (jaw jerk), and palm (palmomental and grasp reflexes). Almost all frontal release signs are normally present in infants. In adults, none of the frontal release reflexes reliably indicates the presence of a pathologic condition. However, if several are detected, a congenital cerebral injury, frontal lobe lesion, or cerebral degenerative condition may be present.

28–39. Define these symptoms or signs and specify the location of the associated lesions:

28. Anosognosia

answer: Anosognosia is the patient's failure to recognize a deficit or disease. The most common example is ignoring a left hemiparesis from a right cerebral infarction. Another example is denial of the sudden onset of blindness (Anton's syndrome) from occipital lobe infarctions. In contrast to these organically based denials, failing to come to grips with serious but non-neurologic illness, such as alcoholism or cancer, is psychogenic, and the term anosognosia would be inappropriate.

29. Aphasia

answer: Aphasia is a disorder of verbal or written language. It almost always results from discrete lesions in the dominant cerebral hemisphere's perisylvian language arc. However, occasionally, degenerative conditions, including Alzheimer's disease, may cause word finding impairments and other language difficulties. Depending on the site and nature of the lesion that causes aphasia, patients may have dysarthria (impairment in pronouncing words). Dysarthria may be the result of lesions in the brainstem, cranial nerves, and even vocal cords, as well as in the cerebral hemispheres.

30. Astereognosis

answer: Astereognosis is the inability to identify objects by touch. It is a variety of cortical sensory loss that is found with lesions of the contralateral parietal lobe.

31. Athetosis

answer: Athetosis is an involuntary movement disorder characterized by slow writhing, sinuous movement of the arm(s) or leg(s). More pronounced in the distal part of the limbs, it is usually the result of basal ganglia damage from perinatal jaundice, anoxia, or prematurity. Although neuroleptics cause jerky or rocking movements (chorea), they do not cause athetosis.

32. Bradykinesia

answer: Bradykinesia is slowness of movement that is usually seen with many basal ganglia diseases and is characteristic of parkinsonism.

33. Chorea

answer: Chorea, another involuntary intermittent disorder, is characterized by random jerking of the limbs, face, or trunk. It may be caused by neurologic medications (e.g., L-dopa), and many basal ganglia diseases, as well as by the long-term use of neuroleptics. The distinction between athetosis and chorea is admittedly artificial. Many patients have movements with both aspects (choreoathetosis).

34. Dementia

answer: Dementia is impairment of memory and judgment, abstract thinking, and other cognitive functions of a degree sufficient to impair social activities or interpersonal relationships. Dementia must not be confused with "forgetfulness of middle age," amnesia, or mental retardation. It usually results from diffuse cerebral structural damage, systemic metabolic aberration, or a single lesion, such as a frontal lobe meningioma, that creates a generalized effect.

35. Dysdiadochokinesia

answer: Dysdiadochokinesia is impairment of rapid alternating movements. It is characteristic of cerebellar injury. When dysdiadochokinesia is unilateral, it is most often due to lesions of the ipsilateral cerebellar hemisphere. Occasionally, lesions of the midbrain that damage the red nucleus cause contralateral dysdiadochokinesia, intention tremor, and other signs of cerebellar damage.

36. Gerstmann's syndrome

answer: Gerstmann's syndrome is the combination of agraphia, finger agnosia, dyscalculia, and inability to distinguish right from left. While finding all elements is extremely rare, the syndrome is attributable to lesions of the dominant hemisphere parietal lobe's angular gyrus.

37. Homonymous hemianopsia

answer: Homonymous hemianopsia is a visual field defect in which the same half of each eye field is lost. The responsible lesion is in the contralateral optic tract or intrahemispheric radiations, but not in the optic nerve. In a right homonymous hemianopsia, the right half of the field is lost:

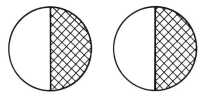

38. Ataxia

answer: Ataxia is incoordination of movement and irregularity of actions. It is a sign of cerebellar injury and is associated with intention tremor, hypotonia, and impaired rapid alternating movements. Ataxia may be confined to the trunk, "truncal ataxia," which is characteristic of midline cerebellar destruction from alcoholism. It may be confined to the arm and leg on one side, "appendicular ataxia," which is characteristic of ipsilateral cerebellar injury found with cerebrovascular accidents, tumor, and single structural lesions.

39. Homonymous superior quadrantanopia

answer: Homonymous superior quadrantanopia is the visual field defect in which the same top quarter is lost bilaterally. This visual field deficit is found with lesions of the temporal or lower occipital lobe.

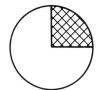 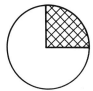 or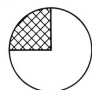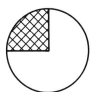

In bitemporal superior quadrantanopia, neither eye appreciates the upper-outer quarter. This visual field deficit indicates lesions of the optic chiasm, such as pituitary adenomas.

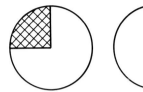

40. Which of the following neurologic diseases are genetically transmitted and, if so, in what manner?

a. Alzheimer's disease
b. Amyotrophic lateral sclerosis (ALS)
c. Cluster headaches
d. Creutzfeldt-Jakob disease
e. Down's syndrome
f. Duchenne's muscular dystrophy
g. Adrenoleukodystrophy
h. Familial amaurotic idiocy (Tay-Sachs)
i. Friedreich's ataxia
j. Guillain-Barré syndrome
k. Huntington's chorea
l. Migraine headaches
m. Sturge-Weber disease
n. Subacute sclerosing panencephalitis (SSPE)
o. Wilson's disease

answer:
a. Nongenetic, except autosomal dominant in certain families
b. Nongenetic, but autosomal dominant in 10 percent of cases
c. Nongenetic
d. Nongenetic in most cases, but autosomal dominant in 10 per cent of cases. This illness probably represents an interaction of genetic vulnerability and an atypical virus infection.
e. Nondysjunction (trisomy 21)
f. Sex-linked recessive
g. Sex-linked recessive
h. Autosomal recessive
i. Autosomal recessive in typical cases
j. Nongenetic (probably infectious)
k. Autosomal dominant
l. Frequently familial, especially in females, but not proven to be genetic
m. Autosomal dominant with variable penetration, but most cases are sporadic
n. Nongenetic (probably infectious)
o. Autosomal recessive

41. After a young man sustains closed head trauma, he has insomnia, fatigue, intellectual and personality changes, and claims that food tastes differently. What is the origin of his symptoms?

answer: He probably has had a contusion of both frontal lobes resulting in a postconcussion syndrome manifested by changes in mentation and personality. The anosmia results from shearing of the thin fibers of the olfactory nerve in their passage through the cribriform plate. Often patients with the postconcussion syndrome have elements of a post-traumatic stress disorder.

42. A middle-aged woman has increasing blindness in the right eye, where the visual acuity is 20/400 and the optic disk is white. The right pupil does not react directly or consensually to light. The left pupil reacts directly, although not consensually. All motions of the right eye are impaired. Where is the lesion?

answer: She evidently has right-sided optic nerve damage. She has right-sided impaired visual acuity, optic atrophy, and loss of direct light reflex in that eye with loss of the indirect (consensual) light reflex in the other. In addition, the complete extraocular muscle paresis indicates oculomotor, trochlear, and abducens nerve damage. Only a lesion located immediately behind the orbit, such as a sphenoid wing meningioma, would be able to damage all these nerves.

43. In what condition do pupils accommodate but not react to light?

answer: Tabes dorsalis with Argyll-Robertson pupils

44. In what condition is a patient in an agitated, confused state with abnormally large pupils?

answer: Atropine, scopolamine, and sympathomimetic intoxications

45. In what condition is a patient in coma with pinpoint-sized pupils?

answer: The combination of coma and miosis is found in heroin, barbiturate, and other overdoses, and in infarctions and hemorrhages in the pons. More important, extensive lower brainstem structural injury and metabolic aberrations that suppress brainstem function both cause life-threatening respiratory depression.

46. What are the most common causes of asymptomatic miosis?

answer: The most common causes of asymptomatic miosis are use of ocular medications for glaucoma and the normal changes of old age.

47. After sustaining a severe head injury, a patient is admitted in coma, with a right pupil dilated and unreactive, right hemiparesis, and bilateral Babinski signs. What well-known catastrophe is happening?

answer: A subdural or intracerebral hematoma is probably causing herniation of the right temporal lobe through the tentorial notch. The mass is compressing the ipsilateral third cranial nerve and the brainstem—transtentorial herniation. Unless the hematoma is evacuated, it will be fatal.

48. On looking to the left, a patient has diplopia. Which nerve is paretic?

answer: Either the left sixth or right third cranial nerve is paretic.

49. Which nerve is responsible when the left eye fails to abduct fully on looking to the left?

answer: The left sixth cranial nerve is impaired.

50. If the right third cranial nerve were injured, how would the eyes appear? In what direction of gaze would diplopia occur?

answer: The right lid would be paretic (ptosis), the right eye would be deviated laterally (abducted), and the pupil would be dilated. The patient would have diplopia on looking forward that would increase on looking to the left.

51. A 15-year-old girl is lethargic and disoriented, walks with an ataxic gait, and has slurred speech. She also has bilateral, horizontal, and vertical nystagmus. What is the most likely cause of her findings?

answer: She may be intoxicated with alcohol, barbiturates, or other drugs. A cerebellar tumor is an unlikely possibility without signs of raised intracranial pressure or corticospinal tract damage. Multiple sclerosis is unlikely because of the lethargy, disorientation, and young age.

52. A young man complains of vertigo, nausea, vomiting, and left-sided tinnitus. He has nystagmus to the right. Where is the lesion?

answer: The unilateral nystagmus, hearing abnormality, nausea, and vomiting are most likely caused by left-sided inner ear disease, rather than by neurologic dysfunction.

53. A 21-year-old soldier has vertical and horizontal nystagmus, mild spastic paraparesis, and ataxia of finger-to-nose motion bilaterally. What process has occurred?

answer: This patient seems to have lesions in the brainstem causing nystagmus; in the cerebellum causing ataxia; and in the spinal cord causing paraparesis. The picture of scattered or "disseminated" lesions is typical of but not diagnostic of multiple sclerosis especially because it is not disseminated in time.

54. A man has developed diplopia when looking to the left. When he looks to the left, the right eye fails to adduct across the midline and the left eye has nystagmus. Both eyes, however, are conjugate while looking ahead and converge while reading. What condition has developed, and what illnesses does it suggest?

>   ***answer:*** The patient has internuclear ophthalmoplegia (INO), which is often called the medial longitudinal fasciculus (MLF) syndrome. In this condition, the third and sixth cranial nerves are uninjured, but their connecting path, the medial longitudinal fasciculus, is damaged. The most common causes are small midline brainstem lesions, such as multiple sclerosis plaques, infarctions, and vascular inflammatory conditions, such as lupus.

55. A 35-year-old man, who has been shot in the back, has paresis of the right leg and loss of position and vibration sensation at the right ankle. Pinprick sensation is lost in the left leg. Where is the lesion?

>   ***answer:*** The gunshot wound has caused hemitransection of the right side of the thoracic spinal cord (the Brown-Sequard syndrome, Fig. 2–16). Occasionally, to alleviate intractable pain, neurosurgeons purposefully sever the lateral spinothalamic tract.

56. A 25-year-old man who has had diabetes mellitus since childhood develops impotence. He has been found previously to have retrograde ejaculation during an evaluation for sterility. Examination of his fundi reveals hemorrhages and exudates. He has absent DTRs at the wrists and ankles, loss of position and vibration sensation at the ankles, and no demonstrable anal or cremasteric reflexes. Why is he impotent?

>   ***answer:*** He has a combination of peripheral and autonomic system neuropathy because of diabetes mellitus. A peripheral neuropathy is suggested by the distal sensory and reflex loss and the absent anal and cremasteric reflexes. Autonomic neuropathy is suggested by the retrograde ejaculation. Other manifestations of autonomic neuropathy that might be sought are urinary bladder hypotonicity, gastroenteropathy, and anhidrosis.

57. A 27-year-old man has a bitemporal hemianopsia. He has had loss of libido for 2 years and mild frontal headaches for the previous 3 months. The optic disks are white and the pupils are large, but they react to light. Aside from a eunuchoid habitus, the routine physical examination reveals no abnormalities. What is the neurologic basis of his symptoms and signs?

>   ***answer:*** He has a tumor pressing against the optic chiasm and the pituitary-hypothalamic region, which most commonly would be a chromophobe adenoma of the pituitary gland, craniopharyngioma, or meningioma. These tumors are detectable with CT or MRI scans. The serum prolactin level is usually elevated with these tumors.

58. An 8-year-old boy with headaches, nausea, and vomiting is found to have papilledema. Examination reveals tremor on intention, ataxia of gait, bilateral hyperreflexia, and bilateral Babinski signs. Where is the lesion, and what are the possible causes?

>   ***answer:*** Most important, on a background of common childhood symptoms, the nausea and vomiting, the papilledema indicates that he has increased intracranial pressure. He also has corticospinal tract and cerebellar dysfunction. Most likely he has obstructive hydrocephalus from a cerebellar tumor, of which the most common is the cystic astrocytoma. This tumor is readily detectable with CT and MRI scans. Lead intoxication, which causes diffuse neurologic dysfunction and cerebral swelling, can mimic a cerebellar tumor.

59. Match the gait abnormalities, which are important neurologic signs, with their descriptions.

a.   Short-stepped, narrow-based with a shuffle
b.   Impaired alternation of feet

c. Broad-based and lurching
d. Seeming to be extraordinarily unbalanced, but without falling
e. Swinging one leg outward with excessive wear on the inner sole
f. Excessively lifting the knees to raise the feet

1. Apraxic
2. Astasia-abasia
3. Ataxic
4. Festinating
5. Hemiparetic
6. Steppage

answer: a-4; b-1; c-3; d-2; e-5; f-6

60. Match the neurologic condition (a–f) with the gait abnormality (1–6) it produces.

a.	Cerebral infarction	1.	Apraxia
b.	Cerebellar degeneration	2.	Astasia-abasia
c.	Parkinsonism	3.	Ataxic
d.	Normal pressure hydrocephalus	4.	Festinating
e.	Hysteria	5.	Hemiparetic
f.	Tabes dorsalis	6.	Steppage

answer: a-5; b-3; c-4; d-1; e-2; f-6. Normal pressure hydrocephalus is characterized by dementia, incontinence, and, most strikingly, apraxia of gait. Gait apraxia is characterized by an inability to alternate leg movements and an inappropriate shifting of weight, such as attempting to lift the weight-bearing foot. The feet are often immobile because the weight is not shifted to the forward foot, and the patient attempts to lift the same foot twice. The feet seem magnetized to the floor (see Fig. 7–7).

Astasia-abasia is a psychogenic pattern of walking in which the patient seems to alternate between a broad base for stability and a narrow, tightrope-like stance, with contortions of the chest and arms that give the appearance of falling (see Fig. 3–2).

Ataxia of the legs and trunk in cerebellar degeneration forces the feet widely apart (in a broad base) to maintain stability. Since coordination is also impaired, the gait has an uneven, unsteady, lurching pattern (see Fig. 2–13).

Festinating gait, also called *marche à petits pas*, a feature of Parkinson's disease, is a shuffling, short-stepped gait with a tendency to accelerate.

Hemiparesis and increased tone (spasticity) from cerebral infarctions force patients to swing (circumduct) a paretic leg from the hip. Circumduction permits hemiparetic patients to walk if they can extend their hip and knee. The weak ankle drags the inner front surface of the foot (see Fig. 2–4).

Patients with tabes dorsalis have impairment of position sense. To prevent their toes from catching, especially when climbing stairs, patients excessively raise their legs.

61. Match the pictures (1,2,3) with the associated characteristics.

a. Cerebral infarction
b. Loss of taste on one side of tongue
c. Idiopathic inflammation
d. Normal
e. Overexposure and drying of eye
f. Loss of the corneal reflex

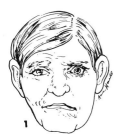
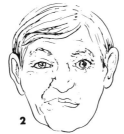
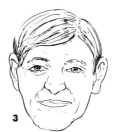

1   2   3

answer: a-2; b-1; c-1; d-3; e-1; f-1. Patient No. 1, who has weakness of his left upper and lower facial muscles, has Bell's palsy. With facial nerve damage, taste sensation is lost in the ipsilateral, anterior two thirds of the tongue. Paresis of the eyelid muscles prevents spontaneous or reflex eyelid closure which results in corneal dehydration and foreign body irritation. Patient No. 2 has weakness of his left lower facial muscles. This pattern of facial weakness is typical of contralateral cerebral injuries and is usually accompanied by arm and leg weakness, i.e., hemiparesis. Patient No. 3 is normal.

62–67. This patient is looking slightly to her right and attempting to raise both arms. Her left eye deviates across the midline to the right, but her right eye cannot abduct.

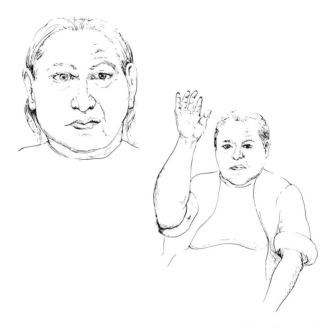

62. Paresis of which extraocular muscle prevents the affected eye from moving laterally?

a. Right superior oblique
b. Right abducens
c. Left abducens

d. Left lateral rectus
e. Right lateral rectus

63. The left face does not seem to be involved by the left hemiparesis. Why might the left side of the face be uninvolved?

a. It is. The left forehead and mouth are contorted.
b. The problem is in the right cerebral hemisphere.
c. The corticospinal tract is injured only after the corticobulbar tract has innervated the facial nerve.
d. The problem is best explained by postulating two lesions.

64. On which side of the body would a Babinski sign most likely be elicited?

a. Right
b. Left

c. Both
d. Neither

65. What is the most likely cause of this disorder?

a. Bell's palsy
b. Hysteria
c. Cerebral infarction

d. Medullary infarction
e. Pontine infarction
f. Midbrain infarction

66. With which conditions might such a lesion be associated?

a. Homonymous hemianopsia
b. Diplopia
c. Impaired monocular visual acuity
d. Intellectual impairment
e. Aphasia if the patient were right cerebral dominant
f. Various nondominant hemisphere syndromes

67. Sketch the region of the damaged brain, inserting the damaged structures and the area of damage.

> ***answer:*** This patient has weakness of the right eye that prevents it from moving laterally, weakness of the right upper and lower face, and paresis of the left arm. She has injury of the right abducens and facial cranial nerves and the cortico-spinal tract before it crosses in the medulla. The lesion is located in the base of the pons and is caused by an occlusion of a small branch of the basilar artery. 62-e; 63-c; 64-b; 65-e (A right pontine infarction would produce this condition); 66-b. Diplopia would be present on right lateral gaze.

PONS

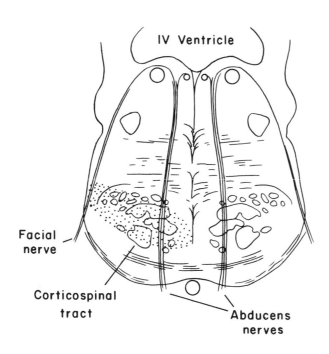

68. Where does the corticospinal tract cross as it descends?

a. Internal capsule
b. Base of the pons
c. Pyramids
d. Anterior horns cells

> ***answer:*** c. Since the corticospinal tracts cross in the pyramids, the tract is often called the "pyramidal tract."

69. Which artery supplies Broca's area and the adjacent corticospinal tract?

a. Anterior cerebral
b. Middle cerebral
c. Posterior cerebral
d. Basilar
e. Vertebral

> ***answer:*** b. The left middle cerebral artery.

70. Which group of illnesses are all suggested by the presence of spasticity, clonus, hyperactive deep tendon reflexes, and Babinski signs?

a. Poliomyelitis, cerebrovascular accidents, spinal cord trauma
b. Bell's palsy, cerebrovascular accidents, psychogenic disturbances
c. Spinal cord trauma, cerebrovascular accidents, congenital cerebral injuries
d. Brainstem infarction, cerebellar infarction, spinal cord infarction
e. Parkinson's disease, cerebrovascular accidents, cerebellar infarction

answer: c. The common denominator is upper motor neuron injury.

71. Which group of illnesses are all suggested by the presence of muscles that are paretic, atrophic, and areflexic?

a. Poliomyelitis, diabetic peripheral neuropathy, traumatic brachial plexus injury
b. Amyotrophic lateral sclerosis, brainstem infarction, psychogenic disturbance
c. Spinal cord trauma, cerebrovascular accidents, congenital cerebral injuries
d. Brainstem infarction, cerebellar infarction, spinal cord infarction
e. Parkinson's disease, cerebrovascular accidents, cerebellar infarction
f. Guillain Barré syndrome, multiple sclerosis, and uremic neuropathy

answer: a. The common denominator is lower motor neuron injury.

72. Match the location of the nerve or lesion (a-k) with its brainstem location (1–3):

a. Cranial nerve nucleus III
b. Cranial nerve nucleus IV
c. Cranial nerve nucleus VI
d. Cranial nerve nucleus VII
e. Cranial nerve nucleus IX
f. Cranial nerve nucleus X
g. Cranial nerve nucleus XI
h. Abducens paresis and contralateral hemiparesis
i. Abducens and facial paresis and contralateral hemiparesis
j. Palatal deviation to one side, contralateral Horner's, and ataxia
k. Miosis, ptosis, anhidrosis

1. Midbrain
2. Pons
3. Medulla

answer:

a-1	g-3
b-1	h-2
c-2	i-2
d-2	j-3
e-3	k-3
f-3	

73. Which of the following illnesses are "motor neuron diseases?"

a. Amyotrophic lateral sclerosis (ALS)   d. Botulism
b. Myasthenia gravis   e. Guillain-Barré syndrome
c. Poliomyelitis (polio)

answer: a, c. All will create paresis, areflexic DTRs, and respiratory impairment; however, only ALS and polio cause the death of motor neurons. Only these cause fasciculations. None directly causes cognitive impairments.

74. Which conditions are attributable to excessive trinucleotide repeats?

a. Psychogenic disturbances   d. Chromosome disorders
b. Infectious illnesses   e. Non-chromosome inherited disorders
c. Storage diseases   f. Down's syndrome and related disorders

answer: d. Excessive trinucleotide repeats are abnormal, unstable segments of autosomal or sexual chromosome DNA. They are thought to be responsible for myotonic dystrophy, fragile X syndrome, and Huntington's disease. Testing for trinucleotide repeats is more accurate than analyzing for restriction length fragments or genetic linkages in diagnosing these illnesses.

75. Which cells produce the covering of cranial nerve II?

a. Schwann
b. Oligodendroglia

c. Neuron
d. Microglia

answer: b. Oligodendroglia cells, which produce the myelin that covers the CNS, produce the myelin that covers cranial nerve II because, unlike other cranial nerves, this nerve is actually an extension of the CNS. Schwann cells produce the myelin that covers peripheral nerves and most cranial nerves. Microglia are supporting cells of the CNS.

76. Which structure separates the cerebrum from the cerebellum?

a. Cerebrospinal fluid (CSF)
b. Foramen magnum

c. Falx
d. Tentorium

answer: d. The tentorium lies above the cerebellum (see Fig. 20–16). Looking at this question another way, the cerebellopontine tracts, which connect these structures, and the fourth ventricle are between these two structures.

77. Which of the structures in Question 76 separate the two cerebral hemispheres?

answer: c. The falx cerebri, which often gives rise to meningiomas, separates the cerebral hemispheres.

78. An 80-year old man sustains an infarction that initially results in the loss of almost all sensation on the left face, trunk, and limbs. Several weeks later, the sensory loss is somewhat less severe, but he begins to develop a continual burning pain in the left face and arm. What is the name of this situation?

a. Trigeminal neuralgia
b. Thalamic pain

c. Temporal arteritis
d. Postinfarction neoplasm

answer: b. The sensory loss indicates that he had sustained a thalamic infarction. The subsequent pain, thalamic pain syndrome, is a frequently occurring late complication.

79. Which will be the pattern of a myelin stain of the cervical spinal cord's ascending tracts several years after a thoracic gunshot wound?

a. The entire cervical spinal cord will be normal.
b. The myelin will be unstained.
c. The fasciculus cuneatus will be black, and the f. gracilis will be unstained.
d. The f. gracilis will be black, and the f. cuneatus will be unstained.

answer: c. Since the f. cuneatus arises from the arms and upper trunk, it will be normal and normally absorb stain, i.e., it will be black. In contrast, the f. gracilis will be unstained because myelin will be lost distal (downstream) from the lesion. The corticospinal tracts will be normally stained (black) because they are normal proximal to the lesion.

80. A 45-year-old man complains of impotence for one year. He has had diabetes since childhood. His neurologic evaluation shows absent DTRs, orthostatic hypotension, and impaired position and vibration sense in the feet and ankles. What is the most likely, specific cause of his impotence?

a. Diabetes
b. Peripheral neuropathy
c. Autonomic neuropathy

d. Spinal cord pathology (myelopathy)
e. None of the above

answer: c. Diabetes damages both the peripheral nervous system and one of its major components, the autonomic nervous system. Autonomic nervous system damage causes orthostatic hypotension, changes in sweating, bladder dysfunction, gastric motility impairment, and sexual dysfunction. Peripheral neuropathy itself does not necessarily cause sexual dysfunction.

81. The patient in Q80 is unable to stand erect, with feet together, and eyes closed. When attempting this maneuver, he tends to topple, but catches himself before falling. What is the name of this sign (a-d), and to which region of the nervous system (1–5) is it referable in this patient?

a. Hoover's
b. Babinski's
c. Chvostek's
d. Romberg's

1. Cerebrum
2. Cerebellum
3. Spinal cord
4. Labyrinthine system
5. Peripheral nerves

> ***answer:*** d, 5. Falling over when standing erect and deprived of visual sensory input suggests a pre-existing loss of joint position sense from the legs. Deprived of visual and joint position senses, people must rely on labyrinthine input, but that system is effective only with rapid or relatively large changes in position. It is activated when people start to fall and prevents their tumbling over.
>
> Romberg's sign was classically described with injury to the posterior columns of the spinal cord because position sense from the feet would not be conveyed to the brain. Now, Romberg's sign is detected most often in people with peripheral neuropathy who have lost position sense and other sensations in their feet and ankles.

82. In which conditions would Romberg's sign be detectable?

a. Tabes dorsalis
b. Multiple sclerosis
c. Combined system disease
d. Alcoholism

e. Diabetes
f. Uremia
g. Cerebellar disease
h. Blindness

> ***answer:*** a–f. Impairment of the peripheral nerves (d–f) or the posterior columns of the spinal cord (a–c) can cause the Romberg sign. However, closing the eyes will not make a person more unstable with either cerebellar disease or blindness.

83. A young adult is suspected of having psychogenic seizures following a routine evaluation, including several EEGs. Which of the following tests will be most valuable?

a. Visual evoked responses
b. Brainstem auditory evoked responses
c. Closed-circuit television
d. EEG averaging

> ***answer:*** c. Simultaneously videotaping episodes of abnormal behavior and the EEG, which may require several days of hospitalization, will often clarify ambiguous situations.

84–92. Which structures are supplied by the vertebral artery or the carotid artery or their branches?

84. Occipital lobe

> ***answer:*** Occipital lobe—vertebral artery

85. Frontal lobe

> ***answer:*** Frontal lobe—carotid artery

86. Cerebellum

> ***answer:*** Cerebellum—vertebral artery

87. Bulb

> ***answer:*** Bulb—vertebral artery

88. Posterior portions of the temporal lobes

> ***answer:*** Posterior portions of the temporal lobes—vertebral artery

89. Posterior portions of the parietal lobes

    answer: Posterior portions of the parietal lobes—vertebral artery

90. Broca's area

    answer: Broca's area—carotid artery

91. Internal capsule

    answer: Internal capsule—carotid artery

92. Vermis

    answer: Vermis—vertebral artery

93–105. Which structures are in the posterior fossa, middle fossa, or neither?

93. Cerebellum

    answer: Cerebellum—posterior fossa

94. Frontal lobes

    answer: Frontal lobes—neither

95. Temporal lobes

    answer: Temporal lobes—middle fossa

96. Parietal lobes

    answer: Parietal lobes—neither

97. Lateral ventricles

    answer: Lateral ventricles—neither

98. Third ventricle

    answer: Third ventricle—neither

99. Fourth ventricle

    answer: Fourth ventricle—posterior fossa

100. Vermis

    answer: Vermis—posterior fossa

101. Bulbar cranial nerves

    answer: Bulbar cranial nerves—posterior fossa

102. The bulb

    answer: The bulb—posterior fossa

103. Carotid artery

    answer: Carotid artery—neither

104. Vertebral artery

    answer: Vertebral artery—posterior fossa

105. Corpus callosum

    answer: Corpus callosum—neither

5 Peripheral Nerve Disorders

Relying on clinical findings, physicians can distinguish peripheral nervous system (PNS) from central nervous system (CNS) disorders. In PNS disorders, damage to one, a group, or all peripheral nerves causes readily identifiable patterns of paresis, deep tendon reflex (DTR) loss, and sensory impairments. Some PNS disorders are associated with mental changes, systemic illness, or a fatal outcome.

ANATOMY

The spinal cord's *anterior horn cells* form the motor neurons of the peripheral nerves. These nerves are the final links that transmit motor commands from the brain through the spinal cord to muscles (Fig. 5–1). Most of the nerves leave the anterior spinal cord as "roots" that mingle within the brachial or lumbosacral plexuses to form the major peripheral nerves, such as the femoral and radial nerves. Even though peripheral nerves are quite long, especially in the legs, they faithfully conduct electrochemical impulses over considerable distances. The impulses are not dissipated because *myelin*, which is a lipid-based sheath made by Schwann cells, surrounds peripheral nerves and acts as insulation.

When stimulated, the nerves release acetylcholine (ACh) packets from storage vesicles at the neuromuscular junction. ACh diffuses across the junction and binds onto receptors on the muscle end plate. The interaction of ACh and receptors depolarizes the muscle membrane and initiates a muscle contraction (see Chapter 6).

Sensory information is also transmitted by peripheral nerves, but from the PNS to the CNS. Impulses from the various types of receptors—pain, temperature, vibration, and position—located in the skin, tendons, and joints flow through peripheral nerves to the spinal cord.

CLINICAL CONDITIONS

Mononeuropathies are disorders of single peripheral nerves that are characterized by flaccid paresis, deep tendon reflex (DTR) loss (*areflexia*), and reduced sensation, particularly pain (*hypalgesia* or *analgesia*; Table 5–1). Sometimes mononeuropathies and other peripheral nerve injuries lead paradoxically to spontaneously occurring painful sensations (*painful paresthesias*) or perversion of neutral stimulation into pain (*dysesthesias*).

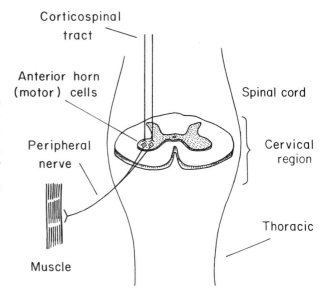

FIGURE 5–1

The corticospinal tracts, as discussed in Chapter 2 and as their name indicates, consist of upper motor neurons (UMNs) that travel from the motor cortex to the spinal cord. They synapse on the spinal cord's *anterior horn cells*, which give rise to the lower motor neurons. These neurons join sensory fibers to form peripheral nerves.

Penetrating and blunt injuries often cause mononeuropathies. Another common nerve injury is compression, especially of those nerves protected only by overlying skin and subcutaneous tissue. People most susceptible to compression injuries are diabetic; those losing weight, which depletes nerves' protective myelin covering; or those found in disjointed positions for long periods because of drug or alcohol use. For example, the radial nerve which is compressed where it winds around the humerus: People in alcohol-induced stupor who lean against their upper arm for several hours are apt to develop a *wrist drop* (Fig. 5–2, left). The *foot drop*, which is the lower extremity counterpart of the wrist drop, is caused by common peroneal nerve compression. In this disorder, the nerve is compressed as it winds around the neck of the fibula by prolonged leg crossing or a constrictive cast.

TABLE 5–1. Major Mononeuropathies

Nerve	Motor Paresis	DTR Lost	Pain or Sensory Loss
Median[a]	Thumb and wrist flexor (thenar atrophy)	None	Thumb, second, and third fingers
Ulnar	Finger and thumb adduction ("claw hand")	None	Fourth and fifth fingers
Radial	Wrist and thumb extensors ("wrist drop")	Brachioradialis[b]	Dorsum of hand
Femoral	Knee extensors	Quadriceps (knee)	Anterior thigh, medial calf
Sciatic	Ankle dorsi- and plantar flexors ("flail ankle")	Achilles (ankle)	Buttock, lateral calf, and most of foot
Peroneal calf	Ankle dorsiflexors and evertors ("foot drop")	None	Dorsum of foot and lateral calf

[a]Carpal tunnel syndrome.
[b]When the radial nerve is damaged by compression in the spiral groove of the humerus, the triceps DTR is spared.

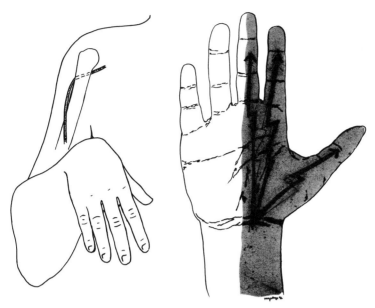

FIGURE 5–2

Left, As the radial nerve winds around the humerus, it is vulnerable to compression. Radial nerve damage leads to the readily recognizable *wrist drop* that results from paresis of the extensor muscles of the wrist, finger, and thumb. *Right,* The usual sensory distribution of the median nerve is the medial palmar surface of the lower forearm and palm, thenar eminence (thumb base), thumb, and adjacent two fingers. In the carpal tunnel syndrome, with median nerve entrapment, pain typically spreads downward from the wrist in the median nerve distribution. However, the pattern is variable within the hand and fingers, and sometimes the paresthesias spread upward (proximal) from the wrist.

A variation on the theme of pressure-induced mononeuropathy is the *carpal tunnel syndrome.* This contemporary hazard results from entrapment of the median nerve as it travels through the carpel tunnel of the flexor surface of the wrist. The median nerve may be injured by repetitive stresses, such as typing, computer programming, assembly-line work, or by fluid retention, especially during pregnancy, which compresses all structures in the tunnel.

In the carpal tunnel syndrome, paresthesias and pain usually shoot from the wrist to the palm, thumb, and adjacent two fingers (Fig. 5–2, right). The symptoms are characteristically worse at night. Pain awakens victims who shake their hands in attempting to find relief. *Tinel's sign* may be elicited by percussing the wrist, which generates electric sensations that spread down into the palm and fingers. Chronic median nerve entrapment leads to thenar (thumb) muscle weakness and atrophy.

Mononeuropathies can also result from systemic illnesses, such as diabetes mellitus, vasculitis (e.g., lupus, polyarteritis nodosa), and lead intoxication. In most of these conditions, the symptoms are painful and sudden in onset, but apt to resolve. Vasculitis and other illnesses can cause stroke-like cerebral insults, as well as PNS injury.

Mononeuritis multiplex is the combination of two or more peripheral injuries that are often accompanied by cranial nerve injuries. For example, a patient with injury of the left radial, right sciatic, and right third cranial nerve would have mononeuritis multiplex. This complex condition is usually the result of a systemic illness, such as diabetes mellitus, vasculitis, or, in Africa and Asia, leprosy.

Polyneuropathy or, for short, *neuropathy* is the most frequently occurring disorder. It is the generalized, symmetric involvement of all peripheral nerves. In certain neuropathies, cranial nerves may also be involved. As though neuropathies affect nerves in proportion to their length, patients' earliest symptoms are usually in the toes and feet, and then in the fingers and hands.

Patients' symptoms reflect both sensory and motor impairment, but in some neuropathies one or the other impairment may predominate. Patients with "sensory neuropathy" usually have numbness and paresthesias in the distal part of their arms or legs and typically describe "burning" or "numbness" in their fingers and toes, i.e. *stocking-glove hypalgesia* (Fig. 5–3). Sometimes the paresthesias cause involuntary leg movements, especially in bed (see Restless Leg Syndrome, Chapter 17). Their weakness is minimal.

Patients with a "motor neuropathy" have weakness in the distal portions of their limbs that impairs fine, skilled movements, e.g., buttoning a shirt. Also, since their ankle and toe muscles are much weaker than their hip muscles, patients have difficulty raising their feet when they walk or climb stairs. Neuropathy usually leads to muscle weakness, atrophy, and flaccidity. It also diminishes wrist and ankle DTRs because of interruption of the lower motor neuron (see Fig. 2–2C).

Common Neuropathies

Most neuropathies are not accompanied by mental status changes, and most patients with neuropathy do not come to the attention of psychiatrists (Table 5–2). Nevertheless, several of these neuropathies should be particularly important to psychiatrists because they are common, exemplify general neurologic principles, and are sometimes associated with mental status changes that only prepared physicians will appreciate.

Guillain-Barré Syndrome. Acute inflammatory demyelinating polyradiculoneuropathy (AIDP) or postinfectious demyelinating polyneuropathy, commonly known as the Guillain-Barré syndrome, is the quintessential PNS illness. Although often idiopathic, this syndrome typically follows an upper respiratory viral infection. Also, in many cases, it is a complication of mononucleosis, Lyme disease, hepatitis, or human immunodeficiency virus (HIV) infection. In Guillain-Barré syndrome, young and middle-aged adults usually first develop paresthesias and numbness in their fingers and toes, and then areflexic, flaccid paresis of their feet and legs. The weakness, which then becomes a much greater problem than the numbness, often ascends to involve the hands and arms. Many patients develop apnea from paresis of the phrenic and intercostal nerves and must be intubated for respirator assistance. If the weakness ascends further, patients develop dysphagia, facial weakness, and ocular immobility. Patients with total paralysis remain conscious in a locked-in syndrome (see Chapter 11). Their cerebrospinal fluid (CSF) contains an elevated protein concentration but few white cells, i.e., the albumino-cytologic dissociation (see Table 20–1).

Most cases resolve within 3 weeks to 3 months as the PNS myelin regenerates. The severity and duration of the paresis can be reduced with plasmapheresis, which seems to filter a toxin, and possibly intravenous administration of human immunoglobulin (HIG).

Guillain-Barré syndrome epitomizes the distinction between diseases of the PNS and CNS. Although paraparesis or quadriparesis might be a common feature, brain or spinal cord injuries (CNS damage) or neuropathies (PNS damage)

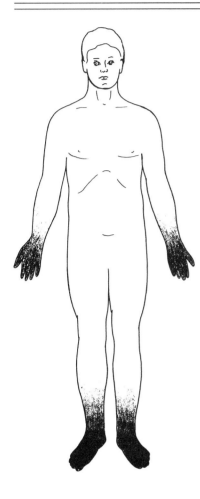

FIGURE 5–3

In polyneuropathy, pain and other sensations are lost symmetrically and most severely in the distal portions of the limbs. The legs are more severely affected than the arms. This disturbance is termed *stocking-glove hypalgesia*.

TABLE 5–2.   **Important Causes of Neuropathy**

Endogenous toxins
  Diabetes mellitus
  Uremia[a]
  Acute intermittent and variegate porphyria[a]
Nutritional deficiencies
  Starvation: dieting, malabsorption, alcoholism[a]
  Combined system disease/pernicious anemia[a]   B12 –
Medicines
  Vitamin B$_6$ (pyridoxine)
  INH, nitrofurantoin, antineoplastic agents
Industrial or chemical toxins[b]
  Nitrous oxide (anesthesia)
  Metals: lead, arsenic, organic and inorganic mercury
  Organic solvents: n-hexane, toluene[a], and others
Infectious/inflammatory conditions
  Vasculitis: systemic lupus, polyarteritis[a]
  Infectious: mononucleosis, hepatitis, Lyme disease[a], idiopathic (Guillain-Barré), leprosy,
    syphilis[a], AIDS[a]
Genetic diseases
  Charcot-Marie-Tooth
  Friedreich's ataxia and other spinocerebellar degenerations
  Metachromatic leukodystrophy[a]

[a]Associated with mental status abnormalities.
[b]May be substances of abuse.

cause different patterns of muscle weakness, change in reflexes, and sensory distribution (Table 5–3). Also, in Guillain-Barré syndrome, as in most neuropathies other than diabetic neuropathy (see below), bladder, bowel, and sexual function are preserved. These pelvic organs might be spared in neuropathies because the nerves innervating them are the relatively short fibers of the autonomic nervous system. With spinal cord disease, in contrast, patients usually have incontinence and impotence at the onset of the injury.

Another distinction is seen between demyelinating diseases of the CNS and PNS. Despite performing a similar insulating function, CNS and PNS myelin differ in chemical composition, antigenicity, and cells of origin. Oligodendrocytes produce CNS myelin, and Schwann cells produce PNS myelin, i.e., oligodendrocytes are to Schwann cells as the CNS is to the PNS. From a clinical viewpoint, although damaged PNS myelin is regenerated and patients with Guillain-Barré syndrome usually recover, damaged CNS myelin is not regenerated and impairments are permanent.

CNS demyelination, as in multiple sclerosis (MS), results in recurring, cumulative deficits referable to several CNS areas, including the optic nerves (see Chapter 15). The partial or even complete recovery that MS patients achieve between episodes results more from the resolution of the inflammatory response rather than the regeneration of myelin. When MS affects large areas of the cerebral CNS myelin, it routinely results in dementia and other mental changes.

From a psychiatric perspective, patients with uncomplicated cases of Guillain-Barré syndrome, despite profound motor impairments, do not develop mental changes because it is a disease of the PNS. However, mental changes do develop in patients who have complications: cerebral anoxia from respiratory insufficiency, "steroid psychosis" from high-dose steroid treatment (which is now outdated), hydrocephalus from impaired CSF reabsorption, fluid and electrolyte imbalance, or sleep deprivation. In other words, look for hypoxia and other serious medical complications in Guillain-Barré patients who develop mental changes. Also, unless the patient is already on a respirator, avoid sedatives and neuroleptics that might further depress respirations.

Diabetes and Other Toxic-Metabolic Neuropathies. Almost all patients who live with diabetes for more than 10 years have loss of sensation and absent DTRs in the feet and ankles, but their strength remains relatively normal. In long-standing diabetic neuropathy, sensation in the fingertips is impaired, pre-

TABLE 5–3. Differences between Central (CNS) and Peripheral Nervous System (PNS) Signs

	CNS	PNS
Motor system	*Upper motor neuron*	*Lower motor neuron*
Paresis	Patterns[a]	Distal
Tone	Spastic[b]	Flaccid
Bulk	Normal	Atrophic
Fasciculations	No	Sometimes
Reflexes		
DTRs	Hyperactive	Hypoactive
Plantar	Babinski sign(s)	Absent
Sensation: areas	Patterns[a]	Hands and feet

[a]Examples: motor and sensory loss of one side or lower half of the body, e.g., hemiparesis or paraparesis, and hemisensory loss.
[b]May be flaccid initially.

venting those diabetics who are blind from "reading" Braille. In addition to having neuropathy, diabetic patients suffer suddenly occurring painful mononeuropathies and mononeuritis multiplex. By a different mechanism—by damaging blood vessels—diabetes can lead to cerebrovascular disease that may cause multi-infarct dementia. (However, if mental aberrations suddenly develop in a diabetic patient, they may be signs of life-threatening hypoglycemia.)

Patients with diabetic neuropathy often suffer from painful paresthesias. Typically they feel a burning sensation in their feet, which is especially distressing at night. Several pain-relieving strategies are helpful (see Chapter 14). Amitriptyline and desipramine, but not fluoxetine, reduce the pain and help people sleep. A skin cream containing capsaicin (Zostrix), which depletes the putative neurotransmitter for pain, substance P, is analgesic.

Patients can also have autonomic nervous system damage that includes impaired gastrointestinal mobility, bladder muscle contraction, ejaculatory function, and erections (see Chapter 16). Strict control of blood glucose through fastidious diets, multiple daily insulin injections, the continuous infusion of insulin, or transplantation of pancrease cells may postpone the onset or reduce the severity of these neurologic complications.

Neuropathies also result from many toxins and metabolic abnormalities. Uremia is a common cause of neuropathy, and it is almost universal in patients undergoing maintenance hemodialysis. Neuropathy also commonly results from various medications, especially those used for chemotherapy of neoplasms, but it has not been a complication of neuroleptic or antidepressant medications.

Aging Neuropathy.   Although the condition is not yet considered a neuropathy and has not yet received a name, elderly people develop sensory loss from peripheral nerve degeneration. Almost all people who are older than 80 years have lost some joint position and vibratory sensation in their feet that is accompanied by absent ankle DTRs. This sensory loss prevents elderly persons from standing with their feet placed closely together. More important, it predisposes them to falling.

NEUROPATHIES ASSOCIATED WITH MENTAL STATUS ABNORMALITIES

Although the neuropathies in the previous section may be painful, incapacitating, or otherwise devastating to the peripheral nervous system, they generally do not cause mental aberrations. Numerous people who are old, diabetic, on hemodialysis, or receiving chemotherapy remain highly intelligent, thoughtful, competent, and cheerful. Mental abnormalities, especially dementia, accompanied by neuropathy, are found with only a few disease categories characterized by both CNS and PNS damage (Table 5–2). This perspective is useful and analogous to the combination of dementia and movement disorders that indicates cerebral cortex and basal ganglia damage (see Table 18–4).

Nutritional Deficiencies

A neuropathy that is predominantly sensory and accompanied by dementia or other mental status abnormality is attributable to absence of a specific vitamin: thiamine (vitamin B_1), niacin (nicotinic acid, B_3), or B_{12}. Vitamin deficiency neuropathies can also result from malabsorption of these vitamins, fats, and other critical substances, such as in starvation, gastrectomy, gastric bypass surgery, and inflammatory bowel disease. Surprisingly few patients with anorexia nervosa or extreme diets develop a neuropathy, possibly because they have a selective, possibly secret, intake of food or vitamins.

Alcohol-induced neuropathy is virtually synonymous with thiamine deficiency because almost all cases result from alcoholics subsisting on alcohol and other carbohydrates devoid of thiamine. Similarly, starvation or malabsorption causes thiamine deficiency neuropathy. Contrary to popular opinion, alcohol itself probably does not cause a neuropathy. Patients with alcohol-induced neuropathy have loss of position sensation and absent DTRs. The disorder is usually asymptomatic until patients walk in the dark when they must rely on position sense generated in the legs and feet. In the infamous *Wernicke-Korsakoff syndrome*, alcohol-induced neuropathy is accompanied by amnesia, dementia, cerebellar degeneration, and, in the acute illness, nystagmus and ocular-motor paresis (see Chapter 7).

Niacin deficiency causes *pellagra*. In this disorder, starved people suffer from dementia, dermatitis, and diarrhea—the "three D's" Although a neuropathy has also often been described in pellagra, it may actually be the result of the deficiency of other vitamins.

Combined system disease (pernicious anemia) or B_{12} deficiency causes a neuropathy that is overshadowed by spinal cord impairment (see Fig. 2–17B), dementia, or anemia. B_{12} deficiency usually results from malabsorption or a strict vegetarian diet. It is diagnosed by determining the serum B_{12} level or by performing a Schilling test. Combined system disease is best known as a "correctable cause of dementia" because B_{12} injections can reverse both the CNS and PNS aspects of the disorder.

One note about the opposite of vitamin deficiency: Several food faddists have developed a profound sensory neuropathy from taking excessive amounts of vitamin B_6 (pyridoxine). Although the normal adult requirement of this vitamin is only 2 to 4 mg daily, those individuals had been consuming several grams daily.

Infectious Diseases

Several common organisms have a predilection for infecting the peripheral nerves, but generally spare the brain. For example, *Herpes zoster* infects a nerve root or a branch of the trigeminal nerve ("shingles"), usually in people with an impaired immune system. It causes an ugly, red vesicular eruption that is excruciatingly painful during and especially after the infection (see Postherpetic Neuralgia, Chapter 14). Leprosy, infection with *Mycobacterium leprae* (Hansen's disease), causes anesthetic, hypopigmented patches of skin, anesthetic fingers and toes, and palpable nerves. The cool portions of the body, such as the nose, ear lobes, and digits, are the most severely affected.

More to the point, some systemic infections involve the CNS, as well as the PNS. Named for the town in Connecticut where it was discovered, *Lyme disease* has become endemic in New England, eastern Long Island, Wisconsin, Minnesota, and the Pacific Northwest. Caused by a spirochete, *Borrelia burgdorferi*, whose vector is a tick, Lyme disease's peak incidence is June through September, when people walk in wooded areas. Reminiscent of the infamous spirochete infection, syphilis, Lyme disease has indolent, multisystem manifestations that include malaise, low-grade fever, cardiac arrhythmias, arthritis, and a pathognomonic bull's-eye-shaped rash, *erythema migrans* (moving red rash), around the tick bite.

PNS involvement, which is the most common neurologic manifestation of Lyme disease, induces facial nerve palsy, similar to Bell's palsy, either unilaterally or bilaterally (see Fig. 4–14). It also causes paresthesias, weakness, and, in extreme cases, a Guillain-Barré syndrome. When the CNS is involved, patients may have dementia and other mental status abnormalities (see Chapter 7), headache, and chronic fatigue (see Chapter 6), but a paucity of physical signs.

With many cases of neurologic involvement, the CSF will have pleocytosis, abnormal protein and glucose concentrations, and Lyme antibodies. Serologic tests for Lyme disease are notoriously inaccurate. Also, because a spirochete is the infectious agent, patients may have biologic false-positive tests for syphilis (see Chapter 7).

The most widespread infection of the CNS and PNS is a*cquired immunodeficiency syndrome (AIDS)*. In AIDS, HIV or cytomegalovirus (CMV) infection or abnormal immune mechanisms produce a variety of debilitating PNS problems that include sensory neuropathy, mixed sensory and motor neuropathy, mononeuropathy multiplex, and Guillain-Barré syndrome. Neuropathy is the most common AIDS-associated peripheral nerve disorder. AIDS also predisposes to the meningovascular varieties of syphilis (acute meningitis or encephalitis), rather than the chronic varieties (dementia or tabes dorsalis). Overall, the neuropathy and the other peripheral nerve disorders associated with AIDS tend to develop with low CD4 cell counts, systemic illness, and advanced illness, when patients are apt to have dementia and other CNS complications (see Chapter 7).

Inherited Metabolic Illnesses

Numerous genetically determined illnesses cause a neuropathy. Although the spinocerebellar degenerations and related disorders cause CNS and PNS dysfunction, few cause mental aberrations.

Acute intermittent porphyria (AIP), the classic autosomal dominant genetic disorder of porphyrin metabolism, causes dramatic attacks of colicky abdominal pain, mental disturbances so bizarre as to be called "psychosis," and quadriparesis. During attacks, the urine turns red and tests, such as the Watson-Schwartz, reveal urinary porphyrins. Although attacks may be exacerbated if the patient is given barbiturates, phenothiazines may be given for psychosis. Despite its prominence in test questions, AIP is rare in the United States.

Metachromatic leukodystrophy (MLD), named for the metachromatic granules that accumulate in many organs, causes both CNS and PNS demyelination (white matter dystrophy). MLD, also rare, is an autosomal recessive illness that most often causes extensive non-neurologic as well as neurologic problems in infants and children (see Chapter 15).

Nevertheless, this illness is important to psychiatrists because in young adults it may present with mental aberrations that can range from personality changes to dementia. The mental aberrations are progressively severe and are eventually accompanied by peripheral neuropathy, but may be overshadowed by signs of CNS demyelination, such as spasticity and ataxia. Moreover, the gallbladder, testicles, retinas, and other organs develop abnormalities.

The activity of arylsulfatase A, a ubiquitous enzyme, is markedly decreased in the urine, leukocytes, serum, and amniotic fluid of patients with MLD. MLD is diagnosed by demonstrating the decreased activity of arylsulfatase A in leukocytes and finding metachromatic lipid material in biopsies of peripheral nerves. Although the pathology is understood, no treatment is effective. In particular, despite great popular expectations, a scientific trial of "Lorenzo's oil" did not benefit patients.

Volatile Substance Exposure

Some sensation-seekers experiment by inhaling nitrous oxide, the common gaseous dental anesthesia, which causes only several minutes of euphoria. However, inhaling nitrous oxide intermittently for several weeks produces neuropathy, but no dementia. Nitrous oxide abuse, with its neurologic side consequences, is apparently an occupational hazard for dentists.

In "glue sniffing," the classic example of volatile substance exposure, the intoxicating component is the common hydrocarbon solvent, n-hexane. Sensation-seekers and industrial workers who may be inadvertently overexposed develop neuropathy because n-hexane damages PNS myelin. Toluene, a component of spray paint and glue, causes damage to CNS myelin. Patients can develop cognitive impairments, pyramidal and cerebellar injury, and even optic nerve damage, which can be visualized on magnetic resonance imaging (MRI). Most importantly, toluene induces dementia in chronic abusers in proportion to the CNS myelin injury.

Ethylene oxide, carbon disulfide, and other industrial products, which have little potential for abuse, attack both the CNS and PNS myelin and cause combinations of neuropathy and dementia. Investigators have not determined whether chronic, industrial-level exposures can lead to permanent personality change, cognitive impairment, or fatigue. Such exposures are much less intense than those to which abusers subject themselves.

One important consideration is the toxicity of Agent Orange, the herbicide that was sprayed extensively in South Vietnam during the war. Agent Orange allegedly produced peripheral neuropathy, cognitive impairments, psychiatric disturbances, and brain tumors in hundreds of the soldiers exposed to it. Although a large scientific review found no evidence that it caused any of those problems, Congress has disregarded the findings and accepted a causal relationship.

AMYOTROPHIC LATERAL SCLEROSIS AND OTHER MOTOR NEURON DISORDERS

Amyotrophic lateral sclerosis (ALS) was known for decades as "Gehrig's disease" because the famous baseball player Lou Gehrig developed this dreadful, untreatable illness at the height of his career. Among neurologists, ALS is known as the classic *motor neuron disease* because both upper and lower motor neurons degenerate while other neurologic systems are spared. In particular, despite the widespread motor neuron degeneration, mental faculties are preserved. The etiology of ALS remains an enigma, but clues include the 5 to 10 per cent of patients with an autosomal dominant (chromosome 21) inheritance pattern, patients with insufficient enzymes to detoxify free radicals, and those with calcium channel antibodies.

People develop ALS at a median age of 66 years, and their first symptoms are weakness, atrophy, and subcutaneous muscular twitching (*fasciculations*) —signs of degenerating anterior horn cells—in one arm or leg (Fig. 5–4).

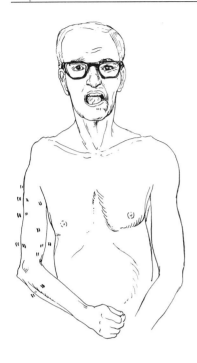
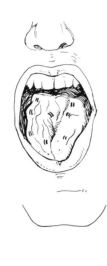

FIGURE 5-4

This elderly gentleman who suffers from ALS has typical (right arm) asymmetric limb atrophy, paresis, and fasciculations. His tongue also has fasciculations and atrophy, as indicated by clefts and furrows.

These signs spread in an asymmetric pattern to other limbs and also the face, pharynx, and tongue (bulbar). Dysarthria and dysphagia develop. Pseudobulbar palsy is superimposed on bulbar palsy. Then speech becomes unintelligible and interrupted by "demonic" laughing and crying (see Chapter 4). Despite extensive motor impairment, ocular muscle control and bladder and bowel function remain normal. Even atrophic muscles have brisk DTRs and Babinski signs—signs of upper motor degeneration—because remaining lower motor neurons are supplied by damaged upper motor neurons.

Patients remain tragically alert, mentally competent, and completely aware of their plight throughout the course of their illness. They have the cognitive capacity to chose their medical care and often refuse mechanical ventilation and resuscitation measures. Death usually occurs within 2 to 4 years from respiratory complications.

Several other motor neuron diseases also cause extensive loss of anterior horn cells while sparing upper motor neurons. An hereditary variety of ALS in infants (Werdnig-Hoffmann disease) and children (Kugelberg-Welander disease) is characterized by an exclusively lower motor neuron involvement: flaccid quadriplegia with atrophic, areflexic muscles.

Poliomyelitis (polio), the most frequently occurring motor neuron disease until development of the Salk vaccine, is a viral infection of the anterior horn (motor neuron) cells of the spinal cord and lower brainstem (the bulb). Polio patients, who were mostly children, developed an acute, febrile illness with ALS-type LMN signs: paresis that was typically asymmetric, muscle fasciculations, and absent DTRs. Those with bulbar polio had respiratory muscle paralysis that forced them to be placed in the "iron lung."

In polio as in ALS, oculomotor, bladder, bowel, and sexual functions are normal (see Chapters 12 and 16). Likewise, polio patients, no matter how devastating their illness, retain normal mental function. For example, Franklin Roosevelt, handicapped by polio-induced paraplegia, served as president of the United States. Unfortunately, some middle-age individuals who had poliomyelitis in childhood tend to develop an ALS-like condition, the *postpolio syndrome*, that causes further weakness and fasciculations.

Benign fasciculations, although they initially strike fear into the heart of medical students and others acquainted with ALS, are an innocent, usually transient phenomena. They are the commonplace muscle twitching precipitated by excessive physical exertion, psychologic stress, use of tobacco, excessive coffee intake, or exposure to some insecticides. Their innocent nature is confirmed by the lack of weakness, atrophy, or reflex changes and their tendency to last for several days or weeks.

A similar, benign disorder consists of fasciculations confined to the eyelid muscles (orbicularis oculi) that create an annoying twitching or jerking movement around one eye. However, if the movements are bilateral, forceful enough to close the eyelids, or have a duration of 1 second, they may represent a facial dyskinesia, such as blepharospasm, hemifacial spasm, or tardive dyskinesia (see Chapter 18).

Orthopedic Disturbances

Cervical spondylosis, which can mimic ALS, is far more common. Osteoarthritis of the vertebrae leads to encroachment on the foramina and narrowing of the spinal canal. Cervical nerve roots are pinched, and sometimes the spinal cord becomes compressed (Fig. 5–5). Cervical nerve compression leads to neck pain with arm and hand paresis, atrophy, hypoactive DTRs, and fasciculations—signs of lower motor neuron injury. Depending on several factors, sensory changes may be present. If spinal cord compression develops, patients will have leg spasticity, hyperreflexia, and Babinski signs— signs of upper motor neuron injury.

Similarly, patients with *lumbar spondylosis* have lumbar nerve compression and low back pain. Although they could not have spinal cord compression (because the spinal cord terminates at the first lumbar vertebra [see Fig. 16– 1]), patients will have signs of lumbar peripheral nerve damage: leg and feet paresis, atrophy, fasciculations, sensory loss, and paresthesias. Unlike ALS, spondylosis is associated with neck or low back pain; sensory loss in the limbs; and normal facial, pharyngeal, and tongue musculature.

Herniated intervertebral disks ("*herniated disks*") usually stem from trauma, strains, poor posture, or obesity that squeezes the gelatinous intervertebral disk material that cushions adjacent vertebral bodies like a shock absorber. Extruded (herniated) disk material presses against the nerve root and other adjacent structures. Over 90 per cent of disk herniations involve the intervertebral disk at either the L4–5 or L5-S1 interspace (Fig. 5–6).

Lumbar herniated disks usually cause low back pain that radiates to the buttocks and down the leg along the compressed nerve. The pain in the but-

FIGURE 5–5

In cervical spondylosis, bony proliferation damages upper and lower motor neurons. Intervertebral ridges of bone (*double arrows*) compress the cervical spinal cord, and narrowing of the foramina (*single arrows*) constrict cervical nerve roots.

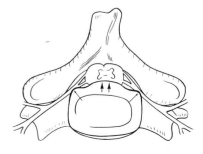

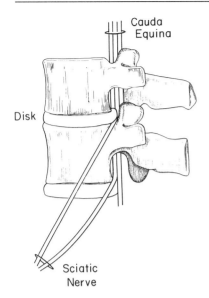

Disk

Cauda
Equina

Sciatic
Nerve

FIGURE 5–6

The cauda equina (horse's tail) is composed of the lumbar and sacral nerve roots in the spinal canal. The nerve roots leave the spinal canal through foramina where they might be compressed by intervertebral disk herniations. Herniated disks usually produce pain in the low back that radiates along the distribution of the sciatic nerve. Common movements that momentarily further herniate the disk, such as coughing, sneezing, or straining at stool, intensify the pain.

tock and leg pain as well as in the low back is characteristically increased by coughing, sneezing, or elevating the straightened leg because these maneuvers press the herniated disk more strongly against the nerve root (Fig. 5–7). Pain that radiates in the distribution of the sciatic nerve, *sciatica*, is indicative of a lumbar herniated disk and distinguishes it from other causes of low back pain. Large herniations can lead to paresis, incontinence, and, rarely, sexual dysfunction.

However, herniated disks are usually not responsible for the pain, disability, and multitude of other symptoms attributed to them. In particular, sexual dysfunction can rarely be attributed to low back pain or a herniated disk without paresis, areflexia, or previous spine surgery. Bulging and desiccated disks, which do not compress nerve roots, certainly cannot be held responsible for those symptoms. Alternative potential causes of low back pain are soft tissue injury, normal degenerative changes of the spine, and retroperitoneal abnormalities, such as endometriosis. As much as in any other neurologic condition, psychologic factors contribute to etiology, disability, and prognosis.

Cervical intervertebral disks are sometimes herniated by trauma, such as a "whiplash" automobile injury. Patients have neck pain that radiates down their arms and sometimes loss of a DTR. As in low back pain, orthopedic and psychologic factors are very important.

For acute low back pain, nonopioid analgesics, anti-inflammatory drugs, and 2 days—no longer than 10 days—of bed rest is usually effective. Sometimes pelvic traction is applied, but the weights usually applied (10 to 20 pounds) produce no benefit other than to enforce bed rest. Hospitalization can provide certain patients a thorough evaluation, intensive physical therapy, and possibly a refuge under the aegis of a hospitalization for medical reasons.

Some patients with chronic low back pain, are best approached by accepting the pain as a chronic illness with the physician attempting to ameliorate but not cure it (see Chapter 14). The goal might be improvement in function, rather than abolishing pain. For example, the goal of treatment could be completing a 6 or 8 hour day of work, swimming 20 laps, or playing 18 holes of golf.

Opioids and surgery should be avoided. Chronic pain alone is not a valid indication for surgery. The Minnesota Multiphasic Personality Inventory

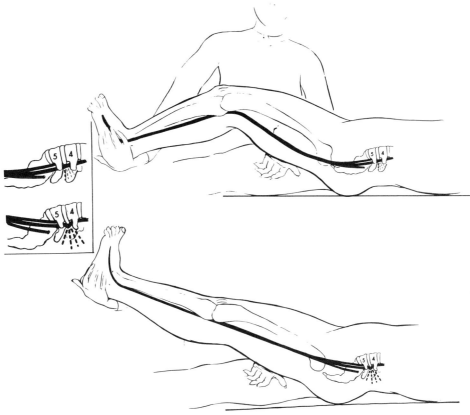

FIGURE 5-7

With herniated disks, the low back pain is intensified and often made to radiate to the buttocks if an examiner raises the patient's *straightened* leg (Lasègue's sign). In this maneuver, the nerve root is compressed and irritated because it is drawn taut against the edge of the herniated disk.

(MMPI) and other psychologic screening tests are unreliable in identifying those patients who will have a good surgical outcome.

Antidepressant medications provide an analgesic effect, even at doses that are smaller than those used for depression. Transcutaneous nerve stimulation (TENS) reduces pain for only a few months, and its benefit may be a placebo effect. Physical therapy is very useful and can become the mainstay of a treatment plan. Finally, physicians and patients should acknowledge, when relevant, that litigation often implicitly promises large amounts of money for *permanent* pain, suffering, and disability. This incentive naturally weighs against accurate reporting, effective treatment, and returning to work.

REFERENCES

Abarbanel JM, Berginer VM, Osimani A, et al: Neurologic complications after gastric restriction surgery for morbid obesity. Neurology *37*:196–200, 1987

Abramowicz M (ed.): Treatment of Lyme disease. Med Lett *34*: 95–97, 1992

Aubourg P, Adamsbaum C, Lavallard-Rousseau MC, et al: A two-year trial of oleic and erucic acids ("Lorenzo's oil") as treatment for adrenomyeloneuropathy. N Engl J Med *329*: 745–752, 1993

Barohn RJ, Gronseth GS, LeForce BR, et al: Peripheral nervous system involvement in a large cohort of human immunodeficiency virus-infected patients. Arch Neurol *50*: 167–171, 1993

Bleeker ML, Bolla KI, Agnew J, et al: Dose-related subclinical neurobehavioral effects of chronic exposure to low levels of organic solvents. Am J Ind Med *19*: 715–728, 1991

Bolla KI, Schwartz BS, Agnew J, et al: Subclinical neuropsychiatric effects of chronic low-level solvent exposure in US paint manufacturers. J Occup Med *32*: 671–677, 1990

Cullen MR, Cherniack MG, Rosenstock L: Occupational medicine. N Engl J Med 322: 675–683, 1990

Dawson DM: Entrapment neuropathies of the upper extremities. N Engl J Med *329*: 2013–2018, 1993

Filley CM, Heaton RK, Rosenberg NL: White matter dementia in chronic toluene abuse. Neurology *40*: 532–534, 1990

Goetz CG, Bolla KI, Rogers SM: Neurologic health outcomes and Agent Orange: Institute of Medicine report. Neurology *44*: 801–809, 1994

Hyde TM, Ziegler JC, Weinberger DR: Psychiatric disturbances in metachromatic leukodystrophy. Arch Neurol *49*: 401–406, 1992

Jensen MC, Brant-Zawadzki MN, Obuchowski N, et al: Magnetic resonance imaging of the lumbar spine in people without back pain. N Engl J Med *331*: 69–73, 1994

Logigian EL, Kaplan RF, Steere AC: Chronic neurologic manifestations of Lyme disease. New Engl J Med *323*: 1438–1444, 1990

Malane MS, Grant-Kels JM, Feder HM, et al: Diagnosis of Lyme disease based on dermatologic manifestations. Ann Int Med *114*: 490–498, 1991

Max MB, Lynch SA, Muir J, et al: Effects of desipramine, amitriptyline, and fluoxetine or pain in diabetic neuropathy. New Engl J Med *326*: 1250–1256, 1992

Merriam AE, Hegarty AM, Miller A. The mental disabilities of metachromatic leukodystrophy. Neuropsychiatry Neuropsychol Behav Neurol *3*: 217–225, 1990

Murata K, Araki S, Yokoyama K, et al: Autonomic and peripheral nervous system dysfunction in workers exposed to mixed organic solvents. Int Arch Occup Environ Health *63*: 335–340, 1991

Omdal R, Henriksen OA, Mellgren SI, et al: Peripheral neuropathy in systemic lupus erythematosus. Neurology *41*: 808–811, 1991

Rahn DW, Malawista SE: Lyme disease: Recommendations for diagnosis and treatment. Ann Intern Med *114*: 472–481, 1991

Rowland LP: Amyotrophic lateral sclerosis: Theories and therapies. Ann Neurol *35*: 129–130, 1994

Ropper AH: Guillain-Barré syndrome. N Engl J Med *326*: 1130–1136, 1992

Russell RW, Flattau PE, Pope AM (Eds.): Behavioral Measures of Neurotoxicity. Washington, DC, National Academy Press, 1990

Sahenk Z, Mendell JR, Couri D, et al: Polyneuropathy from inhalation of N$_2$O cartridges through a whipped-cream dispenser. Neurology *28*: 485–487, 1978

Schaumburg HH, Berger AB, Thomas PK: Disorders of Peripheral Nerves (2nd ed). Philadelphia, F.A. Davis, 1992

QUESTIONS and ANSWERS: CHAPTER 5

1. After recovering from an overdose, a 21-year-old heroin addict has paresis of his right wrist, thumb, and finger extensor muscles. All DTRs are normal except for a depressed right brachioradialis reflex. Where is the lesion and what is the cause?

> *answer:* The patient has a wrist drop from compression of the radial nerve as it winds around the humerus. This is a common problem for drug addicts and alcoholics who lean against their arm while stuporous. Drug addicts are also liable to develop brain abscesses, AIDS, and cerebrovascular accidents—but these are all diseases of the CNS that cause hyperactive DTRs, a different pattern of weakness, and since the *right* arm is involved, aphasia.

2. An 18-year-old waitress has fatigue, a low-grade fever, and "tingling" in her fingers and toes. She has splenomegaly; paresis of the ankle, knees, and wrists; absent DTRs; and hypalgesia in the feet. What process is evolving?

> *answer:* She has symptoms and signs of peripheral neuropathy: paresthesias, distal weakness, areflexia, and sensory loss. In view of her symptoms, she may have a systemic illness, such as mononucleosis or hepatitis. Lyme disease is possible, but it does not cause splenomegaly.

3. A 24-year-old woman has the sudden onset of low back pain with inability to dorsiflex and evert her right ankle. Raising her straightened right leg produces back pain that radiates down the lateral leg. Sensation is diminished on the dorsum of her right foot. No alteration in DTRs is detectable. What is her problem?

answer: The paresis, pain on straight leg raising (Lasegue's sign), and sensory loss indicate that the low back pain involves nerve root injury, rather than merely muscle strain, degenerative spine disease, or retroperitoneal conditions, such as endometriosis. She probably has an L4-5 herniated intervertebral disk compressing the L5 nerve root.

4. A 54-year-old man with pulmonary carcinoma has experienced 2 weeks of mid-thoracic back pain. He complains of the sudden onset of abnormal sensation in his legs and difficulty walking. He has weakness of both legs, which are areflexic, and hypalgesia from the toes to the umbilicus. What process is evolving?

answer: He has an acute spinal cord compression from a metastatic tumor with paraparesis, sensory loss below T10, and areflexia from "spinal shock." His problem is not a neuropathy because of the absence of symptoms in the upper extremities, the presence of a sensory level (rather than a stocking-glove sensory loss), and his localized back pain.

5. After recovering consciousness while still sitting on a toilet, a 27-year-old drug addict is unable to walk. He has paresis of the knee flexor (hamstring) muscles and all ankle and toe muscles. His knee DTRs are normal, but the ankle DTRs and plantar reflexes are absent. Sensation is absent below the knees. Where is (are) the lesion(s) and what is the cause?

answer: He has sustained bilateral sciatic nerve injury, which often happens to drug addicts who take an overdose when sitting on a toilet. This injury, the toilet seat neuropathy, is the lower extremity counterpart of the wrist drop (see Question 1).

6. A 58-year-old carpenter complains of weakness of his right arm and hand. He has fasciculations and atrophy of the hand and triceps muscles and no triceps reflex. There is mild sensory loss along the medial surface of his right hand. What process is occurring?

answer: He has symptoms and signs of cervical spondylosis with nerve root compression, which is an occupational hazard among laborers. Cervical spondylosis resembles ALS because of the atrophy and fasciculations, but the sensory loss precludes that diagnosis. In cervical spondylosis, depending on the degree of foraminal compression, DTRs may be either hyperactive or hypoactive. In ALS, despite the loss of anterior horn cells, DTRs are almost always hyperactive.

7. A 30-year-old computer programmer complains of painful tingling in most of her palms and all her fingers that often wakes her from sleep. Also, she frequently drops small objects. She has mild paresis of her thumb (thenar) flexor and opposition muscles. Percussion of the wrist recreates the paresthesias. DTRs are normal. Where is (are) the lesion(s) and what is the cause?

answer: Despite the mild and indefinite symptoms, she has bilateral carpal tunnel syndrome, i.e., median nerve compression at the wrist. She has sensory disturbances, which typically do not strictly conform to the textbook median nerve's region and an almost pathognomonic Tinel's sign (percussion of the flexor surface of the wrist creates a tingling sensation in the median nerve distribution). The carpal tunnel syndrome frequently occurs when there is fluid accumulation in the carpal tunnel, e.g., during pregnancy, before menses, and after trauma to the wrist, including "repetitive stress injuries," such as assembly-line hand work, word processing, knitting, gardening, etc. Acromegaly or hypothyroidism also leads to tissue or fluid accumulation in the carpal tunnel, but those conditions are rare. The diagnosis in this case, and in most others, is based on the occupation, sensory symptoms, and Tinel's sign. Weakness and atrophy of the thenar muscles develop inconsistently but usually late in the disorder. Nerve conduction velocity studies that demonstrate slowing across the flexor surface of the wrist confirm the diagnosis.

8. A young woman develops confusion and hallucinations, flaccid paresis, and abdominal pain. Her urine has turned red. What is the diagnosis and which test would confirm it?

answer: She has acute intermittent porphyria, which may be confirmed with a Watson-Schwartz test or determination of total urinary porphyrins. Phenothiazines may be used for the mental aberrations, but barbiturates are contraindicated.

9. A 31-year-old neurosurgeon has the sudden onset of inability to elevate and evert her right ankle. Her DTR and plantar reflexes are normal, but she has hypalgesia on the lateral aspect of the calf and dorsum of the foot. Where is the lesion and what are possible causes?

answer: She has had the sudden, painless onset of a peroneal nerve injury. It commonly results from nerve compression by crossing the legs, leaning against furniture, or wearing a cast. The nerve is injured at the lateral aspect of the knee where it is covered only by skin and subcutaneous tissue. When patients lose weight, the nerve is vulnerable to compression because subcutaneous fat is depleted. Sometimes diabetes, Lyme disease, or a vasculitis causes nerve injury.

10. Several workers in a chemical factory complain of tingling of their fingers and toes and weakness of their feet. Each worker has a stocking-glove hypalgesia and absent ankle DTRs. Which objective finding suggests that they suffer from a neuropathy? What are the common causes of industrial neuropathies?

answer: The loss of ankle DTRs is objective. While the hypalgesia and other symptoms and signs can be mimicked, areflexia cannot. Heavy metals, organic solvents, N-hexane, and other hydrocarbons are industrial toxins that cause neuropathies.

11. A 29-year-old woman, recently found to have hypertension, rapidly develops a paresis of the dorsiflexors and evertors of the right foot, paresis of the extensors of the wrist and thumb of the left hand, and paresis of abduction of the right eye. Where is (are) the lesion(s) and what are the possible causes?

answer: Since several different nerves are abnormal—the right common peroneal, left radial, and right abducens nerve—she has mononeuritis multiplex, which usually results from vasculitis, diabetes, or leprosy.

12. A 17-year-old man, after a (losing) fistfight, complains of an inability to walk or feel anything below his waist. He has a complete inability to move his legs, which have normally active DTRs and plantar responses. He has no response to noxious (pinprick) stimulation below his umbilicus, but sensation of position, vibration, and temperature is preserved. Where and what is the lesion?

answer: This is neither a peripheral neuropathy nor a spinal cord lesion. There is no objective evidence of neurologic disease in this man, such as changes in the DTRs or the presence of Babinski signs. Moreover, he is able to feel temperature change but not pinprick, even though both sensations are carried by the same neurologic pathway.

13. A 68-year-old diabetic man has the sudden onset of pain in the anterior right thigh. He has weakness of knee extension, an absent (quadriceps) knee DTR, and hypalgesia of the anterior thigh on the right. Where is the lesion and what is its cause?

answer: The knee weakness and especially the loss of its DTR indicate that the femoral nerve, rather than any CNS injury, has led to his deficits. Diabetes causes infarctions most often of the femoral, sciatic, peroneal, oculomotor, and abducens nerves.

14. A 34-year-old man with chronic low back pain has a sudden exacerbation while raking leaves. He has difficulty walking and pain that radiates from the low back down the left posterior thigh to the lateral ankle. He has paresis of plantar flexion of the left ankle and an absent ankle DTR. He has an area of hypalgesia along the left lateral foot. What has happened to him?

answer: He probably has a herniated L5-S1 intervertebral disk that compresses the S1 root on the left. The radiating pain, paresis, and loss of an ankle DTR characterize an S1 nerve root compression that usually results from a herniated disk. In contrast, compression of the L5 nerve root does not lead to an absent ankle DTR.

15.   A 62-year-old man experiences the gradual onset of weakness of both arms and then the left leg. On examination he is alert and oriented but has dysarthria. His jaw jerk is hyperactive and his gag reflex is absent. The tongue is atrophic and has fasciculations. The muscles of his arms and left leg have atrophy and fasciculations. All DTRs are hyperactive, and Babinski signs are present. Sensation is intact.

- What disease process is occurring?
- How extensive is it?
- What is the chance that one of his parents had had this illness?

  answer: He obviously has ALS with bulbar and both pseudobulbar palsy and wasting of his limb as well as cranial muscles. The corticobulbar and corticospinal tracts, brainstem nuclei, and spinal anterior horn cells are all involved. Characteristically, he has normal ocular movements and mental faculties. Approximately 10 per cent of ALS cases are familial.

16.   A 47-year-old watchmaker has become gradually unable to move his thumbs and fingers. He has sensory loss of the fifth and medial aspect of the fourth fingers, but no change in reflexes. Where is (are) the lesion(s) and what is the cause?

  answer: He has bilateral "tardy" (slowly developing) ulnar nerve palsy, which is an injury caused by pressure on the ulnar nerves at the elbows. Tardy ulnar palsy is an occupational hazard of watchmakers, draftsmen, and other workers who must continuously lean on their elbows. (See Question 7 for occupations that predispose to median nerve compression [carpal tunnel syndrome]).

17.   An elderly man with chronic lumbar back pain radiating down both posterior thighs has paresis and atrophy of the calf muscles. Both ankle and plantar reflexes are absent. His calf muscles have fasciculations. The toes and dorsum of one foot are analgesic. Does he have ALS?

  answer: Clearly ALS should be considered because of the atrophy and fasciculations. Lumbar spondylosis is the most likely disorder because the back pain and sensory loss are inconsistent with ALS and spondylosis is the most common disorder affecting this part of the nervous system.

18.   A 42-year-old schoolteacher has weight loss, burning paresthesias of the feet, jaundice, and a convulsion. Her sclerae are mildly icteric, and she has hepatosplenomegaly. She also has memory impairment, areflexia of the ankle and brachioradialis DTRs, and a stocking-glove hypalgesia. What areas of the nervous system are involved and what are the possible causes?

  answer: The memory impairment and convulsion indicate that she has involvement of the cerebral cortex. The dysesthesia, distal sensory loss, and areflexia indicate a neuropathy. The organomegaly, jaundice, and weight loss suggest a systemic illness, such as malignancies, hepatitis, and toxins. However, alcoholism is the most common cause of this memory impairment and the other symptoms, i.e., Wernicke-Korsakoff syndrome.

19.   A 24-year-old man who distills and drinks moonshine (illegal whisky) suddenly develops an inability to extend his right wrist, thumb, and fingers. He is not aphasic. His DTRs remain intact. What is the problem?

  answer: He has sustained a "wrist drop" from a radial nerve injury. During a drunken stupor, he may have compressed his radial nerve as it winds around the humerus. Alternatively, he may have developed a mononeuropathy from the lead used in the pipes in illegal distillation. (In children, lead intoxication usually results from their eating paint chips or other lead-containing substances [pica]. In them, lead ingestion causes mental retardation and seizures.)

20.   Over the past 3 years, 25-year-old twins have developed a broad-based gait, dysmetria on finger-nose and heel-shin movements, and scanning speech. They have atrophy of the foot, calf, and hand muscles with absent plantar and DTRs. Their position and vibratory sensation at the ankles are impaired, but pain and light touch sensations are preserved. What areas of the nervous system are involved? What type of disease is it?

> *answer:* Their gait ataxia, dysmetria, and dysarthria indicate impairment of the cerebellum. Their atrophy and areflexia indicate impairment of the peripheral nerves. The loss of only position and vibratory sensation indicates impairment of the posterior columns of the spinal cord rather than generalized sensory deficit indicating a peripheral neuropathy. These are the classic signs of spinocerebellar degeneration, e.g., Friedreich's ataxia.

21–25.   Match the cause with the illness.

a.   Genetic abnormality
b.   Glue sniffing
c.   Spirochete infection
d.   Dental anesthetic abuse
e.   Arsenic poisoning

21.   White lines of the nails (Mees' lines)

> *answer:*   e

22.   Lyme disease

> *answer:*   c

23.   Nitrous oxide neuropathy

> *answer:*   d

24.   N-Hexane neuropathy

> *answer:*   b

25.   Metachromatic leukodystrophy (MLD)

> *answer:*   a

26–36.   Which conditions are associated with fasciculations? (Yes or No)

26.   Guillain-Barré

> *answer:*   No

27.   Spinal cord compression

> *answer:*   No

28.   Amyotrophic lateral sclerosis (ALS)

> *answer:*   Yes

29.   Insecticide poisoning

> *answer:*   Yes

30.   Werdnig-Hoffmann

> *answer:*   Yes

31.   Fatigue

> *answer:*   Yes

32.   Porphyria

> *answer:*   No

33.   Psychologic stress

> *answer:*   Yes

34. Cervical spondylosis

answer: Yes

35. Post-polio syndrome

answer: Yes

36. Poliomyelitis

answer: Yes

37. Found with a suicide note, a 42-year-old man is brought to the hospital in coma with cyanosis, bradycardia, and miosis; flaccid, areflexic quadriplegia; and pronounced muscle fasciculations. How has he attempted suicide, and how should he be treated?

> *answer:* Most likely he has taken a common anticholinesterase-based insecticide that might be reversed with atropine. Timely treatment is essential because cerebral anoxia may develop. Most insecticides block neuromuscular transmission and create generalized paralysis, which mimics an acutely developing neuropathy, However, they characteristically also cause fasciculations and increased parasympathetic activity (miosis and bradycardia).

38. Which of the following conditions are associated with sexual dysfunction?
a. Peroneal nerve palsy
b. Carpal tunnel syndrome
c. Diabetes
d. Poliomyelitis
e. Multiple sclerosis
f. Post-polio syndrome
g. ALS
h. Myasthenia gravis

> *answer:*
>
> a. No
> b. No
> c. Yes
> d. No
> e. Yes
> f. No
> g. No
> h. No

39. A 40-year-old man with rapidly advancing Guillain-Barré syndrome develops confusion, overwhelming anxiety, and then agitation. Which of the following statements are correct?
a. He should be treated with sedation.
b. He should be treated with tranquilizers.
c. He may be developing hypoxia, hypercapnia, or both because of chest and diaphragm muscle paresis.
d. He probably has "ICU psychosis."
e. Guillain-Barré syndrome is generally not associated with CNS complications.

> *answer:* c and e. Guillain-Barré syndrome is not directly associated with central nervous system dysfunction. However, respiratory insufficiency, a common complication, might cause anxiety and agitation. Other complications that can induce mental changes are metabolic aberrations, pain, sleep deprivation, or an adverse reaction to a medication; however, these complications are not immediately life-threatening. (Treatment with sedatives or tranquilizers might completely inhibit respirations. These patients are usually intubated.)

40. After admission to the hospital for several months of progressively severe polyneuropathy, a 43-year-old man develops agitation, hallucinations, and disorientation. Of the various causes of neuropathy, which one leads to mental changes after hospitalization?

answer: Alcoholic neuropathy is associated with delirium tremens (DTs) when hospitalized alcoholic patients are deprived of their usual alcohol consumption. They may also develop alcohol withdrawal seizures that precede DTs.

41. Why is "glue sniffing" associated with neuropathy and occasionally with cognitive impairment?

answer: "Glue sniffing," the chronic inhalation of vapors from cements or paint thinners, leads to neuropathy because these substances contain n-hexane, toluene, and other solvents. Since these chemicals are lipophilic, they damage the lipid-rich myelin coat of peripheral nerves. In addition, dementia accompanied by cerebellar signs may develop if toluene or certain other solvents are inhaled for periods of at least 2 months.

42-45. A 60-year-old man who has had mitral valve stenosis and atrial fibrillation suddenly developed quadriplegia with impaired swallowing, breathing, and speaking. He required tracheostomy and a nasogastric feeding tube during the initial part of his hospitalization. Four weeks after the onset of the illness, although quadriplegic with hyperactive DTRs and Babinski signs, he appears alert, establishes eye contact, and blinks appropriately to questions. His vision is intact.

42. What findings indicate that the problem is caused by CNS injury?

answer: The hyperactive DTRs and Babinski signs indicate that there is CNS rather than PNS damage.

43. Is it possible to determine if the lesion is within the cerebral cortex or the brainstem?

answer: A brainstem injury has caused oculomotor paresis, quadriparesis, and apnea. This injury spared his mental, visual, and upper brainstem functions, such as blinking his eyes. He has the well known "locked-in syndrome" (see Chapter 11) and should not be mistaken for being comatose, demented, or vegetative.

44. Does the localization make a difference?

answer: If the lesion is confined to the brainstem, as in this case, intellectual function is preserved. With extensive cerebral damage, he would have had irreversible dementia. Overall, the presence or absence of mental function determines the patient's capacity to make determinations, the appropriate level of care, and expectations for rehabilitation.

45. Which neurologic tests would help distinguish brainstem from extensive cerebral lesions?

answer: Although a CT scan might be performed to detect or exclude a cerebral lesion, only an MRI is sensitive enough to detect a brainstem lesion. An EEG in this case would be a valuable test because, since the cerebral hemispheres are intact, it would show a relatively normal pattern. Visual evoked responses (VERs) will determine the integrity of the entire visual system. Brainstem auditory evoked responses (BAERs) will determine the integrity of the auditory circuits, which are predominantly brainstem pathways.

46–60. Which conditions are associated with multiple sclerosis, Guillain-Barré syndrome, both, or neither?

   a.   Multiple sclerosis
   b.   Guillain-Barré syndrome
   c.   Both
   d.   Neither

46. Areflexic DTRs

answer: b

47. Typically follows an upper respiratory tract infection

> *answer:* b

48. Unilateral visual loss

> *answer:* a

49. Paresthesias

> *answer:* c

50. Internuclear ophthalmoplegia

> *answer:* a

51. Paraparesis

> *answer:* c

52. Cognitive impairment early in the course of the illness

> *answer:* d

53. Mimicked by Lyme disease

> *answer:* b

54. Quadriparesis

> *answer:* c

55. Recovery through remyelination

> *answer:* c

56. Leads to pseudobulbar palsy

> *answer:* a

57. Leads to bulbar palsy

> *answer:* b

58. Where emotional lability of pseudobulbar palsy is frequently mistaken for "euphoria"

> *answer:* a

59. Typically a monophasic illness that lasts several weeks

> *answer:* b

60. Sexual dysfunction can be the only or primary persistent deficit

> *answer:* a

61. A 16-year-old waitress, who has been subsisting on minimal quantities of food and megavitamin treatments, develops symptoms and signs of a neuropathy. In what way can the neurologic picture be ascribed to an eating disorder?

> *answer:* Teenagers who develop a neuropathy may have any of the usual causes (Table 5–2), but several might be given special consideration. Mononucleosis, a common condition of young adults, may be complicated by the development of a neuropathy that is akin to Guillain-Barré syndrome. The abuse of glue, paint thinners, or nitrous oxide might be responsible, particularly when neuropathy develops concurrently in several teenagers. Similarly, alcoholism might be responsible, especially in restaurant personnel. Excessive consumption of pyridoxine (vitamin B_6) should be considered as a potential cause of neuropathy.

62. After gastric partitioning for morbid obesity, a 30-year-old man seems depressed and has signs of a neuropathy. Which conditions might be responsible?

answer: Surgical resection of the stomach or duodenum for either morbid obesity or ulcers may be complicated by Wernicke-Korsakoff syndrome (thiamine deficiency), combined-system disease (B_{12} deficiency), or electrolyte imbalance. Thus, a postoperative change in mental status may be a manifestation of a potentially fatal metabolic aberration.

63. A 29-year-old lifeguard at Cape Cod developed profound malaise for one week and then bilateral facial weakness (facial diplegia). Blood tests for mononucleosis, Lyme disease, AIDS, and other infective illnesses were negative. What should be the next step?

answer: The patient has a typical history and neurologic findings for Lyme disease. Serologic tests are notoriously inaccurate for Lyme disease. Blood tests are frequently negative early in the illness and even throughout its course. Another possibility is that she has Guillain-Barré illness that began, as a small fraction do, with involvement of the cranial nerves rather than with the lower spinal nerves. Myasthenia gravis is a possibility, but it is unlikely because of the absence of oculomotor paresis. Sarcoidosis is a rare cause of facial diplegia. It can be diagnosed by chest x-ray. The next steps would be to perform a lumbar puncture to test the CSF for Lyme disease, to look for the characteristic protein elevation of Guillain-Barré illness, and to obtain a chest x-ray. If the diagnosis remains unclear, the best course would be to treat for Lyme disease.

64. In which ways are CNS and PNS myelin similar?
a. They both derive from the same cells.
b. They possess the same antigens.
c. They insulate electrochemical transmissions.
d. They are affected by the same illnesses.

answer: c

65. Which is the correct relationship?
a. Oligodendrocytes are to glia cells as CNS is to PNS
b. Oligodendrocytes are to Schwann cells as PNS is to CNS
c. Oligodendrocytes are to Schwann cells as CNS is to PNS
d. Oligodendrocytes are to neurons as CNS is to PNS

answer: c

66. Which part of the nervous system is contained in the cauda equina?
a. CNS
b. PNS
c. Autonomic
d. None of the above

answer: b. The cauda equina (horse's tail) consists of the nerves that emanate from the lower portion of the spinal cord and travel in the lumbar spine to supply the legs, pelvic organs, and related structures (Fig. 5–6).

67–70. Match the illness with the skin lesion.
a. Bellagra   c. Herpes zoster
b. Lyme disease   d. Leprosy

67. Erythema migrans
answer: b

68. Dermatitis
answer: a

69. Depigmented, anesthetic areas on ears, fingers, and toes
answer: d

70. Vesicular eruptions in the first division of the trigeminal nerve
answer: c

71. The wife of a homicidal neurologist enters psychotherapy because of several months of fatigue and painful paresthesias. She also describes numbness in a stocking-glove distribution, darkening of her skin, and the appearance of white lines across her nails (Mees' lines). In addition to a general medical evaluation, which specific test should be performed?

> ***answer:*** The astute psychiatrist suspected arsenic poisoning and ordered analysis of hair and nail samples.

72. Which is the most common PNS manifestation of AIDS?

a. A Guillain Barré-like illness
b. Myopathy
c. Neuropathy
d. Myelopathy

> ***answer:*** c

6 Muscle Disorders

Disorders related to muscles must be distinguished from central and peripheral nervous system (CNS and PNS) disorders (Table 6–1). Then, diseases of the neuromusclar junction must be distinguised from those of the muscles themselves, *myopathies* (Table 6–2). Myopathies and neuromuscular disorders generally cause weakness, but only certain ones cause mental impairments. Many of them result from impaired *acetylcholine (ACh)* neuromuscular transmission and other well-established abnormalities. Several result from newly described, novel abnormalities, such as autoanitbody production, progressively greater genetic abnormalities in successive generations, and abnormal mitochondrial DNA.

NEUROMUSCULAR JUNCTION DISORDERS

Myasthenia Gravis

Neuromuscular Transmission Impairment.   Normally, discrete amounts—packets or *quanta*—of ACh are released across the neuromuscular juction (Fig. 6–1). After triggering a muscle contraction, ACh is metabolized and thus inactivated by *acetylcholinesterase (AChE)* enzymes or *cholinesterases.*

Almost all patients with myasthenia gravis, which is the classic neuromuscular junction disorder, produce antibodies to their own ACh receptors (Fig. 6–2). Because these autoantibodies block or destroy ACh receptors, accelerate ACh metabolism, or in other ways interfere with neuromuscular transmission, ACh packets produce relatively brief and weak muscle contractions.

Standard medicines for myasthenia gravis, such as edrophonium (Tensilon) and pyridostigmine (Mestinon), inhibit AChE and thus retard ACh metabolism. By prolonging ACh activity, these *anticholinesterases* (antiAChE medicines) restore strength. In another line of treatment, plasmapheresis and infusions of human immunoglobulin deactivate antibodies to ACh receptors. Steroids and other immunosuppressants are also used in cases when simpler treatments are unsatisfactory.

Changes in ACh neuromuscular transmission may be caused by many other illnesses or may be purposefully induced by medications. Botulinum toxin, as both a naturally occurring food poison and a medication, blocks the release of ACh packets from the presynaptic membrane and causes paresis (see below). Succinylcholine, the muscle relaxant often used in conjunction with electroshock therapy (ECT), relaxes muscles by binding to the neuromuscular junction ACh receptors. Like ACh, succinylcholine depolarizes the muscle membrane until AChE deactivates it.

Before discussing the clinical features of myasthenia, the role of ACh at the neuromuscular junction must be placed in context. Unlike dopamine and se-

TABLE 6–1.   Signs of CNS, PNS, and Muscle Disorders

	CNS	PNS	Muscle
Paresis	Pattern[a]	Distal	Proximal
Muscle tone	Spastic	Flaccid	Sometimes tender or dystrophic
DTRs	Hyperactive	Hypoactive	Normal or hypoactive
Babinski signs	Yes	No	No
Sensory loss	Hemisensory	Stocking-glove	None

[a]Hemiparesis, paraparesis, etc.

TABLE 6–2.   Common Muscle Disorders

I. NEUROMUSCULAR JUNCTION DISORDERS
   A. Myasthenia gravis
   B. Botulism
   C. Tetanus
   D. Nerve gas
   E. Chronic fatigue syndrome
II. MUSCLE DISEASES (MYOPATHIES)
   A. Inherited dystrophies
      1. Duchenne's muscular dystrophy
      2. Myotonic dystrophy
   B. Polymyositis
      1. Polymyositis
      2. Eosinophilia-myalgia syndrome
      3. Trichinosis
      4. AIDS myopathy
   C. Metabolic
      1. Steroid myopathy
      2. Hypokalemic myopathy
      3. Alcohol myopathy
   D. Mitochondrial myopathies
      1. Primarily mitochondrial myopathies
      2. Progressive ophthalmoplegia
      3. MELAS and MERRF
   E. Neuroleptic malignant syndrome
      1. Malignant hyperthermia
III. LABORATORY TESTS FOR NERVE AND MUSCLE DISORDERS
   A. Nerve conduction velocities
   B. Electromyography
   C. Serum enzyme determinations
   D. Muscle biopsy
   E. Thermography

FIGURE 6–1

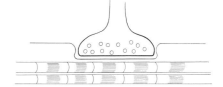

Peripheral nerve endings contain discrete *packets* or *quanta* of acetylcholine (ACh). Nerve impulses release the ACh packets across the neuromuscular junction.

rotonin, ACh is a transmitter at the neuromuscular junction, as well as in the CNS, and its action is terminated predominantly by metabolism instead of by reuptake. In addition, although ACh neuromuscular transmission is impaired in myasthenia, ACh transmission in the CNS is normal. This distinction between neuromuscular and CNS ACh function is illustrated by myasthenia patients' profound weakness in the face of normal cognitive capacity. Moreover,

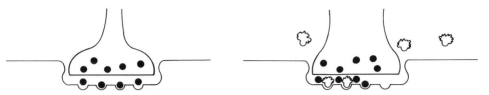

FIGURE 6–2

Left, Normally, ACh packets (*darkened circles*) bind into specific muscle endplate ACh receptors. ACh depolarizes the muscle membrane and triggers a muscle contraction. *Right*, In myasthenia gravis, autoantibodies (*tufted circles*) bind to the ACh receptors, reduce the effect of ACh, and cause weakness.

most antiAChE myasthenia medications have no effect on CNS ACh activity or cognitive capacity because they do not penetrate the blood-brain barrier. An exception, physostigmine, an antiAChE occasionally used for myasthenia, penetrates into the CNS and increases ACh activity. Physostigmine has been proposed as a treatment for conditions with low CNS ACh levels, such as Alzheimer's disease. (In various experiments in Alzheimer's disease patients, however, physostigmine raised the abnormally low cerebral ACh concentrations, but it produced virtually no clinical benefit [see Chapter 7].)

Clinical Features. Myasthenia is characterized by intermittent, asymmetric weakness of the extraocular, facial, and bulbar muscles. Almost 90 per cent of myasthenia patients, who are typically young women and older men, first complain of diplopia and ptosis. These symptoms result from extraocular muscle paresis. Because of facial and neck muscle weakness, patients grimace when attempting to smile (Fig. 6–3) and have nasal speech. In moderately advanced cases, the neck, shoulder, and swallowing and respiratory muscles become weak, i.e., they have bulbar palsy (see Chapter 4). In severe cases, patients develop apnea, quadriplegia, and an inability to speak (anarthria): they can become "locked-in" (see Chapter 11). In contrast to the physical incapacity, neither the disease nor the medications directly produce mental changes.

The absence of certain physical findings is also important. Although extraocular muscles may be paretic, intraocular muscles are spared. Thus, patients may have complete ptosis and no eyeball movements, but their pupils are

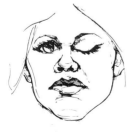 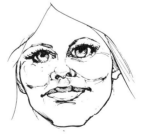

FIGURE 6–3

Left, This young woman with myasthenia gravis has ptosis from a weakened left eyelid following several days of intermittent double vision. In addition, she has typical bilateral facial muscle weakness, which is especially evident in the loss of the contour of the right nasolabial fold and a sagging lower lip. *Right*, After a Tensilon test, in which edrophonium (Tensilon), 10 mg, was administered intravenously, she had a brief (60 seconds) but dramatic restoration of eyelid, ocular, and facial strength. Edrophonium (Tensilon) intensifies ACh activity by inhibiting cholinesterase.

normal in size and reactivity to light. Even though patients may be quadriparetic, their bladder and bowel sphincters will be normal. Unlike other muscle disorders, their DTRs are normal. Of course, there is no sensory loss.

The clinical diagnosis of myasthenia gravis can be confirmed by doing a Tensilon test (Fig. 6–3), detecting serum antibodies to ACh receptors, or performing electromyograms (EMGs). About 5 per cent of patients have underlying hyperthyroidism and 10 per cent a mediastinal thymoma. If these conditions are detected and treated, their myasthenia will be improved.

Differential Diagnosis. Lesions of cranial nerve III, which result from midbrain infarctions (see Fig. 4–4) or compression by posterior communicating artery aneurysms, can also cause extraocular muscle paresis. These disorders are identifiable by a subtle but important difference: The pupil will be widely dilated and unreactive to light because of the intraocular (pupillary) muscle paresis (see Fig. 4–5). Although many illnesses cause facial or bulbar palsy— amyotrophic lateral sclerosis (ALS), Guillain-Barré syndrome, Lyme disease, Bell's palsy, botulism, and brainstem lesions—only myasthenia gravis consistently responds to the Tensilon test.

Botulism

Botulism, a potentially fatal disorder that is superficially related to myasthenia, is caused by a paralytic toxin elaborated by *Clostridium botulinum* spores. As in myasthenia, ACh neuromuscular transmission is impeded, but botulinum toxin blocks the release of ACh from the presynaptic membrane. Botulism victims develop oculomotor, bulbar, and respiratory paralyses that superficially resemble myasthenia, as well as Guillain-Barré syndrome. However, the symptoms arise explosively 18 to 36 hours after ingesting contaminated food. Often several members of a family who eat poorly preserved food simultaneously develop the disease, but occasionally commercially prepared canned food is responsible.

Neurologists are able to turn this botulinum-induced paresis into an advantage. They inject pharmaceutically prepared botulinum toxin to treat head and neck dyskinesias characterized by muscle spasms, such as blepharospasm, hemifacial spasm, and spasmodic torticollis (see Chapter 18).

Tetanus

In contrast to botulism, no benefit can come from tetanus. In this disorder, a *Clostridium tetani* toxin blocks the presynaptic release of inhibitory neurotransmitters, such as glycine, and other neurotransmitters. Uninhibited muscle contractions cause trismus, facial grimacing, an odd but characteristic smile ("risus sardonicus"), and bodily muscle spasms. Especially in drug addicts and others with open wounds, the differential diagnosis of acutely developing facial or jaw muscle spasmodic contractions includes tetanus, neuroleptic-induced dystonia, strychnine poisoning, hypocalcemia, and rabies.

Nerve Gas. Nerve gases, which threatened American troops in the Persian Gulf War, are poisonous because they interfere with ACh. The common gases—GA, GB, GD, and VX—and some insecticides are organophosphates that bind and inactivate AChE. Their antiAChE activity causes excessive cholinergic stimulation that produces tearing, pulmonary secretions, and muscle weakness and fasciculations. Pyridostigmine (Mestinon), if taken before exposure to these gases, protects ACh transmission by temporarily occupying the site on AChE. After exposure and attempts to wash exposed skin, victims are treated with atropine, which blocks the excessive cholinergic stimulation.

Chronic Fatigue Syndrome—A Dubious Relationship. Myasthenia and other muscle disorders are sometimes invoked as an explanation of one of the most vexing problems confronting clinicians: *chronic fatigue syndrome.* Individuals with this condition typically describe a generalized sense of weakness that may have been preceded by flu-like symptoms with myalgias. However, their weakness never affects the extraocular muscles or appears in an asymmetric pattern. Their manual muscle testing typically elicits an unexpectedly brief and weak force. Laboratory values are normal.

Chronic fatigue syndrome—as a distinct entity—does not seem to result from a particular infectious agent or endocrine imbalance. Nevertheless, several neurologic illnesses are complicated by fatigue, lassitude, debility, weariness, and related disturbances: myasthenia, Lyme disease, acquired immune deficiency syndrome (AIDS), mononucleosis, multiple sclerosis, sleep disturbances, eosinophilia-myalgia syndrome, and deconditioning from impaired physical activity. When chronic fatigue complicates these conditions, the underlying disease is evident on clinical grounds.

MUSCLE DISEASE (MYOPATHY)

As would be expected, patients with a myopathy complain primarily of weakness. Although myopathies rarely involve particular regions of the body, most patients' large shoulder and hip girdle muscles—their "proximal" muscles—are affected first, most severely, and often exclusively. Patients have difficulty performing tasks that depend on these muscles: standing, walking, climbing stairs, combing their hair, and reaching upward. Even when the weakness is extensive and severe, patients usually have no oculomotor or sphincter paresis, and they retain the use of their hands and feet. (Hand and feet muscles are "distal" and are affected by neuropathies.)

Acute, inflammatory myopathies cause muscle aches, *myalgias*, and tenderness. Eventually, both inflammatory and noninflammatory myopathies lead to muscle atrophy, *dystrophy*. DTRs are hypoactive roughly in proportion to the weakness. Patients do not have Babinski signs or sensory loss because the corticospinal tracts and sensory systems are not involved. With most myopathies, serum concentrations of muscle-based enzymes, such as creatine phosphokinase (CPK), are elevated and electromyograms (EMGs) are abnormal (see below). Finally, with rare exceptions (see below), myopathies are not associated with mental aberrations.

Inherited Dystrophies

Duchenne's Muscular Dystrophy. Better known as *muscular dystrophy*, *Duchenne's muscular dystrophy* is the most frequently occurring myopathy. In technical terms, a sex-linked genetic illness with expression in childhood, muscular dystrophy is commonly known as a chronic, ultimately fatal illness that develops in boys whose mothers carried the abnormal gene.

Muscular dystrophy, which typically first affects boys' thighs and shoulders, usually becomes evident in early childhood as trouble with standing and walking. In a characteristic finding, *muscle pseudohypertrophy*, affected muscles increase in size because they are infiltrated with fat cells and connective tissue, but paradoxically those apparently excellently developed muscles are drastically weak (Fig. 6–4, Top). As the weakness increases, the boys can arise from sitting only by pulling themselves upward or climbing up their own legs, *Gower's maneuver* (Fig. 6-4, Bottom). Usually by 12 years of age, when their musculature can no longer support their maturing frame, boys become wheelchairbound. They finally develop respiratory insufficiency.

As one of the myopathies associated with mental impairments, muscular dystrophy is accompanied by psychomotor retardation and, in one third to one half of the patients, mental retardation. The children's mental disabilities can overshadow their weakness. Of course, some cognitive, psychologic, social impairments are attributable to isolation, lack of education, and having a progressive handicap. No cure is available, but investigations include the transplantation of muscle cells (myoblast transfer), intramuscular injections of genes, and steroid therapy.

GENETIC STUDIES. Using Duchenne's dystrophy and Huntington's disease (see Chapter 18) as a proving ground, molecular genetic studies have distinguished similarly appearing illnesses, found chromosome markers for numerous illnesses, and greatly increased genetic counseling's reliability. For Duchenne's dystrophy, the abnormal gene's location on the X chromosome had long been assumed because only boys developed the illness. Sophisticated, highly technical *gene positional mapping* by detecting *restriction fragment length polymorphisms (RFLPs)* has isolated the genetic defect—a deletion in most cases—to the short arm of the X chromosome.

RFLP has been the primary technique in identifying the abnormal gene in numerous neurologic illnesses, including myotonic as well as Duchenne's dystrophy. It is based on detecting markers, *genetic polymorphisms*, that adhere closely to the abnormal genes. Using the famous *Southern blot technique*, which is named after a Dr. Southern rather than a region of the country, DNA, cleaved in predictable patterns by enzymes, is separated so that DNA probes can identify the markers (see Appendix 3).

Duchenne's dystrophy causes a pathognomonic absence of a particular muscle-cell membrane protein, *dystrophin*. The relatively benign variant of Duchenne's dystrophy that results from an abnormality in the same gene, *Becker's dystrophy*, causes abnormal dystrophin. In the *dystrophin test*, muscle biopsies are tested for dystrophin to distinguish between these conditions and exclude others that might mimic them.

Reliable diagnoses of Duchenne's dystrophy can be based on finding DNA deletions or absent dystrophin. Affected fetuses can be identified and aborted. Females who carry the gene (and those who do not) can be identified. These techniques have led to a marked decrease in Duchenne's dystrophy.

Myotonic Dystrophy. The most frequently occurring myopathy of adults is *myotonic dystrophy*. Although also an inherited muscle disorder, myotonic dystrophy differs in several respects from Duchenne's dystrophy. In myotonic dystrophy, the median age of onset of symptoms is 20 to 25 years, and women are equally affected. Also, rather than having proximal muscle weakness and pseudohypertrophy, patients develop facial and distal limb muscle weakness and wasting, i.e., dystrophy. Myotonic dystrophy is named after its unique characteristic, *myotonia*: After voluntary effort or percussion, muscles have prolonged contractions. For example, patients are unable to release their grip for several seconds after opening a door or shaking hands. Also, their tongue and palm muscles have long-lasting ridges if tapped with a reflex hammer.

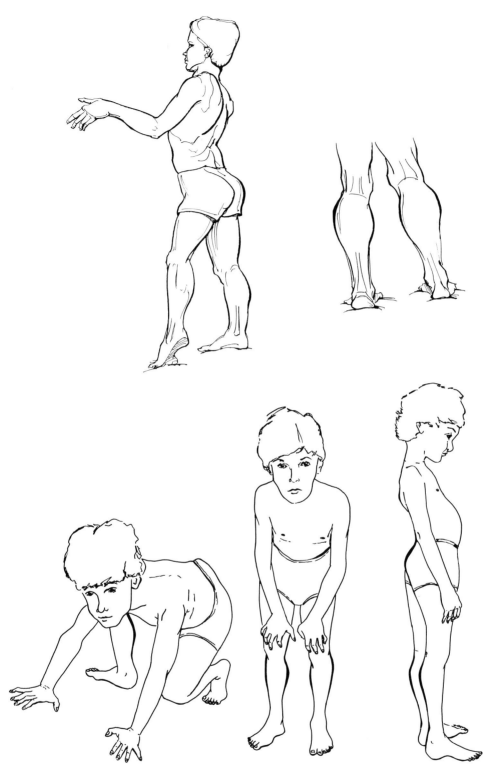

FIGURE 6–4

Top, This 10-year-old boy with typical Duchenne's muscular dystrophy has a waddling gait and inability to raise his arms above his head because of weakness of the shoulder and pelvic girdle muscles. His calves and other weakened muscles are characteristically enlarged because of fat and connective tissue infiltration, not by exercise (*pseudohypertrophy*). There is also a typical exaggeration of the normal inward curve of the lumbar spine, *hyperlordosis.* Duchenne's muscular dystrophy children are frequently pictured on fund-raising posters. *Bottom, Gower's maneuver,* a classical sign of Duchenne's dystrophy, consists of young boys pushing or pulling themselves to a standing position. They must employ their arms and hands because their hip and thigh muscles are weakened early in the disease.

Other unique features are patients' facial appearance and other non-neurologic manifestations. Patients typically lose hair over their temples and develop facial muscle atrophy, which gives them a sunken and elongated face, ptosis, and a prominent forehead (Fig. 6–5). Other manifestations include cataracts, cardiac conduction system disturbances, and endocrine organ failure, such as testicular atrophy, diabetes, and infertility. Treatment is limited to replacement of endocrine deficiencies and reducing myotonia with quinine or other medications.

As with Duchenne's dystrophy, myotonic dystrophy is associated with mental status abnormalities. Duchenne's muscular dystrophy patients often have mental retardation, which is a static cognitive deficit. In contrast, many patients with myotonic dystrophy have a limited intelligence, progressive decline in intellectual function (dementia), and changes in their personality characterized by lack of initiative and progressive blandness. However, although their facial appearance and dysarthria suggest that all myotonic patients have mental impairments, less than 25 per cent of carefully studied patients have shown low intelligence or a deterioration in perceptual-motor functions. Also, cognitive impairments correlate with early age of symptoms and inheritance from the mother, but not with the severity of the dystrophy.

GENETICS. Although patients' manifestations may vary, myotonic dystrophy is a traditional autosomal dominant genetic disorder carried on chromosome 19. The genetic abnormality may be diagnosed by a muscle biopsy that demonstrates abnormal dystrophin, or by disease-specific DNA probes. The abnormal gene is characterized by an excessive number of a certain nucleotide base triplet (*trinucleotide repeat*) in its DNA. The abnormal genes in fragile X syndrome and Huntington's disease are also trinucleotide repeats (see Chapter 18).

The myotonic dystrophy gene is particularly unstable. In a distinctive phenomenon, *amplification*, the genetic abnormality multiplies each time it is reproduced. Succeeding generations are doubly plagued as myotonic dystro-

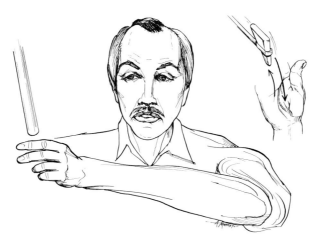

FIGURE 6–5

This 25-year-old man with myotonic dystrophy has the typically elongated face caused by temporal and facial muscle wasting, frontal baldness, and ptosis. Because of myotonia, when his thenar eminence muscle is struck with a percussion hammer, it undergoes a forceful, sustained contraction that pulls the thumb for 3 to 10 seconds. Myotonia also prevents him from rapidly releasing his grasp.

phy appears at a younger age (*anticipation*) and its manifestations are more severe.

Polymyositis

Infectious and inflammatory illnesses occasionally affect muscles either primarily or exclusively. They cause weakness accompanied by myalgias, as in the common "flu," but rarely mental status changes. However, some of them afflict millions of people and create terrible disability.

Polymyositis is a nonspecific, generalized muscle inflammation or infection characterized by myalgia and weakness that are sometimes overshadowed by systemic symptoms, such as fever and malaise. It is most often caused by a benign, self-limited systemic viral illness, but may be a complication of polymyalgia rheumatica, polyarteritis nodosa, and other inflammatory diseases. When polymyositis is accompanied or preceded by a rash on the face and extensor surfaces of the elbows, it is called *dermatomyositis*, which, in adults, is associated with underlying pulmonary or gastrointestinal malignancies.

Trichinosis is a variety of polymyositis that is caused by a *Trichinella* infection of muscles. This illness stems from eating undercooked pork or game and is endemic in South and Central America. In this country, trichinosis is not confined to poor regions, but found in unfortunate diners, hunters who eat their own kills, and recent immigrants.

The *eosinophilia-myalgia syndrome*, which is an inflammatory disorder, has been attributed to tryptophan or contaminants in tryptophan-containing products. These products are taken by insomniacs or health food devotees. The disorder consists of the several-day development of severe myalgias and a markedly elevated number and proportion of eosinophils in the blood. Patients often have other manifestations: fatigue, rash, neuropathy, and cardiopulmonary impairments. Physical symptoms may last more than a year.

More than half the patients with eosinophilia-myalgia syndrome display mild neuropsychologic impairments that are not correlated with physical impairments, eosinophil counts, or concurrent psychiatric disorders. These patients are in danger of being mislabeled as having the chronic fatigue syndrome because of their premorbid lifestyle, variable symptoms, and, except for the eosinophilia, lack of objective findings.

An *AIDS myopathy* causes myalgia and weakness associated with weight loss and fatigue. In most patients, the myopathy results from an infection with human immunodeficiency virus (HIV). Alternatively, in AIDS patients, the myopathy is caused by zidovudine (usually called AZT). In these patients, muscle biopsies often show abnormalities in mitochondria. Withdrawing the medicine leads to partial improvement.

Metabolic Myopathies

Muscles require a delicate balance of hormones, electrolytes, and energy-producing enzymes. These systems are usually independent of cerebral metabolism, but some disorders induce combinations of muscle and cerebral impairment.

Prolonged steroid treatment—for organ transplantation, brain tumors, vasculitis, or asthma—frequently produces *steroid myopathy*. In this disorder, proximal muscle weakness and eventually wasting are accompanied by signs of Cushing's disease, such as a round face, acne, and an obese body with spindly limbs. In high doses, steroids can cause mood changes, agitation, and irrational behavior—loosely termed "steroid psychosis." These mental changes are most apt to occur, of course, in patients with brain tumors and other neurologic illnesses. People who surreptitiously take steroids, such as athletes and body-builders, subject themselves to steroid psychosis and sometimes, to their surprise, muscle weakness.

Another example of the delicate nature of muscle metabolism is that a low serum potassium concentration (hypokalemia) leads to profound weakness, *hypokalemic myopathy*, and cardiac arrhythmias. Hypokalemic myopathy, like steroid myopathy, is an iatrogenic condition because diuretics administered without potassium supplement are its most common cause. Nevertheless, even marked hypokalemia does not alter the mental status. (Sodium depletion [hyponatremia], on the other hand, causes stupor and seizures.)

An interesting variety of hypokalemic myopathy is *periodic paralysis*, in which patients have dramatic episodes, lasting several hours to 2 days, of areflexic quadriparesis associated with hypokalemia. Despite the widespread paralysis, they remain alert and fully cognizant, breathing normally and purposefully moving their eyes. Transmitted in an autosomal dominant pattern, this disorder becomes apparent in adolescent boys and is relatively frequent in Asians, in whom it is associated with hyperthyroidism.

Attacks of periodic hypokalemic paralysis follow exercise, sleep, or large carbohydrate meals. They tend to occur every few weeks, but contrary to the illness' name, the timing is irregular, i.e., periodic paralysis does not occur in a "periodic" pattern. Episodes resemble sleep paralysis and cataplexy, but they have a longer duration and a diagnostic electrolyte disturbance. (All of these conditions differ from psychogenic episodes by their areflexia.)

Other common myopathies sometimes have indirectly related mental status changes. For example, alcoholism leads to limb and cardiac muscle wasting (alcohol cardiomyopathy). In *hyperthyroid myopathy*, weakness develops as part of obvious hyperthyroidism. As a general rule, metabolic myopathies resolve when normal metabolism is restored.

Mitochondrial Myopathies

Whereas the chromosomes' DNA is derived from an equal combination of the DNA of maternal and paternal chromosomes, mitochondrial DNA is derived entirely from maternal mitochondrial DNA. Thus, mitochondrial DNA and its disorders do not conform to standard, Mendelian (chromosomal) inheritance patterns.

Mitochondria contain enzymes for the high-energy cytochrome cycle and lipid metabolism. Their vital energy-producing enzymes are delicate and easily poisoned. Cyanide, an infamous mitochondrial poison, is used for executions in gas chambers and ingested by individuals committing suicide, including several hundred people in the murder-suicide massacre in Jonestown, Guyana in 1978.

Mitochondria DNA (*mtDNA*) abnormalities can produce a tragic but newly elucidated, fascinating group of illnesses, including myopathies, encephalopathies, and possibly Parkinson's disease. These disorders, termed *mitochondrial myopathies*, are characterized by combinations of impaired muscle metabolism, abnormal lipid storage, and brain injury. Muscle mitochondria are unusually numerous, misshaped, or filled with "ragged-red fibers."

Although some overlap occurs, mitochondrial disorders can be divided into three groups. The *primarily mitochondrial myopathies*, which result from deficiencies of lipid storage enzymes and cytochrome oxidase, cause weakness and exercise intolerance, short stature, epilepsy, and lactic acidemia. *Progressive ophthalmoplegia* and related disorders cause ptosis and other extraocular muscle palsies along with numerous non-neurologic manifestations: retinitis pigmentosa, short stature, cardiomyopathy, and endocrine abnormalities. Patients' mental status in both of these varieties may be normal.

The group of mitochondrial disorders characterized by progressively severe encephalopathy has two infamous varieties known best by their acronyms. Both tend to appear between infancy and 12 years. They produce seizures, strokes, and other frank brain injuries and also cause mental retardation, "cognitive regression," dementia, and focal cognitive deficits, such as aphasia.

- *MELAS*: mitochondrial encephalomyelopathy, lactic acidosis, and stroke-like episodes.

- *MERRF*: myoclonic epilepsy and ragged-red fibers

Neuroleptic Malignant Syndrome

The neuroleptic malignant syndrome (NMS), usually a complication of neuroleptics, is characterized by muscle rigidity so intense that it crushes muscles and leads to *rhabdomyolysis* (muscle necrosis), hyperthermia, mental status changes, and cardiovascular collapse. Patients, already suffering from major psychiatric disorders, develop agitation, confusion, or stupor. They also develop autonomic dysfunction with tachycardia, diaphoresis, and hyperthermia. The rhabdomyolysis may lead to myoglobinuria and subsequent renal failure. Body temperatures reaching 107°F cause cerebral cortex damage. Not surprisingly, the mortality rate is 15 to 20 per cent.

NMS has been described most often in patients who have received dopamine-blocking psychotropics, but other dopamine-blocking medications, such as metoclopramide (Reglan), have been implicated as well. It has also been associated in case reports with lithium, desipramine, clozapine, and fluoxetine. The abrupt withdrawal of dopamine precursors, such as levodopa (Sinemet), which creates an effect similar to instituting dopamine-blocking neuroleptics, has also caused NMS.

No explanation accounts for all cases. However, in view of the context in which many NMS cases develop, one credible theory is that NMS is an acute, extreme Parkinson-like reaction to sudden dopamine deficiency in the brain (see Parkinson's disease, Chapter 18). Basal ganglia dopamine deficiency would produce intense muscular rigidity, and hypothalamus deficiency would impair body heat dissipation. Alternatively, dopamine-blocking and other psychotropics might interact with muscle cells and alter their calcium distribution.

In any case, dehydration and renal failure cause an increased concentration of blood urea nitrogen (BUN), and rhabdomyolysis causes a markedly elevated concentration of CPK. The EEG is normal or has only diffuse slowing, which is a mild and nonspecific abnormality indicative either of a toxic disorder or the use of psychotropic medicines (see Chapter 10). Recommended treatment has included ECT, L-dopa, and the dopamine agonist bromocriptine (Parlodel), which all restore dopamine-like activity. Dantrolene (Dantrium) has also been advocated because it restores intracellular calcium distribution.

Other Causes of Muscle Rigidity and Necrosis, Hyperthermia, and Altered Mental States.   *Malignant Hyperthermia* (*MH*) is precipitated by general anesthesia or by the muscle relaxant succinylcholine. Like NMS, MH leads to muscle rhabdomyolysis, hyperthermia, brain damage, and death. However, a tendency to MH, inherited on chromosome 19, may result from an abnormality in a muscle protein receptor for ryanodine. Under certain circumstances, the abnormality leads to a fatal increase in calcium concentration in muscle cells. Especially since MH is an inherited condition, the family history of patients should be reviewed before ECT when succinylcholine is to be administered. Dantrolene may be an effective treatment. Other causes of the sequence, except for the rigidity, are hallucinogen ingestion, heat stroke, delirium tremens (DTs), alcohol intoxication, and general medical conditions, particularly pneumonia.

LABORATORY TESTS FOR NERVE AND MUSCLE DISEASE

Nerve Conduction Velocity (NCV) Studies

The NCV study can determine the site of nerve damage, confirm a clinical diagnosis of polyneuropathy, and distinguish polyneuropathy from myopathy. The NCV is normally 50 to 70 m/sec (Fig. 6–6). When a nerve is damaged, the NCV is slowed at the point of injury, which can be located by proper placement of the electrodes, e.g., across the carpal tunnel. In a polyneuropathy, the NCV of all nerves is slowed, typically to 30 m/sec. In a myopathy, in contrast, the NCV is normal.

Electromyography (EMG)

Electromyographic (EMG) studies are performed by inserting fine needles into selected muscles. The examiner observes the consequent electrical discharges on an oscilloscope during complete muscle rest, voluntary contractions, and stimulation of the innervating peripheral nerve. In a myopathy, muscles produce abnormal, *myopathic*, EMG patterns. Several diseases—myasthenia, ALS, and myotonic dystrophy—produce distinctive EMG patterns.

Abnormal EMG patterns may also be found with mononeuropathies and peripheral neuropathy because muscles deteriorate if the nerves that innervate them are damaged. The EMG can determine which peripheral nerve or nerve

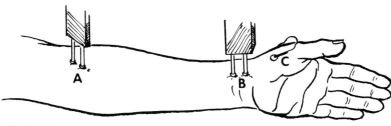

FIGURE 6–6

In determining nerve conduction velocity (NCV), a stimulating electrode that is placed at two points (*A* and *B*) along a nerve excites the appropriate muscle (*C*). The distances between the electrode and the responding muscle and the time intervals between nerve stimulation and muscle response are calculated to provide the NCV, which is normally 50 to 70 m/sec.

root, if any, is damaged. It is particularly useful in cases of lumbar or cervical pain when attempting to document nerve damage from herniated disks.

Serum Enzyme Determinations

Lactic dehydrogenase (LDH), serum glutamic-oxaloacetic transaminase (SGOT), and CPK are enzymes concentrated within muscle cells that escape into the bloodstream when muscles are damaged. Increases in their serum concentration are roughly proportional to the severity of muscle damage and are greatest in NMS. Elevated CPK concentrations are characteristic in Duchenne's dystrophy patients and affected fetuses and assist in the prenatal diagnosis. Patients with peripheral neuropathy, of course, have normal enzyme concentrations. Therefore, for patients with unexplained, ill-defined weakness, as well as ones with myopathy or neuroleptic malignant syndrome, one of the first laboratory tests should be a determination of serum CPK, LDH, and SGOT concentrations.

Muscle Biopsy

In expert hands, the microscopic examination of muscle is useful when muscular atrophy might be the result of a neuropathy, ALS, or certain myopathies. Specific muscle disorders that might be diagnosed in this way include polymyositis, trichinosis, collagen-vascular diseases, and the rare glycogen-storage diseases. Electron microscopy is necessary to diagnose the mitochondrial disorders. A nerve biopsy is useful in uncovering only a few rare diseases.

Thermography

Although infrared thermography is often performed on the head, neck, lower spine, and limbs for a variety of conditions, it has little or no value. In particular, thermography provides little or no reliable information for the diagnosis of nerve root injury from herniated disks in the neck or low back, headache, or cerebrovascular disease. It may have a role in reflex sympathetic dystrophy.

REFERENCES

Caroff SN, Mann SC: Neuroleptic malignant syndrome. Med Clin North Am *77*: 185–202, 1993
Dalakas MC: Polymyositis, dermatomyositis, and inclusion-body myositis. New Engl J Med *325*: 1487–1498, 1991
Drachman DB: Myasthenia gravis. N Engl J Med *330*: 1797–1810, 1994
Engel AG: Gene therapy for Duchenne dystrophy. Ann Neurol *34*: 3–4, 1993
Franzese A, Antonini G, Iannelli M, et al: Intellectual functions and personality in subjects with noncongential myotonic muscular dystrophy. Psychol Rep *68*: 723–732, 1991
Grau JM, Masanés F, Pedrol E, et al: Human immunodeficiency virus Type 1 infection and myopathy: Clinical relevance of zidovudine therapy. Ann Neurol *34*: 206–211, 1933
Gunderson CH, Lehmann CR, Sidell FR, et al: Nerve agents: A review. Neurology *42*: 946–950, 1992
Harper CM, Low PA, Fealy RD, et al: Utility of thermography in the diagnosis of lumbosacral radiculopathy. Neurology *41*: 1010–1014, 1991
Hedberg K, Urbach D, Slutsker L, et al: Eosinophilia-myalgia syndrome. Natural history in a population-based cohort. Arch Intern Med *152*: 1889–1892, 1992
Huber SJ, Kissel JT, Shuttleworth EC, et al: Magnetic resonance imaging and clinical correlates of intellectual impairment in myotonic dystrophy. Arch Neurol *46*: 535–540, 1989

Karpati G, Ajdukovic D, Arnold D, et al: Myoblast transfer in Duchenne dystrophy. Ann Neurol 34: 8–17, 1993

Kartsounis LD, Troung DD, Morgan-Hughes JA, et al: The neuropsychological features of mitochondrial myopathies and encephalomyopathies. Arch Neurol 49: 158–160, 1992

Koo B, Becker LE, Chuang S, et al: Mitochondrial encephalopathy, lactic acidosis, stroke-like episodes (MELAS): Clinical, radiological, pathological, and genetic observations. Ann Neurol 34: 25–32, 1993

Krup LB, Masur DM, Kaufman LD: Neurocognitive dysfunction in the eosinophilia-myalgia syndrome. Neurology 43: 931–936, 1993

Miller RG, Carson PJ, Moussavi RS, et al: Fatigue and myalgia in AIDS patients. Neurology 41: 1603–1607, 1991

Rosebush P, Stewart T: A prospective analysis of 24 episodes of neuroleptic malignant syndrome. Am J Psychiatry 146: 717–725, 1989

Rosenberg RN: Amplification signals anticipation—Less DNA is better. Neurology 42: 1857–1858, 1992

Rowland LP: The first decade of molecular genetics in neurology. Ann Neurol 32: 207–214, 1992

Sewell DD, Jeste DV: Distinguishing neuroleptic malignant syndrome (NMS) from NMS-like acute medical illnesses: A study of 34 cases. J Neuropsychiatry Clin Neurosci 4: 265–269, 1992

Shelbourne P, Davies J, Buxton J, et al: Direct diagnosis of myotonic dystrophy with disease-specific DNA marker. N Engl J Med 328: 471–475, 1993

Simpson DM, Citak KA, Godfrey E, et al: Myopathies associated with human immunodeficiency virus and zidovudine. Neurology 43: 971–976, 1993

QUESTIONS and ANSWERS: CHAPTER 6

1–3. A 17-year-old woman complains of occasional double vision when looking to the left, but with each eye alone, her visual acuity is normal. She has right-sided ptosis and difficulty keeping her right eye adducted. Her pupils are 4 mm, round, and reactive. Her speech is nasal, and her neck flexor muscles are weak. There is no paresis or reflex abnormalities of the limbs.

1. Which diseases might explain the ocular abnormalities?

a. Multiple sclerosis
b. Psychogenic weakness
c. Myasthenia gravis
d. Right posteriar communicating artery aneurysm

> ***answer:*** c. This is a classical case of myasthenia gravis with ocular, pharyngeal, and neck flexor paresis, but no pupil abnormality. In contrast, this pattern of neck flexor paresis, ocular muscle weakness, and ptosis does not occur in multiple sclerosis (MS). Although internuclear ophthalmoplegia does occur frequently in MS, it is causes nystagmus in the abducting eye as well as paresis of the adducting eye (see Chapters 12 and 15). As for psychogenic disturbances, people cannot mimic paresis of one ocular muscle or ptosis. Aneurysmal compression of the third cranial nerve produces ptosis and paresis of adduction, but it has a painful onset, and the pupil becomes large and unreactive to light. Furthermore, the bulbar palsy could not be explained by an aneurysm.

2. Which tests are helpful?

a. AChr antibodies
b. Nerve conduction velocities (NCV)
c. Electromyograms (EMG)
d. Tensilon test
e. Muscle enzymes: CPK, LDH, SGOT

> ***answer:*** a, c, d

3. Which conditions may underlie the main problem?

a. Hypothyroidism
b. Hyperthyroidism
c. Bell's palsy
d. Thymoma

> ***answer:*** b, d. Correction of coexistent hyperthyroidism or thymoma will improve or eliminate myasthenia.

4–5. An 18-year-old dancer develops progressive weakness of her toes and ankles. On examination she has loss of the ankle reflexes, unresponsive plantar reflexes, and decreased sensation in the toes and feet.

4. Which diseases might explain her symptoms and signs?

a. Myasthenia gravis
b. Toxic polyneuropathy
c. Polymyositis
d. Guillain-Barré syndrome
e. Thoracic spinal cord tumor

> *answer:* b or d. She has distal lower extremity paresis, areflexia, and hypalgesia, which indicate a polyneuropathy. Common causes are alcohol, chemicals, and inflammation, e.g., Guillain-Barré syndrome. Myasthenia rarely affects the legs alone and does not cause a sensory loss. Likewise, the sensory loss and pattern of distal paresis preclude a diagnosis of muscle disease. A spinal cord tumor is unlikely because her ankle reflexes are not hyperactive, Babinski signs are not present, and she has no "sensory level" or urinary incontinence.

5. Which tests would be most likely to be helpful in making a diagnosis?

a. EEG
b. NCV
c. EMG
d. Tensilon test
e. Muscle enzymes: CPK, LDH, SGOT

> *answer:* b. NCV will probably confirm the presence of a peripheral neuropathy, but it will not suggest a particular cause.

6–11. A 5-year-old boy is beginning to have difficulty standing upright. He has to push himself up on his legs in order to stand. He cannot run. A cousin of the same age has a similar problem. The patient seems to be unusually muscular and has a normal examination aside from paresis of his upper leg muscles and decreased quadriceps (knee) reflexes.

6. What disease is the patient likely to have?

a. Porphyria
b. Peripheral neuropathy
c. Spinal cord tumor
d. Duchenne's muscular dystrophy
e. A psychogenic disorder

> *answer:* d. The boy and his cousin probably have Duchenne's muscular dystrophy because he has the typical findings: Gower's sign (pushing against one's own legs to stand), pseudohypertrophy, and areflexia of weak muscles.

7. What tests will help diagnose the case?

a. Muscle dystrophin tests
b. NCV
c. EMG
d. Tensilon test
e. Muscle enzymes

> *answer:* a, c, e. Muscle dystrophin will be absent, which is a definitive finding. In the variant, Becker's dystrophy, dystrophin will be abnormal. EMGs will show abnormal (myopathic potential) patterns, and the CPK will be markedly elevated.

8. What is the sex of the cousin?

a. Male
b. Female
c. Either

> *answer:* a. Duchenne's muscular dystrophy is a sex-linked trait. Becker's dystrophy, which is probably carried on an allele of the Duchenne's gene, is then also a sex-linked trait. In contrast, myotonic dystrophy is an autosomal dominant trait that is inherited through the chromosomes in a classic Mendelian pattern of transmission. Progressive external ophthalmoplegia is probably inherited

through mitochondrial DNA (mtDNA), which is derived entirely from the mother: this is non-Mendelian inheritance.

9. Who is the carrier of this condition?

a. Father
b. Mother
c. Either
d. Both

answer: b

10. How can a sister of the patient know if she is a carrier?

answer: She can have the serum CPK level measured. An elevation will suggest that she is a carrier. DNA probes will soon be available.

11. What percentage of a carrier's children will also be carriers or have the disease?

answer: One half of the boys and one half of the girls will inherit the abnormal X chromosome. The boys who inherit it will develop the disease, but the girls who inherit it will only be carriers. Therefore, 25 per cent of the children (one half of the boys) will have the disease and 25 per cent of the children (one half of the girls) will be asymptomatic carriers. No boy will be an asymptomatic carrier. One half of the girls and one half of the boys will have normal genes.

12–15. A 68-year-old man has aches and tenderness of the shoulder muscles. He is unable to lift his arms above his head. There is a blotchy red rash about his head, neck, and upper torso.

12. What diseases should be considered?

a. Steroid myopathy
b. Dermatomyositis
c. Polyneuropathy
d. Periodic paralysis
e. Myasthenia
f. Trichinosis

answer: b, f. The muscle pain, tenderness, and paresis suggest an inflammatory myopathy. Steroid myopathy and most other metabolically induced myopathies are painless.

13. Which tests are most likely to confirm the diagnosis?

a. EEG
b. NCV
c. EMG
d. Tensilon test
e. Muscle enzymes
f. Skin and muscle biopsy
g. Nerve biopsy

answer: e, f. There will be a marked elevation in concentrations of muscle enzymes in the serum CPK, LDH, and SGOT. A biopsy will permit the diagnosis of dermatomyositis, vasculitis, and trichinosis.

14. Which conditions are associated with dermatomyositis in the adult?

a. Dementia
b. Pulmonary malignancies
c. Diabetes mellitus
d. Gastrointestinal malignancies
e. Delirium
f. Polyarteritis nodosa

answer: b, d, f

15. Which of the above conditions are associated with polymyositis in the child?

answer: None. In children, polymyositis is associated only with viral illnesses.

16–24. Which medications are associated with (a) neuropathy, (b) myopathy, (c) neither, or (d) both?

16 Prednisone

answer: b

17. Chlorpromazine

answer: c

18. Nitrofurantoin

answer: a

19. Isoniazid (INH)

answer: a

20. Hydrochlorothiazide

answer: b (via hypokalemia)

21. Amitriptyline

answer: c

22. Thyroid extract

answer: b (hyperthyroid myopathy)

23. Lithium carbonate

answer: c

24. Vitamin B_6

answer: a

25–27. A 50-year-old man has developed low thoracic back pain and difficulty walking. He has mild weakness in both legs, a distended bladder, diminished sensation to pinprick below the umbilicus, and equivocal plantar and DTRs. He has tenderness of the midthoracic spine.

25. With which conditions are his symptoms and signs most consistent?

a. Polymyositis
b. Herniated lumbar intervertebral disk
c. Idiopathic polyneuropathy
d. Thoracic spinal cord compression

answer: d. The patient has spinal cord compression at T10. The reflexes are equivocal because in acute spinal cord compression reflexes are diminished in a phenomenon called "spinal shock." The level is indicated by the sensory changes at the umbilicus. Metastatic tumors are the most frequent cause of spinal cord compression, but herniated thoracic intervertebral disks, multiple sclerosis, tuberculous abscesses, and trauma are sometimes responsible. In contrast, polymyositis affects the arms as well as the legs and does not involve the bladder muscles, produce loss of sensation, or cause spine pain or tenderness.

26. If the routine history, physical examination, and laboratory tests, including a chest x-ray, were normal, which of the following tests should be performed next?

a. Computed tomography (CT) scan of the spine
b. X-rays of the lumbosacral spine
c. Nerve conduction velocities
d. Tensilon test
e. Magnetic resonance imaging (MRI) of the spine

answer: e. MRI is usually the first test, but sometimes CT-myelograms are performed.

27. The diagnostic test confirms the clinical impression. If the condition does not receive prompt, effective treatment, which complications might ensue?

a. Sacral decubitus ulcers
b. Urinary incontinence

c.   Permanent paraplegia
d.   Hydronephrosis and urosepsis

answer: a, b, c, d

28.   Which of the following are complications of excessive or prolonged use of steroids?

a.   Obesity, especially of the face and trunk
b.   Steroid myopathy
c.   Compression fractures of the lumbar spine
d.   Opportunistic lung and CNS infections
e.   Gastrointestinal bleeding
f.   Easy bruisability

answer: a–f

29.   A 31-year-old woman, who has systemic lupus erythematosus (SLE), has been treated for 10 months with prednisone (40 mg daily). She has developed agitation, hallucinations, confusion, and a temperature of 100.5°F. The routine history, general physical examination, neurologic examination, and laboratory tests do not reveal the cause of the mental changes or a source of the fever. Which of the following tests or procedures should be attempted and in which order should they be performed?

a.   Stop the steroids
b.   Begin haloperidol or another major tranquilizer
c.   Do a CT scan of the head
d.   Perform a lumbar puncture
e.   Raise the steroid dosage

answer: b, e, c, d. The real problem is determining whether the patient suffers from too much or too little steroids, i.e., steroid psychosis versus lupus cerebritis. Also, the use of steroids may have been complicated by the development of an opportunistic CNS infection, such as tuberculous or cryptococcal meningitis. While diagnostic tests are being undertaken, psychosis must be controlled with major tranquilizers. The question of stopping or raising steroids is best answered by raising them because lupus cerebritis is more common than steroid psychosis, and prednisone at only 40 mg daily is unlikely to cause steroid psychosis. Moreover, since the patient is under physical and psychiatric stress, she might develop adrenal crisis if a long-standing steroid medication were abruptly stopped.

A CT or MRI scan should be performed to exclude an intracranial mass lesion, such as an abscess or a subdural hematoma. If no mass lesion is detected, a lumbar puncture should be performed to examine the CSF for evidence of infection and other abnormalities.

30.   A 75-year-old woman is hospitalized for congestive heart failure, placed on a low-salt diet, and given a potent diuretic. Although her congestive heart failure resolves, she develops somnolence, disorientation, and generalized weakness. What is the most likely explanation of her mental status change?

a.   Hypokalemia
b.   A cerebrovascular infarction
c.   A subdural hematoma
d.   Cerebral hypoxia from congestive heart failure
e.   Dehydration, hyponatremia, and hypokalemia

answer: e. Administration of potent diuretics to patients on low-salt diets eventually leads to hyponatremia and dehydration. Diuretics often cause obtundation and confusion, especially in the elderly. A low potassium concentration (hypokalemia) alone, however, does not cause mental abnormalities.

31.   Which myopathies are associated with mental impairment?

a.   Polymyositis
b.   Duchenne's muscular dystrophy
c.   Carpal tunnel syndrome

d.   Myotonic dystrophy
e.   Periodic paralysis

answer: b, d. These conditions are associated with congenital intellectual impairments. Myotonic dystrophy is associated with declining intellectual function and personality changes. Moreover, the mental symptoms appear in younger individuals in succeeding generations with myotonic dystrophy.

32–37.   Match the illness with its probable or usual cause:

a.   Autosomal inheritance
b.   Sex-linked inheritance
c.   mtDNA abnormality
d.   Viral illness

e.   Underlying malignancy
f.   ACh receptor antibodies
g.   Medications
h.   None of the above

32.   MERRF

answer: c

33.   Cytochrome oxidase deficiency

answer: h

34.   Progressive ophthalmoplegia

answer: c

35.   Trichinosis

answer: c

36.   Primary mitochondrial myopathies

answer: b

37.   Periodic paralysis

answer: a

38–50.   Match the illness or condition with the appropriate diagnostic test(s):

a.   NCV
b.   EMG
c.   CPK, LDH, and SGOT determinations
d.   MRI
e.   Muscle biopsy
f.   None of the above

38.   Carpal tunnel syndrome

answer: a. NCV studies will show a block of the median nerve at the affected wrist.

39.   Spinal cord compression

answer: d

40.   ALS

answer: b. EMG studies will reveal fibrillations, which are roughly the electrical counterpart of fasciculations. A muscle biopsy may be helpful.

41.   Porphyria (acute intermittent)

answer: NCVs might show nonspecific slowed conduction. The definitive test would be a Watson-Schwartz or other test for urinary porphobilinogens.

42.   Polymyositis

answer: c, e

43. MERRF

answer: e. Muscle tissue will reveal ragged red fibers.

44. Herniated lumbar intervertebral disk

answer: d. Many cases are studied with EMGs to look for nerve root compression, which is often associated with herniated disks.

45. Trichinosis

answer: e

46. Uremic polyneuropathy

answer: a. NCVs will reveal slowing.

47. Myotonic dystrophy

answer: b. EMGs will reveal characteristic electrical discharges associated with myotonia.

48. Duchenne's muscular dystrophy

answer: e and c. Muscles enzymes are elevated, but the increase can be found in other conditions, such as polymyositis. Muscle biopsy showing the lack of dystrophin is diagnostic. DNA probes will be available soon.

49. Guillain-Barré syndrome

answer: a. Guillain-Barré syndrome is a clinical diagnosis confirmed by an elevated CSF protein concentration. In addition, NCVs show slowing.

50. Tetanus

answer: f. Tetanus is virtually an entirely clinical diagnosis. In only 30 per cent of cases will wound cultures reveal clostridial organisms.

51–56. Match the myopathy with the phenomenon:

a. Myasthenia gravis
b. Duchenne's dystrophy
c. Myotonic dystrophy
d. Polymyositis

51. Unilateral ptosis

answer: a

52. Facial rash

answer: d

53. Waddling gait

answer: b

54. Inability to release a fist

answer: c

55. Pseudohypertrophy of calf muscles

answer: b

56. Premature balding and cataracts

answer: c

57. Myasthenia gravis is a disorder in which antibodies damage the postsynaptic neuromuscular ACh receptor. Which of the following therapies are helpful?

a. Giving steroids to reduce the abnormal immunologic reaction
b. Performing plasmapheresis to extract ACh antibodies from the bloodstream

   c. Giving medications that enhance cholinesterase
   d. Giving medications that impair cholinesterase
   e. Giving medications that cross the blood-brain barrier
   f. Performing a thymectomy whether or not a thymoma is detected

> ***answer:***
> a. Giving steroids in large doses is a powerful, effective treatment.
> b. Plasmapheresis can be effective even when all other modalities have failed.
> c. No. They would reduce the concentration of ACh at the neuromuscular junction.
> d. By reducing the effectiveness of cholinesterase, the concentration of ACh would increase. Muscle strength would increase as ACh receptors were stimulated by more ACh.
> e. Being a disorder of the neuromuscular junction, myasthenia gravis does not involve the brain. The anticholinesterases in common use, such as Mestinon (pyridostigmine), do not cross the blood-brain barrier and do not precipitate mental abnormalities.
> f. Removal of thymomas or even persistent, but otherwise normal, thymus tissue improves myasthenia gravis patients.

   58. A 50-year-old man complains of impotence. He had had poliomyelitis as a child, which caused a scoliosis and atrophy of his right leg and left arm. Deep tendon reflexes are absent in the affected limbs. What role do the polio-induced physical deficits play in his chief complaint?

> ***answer:*** The polio-induced muscle weakness and atrophy are typically confined to the voluntary muscles of the trunk and limbs. Polio victims have no sensory loss, autonomic dysfunction, or sexual impairment. Although polio survivors sometimes develop a "postpolio," ALS-like syndrome in middle age, it does not cause sensory, autonomic, or sexual dysfunction. This patient's impotence must have an explanation other than polio.

   59. A corporation's chief executive officer develops ALS. His left arm begins to weaken. Then a hostile takeover bid is initiated by a multinational conglomerate that claims the executive is losing his mental capabilities. Can this contention be supported by the facts known about ALS?

> ***answer:*** ALS is strictly a motor neuron disease. No intellectual deterioration can be attributed to ALS. Although this illness can cause dysarthria and apparent loss of emotional control because of pseudobulbar palsy, ALS does not cause cognitive impairment.

   60. A 30-year-old woman is admitted to an intensive care unit for exacerbation of myasthenia gravis. She has been treated with high-dose anticholinesterase medications, e.g., Mestinon. Plasmapheresis and high-dose steroid treatment are initiated. Nevertheless, the next day, she becomes confused and agitated. What are the likely causes of her mental aberration?

> ***answer:*** Myasthenia gravis is basically a disorder of the ACh receptors of the voluntary muscles. ACh receptors in the brain are not involved. Mental aberrations that occur in myasthenia gravis are not attributable either to the illness or to anticholinesterase medications. However, ventilator failure could cause cerebral hypoxia, high dose steroids could create psychotic behavior, or being confined to an intensive care unit may create a psychologically stressful situation that, superimposed upon medical illnesses, might precipitate "ICU psychosis."

   61. Match the process with its terminology:

   a. Breakdown of muscle cells
   b. Determination of abnormal gene location
   c. Arising from lying position by pushing against one's own thighs

   1. Restriction fragment length polymorphism (RFLP)
   2. Rhabdomyolysis
   3. Gower's maneuver

> ***answer:*** a-2, b-1, c-3

62. Which of the following are features *not* common to neuroleptic malignant syndrome and malignant hyperthermia?

a. Fever
b. Muscle rigidity
c. Brain damage

d. Elevated CPK
e. Tachycardia
f. Familial tendency

> *answer:* f

63. Which of the following is a neurotransmitter at the neuromuscular junction as well as CNS?

a. Dopamine
b. Serotonin

c. GABA
d. Acetylcholine

> *answer:* d

64. Which of the following is deactivated more by metabolism than reuptake?

a. Dopamine
b. Serotonin

c. GABA
d. Acetylcholine

> *answer:* d

65. In myasthenia gravis, against which site are antibodies directed?

a. Orbicularis oculi
b. All acetylcholine (ACh) receptors

c. Nerve endings
d. Neuromuscular junction ACh

> *answer:* d

66. In which condition is dystrophin absent, present but abnormal, and probably normal?

a. Myasthenia gravis
b. Duchenne's dystrophy
c. Becker's dystrophy
d. Myotonic dystrophy

> *answer:*
> Absent: Duchenne's dystrophy
> Abnormal: Becker's dystrophy
> Probably normal: Myasthenia gravis and myotonic dystrophy

67. Which are characteristics of myotonic dystrophy, but not of Duchenne's dystrophy?

a. Dystrophy
b. Cataracts
c. Baldness
d. Myotonia
e. Infertility

f. Autosomal inheritance
g. Dementia
h. Distal muscle weakness
i. Pseudohypertrophy

> *answer:* b-f, h

68. Which conditions are associated with episodic quadriparesis in teenage boys?

a. Low potassium
b. REM activity
c. Hypnopompic hallucinations

d. Hypnagogic hallucinations
e. Hyponatremia

> *answer:* a-d. Hypokalemic periodic paralysis and narcolepsy-cataplexy syndrome cause episodic quadriparesis. Hypokalemia causes episodes lasting many hours to days, rather than a few minutes. Hyponatremia, when severe, causes stupor and seizures, but not quadriparesis.

69. Which statements concerning mitochondria are true?

a. They contain the essential elements of respiratory energy.
b. Their DNA is inherited exclusively from the mother.
c. Abnormalities may affect the brain, as well as muscles.

d. Abnormalities often produce combinations of myopathy, lactic acidosis, lipid storage, and the virtually pathognomonic ragged red fibers.

answer: a-d

70. On which of the following can the diagnosis of Duchenne's dystrophy can be based?

a. Elevated serum CPK
b. Deletion in the DNA of the short arm of the X chromosome
c. Deletion in the DNA of the short arm of the Y chromosome
d. Deletion in mtDNA
e. Absent dystrophin
f. Abnormal dystrophin

answer: a, b, e

71. Which of the following statements are true regarding dystrophin?

a. Dystrophin is located in the muscle surface membrane.
b. Dystrophin is absent in Duchenne's dystrophy.
c. Dystrophin is absent in myotonic dystrophy.
d. Dystrophin absence is a reliable marker of Duchenne's dystrophy.
e. Dystrophin is present but abnormal in Becker's dystrophy, which results from the same gene as Duchenne's dystrophy.
f. Dystrophin is present but abnormal in myotonic dystrophy, which results from the same gene as Duchenne's dystrophy.

answer: a, b, d, e

72. In regard to the genetics of myotonic dystrophy, what are the consequences of its particularly unstable gene?

a. Females as well as males are likely to develop the illness.
b. Mitochondrial DNA might be affected.
c. In successive generations, the disease becomes apparent at an earlier age, i.e., genetic anticipation.
d. In successive generations, the disease is more severe.
e. Theoretically, at least, the gene might self destruct as it prevents young, severely affected individuals from reproducing.

answer: c, d, e

73. Which system do common nerve gases poison?

a. Glycine
b. GABA
c. Serotonin
d. Acetylcholine

answer: d. Nerve gases, by inactivating acetylcholinesterase (AChE), cause excessive ACh activity. Tetanus blocks the release of the inhibitory neurotransmitter, glycine. Botulinum toxin blocks the release of acetylcholine.

74. Which of the following may be the result of body-builders taking steroids?

a. Muscle atrophy
b. Muscle development
c. Mood change
d. Euphoria
e. Depression
f. Acne
g. Compression fractures in the spine

answer: a-g. If taken in excess, steroids produce myopathy, mental changes, and signs of Cushing's disease.

75–79. Match the muscle disorder and its cause

a. Trichinosis
b. Eosinophilia-myalgia syndrome
c. AIDS-associated myopathy
d. Organ-rejection treatment
e. Cardiac myopathy

75. Steroids

answer: d

76. HIV infection

answer: c

77. Tryptophan-containing products

answer: b

78. Alcohol

answer: e

79. Trichinella

answer: a

80. Which of the following statements are true regarding restriction fragment length polymorphism (RFLP) testing?
a. It is useful in detecting Duchenne's and myotonic dystrophies.
b. In detecting myotonic dystrophy, the better test is determining trinucleotide repeats.
c. It is useful in detecting autosomal dominant manic-depressive disease.
d. It is occasionally flawed by DNA crossover and mutations.
e. It is useful in detecting MELAS.

answer: a-d

MAJOR NEUROLOGIC SYMPTOMS

Introduction

The second half of this book focuses on symptoms that are common, illustrate neurologic principles, or indicate serious illnesses. Many are likely to be encountered by psychiatrists because they produce neuropsychologic changes; however, several are included specifically because, possibly contrary to expectations, they are not associated with such changes. Psychiatrists familiar with this material will be better able to perform evaluations that are reliable, effective, and helpful.

Each chapter is devoted to a single symptom's or illness' clinical features, routine laboratory tests, and differential diagnosis. Discussions stress their neuropsychologic aspects, related conditions, and underlying neuroanatomy. The discussions are not meant to represent a comprehensive review or encyclopedic approach. Textbooks offering such approaches are listed in "Notes About the References" (Preface). A list of references for each chapter includes comprehensive textbooks and, where appropriate, textbooks written for patients and their families.

Questions at the end of chapters summarize the material. Those at the end of the book compare information presented in several chapters. In keeping with the current "problem-based" method of teaching medical students, the question-and-answer method helps readers deduce general knowledge and principles from individual cases.

Self-help groups for each illness are listed in Appendix 1. The costs of the diagnostic tests, which can be considerable, are listed in Appendix 2. Although recommendations are offered regarding testing, medications, and other treatments, they do not necessarily pertain to individual patients. Physicians must heed the warnings in this book's preface, package inserts, and other references for indications, dosages, potential complications, and alternatives, including doing nothing.

7 Dementia

Dementia, which is a clinical condition or syndrome rather than an illness itself, consists of the development of cognitive decline. Its chief feature is progressive impairment in memory accompanied by impairments in at least one other cognitive sphere, such as abstract thinking, judgment, or language. The cognitive decline must be sufficiently severe to interfere with an individual's functioning in such areas as work, social activities, or interpersonal relationships. An exception might be that, in a retirement community or nursing home, an individual might develop cognitive impairments, but not suffer functional impairments. In any case, patients in the early stages of dementia must be fully alert. This descriptive definition of dementia differentiates it from related disorders, normal aging, and toxic-metabolic encephalopathies or delirium. Generally used by neurologists, the essentials of this definition have been adopted by the *Diagnostic and Statistical Manual (DSM) IV.*

DISORDERS RELATED TO DEMENTIA

Mental Retardation

In contrast to dementia, mental retardation consists of stable intellectual impairments that have been present since infancy or childhood. Especially when profound, mental retardation is often accompanied by two other signs of cerebral injury: seizures and "cerebral palsy" (see Chapter 13). In cases of genetic anomalies, mental retardation is accompanied by abnormalities in the skeleton, facial structure, skin, and other non-neurologic organs.

Diagnostic criteria for mental retardation are a general intelligence quotient (IQ) of 70 or less and the impairment of adaptive functions, such as social skills and personal independence. Of course, mentally retarded children may, in later life, develop dementia. The most important example of this phenomenon is that individuals who have been mentally retarded as a result of Down's syndrome characteristically develop dementia in their fourth or fifth decades (see below).

Frontal Lobe Syndrome

The frontal lobes are integrally related to the generation of personality, emotions, and executive decisions. They also house inhibitory systems for controlling certain behavior, including bladder and bowel release. Impairment in those functions, loosely termed the *frontal lobe syndrome*, is not strictly speaking a form of dementia because memory, simple calculation ability, and visual-spatial perception are often preserved. Indeed, IQ test results may be normal.

No specific frontal lobe syndrome exists, but at least two varieties, the orbital syndrome and the dorsolateral syndrome, have been described. Physicians need to identify only the general features of frontal lobe damage.

Patients with frontal lobe damage typically speak slowly and, lacking spontaneity, only in response to requests. In severe cases, they are virtually mute, i.e., have *abulia*. Likewise, they have a poverty of thought and emotion. They seem to be indifferent to their surroundings and underlying illness.

On the other hand, impaired inhibitory systems occasionally release flighty and inappropriate speech, emotions, thoughts, and behavior, including incontinence. Uninhibited patients characteristically display a superficial, odd jocularity or facetiousness (*witzelsucht*).

Just like patients' thinking, their movements are awkward, slow, or absent (bradykinetic or akinetic). Their walking is slow and uncertain (frontal ataxia or gait apraxia [see below]). Physicians can elicit frontal release signs (see below). The combination of slowed thinking and movement, *psychomotor retardation*, is characteristic. Psychomotor retardation and abulia naturally appear in conjunction with other signs of frontal lobe injury: pseudobulbar palsy, nonfluent aphasia, and incontinence.

The frontal lobe syndrome is usually caused by discrete lesions, typically penetrating head wounds, a glioblastoma multiforme, metastatic tumors, or infarction of both anterior cerebral arteries. Although one degenerative disease, Pick's disease (see below), may cause relatively isolated frontal lobe damage, Alzheimer's disease and multi-infarct dementia[1] are not usually responsible because they affect the entire cerebral cortex and create generalized cognitive impairment. The infamous *frontal lobotomy*, a neurosurgical procedure in which surgeons resected patients' frontal lobes or severed their large white matter tracts, produced a modified version of the frontal lobe syndrome (see Fig. 20–14).

Amnesia

Another condition closely related to dementia is the *amnestic syndrome*, or simply *amnesia*, which is memory loss with otherwise preserved intellectual function. The distinction is based on the dictum that *memory loss alone is not dementia*. Amnesia is usually attributed to injury or dysfunction of the *hippocampus* and other portions of the limbic system (see Fig. 16–5).

Transient amnesia—suddenly developing amnesia in previously healthy individuals with a duration of several minutes to several hours—is a relatively common, important disorder that might be mistaken for a psychogenic lapse (Table 7–1). In addition, transient amnesia almost invariably results from electroconvulsive therapy (ECT). Post-ECT amnesia impairs memories acquired shortly before and after treatment. The amnesia is more pronounced with high electrical dosage and with bilateral rather than unilateral treatment (see Chapter 10).

In contrast to transient amnesia, head trauma may cause amnesia that lasts for months or is permanent (see Chapter 22). Post-traumatic amnesia probably stems from contusion of the frontal and temporal lobes' anterior surfaces after they are thrown against the inner surfaces of the frontal and middle fossae. The amnesia's duration is roughly proportional to the presence and depth of

---

[1]Multi-infarct dementia is a major component of "vascular dementia," according to the DSM (Diagnostic and Statistical Manual) IV. For practical purposes, the terms are interchangeable.

**TABLE 7–1. COMMONLY CITED
CAUSES OF TRANSIENT AMNESIA**

Alcohol abuse
  Wernicke-Korsakoff syndrome
  Alcoholic blackouts
Head trauma, e.g., concussion
Medications
Partial complex seizures
Transient global amnesia

post-traumatic coma. With severe and extensive head trauma, the amnesia is accompanied by epilepsy and physical deficits, such as hemiparesis, ataxia, and pseudobulbar palsy (see Chapter 22).

Many individuals with Alzheimer's disease, especially at its onset, have amnesia as their only symptom. Until other cognitive deficits develop, these people do not fulfill the criteria for dementia. Amnesia is also a prominent feature of *Herpes simplex* encephalitis, which is the most common, sporadically occurring (nonepidemic) viral encephalitis. (HIV encephalitis is, of course, epidemic.) Presumably entering through the nasopharynx, *Herpes simplex* has a predilection for the undersurface of the frontal and temporal lobes. Temporal lobe destruction can be so severe that amnesia may be accompanied by other manifestations of temporal lobe damage, such as the Klüver-Bucy syndrome, personality changes, and partial complex seizures. More extensive cerebral *Herpes* infection causes dementia. A remote effect of cancer, *paraneoplastic limbic encephalitis*, causes inflammation in the temporal lobe (see Chapter 19).

A certain degree of persistent amnesia is a common, benign condition in people older than 40 years and is called *benign senescence, forgetfulness of old age*, or *age-associated memory impairment*. This variety of amnesia is characterized by forgetfulness for the names of people and other isolated facts; however, judgment, intellect, language function, and learning capacity are preserved. It probably reflects the slowed retrieval of specific information (see below) and, although troublesome, is not incapacitating.

Patients may seem to have amnesia because of psychiatric disturbances, including depression or malingering. Characteristics of malingering-induced "amnesia" are an inability to recall personal information (which is normally deeply embedded) and inconsistent results on memory testing. Amytal infusions may temporarily reverse memory impairments from conversion disorders.

Neuropsychologic Conditions

Amnesia is frequently associated with *confabulation*—a neuropsychologic condition that could easily be mistaken for dementia or a psychiatric disorder. Patients with confabulation offer implausible answers in a sincere, forthcoming, and typically jovial manner. They are not being malicious, but are only concealing their memory impairments. Confabulation is a well-known aspect of a variety of conditions: Wernicke-Korsakoff's syndrome, Anton's syndrome (see cortical blindness, Chapter 12), and anosognosia (see Chapter 8). Because confabulation is associated with these conditions, which are referable to entirely different regions of the brain, it lacks a consistent anatomic correlation.

Aphasia, anosognosia, apraxia, and other neuropsychologic disorders may impair mentation or communication and occur within the spectrum of impediments found in dementia; however, each represents a intellectual deficit that alone does not meet the criteria for dementia (see Chapter 8). Also unlike dementia, these neuropsychologic disorders are usually caused by discrete cerebral lesions. Nonfluent aphasia is the neuropsychologic condition most likely to be confused with dementia because both cause poor performance on routine mental status tests. Moreover, these disorders often cause apathy, abulia, and other symptoms of frontal lobe damage. Of course, several illnesses, such as multiple infarctions or metastatic tumors, can simultaneously cause both dementia and any of these neuropsychologic disorders. Physicians must use skillful testing, which may require nonverbal components, to identify these disorders and detect cases where they coexist with dementia.

NORMAL AGING

Dementia frequently must be distinguished from the cognitive and other neurologic changes that accompany aging. Age-related changes set in with great variability, but people are arbitrarily considered "older" at 65 years. As people become older, they develop a shorter attention span, slower learning (acquisition of new information), and a decreased ability to perform complex tasks, in addition to the memory impairments previously discussed. Their general intelligence declines slightly, as measured by the *Wechsler Adult Intelligence Scale Revised* (*WAIS-R*). In contrast, they have little or no loss of vocabulary, language ability, reading comprehension, or general information. In other words, people older than 65 years tend to remain well spoken, well read, and knowledgeable, although somewhat forgetful.

Another aspect of normal aging is that sleep is fragmented, sleep and awakening times are phase-advanced, and there is less stage 4 NREM sleep (see Chapter 17). Older people usually lose deep tendon reflex (DTR) activity in their ankles, perception of vibration sensation in their legs, and some strength in their limbs. They also have impaired postural reflexes and loss of balance.

These neurologic changes, especially when combined with age-related musculo-skeletal changes, lead to the common standing and walking pattern of older people known as "senile gait." This gait impairment, which is largely compensatory and nonspecific, is characterized by increased flexion of the trunk and limbs, diminished arm swing, and short steps ("shorter or reduced stride"). Many older individuals instinctively compensate by using a cane.

This and other gait impairments lead to falls. In the elderly, falls are a major threat to health because they are incapacitating and potentially fatal. Cognitive impairments, use of sedatives, and a history of a fall are other major risk factors for falling.

Deterioration that occurs in sensory organs impairs hearing and vision. These senses must be tested carefully in elderly patients with mental aberrations because their loss can give the appearance of dementia and can accentuate other physical disabilities. In the extreme, their loss leads to sensory deprivation and its complications, including hallucinations.

The electroencephalogram (EEG) typically shows slowing of the normal background alpha activity (8 to 12 Hz). The dominant background rhythm in older individuals is frequently in the slower frequencies of alpha activity or even slightly slower. Computer tomography (CT) and magnetic resonance imaging (MRI) may be normal, but often these studies reveal decreased volumes of the cerebral hemispheres, atrophy of the cerebral cortex, expansion of the sylvian fissure, and increased volumes of the lateral and third ventricles (see Figs. 20–2, 20–3, and 20–16). In addition, MRIs reveal white matter hyperintensities in many older people. Such abnormalities, although often striking, do not indicate early Alzheimer's disease.

With advancing age, brain weight decreases to about 85 per cent of normal. Age-associated histologic changes include the loss of large cortical neurons and the presence of lipofuscin granules, granulovacuolar degeneration, senile plaques that contain amyloid, and a limited number of neurofibrillary tangles. These changes affect the frontal and temporal lobes more than the parietal lobe.

DEMENTIA

Causes and Classifications

A seemingly endless number of illnesses can cause dementia. The traditional classification by etiology is only slightly more enlightening than an alphabetical list. Classifications based on salient clinical features, although overlapping, are more practical and easier to learn. Classification schemes of commonly cited causes of dementia are based on the following features:

- *Their prevalence*: The most common causes of dementia are Alzheimer's disease and multiple infarctions (multi-infarct or vascular dementia).

- *The patient's age at the onset of dementia*: For people older than 65 years, dementia is most often caused by Alzheimer's disease or multiple infarctions (multi-infarct dementia); people 21 to 65 years, acquired immunodeficiency disease (AIDS), drugs and alcohol abuse, head trauma, multiple sclerosis, and other demyelinating diseases; adolescents (Table 7–2); and younger children (see Chapter 13).

- *Accompanying physical manifestations*: Dementia can be associated with gait apraxia (see below), myoclonus (see below), peripheral neuropathy (see Table 5–2), chorea and other involuntary movement disorders (see Table 18–4), and lateralized signs in brain tumors and head trauma.

- *Genetics*: Dementia is transmitted in an autosomal dominant pattern in Huntington's disease and in some families with Alzheimer's and Creutzfeldt-Jakob's diseases; in an autosomal recessive pattern in Wilson's disease; and in unclear patterns in Pick's disease.

TABLE 7–2. COMMONLY CITED CAUSES OF DEMENTIA THAT AFFECT ADOLESCENTS

Metabolic abnormalities
  Wilson's disease
  Drug and alcohol abuse
Degenerative illnesses
  Huntington's disease
  Metachromatic leukodystrophy
  Other rare, usually genetically transmitted illnesses
Infections
  Subacute sclerosing panencephalitis (SSPE)
  AIDS dementia

- *Reversibility*: The most common reversible causes of dementia are medications, depression, hypothyroidism, and other metabolic abnormalities. Dementia due to some other conditions, such as subdural hematomas and normal pressure hydrocephalus, is theoretically reversible, but substantial, sustained improvement is unusual. In fact, only 8 per cent of dementia cases are partially reversible, and even less—3 per cent—are fully reversible. Also, most reversible situations consist of only mild cognitive impairment lasting less than 2 years.

- *A grouping of "cortical" and "subcortical" dementias*: Cortical dementias are accompanied by other signs of cortical injury, typically aphasia, agnosia, and apraxia. Because the deeper areas of the brain are relatively untouched, patients remain alert, attentive, and ambulatory. The prime examples of cortical dementia are Alzheimer's and Pick's diseases. In contrast, subcortical dementias are typified by less severe intellectual and memory dysfunction and prominent apathy, affective changes, slowed mental processing, and gait abnormalities. Prime examples of subcortical dementia are Huntington's disease, Parkinson's disease, normal pressure hydrocephalus, multi-infarct dementia, and AIDS dementia. This classification has been slipping into disuse because of inconsistencies in individual patients and prominent exceptions inherent in several illnesses, which have included subcortical pathology in Alzheimer's disease and cortical abnormalities in Huntington's disease.

This chapter discusses Alzheimer's disease and other commonly occurring or otherwise important neurologic illnesses that cause dementia. Subsequent chapters will discuss certain illnesses that also cause dementia, but are characterized by different features, such as multi-infarct dementia (see Chapter 11); several childhood illnesses (see Chapter 13); Huntington's, Parkinson's, and Wilson's diseases (see Chapter 18); brain tumors (see Chapter 19): and head trauma (see Chapter 22).

Mental Status Testing

Screening tests, which can be administered in 5 to 10 minutes, are useful in detecting and estimating the severity of cognitive deficits. However, screening tests are limited in several respects. They provide only a coarse measurement that tends to indicate dementia in people who have been isolated or poorly educated. Likewise, well-educated people do better. Most tests are unreliable in distinguishing mild dementia from age-related memory impairments and depression. Since most tests have been developed to detect the dementia associated with Alzheimer's disease, they may be unreliable in detecting dementia associated with other illnesses. From a clinical viewpoint, these tests cannot substitute for a thorough evaluation.

The *Blessed Mental Status Test* has been well validated (Fig. 7–1). Increased cognitive deficiency, as measured by this test, had been correlated with greater neuritic plaque concentration. (Even though recent studies have not confirmed the correlation of plaques and dementia, the Blessed test remains widely and reliably used.)

The Mini-Mental State Examination (MMS), which gives results consistent with those of the Blessed test, also correlates cognitive impairment with plaques (Fig. 7–2). Unlike the Blessed, the MMS tests visual-spatial relationships and language function. However, it is "too easy." Mild dementia may escape detection. The Blessed Test is more sensitive.

Scores on both tests decline unevenly from year to year, which suggests that the progression of dementia is neither linear nor predictable. Successive testing in two situations may cast doubt on a diagnosis of Alzheimer's disease. If

Patient Initials

F   M   L

(1) Observation Date

Month / Day / Year

(2) Patient Study Number

Score each item 0 if correct, 1 if wrong.   Starting Time _____

Name _____

Correct Name, if wrong _____

Age _____ (D.O.B. _____)

When born? _____ (Month, Year)

Where born? _____ Say: Some questions will be easy, some will be hard.

Name of this place _____

What street is it on? _____

How long are you here? _____ (How long today?)

Name of this city? _____

Today's date? _____ (Within a day)

Month _____

Year _____

Day of Week _____

Part of Day _____

Time? (best guess) _____ (Time: (Within 1 hour)

Season _____

Something to remember (Score: immediate repetition-0; phrase by phrase-1; word by word-2; no repetition-3)

____ John   ____ Brown   ____ 42   ____ Market St.   ____ Chicago   Repetition Score _____

Mother's first name _____ (Any sensible response)

How much schooling did you have? _____

Name of one specific school _____

What kind of work have you done? _____

Who is the president <u>now</u>? _____

Who was the last president? _____

Date of WW I (1914-18) _____   Date of WW II (1938-45) _____

Next 3 items: For uncorrected errors, score 2; for corrected errors, score 1.

Months of the year, backwards. Start with December . . . .

D   N   O   S   A   Jl   Jn   M   Ap   Mch   F   Ja

Count 1–20

Count 20–1 (20 19 18 17 16 15 14 13 12 11 10 9 8 7 6 5 4 3 2 1)

Recall name & address __ J __ B __ 42 __ M __ C (Cue with "John Brown" only. Score up to 5 errors.)

TOTAL BLESSED   Finishing Time _____

FIGURE 7–1

Blessed Mental Status Test. Each incorrect answer adds one point to the dementia score. The scores for normal middle-aged adults are 3 points or less. Studies have shown that older individuals with these scores have little probability of developing dementia. People with scores of 5 to 7 have approximately a 50 per cent chance of developing dementia within 2 years. The scores for people with dementia are 8 points or more. When they die, their brains have increased numbers of neuritic plaques. The critical questions are those requiring the repetition of the John Brown phrase, which requires recall of five items, and saying the months backward. Note that the dates of World Wars I and II are those of Britain's participation, and thus, with time and increasing cultural differences, the test will become less valid. (Reprinted from Blessed G, Tomlinson BE, Roth M: The association between quantitative measures of dementia and senile change in the cerebral gray matter of elderly subjects. Br J Psychiatry *114*: 797–811, 1968. With permission of Dr. Blessed and The British Journal of Psychiatry.)

Patient . . . .
Examiner . . . .
Date . . . .

Maximum
Score   Score

ORIENTATION

5   ( )   What is the (year)(season)(date)(day)(month)?
5   ( )   Where are we: (state)(county)(town)(hospital)(floor).

REGISTRATION

3   ( )   Name 3 objects: 1 second to say each. Then ask the patient all 3 after you have said them.
                            Give 1 point for each correct answer. Then repeat then until he learns all 3.
                            Count trials and record.
                         Trials

ATTENTION AND CALCULATION

5   ( )   Serial 7's. 1 point for each correct. Stop after 5 answers. Alternatively spell "world" backwards.

RECALL

3   ( )   Ask for the 3 objects repeated above. Give 1 point for each correct.

LANGUAGE

9   ( )   Name a pencil, and watch (2 points)
          Repeat the following "No ifs, and, or buts." (1 point)
          Follow a 3-stage command:
              "Take a paper in your right hand, fold it in half, and put it on the floor" (3 points)
          Read and obey the following:

CLOSE YOUR EYES (1 point)

          Write a sentence (1 point)
          Copy design (1 point)
_____   Total score
          ASSESS level of consciousness along a continuum_____
                                       Alert   Drowsy   Stupor   Coma

INSTRUCTIONS FOR ADMINISTRATION OF
MINI-MENTAL STATE EXAMINATION

ORIENTATION

1. Ask for the date. Then ask specifically for parts omitted, e.g., "Can you also tell me what season it is?" One point for each correct.
2. Ask in turn "Can you tell me the name of this hospital?" (town, county, etc.). One point for each correct.

REGISTRATION

Ask the patient if you may test his memory. Then say the names of 3 unrelated objects, clearly and slowly, about one second for each. After you have said 3, ask him to repeat them. This first repetition determines his score (0–3) but keep saying them until he can repeat all 3, up to 6 trials. If he does not eventually learn all 3, recall cannot be meaningfully tested.

ATTENTION AND CALCULATION

Ask the patient to begin with 100 and count backwards by 7. Stop after 5 subtractions (93, 86, 79, 72, 65). Score the total number of correct answers.

If the patient cannot or will not perform this task, ask him to spell the word "world" backwards. The score is the number of letters in correct order, e.g. dlrow = 5, dlorw = 3.

RECALL

Ask the patient if he can recall the 3 words you previously asked him to remember. Score 0–3.

LANGUAGE

Naming: Show the patient a wrist watch and ask him what it is. Repeat for pencil. Score 0–2.
Repetition: Ask the patient to repeat the sentence after you. Allow only one trial. Score 0 or 1.
3-State command: Give the patient a piece of plain blank paper and repeat the command. Score 1 point for each part correctly executed.
Reading: On a blank piece of paper print the sentence "Close your eyes" in letters large enough for the patient to see clearly. Ask him to read it and do what it says. Score 1 point only if he actually closes his eyes.
Writing: Give the patient a blank piece of paper and ask him to write a sentence for you. Do not dictate a sentence, it is to be written spontaneously. It must contain a subject and verb and be sensible. Correct grammar and punctuation are not necessary.
Copying: On a clean piece of paper, draw intersecting pentagons, each side about 1 in., and ask him to copy it exactly as it is. All 10 angles must be present and 2 must intersect to score 1 point. Tremor and rotation are ignored.

Estimate the patient's level of sensorium along a continuum, from alert on the left to coma on the right.

FIGURE 7–2
_____

Mini-mental State Examination. Points are assigned for correct answers. Scores of 20 points or less indicate dementia, delirium, schizophrenia, or affective disorders alone or in combination. Such scores are not found in normal elderly people or in those with neuroses or personality disorders. (Reprinted from Folstein MF, Folstein SE, McHugh PR; "Mini-mental state": A practical method for grading the cognitive state of patients for the clinician. J Psychiatr Res *12*: 189–198, 1975, with permission.)

the scores remain stable for 2 years, the diagnosis of Alzheimer's disease should be reconsidered because it almost always causes a progressive decline. If the scores decline precipitously, such as a fall in a MMS score of 20 points in 6 months, an illness that causes a rapidly advancing dementia, such a glioblastoma or Creutzfeldt-Jakob disease (see below), is more likely than Alzheimer's disease.

For patients who were highly intelligent and well educated before the onset of their illness, the *Graduate Record Examination*, might be administered and, if possible, compared to prior test results.

Extensive neuropsychologic testing is indicated when a diagnosis of dementia remains uncertain, a quantitative measure of the severity of dementia is required, or a coexisting aphasia or other neuropsychologic deficit is suspected. In early dementia, performance scales on the WAIS-R are lower than verbal scales, and intelligence is decreased from estimated premorbid levels.

Although neurologists and psychiatrists rely on traditional neuropsychologic tests, a complementary format evaluates the *functional status* of patients. These assessments measure patients' performance of daily activities that require judgment, memory, and attentiveness. Several apparently hierarchical activities reflect functional status (Fig. 7–3).

Laboratory Evaluation

When no particular cause of dementia is suggested by the clinical evaluation, neurologists generally request a series of screening laboratory tests (Table 7–3). Even though these tests are expensive and, as previously suggested, unlikely to disclose a correctable cause of dementia, they are cost effective compared to the huge annual charge for nursing home care (see Appendix 2).

A CT scan is reliable in detecting most structural abnormalities, including brain tumors, subdural hematomas, and normal-pressure hydrocephalus. An MRI scan is superior in certain respects: It is better able to diagnose multiple infarctions, demyelinating diseases, and small lesions. However, neither CT nor MRI can diagnose Alzheimer's disease because cerebral atrophy, which is virtually the only abnormality evident on CT or MRI, is also present in people with normal age-related changes, Down's syndrome, alcoholic dementia, AIDS dementia, some varieties of schizophrenia, and numerous other conditions.

Although the EEG will eventually be abnormal in most cases of dementia, its diagnostic value is limited to moderately severe Alzheimer's disease and a few other illnesses. Slowing of the EEG background activity, which is char-

FUNCTIONAL CAPACITY ASSESSMENT

Fulfills professional/occupational responsibilities
Continues hobbies
Shops, keeps house, cooks
Maintains financial records: checkbook, credit accounts, etc.
Travels independently to work, friends, or relatives

FIGURE 7–3

The Functional Capacity Assessment is not a quantitative assessment, but a survey. The health care worker should determine whether the patient performs or at least tolerates these common activities. If an activity cannot be performed, the worker should determine if the reason is impaired intellectual ability, emotional disturbance, social isolation, or physical incapacity, including impaired special senses.

**TABLE 7–3. SCREENING LABORATORY TESTS FOR
DEMENTIA**

Routine tests
  Chest x-ray
  Electrocardiogram
  Complete blood count
  Chemistry profile
  Urine analysis
Specific blood tests
  Thyroid function, e.g., T_4
  Syphilis test[a]
  B_{12} level[b]
  Human immunodeficiency virus (HIV) antibodies[c]
  Lyme titers[c]
Neurologic tests
  Electroencephalogram (EEG)
  Computed tomography (CT)
  Magnetic resonance imaging (MRI)[d]

[a]In testing for neurosyphilis, either the FTA-ABS or MHA-TP test
is preferred to the VDRL or RPR (see text).
[b]Serum folate level determinations are indicated only if patients
have anemia or nutritional impairments.
[c]For individuals in risk groups.
[d]The MRI is not standard because the CT is usually sufficient.

acteristic of early Alzheimer's disease, may be indistinguishable from normal age-related EEG changes. In more advanced Alzheimer's disease, the EEG shows unequivocal, but nonspecific, slowed and disorganized background activity (see below). In Creutzfeldt-Jakob disease and subacute sclerosing panencephalitis (SSPE), the EEG shows "periodic complexes" or "burst-suppression patterns" (see Fig. 10–6).

The EEG can make an unequivocal contribution to the diagnosis of pseudodementia. In this disorder, a patient's poor performance on mental status tests contrasts with the EEG showing normal activity or only mild background slowing.

A lumbar puncture (LP) is not a routine test because it adds nothing to the diagnosis of Alzheimer's disease or multi-infarct dementia. The LP should be performed to inspect the cerebrospinal fluid (CSF) when patients with dementia have signs of infection or indications of neurosyphilis, chronic meningitis, SSPE, or sometimes AIDS dementia.

Many tests should be reserved for particular indications. For instance, if adolescents or young adults develop dementia, the evaluation might include testing for AIDS; serum ceruloplasmin determination and slit-lamp examination for Wilson's disease; urine toxicology screens for drug abuse; and, rarely, urine analysis for metachromatic granules and arylsulfatase-A activity for metachromatic leukodystrophy (see Chapter 5). Likewise, systemic lupus erythematosus (SLE) preparations, serum Lyme disease titer determinations, and other tests for systemic illness should be judiciously performed.

ALZHEIMER'S DISEASE

Since a "definite" diagnosis of Alzheimer's disease requires histologic examination of brain tissue, this criterion is rarely met in clinical practice. Instead, a "probable" diagnosis, which is accepted for clinical purposes and is consistent with psychiatric criteria, is offered if (a) adults have the insidious onset of a progressively worsening dementia and (b) clinical and laboratory evaluations (Table 7-3) have excluded other neurologic and systemic illnesses that could account for the dementia. These criteria yield a diagnostic accuracy of 90 per cent.

Clinical Features

Alzheimer's disease typically runs a progressive, relentless course, but its rate of progression and some clinical features can differ among individuals. Also, in many individuals the decline is uneven, and in about 10 per cent the course plateaus for several years. Nevertheless, three progressive stages, based on the severity of intellectual deterioration, can be discerned. In the early stage, patients may be conversant, sociable, and physically intact. However, they may be disoriented either at night or when they are moved to new surroundings. Testing reveals impaired judgment and memory. When evaluated casually, their impairments are liable to be misinterpreted as depression or age related.

The middle stage of Alzheimer's disease is marked by overt memory loss accompanied by impairment in language and visual-spatial functions. Language impairments include a decrease in spontaneous verbal output, an inability to find words (anomia), and the use of incorrect words (paraphasic errors)—which are elements of aphasia (see Chapter 8). Impairments in speaking are followed by a decline in comprehension of all communications that eventually leads to mutism. Aphasia is a frequently occurring manifestation of Alzheimer's disease; however, it is more closely associated with cerebral infarctions and multi-infarct dementia.

Another major symptom is constructional apraxia, which is caused by deterioration of visual-spatial abilities (see Chapter 8). Evidence of constructional apraxia in patients' drawing includes simplification, impaired perspective, and sloppiness. Impairments in language and construction, which are cortical functions, have given rise to consideration of Alzheimer's disease as the quintessential cortical dementia.

Patients commonly develop hallucinations that are mostly visual, but are sometimes auditory or olfactory. Hallucinations are associated with delusions and behavioral disturbances, a rapid decline of cognitive function, more severely abnormal EEGs, and a poor prognosis.

Delusions are also common and are associated with a rapid cognitive decline. A substantial minority of patients have prominent paranoid ideation that sometimes reaches psychotic proportions. However, unlike several other illnesses characterized by progressive dementia, such as Huntington's disease and AIDS dementia, Alzheimer's disease is not associated with an unusually high suicide rate.

More than in normal elderly people, Alzheimer's patients lose their normal, circadian sleep-wake pattern, and their sleep becomes fragmented throughout the day (see Chapter 17). Also, in a phenomenon known as "sundowning," thought and behavioral disturbances appear during the early evening hours. It is commonly attributed to the loss of environmental visual and time-based signposts, but this rational and popular explanation has never been proved. Similarly, disorientation plagues patients who are moved to a new environment, such as a vacation or nursing home.

Another important problem is a tendency for Alzheimer's patients who drive to be involved in motor vehicle accidents. Their accident rate is greater than comparably aged individuals, and it increases with the duration of their illness. (Yet, the more striking comparison is with young men who have an even higher rate of motor vehicle accidents than Alzheimer's patients!)

In the late stages, a patient might have frontal release signs (Fig. 7–4), increased jaw jerk reflex (see Fig. 4–12), and Babinski signs. Although dementia signifies extensive cerebral destruction, patients typically have relatively few physical deficits. In particular, patients with Alzheimer's disease, unlike those with multi-infarct dementia, do not have lateralized signs, such as a hemiparesis or homonymous hemianopsia. Until the late stage of the illness, Alzheimer's disease patients are ambulatory. The common sight of a patient wandering aimlessly, but steadily, through a neighborhood characterizes the disparity between intellectual and motor deficits.

In the late stage, physical as well as cognitive deficits become profound. Patients become mute, unresponsive to verbal requests, and bedridden in a decorticate (fetal) posture. They can slip into the persistent vegetative state (see Chapter 11).

Clinical Variants

Alzheimer's disease occasionally follows a familial, autosomal dominant pattern; however, variations among affected families indicate heterogeneity

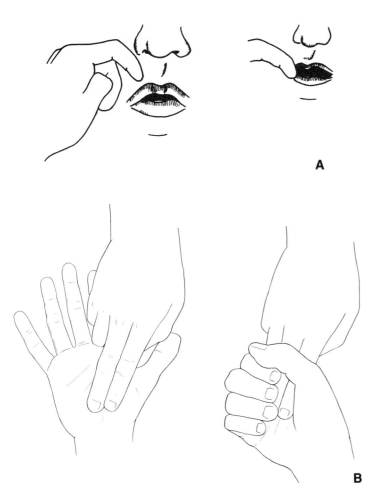

A

B

FIGURE 7–4

The frontal lobe release reflexes that are found frequently in elderly individuals with severe dementia are the snout and grasp reflexes. A, The snout reflex is elicited by tapping the patient's upper lip with a finger or a percussion hammer. This reflex causes the patient's lips to purse and the mouth to pout. B, The grasp reflex is elicited by stroking the patient's palm crosswise or the fingers lengthwise. The reflex causes the patient to grasp the examiner's fingers and fail to let go despite requests.

even within familial Alzheimer's disease. In "early-onset" familial Alzheimer's disease, the symptoms appear in relatively young patients—in their fifth and sixth decade—and run a fulminant course. In "late-onset" Alzheimer's disease, the symptoms appear after age 65 and are similar to sporadically occurring cases.

Given the genetics, the incidence among first-degree relatives of *familial* Alzheimer's disease patients eventually approaches 50 per cent. If both parents have Alzheimer's disease in its sporadic or familial form, about 20 per cent of their offspring will have the illness. Monozygotic twins can develop symptoms at greatly different times.

A disorder that is akin to Alzheimer's disease is *diffuse Lewy body disease.* In fact, it may account for up to 25 per cent of cases initially diagnosed as Alzheimer's disease. Diffuse Lewy body disease is characterized by the rapid development in older individuals of progressive dementia accompanied by mild Parkinson-like features, such as masked face and bradykinesia. Its histologic feature is the diffuse distribution of Lewy bodies throughout the cerebral cortex. Ordinarily, Lewy bodies are characteristic of Parkinson's disease, where they are mostly confined to the substantia nigra (see Chapter 18).

Tests

The EEG can be normal in early Alzheimer's disease, when the clinical diagnosis is most difficult. As previous noted, although over 80 per cent of patients eventually have EEG background slowing, early EEG changes are difficult to distinguish from the slowing that normally occurs in elderly individuals. Moreover, when the EEG is slow and disorganized in a patient with dementia, it provides little specific diagnostic information. In the future, more sophisticated electrophysiologic testing, such as spectral frequency analysis and evoked responses (see Chapter 15), might be able to pinpoint the onset of this disease.

In Alzheimer's disease, CT and MRI both frequently show atrophy first of the hippocampus, then of the temporal and parietal lobes, and eventually of the frontal lobes. The cerebral parenchymal atrophy is accompanied by widening of the third ventricle. Compared to CT, MRI is the more sensitive in detecting cerebral *cortex* atrophy, enlargement of the ventricles, and *leukoariosis*, which is a nonspecific, probably ischemic abnormality in the white matter. However, these changes are absent in many patients with Alzheimer's disease, but are present in many individuals who are normal, highly intelligent, or suffering from any of a number of neurologic illnesses. In any case, when cerebral atrophy accompanies Alzheimer's disease, it has no predictive value.

Positron emission tomography (PET), in about one half of Alzheimer's patients, shows decreased cerebral oxygen and glucose metabolism in the parietal, temporal, and sometimes the frontal lobes' cortex. As the disease progresses, areas of hypometabolism increase. In contrast, multi-infarct dementia causes multiple focal areas of hypometabolism. Nevertheless, PET remains unsuitable for routine clinical use (see Chapter 20).

Single-photon emission computed tomography (SPECT) is a simpler, less expensive version of PET that produces similar results. SPECT has the potential to become a clinically useful test for the diagnosis and management of Alzheimer's disease.

Cerebral cortex biopsies for diagnostic purposes are rarely indicated—mostly because the clinical evaluation is over 90 per cent reliable. Although the histologic findings in Alzheimer's disease differ quantitatively rather than qualitatively from age-related changes, a biopsy might be appropriate in patients suspected of having Creutzfeldt-Jakob disease or familial Alzheimer's disease.

Pathology

Compared with age-matched controls, the brains of patients with Alzheimer's disease are more atrophic. The atrophy is pronounced in the cerebral cortex association areas, such as the parietal-temporal junction, and the limbic system, especially the hippocampus. In contrast, the cortex governing primary motor, sensory, or visual functions is relatively spared. The lateral and, more characteristically, the third ventricles are dilated.

"Plaques and tangles" are a feature of Alzheimer's disease, but are not diagnostic of it. Similar lesions are found in aging and other conditions. Their diagnostic importance in Alzheimer's disease rests on both their density and, like the atrophy, distribution in the cortex association areas and limbic system, especially the hippocampus.

Neurofibrillary tangles are composed of paired, helical filaments of abnormal protein within neurons. In Alzheimer's disease, they are numerous, concentrated in the hippocampus, and, most importantly, parallel the duration and severity of the dementia. Although they are closely associated with Alzheimer's disease, they are also found in other illnesses, such as dementia pugilistica and SSPE, where they affect different populations of neurons.

Senile plaques are extracellular aggregates composed of an amyloid core surrounded by abnormal axons and dendrites (*neurites*). Contradicting preliminary investigations, plaques are not correlated with the presence or degree of dementia: Neurofibrillary tangles correlate much more closely than plaques with dementia.

The *amyloid* found in senile plaques is *beta-amyloid*, which is cleaved from *amyloid precursor protein* by enzymes encoded on chromosome 21. Beta-amyloid differs from amyloid deposited in viscera as the result of various systemic illnesses, such as multiple myeloma and amyloidosis. An alternative to the proposition that beta-amyloid contributes to cell death is that it is deposited in response to cell death or the loss of synapses.

Loss of neurons in the frontal and temporal lobes and particularly in the *substantia innominata* (the *nucleus basalis of Meynert*)—a group of large neurons located near the septal region beneath the globus pallidus—is characteristic of Alzheimer's disease. Loss of synapses and reduction in ACh concentration strongly correlate with cognitive decline. The correlation is postulated to result from the loss of ACh that normally modulates synapses associated with learning.

Biochemical Abnormalities. Substantia innominata neurons normally project upward to virtually the entire cerebral cortex, providing extensive cholinergic (*acetylcholine [ACh]*) innervation. The importance of losing these neurons is that cerebral cortex concentrations of ACh and the enzyme required for its synthesis, *choline acetyltransferase (ChAT)*, are markedly reduced.

ACh is synthesized from acetylcoenzyme-A (acetylCoA) and choline:

$$\text{Acetyl CoA} + \text{Choline} \xrightarrow{\text{ChAT}} \text{ACh}$$

Cerebral cortical ACh concentrations are consistently decreased in Alzheimer's disease compared to aged-matched controls. Decreased concentrations of other neurotransmitters are more variable.

Another characteristic biochemical abnormality in Alzheimer's disease is a pronounced reduction in the peptide neurotransmitter, *somatostatin*; however, unlike ACh reduction, somatostatin reduction does not closely correlate with dementia. Other putative neurotransmitters that are depleted in Alzheimer's disease, but to a much lesser extent, are substance P, norepinephrine, vasopressin, and several other polypeptides.

Drawn from the biochemical observations, the "cholinergic hypothesis" postulates that dementia in Alzheimer's disease results from reduced cholinergic activity. This hypothesis is supported by the demonstration that scopolamine, which has central anticholinergic activity, induces brief Alzheimer-like cognitive impairments that can be reversed with physostigmine (Fig. 7–5). Even the transdermal absorption of scopolamine from motion sickness patches can induce transient amnesia.

Although the ChAT deficiency is striking, it is not peculiar to Alzheimer's disease. Pronounced ChAT deficiencies are also found in the cortex of brains in Down's syndrome, and Parkinson's disease dementia, but not Huntington's disease.

Etiology

Many statistically significant associations (risk factors)—but not causal relationships—have been noted between Alzheimer's disease, other condi-

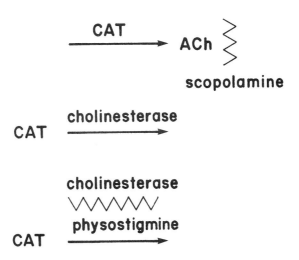

FIGURE 7–5

Top, Choline acetyltransferase (ChAT) is the enzyme that catalyzes acetylcholine (ACh) synthesis. Scopolamine, unlike most other anticholinergic substances, can cross the blood-brain barrier to block ACh. Atropine also blocks ACh, but unless large quantities are administered, it does not cross the blood-brain barrier. *Middle,* ACh is metabolized and deactivated by cholinesterases. *Bottom,* Anticholinesterases, or cholinesterase inhibitors, block the enzyme and preserve ACh concentrations. Anticholinesterases, such as edrophonium (Tensilon) and pyridostigmine (Mestinon), are used in the treatment of myasthenia gravis, where they preserve neuromuscular junction ACh (see Fig. 6–2). For this reason, anticholinesterases are also widely used in insecticides, which cause paralysis by creating prolonged ACh activity at neuromuscular junctions. Physostigmine, a powerful anticholinesterase that can cross the blood-brain barrier, is administered to correct purported ACh deficits in Alzheimer's disease and tardive dyskinesia (see Chapter 18). It is also used to counteract excessive anticholinergic activity in tricyclic antidepressant overdose.

tions: advanced age, family history of Alzheimer's disease and Down's syndrome, and head trauma. Weak associations have been found between Alzheimer's disease and myocardial infarction, episodic depression, personality disorder, hypertension, hyperthyroidism, and increased cerebral concentrations of aluminum silicate.

A newly established risk factor is *apolipoprotein E (Apo-E)*, which is cholesterol-carrying protein produced in the liver and brain that binds amyloid. Apo-E is encoded on chromosome 19 in three isoforms: Apo-E2, Apo-E3, and Apo-E4. Having two genes (being homozygote) for Apo-E4 increases the risk of Alzheimer's disease.

Although the Apo-E data and other information implicate chromosome 19, chromosome 21 abnormalities have also received consideration as a possible etiology for at least three reasons: (1) The gene for amyloid precursor protein, which is associated with plaques, is situated on chromosome 21. (2) A few cases of early-onset *familial Alzheimer's disease* are traceable to chromosome 21. (3) About 95 per cent of individuals who have trisomy 21 (Down's syndrome) develop the pathologic manifestations of Alzheimer's disease by the time that they are 40 years old (see below).

In addition, most early-onset familial Alzheimer's disease is linked to chromosome 14. Therefore, three chromosomes—14, 19, and 21—have individually been suspected of transmitting or rendering people susceptible to Alzheimer's disease. The multiple potential genetic causes suggest that Alzheimer's disease may not be a single disorder.

Treatment

Attempts to Reverse Alzheimer's Disease Dementia.   Despite compelling logic, treatments based on the cholinergic hypothesis have been disappointing. In attempting to restore normal ACh concentrations, researchers first administered ACh precursors, such as choline and lecithin (phosphatidyl choline), but theses substances produced no benefit. A complementary strategy increased ACh concentrations by reducing its metabolism with centrally acting anticholinesterases, such as physostigmine and tetrahydroacridine (tacrine [Cognex]).

Tacrine, which is a long-acting, orally administered anticholinesterase, has retarded cognitive decline and thus preserved functional capacity for about 6 to 12 months. It produced dose-related improvements on performance-based tests, "global evaluations," and measurements of quality of life. However, tacrine is effective only in a minority of patients, and patients who are initially helped resume their decline. Moreover, its use is frequently complicated by moderately severe, but transient, liver impairments.

Another ACh strategy has been to provide ACh agonists, such as arecoline, oxotremorine, and bethanechol, by intraventricular as well as traditional routes. ACh release from cerebral neurons has been stimulated by piracetam and praxilene. All of these treatments have been completely unsuccessful.

Other ineffective approaches have been to replace somatostatin, vasopressin, and other polypeptides. Although reduced cerebral blood flow is a result, not a cause, of Alzheimer's disease, attempts have been made to restore normal blood flow with cyclospasmol and hydergine. A minimal improvement following hydergine, which is an ergot alkaloid, is attributable to its antidepressant properties.

Ameliorating Other Symptoms. Because depression may complicate dementia or sometimes be the root of the problem (pseudodementia, see below), trials of antidepressants have been freely given. Likewise, agitation, delusions, nocturnal behavioral disturbances, and psychotic behavior often require neuroleptics.

Although few studies have compared specific psychotropic medications used in Alzheimer's disease, several rules seem sensible. In view of the ACh deficiency, psychotropics should theoretically have minimal anticholinergic activity. Also, as though atrophied brains require less medication, only low doses should be prescribed. Physicians should periodically reassess the need for psychotropics because, as the disease progresses, symptoms change or even disappear. Moreover, these medications may themselves cause disabling or disconcerting side effects.

Sleep disturbances may be reduced by daytime exercise, exposure to sunlight, and restricted naps. When thought disorders appear predominantly during the night, tranquilizers or sedatives should be given pre-emptively in the early evening. Hallucinations and potentially harmful behavior justify major tranquilizers.

Disruptive behavior—not cognitive decline—is the most compelling reason for families to place Alzheimer's disease patients in nursing homes. The other reasons are incontinence and night-time disruptions.

Neurologists and psychiatrists are often called upon to decide whether a patient must be placed in a nursing home. The physician, accepting the role of the "Bad Guy," can help families by keeping their expectations realistic, preserving their resources, and securing help from social service agencies. Support groups assist the family, as well as the patient.

RELATED DISORDERS

Down's Syndrome

Almost all individuals with Down's syndrome, which is the result of chromosome 21 trisomy, develop an Alzheimer-like dementia superimposed on their mental retardation if they live to 40 years. Moreover, their brains have Alzheimer's disease changes: atrophy, cholinergic depletion, amyloid plaques, neurofibrillary tangles, and loss of neurons in the nucleus basalis. CT, MRI, and PET changes are similar. The striking similarities between Down's syndrome and Alzheimer's disease suggest that in certain families Alzheimer's disease results from an abnormality in chromosome 21.

Pick's Disease

Pick's disease, like Alzheimer's disease, causes a progressive, untreatable dementia. However, rather than having a progressively greater incidence as age increases, the incidence of Pick's disease peaks in the late sixth decade and declines thereafter. Most cases develop in individuals younger than 65 years. Other differences are that Pick's disease is rare, and although genetic etiology has yet not been proven, it has a strong familial tendency.

This disease's gross and microscopic histologic changes are characteristic. The frontal and anterior temporal lobes, but not the parietal lobes, are atrophic. Neurons contain argentophilic (silver-staining) inclusions (*Pick bodies*).

In Pick's disease, selective degeneration of the various cerebral lobes, except for the parietal lobe, produces neuropsychologic symptoms. However, only subtle, evanescent, clinical differences distinguish Pick's disease from Alzheimer's disease. Frontal lobe degeneration causes prominent and early occurring personality changes and relatively uninhibited behavior, thus qualifying Pick's disease as a cause of the frontal lobe syndrome. Temporal lobe degeneration causes language impairment and elements of the Klüver-Bucy syndrome, such as "hyperorality" (see Chapters 12 and 16). In contrast, because the parietal lobe is spared, visual-spatial ability is relatively preserved.

CT and MRI changes, which are predictable in view of the gross pathology, consist of frontal and temporal lobe atrophy with relatively normal-sized parietal lobes (see Fig. 20–10A). By way of contrast, CT and MRI changes in Alzheimer's disease, when atrophy is present, affect all the lobes.

NON-ALZHEIMER'S CAUSES OF DEMENTIA

Multi-Infarct (Vascular) Dementia

After Alzheimer's disease, multiple cerebral infarctions are the most common cause of dementia (see Chapter 11). From a technical viewpoint, multi-infarct dementia is a subset of vascular dementia. In any case, one or more infarctions may complicate Alzheimer's disease and produce a mixed clinical picture.

In multi-infarct dementia, unlike Alzheimer's disease, patients sustain multiple cerebrovascular accidents (CVAs) that characteristically produce a *stepwise* intellectual deterioration. Another distinguishing feature is that multi-infarct dementia is accompanied by focal or lateralized physical signs, such as hemiparesis, visual field cuts, and ataxia. In addition, pseudobulbar palsy and aphasia are often superimposed on the dementia and alter its appearance.

To confound the clinical picture further, multi-infarct dementia patients frequently have underlying renal and cardiac disease. These conditions and the medications used to treat them can cause additional symptoms and exacerbate cognitive impairments.

Wernicke-Korsakoff Syndrome

Chronic, excessive alcohol consumption is complicated by intellectual deterioration and other signs of central nervous system (CNS) and peripheral nervous system (PNS) damage. Although any particular neurologic complication may predominate, virtually all are elements of the *Wernicke-Korsakoff syndrome*.

The Wernicke-Korsakoff syndrome is probably the result not of a toxic effect of alcohol, but of a nutritional deficiency because it is also found in nonalcoholic people who have undergone starvation, dialysis, or chemotherapy. The Wernicke-Korsakoff syndrome is attributable to a profound deficiency in thiamine (vitamin B_1), which is an essential co-enzyme in carbohydrate metabolism.

Cognitive impairments evolve. They begin with a *global confusional state*, in which patients are apathetic, slow, oblivious to their surroundings, and impaired by a characteristic and prominent memory impairment (amnesia). Subsequently, patients become fully alert, attentive, and even jovial, but they typically have a clear-cut amnesia for previously known facts (retrograde amnesia) coupled with an inability to learn new ones (anterograde amnesia).

Moreover, the amnesia impairs various memory-based cognitive functions, especially learning. Eventually, most cognitive functions deteriorate. Although confabulation has often been considered a hallmark, it is usually absent or inconspicuous.

In acute stages, patients may have ataxia and ocular motility abnormalities that include conjugate gaze paresis, abducens nerve paresis, and nystagmus (see Chapters 4 and 12); however, only a minority of patients have all these findings. In addition to the dementia, chronic alcoholics have peripheral neuropathy (see Chapter 5) and cerebellar atrophy, particularly of the vermis (see Chapter 2), which leads to the distinctive gait ataxia (see Fig. 2–13).

CT and MRI scans may be normal or show only cerebral atrophy. The EEG is usually normal. The mamillary bodies and the structures surrounding the third ventricle and the aqueduct of Sylvius (see *periaqueductal gray matter*, Fig. 18–2) have petechial hemorrhages. Since these structures are elements of the limbic system—the cornerstone of memory—their injury is responsible for the characteristic amnesia (see Fig. 16–5).

Thiamine can abort the injury. It should be administered as soon as possible in equivocal as well as clear-cut cases. However, only 25 per cent of patients recover from dementia, and pathologic changes are irreversible.

Although the Wernicke-Korsakoff syndrome had been used interchangeably with "alcoholic dementia," that condition is no longer recognized because it has no distinct clinical or pathologic features. Dementia in alcoholics is attributable to the Wernicke-Korsakoff syndrome alone or in combination with the other, common causes of dementia and certain conditions to which they are vulnerable. They frequently sustain head trauma that causes contusions and sometimes subdural hematomas. They are often involved in motor vehicle accidents (MVAs) because of impaired judgment, slowed physical responses, and a tendency to fall asleep while driving. Those with Laennec's cirrhosis are liable to develop hepatic encephalopathy, especially after gastrointestinal bleeding. Rarely, but interestingly, alcoholics can have degeneration of the corpus callosum that causes a "split brain syndrome" (see Marchiafava-Bignami syndrome, Chapter 8). They have seizures from either excessive alcohol or alcohol withdrawal. In either case, because the seizures result from metabolic aberrations, they are more likely to be generalized, tonic-clonic than partial complex (see Chapter 10). Finally, infants of severely alcoholic mothers are often born with the *fetal alcohol syndrome*, which includes facial abnormalities, a low birth weight, microcephaly, and tremors.

Medication-Induced Dementia

Although medications often induce mental aberrations and lethargy, they sometimes cause cognitive impairments that mimic dementia. Iatrogenic cognitive impairments are one of the few readily correctable varieties of dementia.

Virtually any medication can be suspected. Some, such as reserpine and levodopa, routinely cause or precipitate impairments. Others, such as cimetidine, do so infrequently and unpredictably. Even medicines that are apparently benign because they are instilled into the eye, inhaled, absorbed transcutaneously, or purchased over-the-counter may be the culprit. In addition, nonpharmacologic treatments, such as cranial radiotherapy, may lead to mental changes.

Neurologists frequently prescribe medications that are designed to act on the CNS, but are frequently complicated by mental aberrations. Those medications that are often responsible are narcotic analgesics, tricyclic antidepressants, anticonvulsants, antiparkinson agents, and steroids.

Normal Pressure Hydrocephalus

Normal pressure hydrocephalus (NPH) is a commonly cited, treatable cause of dementia that clinicians might be able to identify by its physical manifestations. However, the actual number of patients that are properly identified and then successfully treated is small because NPH's clinical and laboratory diagnoses are not totally reliable and its treatment is hazardous and inconsistently effective.

NPH is a clinical syndrome that consists of dementia, urinary incontinence, and *gait apraxia*. The hydrocephalus is caused by the combination of reduced CSF absorption through the arachnoid villi overlying the brain and continued CSF production (Fig. 7–6). Meningitis, subarachnoid hemorrhage, or, most often, an unknown injury seems to "plug up" the villi and produce NPH.

The NPH dementia is unusual. It is characterized as much by psychomotor retardation as by cognitive impairments. Also, it is accompanied or overshadowed by the accompanying physical features. Gait apraxia is usually the first and most prominent symptom of NPH (Fig. 7–7). Its severity is proportional to the degree of hydrocephalus. With treatment, gait apraxia is similarly the first and most likely symptom to improve. The urinary incontinence initially consists of urgency and frequency, but in severe cases total incontinence. The presence of gait abnormality and urinary incontinence at the onset of dementia distinguishes NPH from Alzheimer's disease where, if these physical problems occur, they are late developments.

CT and MRI scans show ventricular dilation, particularly of the temporal horns (hydrocephalus; see Figs. 20–4 and 20–15). The large ventricles are accompanied by minimal or no cerebral atrophy and sometimes evidence of CSF reabsorption across ventricular surfaces. However, the identification of NPH by CT and MRI scans is uncertain because this pattern is nonspecific and it resembles cerebral atrophy with resultant hydrocephalus, *hydrocephalus ex vacuo* (see Fig. 20–3). The CSF pressure and its protein and glucose concentrations are normal. The EEG is not helpful in making a diagnosis.

A common test is simply a therapeutic trial of repeated lumbar punctures: CSF withdrawal might reduce hydrocephalus. Clinical improvement after several lumbar punctures indicates NPH and predicts benefits from permanent CSF drainage.

NPH can be relieved—at least theoretically—by the placement of a thin plastic tube (shunt) into a lateral ventricle that diverts CSF into the chest or abdominal cavity for absorption. However, a clinically beneficial response to shunt installation is as low as 15 to 35 per cent. Moreover, despite the apparent simplicity of the procedure, neurosurgical complications, which can be devastating, occur in 13 to 28 per cent of patients.

INFECTIONS

Neurosyphilis

Neurosyphilis, which is caused by persistent *Treponema pallidum* infection, had been largely of historic interest until the late 1980s when it began to

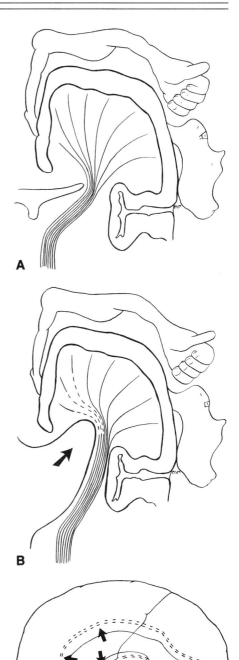

FIGURE 7-6

A, B, Ventricular expansion, as in normal pressure hydrocephalus, results in compression of brain parenchyma and stretching of the myelinated tracts of the internal capsule (see Fig. 18-1). Gait impairment (apraxia) and urinary incontinence are prominent symptoms because the tracts that govern the legs and the voluntary muscles of the bladder are the most stretched. *C,* Also, because the CSF exerts force equally in all directions, pressure on the frontal lobes leads to dementia and psychomotor retardation.

be diagnosed in many AIDS patients. In its secondary stage, syphilis causes *acute syphilitic meningitis*, but only a small fraction of patients with secondary syphilis eventually develop meningovascular syphilis or neurosyphilis-induced dementia, which are tertiary-stage symptoms.

Mental aberrations induced by neurosyphilis may initially consist of only mild, nonspecific personality changes and amnesia, but they then evolve into

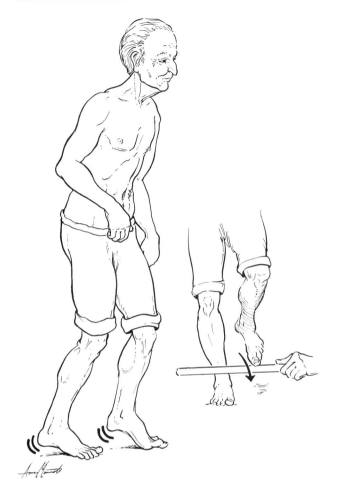

FIGURE 7–7

Gait apraxia, which is a cardinal manifestation of normal pressure hydrocephalus, is one of several gait abnormalities indicative of certain illnesses (see Table 2–4). Patients with gait apraxia fail to alternate their leg movements and do not shift their weight to the forward foot. They tend to pick up the same leg twice in a row or elevate the weight-bearing foot. When their weight remains on the foot that they attempt to raise, that foot appears to be stuck or "magnetized" to the floor.

Gait apraxia is most pronounced when patients start to walk or begin a turn. However, they can sometimes step over a stick or other obstacle because their stepping reflex is relatively preserved.

authentic dementia. Delusions of grandeur, despite their notoriety, occur rarely. Patients with advanced neurosyphilis often have Babinski signs, dysarthria, tremors, Argyll-Robertson pupils (see Chapter 12), tabes dorsalis, and optic atrophy.

In AIDS patients, neurosyphilis is generally more aggressive and difficult to diagnose because, in part, patients cannot mobilize the immunologic responses, which serve as markers, that are required to fight the infection. Also, in these patients, neurosyphilis is often accompanied by ocular involvement.

CT scans typically reveal cerebral atrophy and rarely gummas. Treatment with penicillin may improve cognitive impairments and reverse CSF abnormalities (see below); however, complete clinical recovery is rare.

A blood *Venereal Disease Research Laboratory (VDRL)* test has been the standard screening procedure for syphilis. About 85 per cent of neurosyphilis patients have positive test results. False-positive results, however, are commonly found in the "3 A's:" old age, addiction, and autoimmune diseases. False-negative blood VDRL results may result from the naturally occurring resolution of serologic abnormalities or from prior, sometimes inadequate, treatment.

The VDRL test is being replaced by the similar *rapid plasma reagin (RPR)* test. The RPR test is easier to perform, but may still produce false-positive results.

Tests that are highly specific and sensitive—"confirmatory" or treponemal tests: the *fluorescent treponemal antibody absorption (FTA-ABS) test* and the *treponemal microhemagglutination assay (MHA-TP)*—are positive in more than 95 percent of neurosyphilis cases. Moreover, false-positive FTA-ABS and MHA-TP tests are exceedingly rare, except in cases of other spirochete infections and in testing the CSF. In fact, when evaluating a patient for dementia that might result from neurosyphilis, rather than first ordering a VDRL or RPR test, simply order a FTA-ABS or MHA-TP.

CSF testing should be done when individuals who develop dementia have clinical evidence of syphilis, test positive on the FTA-ABS or MHA-TP, or have AIDS. The VDRL is the only currently available CSF test. In about 60 per cent of neurosyphilis cases, the CSF has an elevated protein concentration (45 to 100 mg/100 ml) and a lymphocytic pleocytosis (5 to 200 cells/ml); however, the CSF has 10 or fewer lymphocytes/ml in 90 per cent of cases.

A potentially confusing point is that the CSF in AIDS patients *without* syphilis often has an elevated protein concentration and a lymphocytic pleocytosis, which might lead to a false-positive diagnosis of syphilis. Moreover, when AIDS patients develop neurosyphilis, the CSF as well as routine serologic tests may, for unclear reasons, be false negative.

One reliable guideline is that a positive CSF VDRL test diagnoses neurosyphilis. However, the CSF VDRL test is false negative in as many as 40 per cent of neurosyphilis cases. Neurosyphilis can nevertheless be diagnosed by the clinical situation and the CSF profile. Another general guideline is to treat patients for neurosyphilis in equivocal cases. Finally, penicillin is the only acceptable treatment for neurosyphilis, and it should be administered even if a penicillin-allergic patient must be desensitized.

Subacute Sclerosing Panencephalitis (SSPE)

SSPE is a rare infectious illness predominantly of children. Its earliest manifestations are poor school work, behavioral disturbances, restlessness, and personality changes. As the illness progresses, the children develop dementia and characteristic *myoclonus* (see Chapter 18). A clinical diagnosis of SSPE may be confirmed by finding an elevated CSF measles antibody titer and, during the initial stage of the illness, periodic complexes or burst-suppression patterns on the EEG (see Fig. 10–6). Although antiviral medications may arrest its course, SSPE is usually fatal in 1 to 2 years.

Several observations point to a defective measles (rubeola) virus as the cause: about 50 per cent of patients contracted measles before 2 years of age, the CSF measles antibody titer is very high in SSPE patients, and almost no children who have been vaccinated against measles have developed SSPE.

Creutzfeldt-Jakob Disease

Creutzfeldt-Jakob disease, like SSPE, causes a distinctive triad of dementia, myoclonus, and periodic EEG complexes. However, Creutzfeldt-Jakob disease usually affects people older than 60 years; causes pyramidal, extrapyramidal, and cerebellar impairment as well as myoclonus; and has a rapidly fatal course of about 6 months.

Another striking feature is that Creutzfeldt-Jakob disease and several variants seem to be caused by genetic susceptibility to a unique infection. The infectious agent is termed a *prion* because it contains protein but not DNA or RNA. (Prion stands for "*pro*teinaceous *in*fective agent.")

In Creutzfeldt-Jakob disease and its variants, *Prion protein (PrP)*, an amyloid protein, accumulates in the cerebral cortex where it can be detected in many cases with special stains. These illnesses are often called "human prion diseases" or, because of the appearance of cerebral biopsies (see below), *spongiform encephalopathies*.

Creutzfeldt-Jakob disease's infectious nature has been established by inoculating animals with brain tissue from human patients. Similarly, this disease has been accidentally transferred to humans by corneal transplantation, intracerebral EEG electrodes, and pathology and neurosurgery specimens. In an iatrogenic tragedy, a group of children contracted Creutzfeldt-Jakob disease from growth hormone extracted from human cadaver pituitary glands.

Although most cases of Creutzfeldt-Jakob disease are sporadic, almost 15 per cent are familial. Those cases and at least one variant, *Gerstmann-Sträussler* disease, follow an autosomal dominant pattern and have an earlier age of onset. Genetic studies suggest that the precursor of PrP is encoded on chromosome 20.

The cerebral cortex has a distinctive microscopic, sponge-like appearance, which leads to the illness' name, spongiform encephalopathy, and, in many cases, the PrP amyloid protein. Despite the infectious nature of the illness, biopsy specimens surprisingly lack inflammatory cells. Cerebral cortex biopsies are performed only in diagnostic dilemmas or when alternative diagnoses are treatable.

Lyme Disease

Neurologic involvement in Lyme disease (*neuroborreliosis*), in its acute stages, causes facial palsy, headache, peripheral neuropathy, and meningitis (see Chapter 5). In a chronic form, presumably because of encephalitis, Lyme disease produces combinations of cognitive impairments, particularly memory difficulties, that may reach the level of dementia; various emotional aberrations that include irritability, depressed affect, and lability; sleep disturbances; and chronic fatigue (see Chapter 6). Although its symptoms can mimic multiple sclerosis or other neurologic illness, the differential diagnosis in practice is more often Lyme disease versus depression, rather than Lyme disease versus another neurologic illness.

Currently available serum and CSF tests for Lyme disease are not definitive in confirming or refuting a clinical diagnosis of Lyme disease. Also, serum and CSF test results do not correlate with memory impairment. To further confuse the issue, reflecting that the infectious agent, *Borrelia burgdorferi*, is a spirochete as in syphilis, serum FTA-ABS and VDRL tests may be positive. In many cases, the CSF will have pleocytosis, elevated protein concentration, reduced glucose concentration, and Lyme antibodies. The EEG, CT, and MRI are not helpful, except to exclude other possibilities.

Lyme disease can be considered a correctable cause of dementia because treatment with several weeks of intravenous antibiotics is effective. (On the other hand, a large group of patients with symptoms and test results indicative of Lyme disease do not respond to treatment because they did not have Lyme disease in the first place.)

AIDS Dementia

Acquired immunodeficiency syndrome (AIDS) results from an infection with the *human immunodeficiency virus* (*HIV*). HIV is a member of a group of RNA viruses, *retroviruses*, that reverse the usual sequence of genetic information so that it flows from RNA to DNA.

The principal target of HIV infection is "helper lymphocytes" with CD4 receptors (*CD4 cells*). In HIV infection, the concentration of CD4 cells declines below the normal value of $\geq 1,400$ cells/cu mm. Patients who have fewer than 500 CD4 cells/cu mm are subject to opportunistic infections and neoplasms.

A second target of HIV is the CNS. CNS involvement leads to encephalitis, myelitis, and meningitis. All parts of the CNS, including the CSF, are potentially infectious.

AIDS dementia, which is also called HIV dementia or, according to the DSM-IV, *dementia due to HIV disease*, is the most frequent neurologic complication of AIDS. It affects 20 per cent of all AIDS patients, including 30 to 60 per cent of those in the late stages of the illness. Reflecting its tendency to be a manifestation of the late stages of AIDS, the dementia is associated with anemia, weight loss, and systemic symptoms. Although dementia is not immediately preceded by a fall in the CD4 count, most patients with AIDS dementia have very low CD4 counts and previously had overt opportunistic infections. AIDS dementia is also disproportionately prevalent in older compared to younger patients. AIDS patients with dementia do not live as long as those without it: After developing dementia, AIDS patients live only about 6 months.

On the other hand, dementia may be a relatively early complication or even the exclusive manifestation of HIV infection. Dementia occurs in only 0.4 per cent of otherwise asymptomatic HIV-positive individuals, but in 3 per cent when AIDS is first diagnosed and in 7 per cent during the following year.

AIDS dementia is usually caused by direct HIV infection of the brain, i.e., *HIV encephalitis.* The cells most clearly infected are the macrophages and the microglia. In some patients, however, cytomegalovirus or toxoplasmic encephalitis may be contributory or responsible.

Manifestations. AIDS dementia causes a decline, over weeks to a few months, in behavior and motor skills, as well as cognitive function. The initial cognitive problems, which appear rapidly if not abruptly, are poor memory and impaired concentration. These cognitive changes are accompanied by psychomotor retardation, apathy, personality changes, and withdrawal from social interactions. Language function is preserved. Neuropsychologic tests confirm the characteristic slowed psychomotor function and impaired nonverbal memory.

Early AIDS dementia mimics depression because patients tend to have blunted affect, social withdrawal, and, because of their illness, vegetative symptoms, such as anorexia and sleeplessness; however, depressive disorders are uncommon in AIDS. The practical implication of this overlap is that if an AIDS patient seems to have depression, first consider dementia.

Likewise, although the rate of suicide is markedly increased (17 to 36 times greater) in AIDS patients, this behavior may also, in part, have a neurologic basis. Suicide ideation is associated with a depressed mood. Moreover, as in other illness causing dementia, such as Huntington's disease, dementia-induced impetuous behavior and impaired judgment can lead to suicide.

At the onset of AIDS dementia, most patients have slow and clumsy walking, ocular mobility abnormalities, and awkward finger movements. A neurologic examination usually can elicit frontal release signs, ataxia, and, in the legs, increased tone, clonus, and hyperactive reflexes. Gait difficulties and slow movements have been so consistent that AIDS dementia is classified by those who value the distinction as a subcortical dementia.

Within a year of the onset of HIV dementia, 80 per cent of patients lose virtually all cognitive function. They often decline into a persistent vegetative state (see Chapter 11), in which they are akinetic (immobile), incontinent, paraplegic, and mute. Their course may be complicated by seizures, myoclonus, and parkinsonism (see Chapter 18). Also, they are beset with systemic or constitutional symptoms, such as weight loss and fevers. Although the purple plaques of Kaposi's sarcoma (Fig. 7–8) are characteristic of AIDS, they are not a marker for dementia.

Zidovudine (AZT [Retrovir]), an antiviral medication that acts by inhibiting reverse transcriptase, was initially believed to slow or possibly reverse AIDS dementia; however, recent studies indicated that it failed to curb dementia; it had harmful side effects, which included mental aberrations, bone marrow suppression, myopathy (see Chapter 6); and it was costly. Stimulants, such as dextroamphetamine and methylphenidate, may help psychomotor retardation, social withdrawal, and fatigue. Depressed patients have been successfully treated with tricyclic antidepressants, serotonin reuptake inhibitors, and, after physicians have scrupulously avoided treating patients with mass lesions, ECT.

Testing.   The standard HIV screening test is an enzyme-linked immunoassay (ELISA); however, the results may remain negative for 6 months after HIV infection is contracted, and the test yields some false-positive results. All patients suspected of having AIDS dementia must have a positive ELISA test and confirmation with the Western blot, PCR, or other highly specific test. They should also have a determination of their CD4 count.

Both CT and MRI scans reveal cerebral atrophy, often basal ganglia abnormalities, and, if they are present, almost all opportunistic infections and neo-

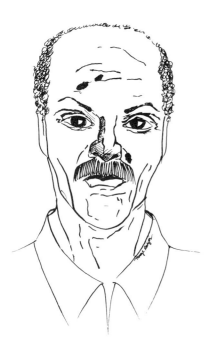

FIGURE 7–8

Kaposi's sarcoma lesions, which appear as small, slightly raised, dry, purple or red-brown patches, indicate but do not prove AIDS. They are most often found in homosexual male AIDS patients.

plasms. MRI scans, but not CT scans, can show nonspecific scattered white matter abnormalities in uncomplicated AIDS-dementia and pathologic large white matter plaques (see below, PML).

The CSF shows a lymphocytic pleocytosis and an elevated protein concentration with, in most cases, an increased IgG content. In a minority of patients, the CSF contains oligoclonal bands, but no myelin basic protein. (Multiple sclerosis, in contrast, typically has CSF with oligoclonal bands and, in periods of exacerbations, myelin basic protein [see Chapter 15].) When opportunistic infections are present, the CSF shows much more pronounced abnormalities. When infected with *Cryptococcus*, the CSF often contains antigens.

Routine EEGs show only mild, nonspecific changes that are not generally helpful in distinguishing dementia from depression. In contrast to the evaluation of patients who develop Alzheimer's disease, a lumbar puncture is usually indicated in evaluating AIDS patients who develop dementia.

Depending on the circumstances, tests might also be conducted for illnesses other than AIDS that are associated with drug abuse or unsafe sex, such as hepatitis, subacute bacterial endocarditis, and syphilis.

At autopsy, the brain is atrophic and pale. Microscopic examination shows perivascular infiltrates, gliosis of cerebral cortex, demyelination, microglial nodules, and multinucleated giant cells. HIV can be isolated from the brains of virtually all AIDS patients with dementia and from many without it. Overall, clinical changes may be more pronounced than histologic abnormalities.

AIDS-Induced Cerebral Lesions. Infectious or neoplastic AIDS-induced cerebral lesions, like other cerebral lesions, cause focal seizures, lateralized signs, and increased intracranial pressure. Moreover, they can exacerbate AIDS dementia.

After HIV, the protozoan *Toxoplasma gondii* is the most common AIDS-related CNS infectious agent. Although a cerebral biopsy is required for definitive diagnosis, bedside decisions are based on the clinical situation and CT scans showing multiple ring-shaped enhancing lesions (see Figs. 20–7 and 20–18). Because toxoplasmosis is so common in AIDS and antibiotics are highly effective, neurologists usually prescribe a therapeutic trial and reserve a cerebral biopsy for patients who do not respond.

Other opportunistic organisms that cause cerebral lesions are fungi, such as *Candida* and *aspergillus*, and viruses, such as CMV and polyoma virus. A polyoma virus, *JC virus,* causes *progressive multifocal leukoencephalopathy (PML)*. As its name suggests, PML produces several widespread, but sometimes confluent, lesions in the white (*leuko*) matter—or myelin—of the brain and spinal cord. Patients develop hemiparesis, spasticity, blindness, and ataxia. Although the neurologic findings and MRI appearance of PML mimic multiple sclerosis (see Chapter 15), which is another demyelinating illness of young adults, the different clinical situations and reliability of HIV testing should eliminate confusion. PML is one of the few conditions where the MRI is clearly superior to CT in detecting the abnormality.

Syphilis and tuberculosis, which both develop in AIDS patients, produce virulent illnesses. Syphilis usually causes acute syphilitic meningitis or meningovascular involvement, but AIDS patients rarely live long enough to develop tertiary neurosyphilis.

The most common cerebral neoplasm complicating AIDS is *primary cerebral lymphoma*. Although this tumor's clinical and CT features are similar to toxoplasmosis, it occurs much less frequently and usually causes only a solitary lesion. Compared to common systemic lymphomas, primary cerebral lymphomas are poorly responsive to radiotherapy, steroids, and other treatment. Gliomas, metastatic Kaposi's sarcoma, and other malignancies are also associated with AIDS.

Other AIDS-Related Conditions.   The spinal cord is also subject to various infections and neoplasms. In particular, spinal cord infection (myelitis) with HIV, *vacuolar myelopathy*, produces paraparesis and other signs of spinal cord injury. The spinal cord damage is similar to combined system disease, but vitamin B_{12} treatments do not help.

AIDS patients with or without dementia may develop meningitis from HIV infection, cryptococcosis, TB, or syphilis. In addition to causing headache, fever, and malaise, meningitis in AIDS patients causes mental aberrations that can mimic or exacerbate dementia.

The PNS is also frequently involved. HIV or CMV infections lead to polyneuropathy, a Guillain-Barré syndrome (see Chapter 5), and mononeuropathies. Many of these PNS infections are extraordinarily painful. AIDS also causes fatigue and a painful myopathy because of infection or medications, such as AZT (see Chapter 6). AZT and other anti-retroviral medicines also cause a neuropathy.

Pseudodementia

Pseudodementia is a condition in which psychiatric disturbances produce cognitive impairments. It is usually caused by depression in the elderly; however, schizophrenia, factitious disorders, or anxiety may be responsible. Unlike patients with dementia from Alzheimer's disease, patients with pseudodementia from depression are typically, but not always, middle-aged people with previous episodes of depression who are beset with affective and vegetative disturbances. More important, their cognitive impairments are brief, fluctuate, and do not include disorientation. Indeed, many patients will perform normally on mental status examinations when encouraged and given additional time. WAIS tests show comparably abnormal performance and verbal scales; however, if psychomotor retardation is present, performance scales may be severely depressed. Allowing for age-related changes, the EEG is usually normal.

A problem for a psychiatrist would be to recognize pseudodementia in individuals older than 65 years. In them, pseudodementia might be overlooked because of prominent—but inconsequential—age-related neurologic factors, such as benign forgetfulness, mild EEG slowing, and CT or MRI scans showing cerebral atrophy. Another problem is that some patients who seem to have had pseudodementia and have responded to antidepressant treatment develop unequivocal dementia 1 to 2 years later.

TOXIC-METABOLIC ENCEPHALOPATHY

Characteristics

Toxic-metabolic encephalopathy causes cognitive impairments that, compared to dementia, have a different course, quality, associated neurologic findings, and etiology. The disorder usually develops over several hours to several days—a relatively brief period. When the underlying abnormality is corrected, the impairments resolve, typically giving the course of the encephalopathy a "bell-shaped curve."

Sometimes, despite an apparently successful treatment, a patient's neurologic condition deteriorates (Fig. 7–9). Another unusual situation is *chronic* encephalopathy, which mimics dementia, from renal, hepatic, or pulmonary insufficiency or the use of certain medications.

Young children and people older than 65 years are particularly susceptible to toxic-metabolic encephalopathy. Also, people with pre-existing dementia are apt to become temporarily stuporous or comatose and, after treatment, have further cognitive deterioration.

The primary features of toxic-metabolic encephalopathy are a change in the level of consciousness that fluctuates, inattention, and disorientation. Most patients are lethargic or stuporous and are unaware of their surroundings; however, a minority are intermittently fully alert (actually manic or "hypervigilant"), apt to misinterpret stimuli, and physically agitated with excessive autonomic activity.

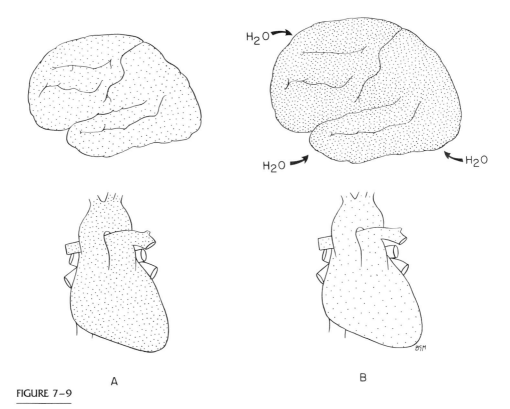

A   B

FIGURE 7–9

A distressing clinical situation occurs when patients deteriorate—that is, develop confusion, lethargy, and other mental symptoms—after correction of certain metabolic abnormalities. For example, in cases of uremia or hyperglycemia, as portrayed in the sketches on the left, a roughly equal concentration of solute is present in the brain and blood. Overly vigorous dialysis or insulin administration will precipitously lower the solute concentration in the blood. Then, the brain's solute concentration will be greater than that of the blood because the solute is cleared more slowly from the brain than the blood. The concentration gradient causes free water to move into the brain, which results in cerebral edema.

Tremors are common and seizures occur occasionally, but these signs have no particular diagnostic value. Characteristic signs may be elicited in several conditions. In Wernicke-Korsakoff syndrome, patients have oculomotor palsies, nystagmus, ataxia, and polyneuropathy (see Chapters 5, 7, and 12); those with hepatic or uremic encephalopathy have *asterixis* (Fig. 7–10); and some with uremia, penicillin intoxication, and other metabolic encephalopathies have myoclonus (see Chapter 18). Narcotic and barbiturate intoxication causes miosis (small pupils), and amphetamines, atropine, and other sympathomimetic drugs cause dilated pupils. As a general rule, patients with a toxic-metabolic encephalopathy have no signs of increased intracranial pressure or lateralized findings.

EEGs show slowing and other nonspecific abnormalities beginning at the onset of mental aberrations and continuing throughout the course of the illness. In hepatic and uremic encephalopathy, the EEG may have characteristic triphasic waves (see Chapter 10). CT and MRI scans, which are performed to exclude coexisting structural lesions, such as a subdural hematoma, are normal. The CSF in meningitis, encephalitis, subarachnoid hemorrhage, and severe hepatic encephalopathy is abnormal, but is normal in most other situations.

Related Conditions

The clinical features that distinguish toxic-metabolic encephalopathy from dementia are a rapid progressive depression of the level of consciousness—from lethargy to stupor to coma—and mental aberrations that fluctuate on an hourly basis. When present, autonomic system hyperactivity is characteristic.

Delirium, as defined in the DSM-IV, is a broader term than toxic-metabolic encephalopathy. It includes postictal states, post-traumatic mental aberrations, and mental effects from tumors in certain areas of the brain.

Neurologists usually reserve the term "delirium" for patients who are mentally excited, physically agitated, and have excessive autonomic activity, i.e., "delirious." These physicians call acutely occurring, fluctuating inattention and disorientation without excessive autonomic activity an "acute confusional state." They use the term "toxic-metabolic encephalopathy," in large part, to indicate that the patient does not harbor a mass lesion. Neurologists apply

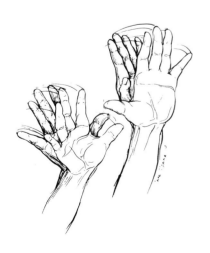

FIGURE 7–10

Asterixis, a sign of a toxic-metabolic encephalopathy, is elicited by having patients extend their arms and hands, as though they were stopping traffic. The hands make a quick downward action and slowly return to their extended position, as though someone were waving "good-bye."

these terms only until they determine the etiology, e.g., postictal confusion, transient global amnesia, and hepatic encephalopathy.

Causes

Especially in older patients, a toxic-metabolic encephalopathy may be the first manifestation of a potentially fatal illness. Innumerable causes are known, but only a few account for most cases in acute care hospitals (Table 7–4). The diagnosis is usually evident in reviewing the patient's history, physical abnormalities, and laboratory tests. While attempting to identify and correct the underlying abnormality, routine medical care consists of providing fluids, electrolytes, nutrition, and often antibiotics. Until the situation is rectified, minor or major tranquilizers might be necessary to make the patient safe, comfortable, and cooperative with testing and treatment.

Only general rules concerning causes can be offered to the practicing physician. Of the hundreds of medications that might cause an encephalopathy, those that are intended to act on the CNS—psychotropic, anti-Parkinsonian, anticholinergic, hypnotic, anesthetic, and narcotic medications—are most likely to act *in an adverse manner* on the CNS. Also, although excessive serum concentrations of the medicines are usually required to produce encephalopathy, it can result from small doses in previously unexposed patients, interactions between otherwise benign medications, administration by ocular or topical routes, or even the withdrawal of certain medications.

Antihypertensive medications also routinely cause adverse neurologic side effects: orthostatic hypotension, which mimics transient neurologic disturbances, sexual impairment, and mental status changes that mimic depression or dementia. The widespread use of antihypertensives, often in combination with several other medications, has made medication-induced dementia common. It is the most common reversible cause of dementia.

A particularly interesting and relatively common variety of toxic-metabolic encephalopathy is *hepatic encephalopathy*. Often, as the liver fails, mental function and consciousness steadily decline into coma. Mild confusion with either somnolence or, less frequently, agitation may precede overtly abnormal liver function tests. The EEG may show triphasic waves. The episodes follow meals with a high protein content or gastrointestinal bleeding.

Hepatic encephalopathy has been traditionally attributed to an elevated concentration of ammonia (NH_3), which is non-ionic (uncharged) and easily able to penetrate the blood-brain barrier. Thus, treatment has been directed at converting NH_3 to ammonium (NH_4^+), which is ionic and unable to penetrate the blood-brain barrier. Current thinking is that, in liver failure, substances

TABLE 7–4. COMMONLY CITED FREQUENT CAUSES OF TOXIC-METABOLIC ENCEPHALOPATHY

Narcotics and alcohol
Medications
Major surgery
Hepatic or uremic encephalopathy
Fluid or electrolyte imbalance, especially dehydration
Pneumonia or other non-neurologic infection

bind to benzodiazepine-GABA receptors and increase GABA activity. Giving a benzodiazepine antagonist briefly reduces hepatic encephalopathy.

REFERENCES

Age Related Changes and Dementia

Applegate WB, Blass JP, Williams TF: Instruments for the functional assessment of older patients. N Engl J Med *322*: 1207–1214, 1990
Clarfield AM: The reversible dementias: Do they reverse? Ann Intern Med *109*: 476–486, 1988
Coffey CE, Wilkinson WE, Parashos IA, et al: Quantitative cerebral anatomy of the aging human brain: A cross-sectional study using magnetic resonance imaging. Neurology *42*: 527–536, 1992
Huber SJ, Shuttleworth EC, Paulson GW, et al: Cortical vs subcortical dementia: Neuropsychological differences. Arch Neurol *43*: 392–394, 1986
Hulette CM, Earl NL, Crain BJ: Evaluation of cerebral biopsies for the diagnosis of dementia. Arch Neurol *48*: 28–31, 1992
Tinetti M, Baker DI, McAvay ASG, et al: A multifactorial intervention to reduce the risk of falling among elderly people living in the community. N Engl J Med *331*: 821–827, 1994
Whitehouse PJ: The concept of subcortical and cortical dementia: Another look. Ann Neurol *19*: 1–6, 1986

Alzheimer's Disease

Abramowicz M ed: Tacrine for Alzheimer's disease. Med Lett *35*: 87–88, 1993
Arriagada PV, Growdon JH, Hedley-Whyte ET, et al: Neurofibrillary tangles but not senile plaques parallel duration and severity of Alzheimer's disease. Neurology *42*: 631–639, 1992
Blessed G, Tomlinson BE, Roth M: The association between quantitative measures of dementia and of senile change in the cerebral gray matter of elderly subjects. Br J Psychiatry *114*: 797–811, 1968
Brugge KL, Nichols SL, Salmon DP, et al: Cognitive impairment in adults with Down's syndrome: Similarities to early cognitive changes in Alzheimer's disease. *Neurology 44*: 232–238, 1994
Claus JL, Harskamp FV, Breteler MMB, et al: The diagnostic value of SPECT with Tc99m HMPAO in Alzheimer's disease. Neurology *44*: 454–461, 1994
Davis KL, Thal LJ, Gamzu ER, et al: A double-blind, placebo-controlled multicentered study of tacrine for Alzheimer's disease. N Engl J Med *327*: 1253–1259, 1992
Drachman DA, Swearer JM: Driving and Alzheimer's disease: The risk of crashes. Neurology *43*: 2448–2456, 1993
Folstein MR, Folstein SE, McHugh PR: "Mini-Mental State": A practical method for grading the cognitive state of patients for the clinician. J Psychiatr Res *12*: 189–198, 1975
Lerner AJ, Koss E, Patterson MB: Concomitants of visual hallucinations in Alzheimer's disease. Neurology *44*: 523–527, 1994
Kirk A, Kertesz: On drawing impairment in Alzheimer's disease. Arch Neurol *48*: 73–77, 1991
Knapp MJ, Knopman DS, Solomon PR, et al: A 30-week randomized controlled trial of high-dose tacrine in patients with Alzheimer's disease. The Tacrine Study Group. JAMA *271*: 985–91, 1994
Kokmen E, Beard CM, Chandra V, et al: Clinical risk factors for Alzheimer's disease. Neurology *41*: 1393–1397, 1991
Lopez OL, Becker JT, Brenner RP, et al: Alzheimer's disease with delusions and hallucinations: Neuropsychological and electroencephalographic correlates. Neurology *41*: 906–912, 1991
Mace NL: Dementia Care: Patient, Family, and Community. Baltimore, The Johns Hopkins University Press, 1990
Mayeux R, Stern Y, Ottman R, et al: The apolipoprotein e4 allele in patients with Alzheimer's disease. Ann Neurol *34*: 752–754, 1993
Schapiro MB, Ball MJ, Grady CL, et al: Dementia in Down's syndrome. Neurology *38*: 938–942, 1988
Terry RD, Katzman R, Bick KL (eds): Alzheimer's Disease. New York, Raven Press, 1994
Vitiello MV, Bliwise DL, Prinz PN: Sleep in Alzheimer's disease and the sundown syndrome. Neurology *42* (suppl 6): 83–94, 1992
Wyper D, Teasdale E, Patterson J, et al: Abnormalities in rCBF and computed tomography in patients with Alzheimer's disease and in controls. Br J Radiol *66*: 23–27, 1993
Yanker BA, Mesulam MM: Beta-amyloid and the pathogenesis of Alzheimer's disease. N Engl J Med 325: 1849–1857, 1991

AIDS-Dementia Complex

Franzblau A, Letz R, Hershman D, et al: Quantitative neurologic and neurobehavioral testing of persons infected with human immunodeficiency virus type I. Arch Neurol 48: 263–268, 1991.

Gelman BB, Guinto FC: Morphometry, histopathology, and tomography of cerebral atrophy in the acquired immunodeficiency syndrome. Ann Neurol 32: 31–40, 1992

Holtom PD, Larsen RA, Leal ME, et al: Prevalence of neurosyphilis in human immunodeficiency virus-infected patients with latent syphilis. Am J Med 93: 9–12, 1992

Marra CM: Syphilis and human immunodeficiency virus infection. Sem Neurol 12: 43–50, 1992

McArthur JC, Selnes OA, Glass JD: HIV dementia. Incidence and risk factors. Res Publ Assoc Res Nerv Ment Dis 72: 251–272, 1994

Miller RG, Carson PJ, Moussavi RS, et al: Fatigue and myalgia in AIDS patients. Neurology 41: 1603–1607, 1991

Price RW, Perry SW (eds): HIV, AIDS, and the Brain. New York, Raven Press, 1994

Siditis JJ, Gatsonis C, Price RW, et al: Zidovudine treatment of the AIDS dementia complex: Results of a placebo-controlled trial. Ann Neurol 33: 343–349, 1993

Other Causes of Dementia

Belman AL, Iyer M, Coyle PK, et al: Neurologic manifestations in children with North American Lyme disease. Neurology 43: 2609–2614, 1993

Berger JR, David NJ: Creutzfeldt-Jakob disease in a physician: A review of the disorders in health care workers. Neurology 43: 205–206, 1993

Brown P, Gibbs CJ, Rodgers-Johnson P, et al: Human spongiform encephalopathy: The National Institutes of Health series of 300 cases of experimentally transmitted disease. Ann Neurol 35: 513–529, 1994

Charness ME, Simon RP, Greenberg DA: Ethanol and the nervous system. N Engl J Med 321: 442–454, 1989

Fradkin JE, Schonberger LB, Mills JL, et al: Creutzfeldt-Jakob disease in pituitary growth hormone recipients in the United States. JAMA 265: 880–884, 1991

Halperin JJ, Volkman DJ, Wu P : Central nervous system abnormalities in Lyme neuroborreliosis. Neurology 41: 1571–1582, 1991

Kaplan RF, Meadows ME, Vincent LC, et al: Memory impairment and depression in patients with Lyme encephalopathy: Comparison with fibromyalgia and nonpsychotically depressed patients. Neurology 42: 1263–1267, 1992

Knopman DS, Christensen KJ, Schut LJ, et al: The spectrum of imaging and neuropsychological findings in Pick's disease. Neurology 39: 362–368, 1989

Krup LB, Masur D, Schwartz J, at al: Cognitive functioning in late Lyme borreliosis. Arch Neurol 48: 1125–1129, 1991

Lindqvist G, Anderson H, Bilting M, et al: Normal-pressure hydrocephalus: Psychiatric findings before and after shunt operation classified in a new diagnostic system for organic psychiatry. Acta Psychiatr Scand 373 (suppl): 18–32, 1993

Mendez MF, Selwood A, Mastri AR, et al: Pick's disease versus Alzheimer's disease: A comparison of clinical characteristics. Neurology 43: 289–292, 1993

Prusiner SB, Hsiao KK: Human prion diseases. Ann Neurol 35: 385–395, 1994

Roberts MC, Emsley RA, Jordaan GP: Screening for syphilis and neurosyphilis in acute psychiatric admissions. S Afr Med J 82: 16–18, 1992

Simon RP: Neurosyphilis. Arch Neurol 42: 606–613, 1985

Steere AC, Taylor E, McHugh GL, et al: The overdiagnosis of Lyme disease. JAMA 269: 1812–1816, 1993

Tan E, Namer IJ, Ciger A, et al: The prognosis of subacute sclerosing panencephalitis in adults: Report of 8 cases and review of the literature. Clin Neurol Neurosurg 93: 205–209, 1991

Vanneste J, Augustijn P, Dirven C, et al: Shunting normal-pressure hydrocephalus: Do the benefits outweigh the risks? A multicenter study and literature review. Neurology 42: 54–59, 1992

Victor M, Adams RD, Collins GH: The Wernicke-Korsakoff Syndrome and Related Neurologic Disorders Due to Alcoholism and Malnutrition (2nd ed.). Philadelphia, F.A. Davis, 1989

Toxic-Metabolic Encephalopathy

Abramowicz M (ed): Drugs that cause psychiatric symptoms. Med Lett 35: 65–70, 1993

Basile AS, Jones EA, Skolnick P: The pathogenesis and treatment of hepatic encephalopathy. Pharmacol Rev 43: 27–71, 1991

Lipowski ZJ: Delirium: Acute Confusional States. New York, Oxford University Press, 1990

Sackeim HA, Prudic J, Devanand DP, et al: Effects of stimulus intensity and electrode placement on the efficacy and cognitive effects of electroconvulsive therapy. N Engl J Med 328: 839–846, 1993

Strub RL, Black FW: The Mental Status Examination in Neurology, 3rd ed. Philadelphia, F.A. Davis, 1993

QUESTIONS and ANSWERS: CHAPTER 7

1. What are these illnesses' features in addition to dementia or delirium?

1. CNS lupus
2. Normal-pressure hydrocephalus
3. Diffuse Lewy body disease
4. Wilson's disease
5. Huntington's disease
6. Bromism
7. Arsenic poisoning
8. Porphyria
9. Wernicke's encephalopathy
10. Myxedema
11. Tuberous sclerosis
12. Hepatic encephalopathy
13. SSPE
14. Crutzfeldt-Jakob disease

a. Akinesia, tremor, and postural reflex abnormalities
b. Acne-like skin rash, headache, and lethargy
c. Amnesia with nystagmus, ocular paresis, and ataxia
d. Tremor, rigidity, and Kayser-Fleischer rings
e. Nonspecific mental dullness and peripheral neuropathy
f. Adenoma of face and seizures, usually beginning in childhood
g. Seizures, strokes, and psychosis (the three S's)
h. Chorea but, in young adults, rigidity
i. Recurrent episodes of delirium, seizures, peripheral neuropathy, and abdominal pain with dark red urine
j. Slow mentation and depression, but sometimes excited confusion ("madness")
k. Lethargy and asterixis
l. Incontinence and gait apraxia
m. Myoclonus with pyramidal or extrapyramidal findings in individuals older than 65 years
n. Myoclonus, usually in rural boys

answer: 1-g, 2-l, 3-a, 4-d, 5-h, 6-b, 7-e, 8-i (acute intermittent porphyria only), 9-c, 10-j, 11-f, 12-k, 13-n, 14-m

2. Which tests (a–l) are used to diagnose the illness (1–16)?

1. Gerstmann-Sträussler disease
2. Combined system disease or subacute combined degeneration
3. Porphyria
4. Arsenic poisoning
5. Lead poisoning
6. Tabes dorsalis
7. SSPE
8. Water intoxication
9. Bromism
10. Subarachnoid hemorrhage
11. Subdural hematomas
12. Creutzfeldt-Jakob disease
13. Wilson's disease
14. Sphenoid wing meningioma
15. Hepatic encephalopathy
16. Cryptococcal meningitis

a. CSF analysis
b. Serum electrolyte determination
c. Serum T_4 level determination
d. CT or MRI
e. Serum heavy metal testing
f. Serum B_{12} level determination
g. Brain biopsy
h. Watson-Schwartz test or urine porphyrin levels
i. Slit-lamp examination
j. Serum ceruloplasmin level
k. EEG
l. Finger nail analysis

answer: 1-g and k (spongiform changes on brain biopsy), 2-f, 3-h, 4-e and l, 5-e, 6-a, 7-a and k (CSF measles antibody and EEG periodic complexes), 8-b, 9-b (an anion gap), 10-a and d (bloody or xanthochromic CSF or a CT or MRI showing blood), 11-d, 12-g and k (spongiform changes on brain biopsy and EEG periodic complexes), 13-i and j, 14-d, 15-k (EEG triphasic waves. Liver function tests may be helpful, but blood ammonia concentrations are inconsistent), 16-a (CSF cryptococcal antigen is the most specific and occasionally the only positive test.)

3. For which illnesses is the EEG usually helpful in making a diagnosis?

a. Alzheimer's disease
b. SSPE
c. Tuberous sclerosis
d. Lead poisoning
e. Uremia
f. Hepatic encephalopathy
g. Creutzfeldt-Jakob disease
h. Neurosyphilis

i. Multi-infarct dementia
j. Diffuse Lewy body disease
k. Valium intoxication
l. Pseudodementia
m. Parkinson's disease
n. Herpes encephalitis
o. Subdural hematoma
p. AIDS dementia

answer: b, c, e, f, g, k, l (lack of abnormality is important), n

4. The diagnosis of normal pressure hydrocephalus (NPH) has received much attention in the literature because installation of a ventricular-peritoneal shunt may correct the dementia.

a. Which conditions predispose a patient to NPH?
b. What approximate percentage of patients thought to have NPH benefit from placement of a shunt?

1. 0%
2. 25%

3. 50 %
4. 100%

answer: (a) Subarachnoid hemorrhage, chronic meningitis, but mostly no evident illness precipitate or cause NPH. (b) 2

5. Is a cerebral cortex biopsy indicated in the routine diagnosis of Alzheimer's disease?

answer: No. Routine histologic examination cannot be diagnostic because plaques and tangles are found in normal aged brains. However, if the studies can be performed, a lowered acetylcholine or choline acetyltransferase level would be virtually diagnostic.

6. With which feature is Alzheimer's disease dementia most closely associated?

a. Large ventricles
b. Increased concentration of plaques
c. Increased concentration of tangles
d. Degree of neuron loss

answer: d. The other changes are more closely associated with age.

7. What medication or therapy (column B) is appropriate for severe intoxication of the following (column A)?

[A]	[B]
1. Lithium	a. Physostigmine
2. Bromide	b. Hypertonic saline or water restriction
3. Heroin	c. Atropine
4. Methadone	d. Dialysis
5. Phenobarbital	e. Saline and diuretics
6. Imipramine	f. Ethyl alcohol 50 percent
7. Valium	g. B_6
8. Water	
9. Lead	h. BAL (dimercaprol)
10. Belladonna	i. Penicillin
11. Methanol	j. Naloxone
12. Arsenic	k. Hypotonic saline
13. Organic phosphates	l. Glucose
14. Phenothiazines	m. Supportive therapy and possibly sedatives or neuroleptics
15. Mercury	n. Propranolol
16. LSD intoxication	o. Benzodiazepine receptor blockers
17. Isoniazid (INH)	
18. Scopolamine	
19. L-dopa	
20. Thyroxine	

answer: 1-d or e, 2-e, 3-j, 4-j, 5-d, 6-a (severe cases), 7-o, 8-b, 9-h, 10-m, 11-f, 12-h, 13-c, 14-m, 15-h, 16-m, 17-g, 18-m, 19-m, 20-n

8. What is the pattern of inheritance (a-d) of the following illnesses (1-4)?

1.	Wilson's disease	a.	Sex-linked recessive
2.	Huntington's disease	b.	Autosomal recessive
3.	Familial Creutzfeldt-Jakob	c.	Autosomal dominant
4.	Familial Alzheimer's disease	d.	None of the above

answer: 1-b, 2-c, 3-c, 4-c

9. Which feature is *not* common to Alzheimer's disease and Down's syndrome?

a. An abnormality referable to chromosome 21
b. Dementia
c. Presence of cerebral plaques and tangles
d. Low concentrations of cerebral acetylcholine
e. Abnormalities in the nucleus basalis of Meynert
f. High incidence of leukemia

answer: f. Alzheimer's disease and Down's syndrome are remarkably similar illnesses. Of the characteristics listed, leukemia is much more closely associated with Down's syndrome.

10. Which of the following are normal, age-related changes?

a. 8-Hz EEG background
b. Forgetfulness of names and isolated facts
c. MRI hyperintense spots in the cerebrum
d. Slower learning
e. Loss of vocabulary
f. Impaired judgment
g. Hypoactive or absent deep tendon reflexes in the legs
h. Impaired vibration sensation and balance
i. Dilated ventricles
j. Plaques and tangles
k. Gummas in the cerebrum
l. Brain weight of 66 per cent of normal
m. Delayed sleep and awakening times
n. More slow-wave sleep

answer: a, b, c, d, g, h, i, j

11. Which of the following diseases routinely cause dementia that develops in individual's sixth decade in a familial pattern?

a. Subacute sclerosing panencephalitis (SSPE)
b. Wilson's
c. Familial Alzheimer's
d. Parkinson's
e. Pick's
f. Gerstmann-Sträussler
g. Huntington's

answer: c, e, f. SSPE and Wilson's disease cause dementia, but in children and teenagers, and SSPE is not a familial illness. Parkinson's disease causes dementia, but it rarely follows a familial pattern, its onset is later, and the dementia develops only after the illness has been present for at least 5 years. Although familial, Huntington's disease becomes symptomatic, on the average, in the fourth decade. (Alcoholism might be added to a list of causes of dementia that occur in families.)

12. Match the histologic finding in Alzheimer's disease with its description.

1. Paired helical filaments
2. Cluster of degenerating nerve terminals with an amyloid core

3. Group of neurons beneath the globus pallidus
a. Neurofibrillary tangles
b. Neuritic plaque
c. Substantia innominata or nucleus basalis of Meynert

answer: 1-a, 2-b, 3-c

13. What is the most common form of dementia accompanied by a peripheral neuropathy?

answer: Wernicke-Korsakoff syndrome

14. Which is the most common EEG finding in patients with early Alzheimer's disease?

a. Theta and delta activity
b. Periodic complexes
c. High-voltage fast activity
d. Normal or slight slowing of the background activity

answer: d

15. In which conditions is cerebral atrophy found on MRI or CT scans?

a. Alzheimer's disease
b. Down's syndrome
c. Normal aging
d. Normal-pressure hydrocephalus
e. Encephalitis
f. Pseudotumor cerebri
g. AIDS dementia
h. Cerebral toxoplasmosis
i. Wernicke-Korsakoff syndrome

answer: a, b, c, g, i

16. With which condition is cerebral atrophy, as detected by CT or MRI, most closely associated?

a. Alzheimer's disease
b. Intellectual impairment
c. Old age

answer: c

17. What are the implications in Alzheimer's disease of the demonstration by positron emission tomography (PET) and other studies of decreased cerebral glucose metabolism, decreased oxygen consumption, and normal oxygen extraction?

a. Alzheimer's disease results from cellular hypoxia.
b. Oxygen consumption is low because cerebral requirements are low.
c. When cerebral metabolism is lowered, oxygen consumption is secondarily lowered.
d. Giving oxygen to Alzheimer's disease patients will reverse the dementia.

answer: b, c

18. From which area of the brain do the majority of cerebral cortex cholinergic fibers originate?

a. Hippocampus
b. Basal ganglia
c. Frontal lobe
d. Nucleus basalis of Meynert

answer: d

19–22. Choline acetyltransferase (ChAT) is the fundamental enzyme in synthesis of acetylcholine (ACh). What is the effect of the following substances on ACh activity?

a. Increases ACh activity
b. Decreases ACh activity
c. Does not change ACh activity

19. Tacrine

answer: a. Tetrahydroacridine (tacrine [Cognex]) is a centrally acting anticholinesterase.

20.   Scopolamine

answer: b. Scopolamine is a centrally acting anticholinergic medication. Atropine is a similar anticholinergic medication, but in normally used doses it does not cross the blood-brain barrier. However, in high doses, atropine causes a toxic psychosis.

21.   Organic phosphate insecticides

answer: a. Organic phosphate insecticides are generally anticholinesterases that paralyze the neuromuscular junction with an overabundance of ACh.

22.   Physostigmine

answer: a. Physostigmine is a centrally acting anticholinesterase.

23.   Which features of multi-infarct dementia are absent in Alzheimer's disease?

a.   Prominent physical impairments, e.g., hemiparesis, spasticity, dysarthria
b.   History of hypertension and cerebrovascular infarctions
c.   Helpfulness of EEG in diagnosis
d.   A CT or MRI scan showing multiple lucencies or frank strokes
e.   Improvement in symptoms with antihypertensive treatment
f.   Multiple abnormal areas on PET scans

answer: a, b, d, f

24.   Which are frequent features of Wernicke-Korsakoff syndrome?

a.   A CT or MRI scan that is normal or shows atrophy
b.   Confabulation
c.   Hemorrhage in portions of the limbic system
d.   Treatment is thiamine
e.   A global confusional state followed by dementia with predominant amnesia

answer: a, c (The mamillary bodies are part of the limbic system.), d, e

25.   Why do some patients with active neurosyphilis have negative blood VDRL or RPR tests?

a.   Autoimmune diseases often cause false-negative tests.
b.   After years, these tests tend to revert to being negative.
c.   Small doses of antibiotics, given for unrelated reasons, treat syphilis partially but inadequately. The VDRL and RPR tests revert to being negative, but neurosyphilis persists.
d.   Very high antibody levels interfere with standard screening tests.
e.   They may have AIDS.

answer: b, c, d (A positive VDRL should be confirmed before doing a lumbar puncture.), e

26.   Possibly 40 per cent of patients with neurosyphilis have a negative CSF VDRL. How should the clinician evaluate the CSF in patients with dementia where neurosyphilis is suspected?

a.   A lumbar puncture should be performed. If CSF pleocytosis or increased protein concentration is present, treat for neurosyphilis despite a negative CSF VDRL.
b.   Perform a lumbar puncture and treat only if the CSF FTA-ABS test is positive.
c.   Perform a lumbar puncture on all patients with dementia.
d.   Perform a lumbar puncture on all patients with dementia who have a positive blood VDRL or RPR.
e.   Perform a lumbar puncture if there is a history of syphilis that was untreated, physical signs indicate neurosyphilis, or a positive blood VDRL or RPR is confirmed by a more specific test.
f.   In patients with risk factors for AIDS, include HIV testing.

answer: a, e, f. Of the various screening and confirmatory tests, only the VDRL is suitable for testing the CSF. Otherwise the VDRL and RPR are equivalent. AIDS and syphilis are both sexually transmitted diseases and frequently coexist.

27. Of the following, which is the most specific blood test for syphilis?

a. VDRL
b. Microhemagglutination assay (MHA-TP)
c. Wassermann
d. Colloidal gold curve
e. RPR

answer: b. The Wassermann and colloidal gold curve tests are outdated tests for syphilis. The VDRL and RPR tests are reagin tests that are nonspecific and have a relatively high false-positive rate. The MHA-TP and the FTA-ABS are specific for spirochetes. These tests may also be positive in Lyme disease and, less often, in spirochete infections.

28. Which are *not* characteristics of Pick's disease?

a. Relatively preserved visuospatial ability
b. Familial tendency
c. Preserved parietal lobe despite otherwise generalized cerebral atrophy
d. Argentophilic intraneuronal bodies
e. Transmissibility to monkeys
f. Easy clinical identification
g. Occasional frontal lobe personality changes, Klüver-Bucy syndrome, or aphasia
h. A steadily increasing incidence after age 55 years

answer: e, f, h

29. Which of the following conditions are complications of professional boxing?

a. Dementia pugilistica
b. Intracranial hemorrhage
c. Parkinsonism
d. Slowed reaction times
e. Progression of dementia after retirement

answer: a, b, c, d, e

30. Which forms of intellectual deterioration are associated with peripheral neuropathy?

a. Alzheimer's disease
b. Wernicke-Korsakoff syndrome
c. Metachromatic leukodystrophy
d. Uremia
e. Acute intermittent porphyria
f. Nitrous oxide abuse
g. Combined system disease (B_{12} deficiency)
h. Polyarteritis
i. AIDS dementia

answer: b, c, d, e, f, g, h, i (Table 5-2)

31. Which movement disorders are associated with cognitive impairments?

a. Choreoathetosis
b. Parkinson's disease
c. Dystonia musculorum deformans (torsion dystonia)
d. Tourette's syndrome
e. Essential tremor
f. Rigid form of Huntington's disease
g. Wilson's disease
h. Spasmodic torticollis

answer: a (associated with mental retardation in many but not all cases), b (in the middle to late stages), f, g

32. A 65-year-old man was brought to the Emergency Room by his wife who said that he suddenly became "confused" during sexual intercourse. On examination, he was fully alert and attentive but distraught. He was unable to recall recent or prior events, the date, or any of three objects after a three-minute delay. His language was normal. At least grossly, his judgment was intact. The symptoms resolved after two hours. Which of the following conditions is this episode most likely to represent?

a. Hysteria
b. Dementia
c. Nondominant hemisphere ischemia

d. Transient global amnesia
e. Transient ischemic attack (TIA)

answer: d. The patient had a two-hour episode of memory impairment with preservation of consciousness, perception, and judgment. Amnesia is usually caused by temporal lobe dysfunction produced by ischemia, infarction, epilepsy, hemorrhage, or metabolic imbalance. In this case, the problem is *transient global amnesia (TGA)*. TGA is attributable to ischemia of the posterior cerebral arteries, which supply the temporal lobe; however, some neurologists believe that it is a variety of seizure. It is most common in individuals older than 65 years, and it may be precipitated by sexual intercourse, physical stress, or strong emotions. Other neurologic causes of transient amnesia are partial complex seizures, Wernicke-Korsakoff syndrome, and use of certain medications, such as scopolamine.

33–35. Match the following conditions, which produce confabulation, with the location of the underlying brain damage:

a. Right parietal lobe
b. Periventricular gray matter, mamillary bodies
c. Occipital lobes, bilaterally

33. Wernicke-Korsakoff syndrome

answer: b

34. Anton's syndrome

answer: c

35. Nondominant hemisphere syndrome

answer: a

36. Which of the following traits is characteristic of normal 65-year-old individuals?

a. Shorter attention span
b. Slower acquisition of new information
c. Decreased ability to perform new tasks
d. Slight decrease in intelligence, as measured by the WAIS-R
e. Significant loss of vocabulary
f. Impairments in language ability
g. Decreased general information

answer: a, b, c, d

37. A 68-year-old man has the onset of dementia. His blood RPR test is positive at a 1:2 dilution, but no other test indicates a specific cause. Should he be treated for syphilis?

a. Yes, and at doses of penicillin suitable for neurosyphilis
b. No
c. Not until a further blood test, such as the FTA-ABS or MHA-TP, confirms the diagnosis. The reactivity of the RPR at a low dilution may be a biologic false-positive result.
d. Perhaps. If the clinical suspicion is high or if a confirmatory blood test is positive, then examination of the CSF is indicated (see Question 26). Of course, he may require treatment for syphilis that has not involved the nervous system.

answer: c, d

38. Match the histologic finding with the disease:

a. Argentophilic intraneuronal inclusions	1. Creutzfeldt-Jakob
	2. Wilson's
b. Prions	3. Pick's
c. Lewy bodies	4. Diffuse Lewy body
d. Neurofibrillary tangles	5. Parkinson's
e. Spongiform encephalopathy	6. Alzheimer's
f. Kayser-Fleisher rings	

answer: a-3, b-1, c-4 and 5, d-6, e-1, f-2

39. Which is the skin malignancy characteristically associated with AIDS?

a. Lymphoma
b. Herpes simples
c. Kaposi's sarcoma
d. Chancre
e. Herpes zoster

answer: c

40. Which of the following descriptions may be applied to patients in the end stages of Alzheimer's disease?

a. Locked-in syndrome
b. Persistent vegetative state
c. Electrocerebral silence
d. Slow wave sleep

answer: b. The persistent vegetative state results from extensive cerebral cortex damage. The locked-in syndrome results from a massive but incomplete lower brainstem injury, but sometimes from extensive cranial and peripheral nerve dysfunction. Electrocerebral silence is the absence of EEG activity that is found in brain death, barbiturate overdose, or deep anesthesia. Slow-wave sleep is normal stage 3 and 4 NREM sleep.

41. What is the cause of AIDS-dementia complex?

a. HIV encephalitis
b. Toxoplasmosis
c. Cerebral lymphoma
d. Unknown

answer: a, occasionally b

42. What is the most common cause of multiple, discrete cerebral lesions in AIDS patients?

a. Lymphoma
b. Kaposi's sarcoma
c. Cryptococcus
d. Toxoplasmosis
e. Tuberculosis

answer: d. Although toxoplasmosis causes the most common mass lesion, the other conditions also form cerebral mass lesions.

43. Which is the most frequently occurring, nonepidemic form of encephalitis?

a. HIV encephalitis
b. *Herpes simplex* encephalitis
c. *Herpes zoster* encephalitis
d. Meningococcal encephalitis

answer: b. HIV and meningococcus are epidemic infections. Meningococcus causes meningitis much more often then encephalitis. *Herpes zoster* rarely invades the brain or spinal cord. *Herpes simplex* typically invades the temporal lobes and causes partial complex seizures, amnesia, and the Klüver-Bucy syndrome.

44. Which are commonly encountered features of Alzheimer's disease?

a. Lewy bodies
b. Neurofibrillary tangles
c. Amyloid plaques
d. Prions
e. Loss of synapses

answer: b, c, e. Lewy bodies are found in Parkinson's disease and diffuse Lewy body disease. Prions are found in Creutzfeldt-Jakob disease.

45. Which of the following illnesses that cause dementia are associated with suicide?

a. Alzheimer's disease
b. AIDS

c. Huntington's disease
d. Creutzfeldt-Jakob disease

answer: b, c

46. Amnesia in Alzheimer's disease may be most closely associated with deficiency of which of the following substances?

a. Dopamine
b. Scopolamine
c. Somatostatin

d. Acetylcholine
e. Serotonin

answer: d

47. Which group of drivers has the highest car crash rate?

a. Healthy individual older than 65 years
b. Alzheimer's disease patients older than 65 years
c. All licensed drivers
d. Men younger than 25 years

answer: d. Individuals older than 65 years have a car crash higher rate than the average driver. Those with Alzheimer's disease have a greater rate than the same-aged drivers, and their rate increases with the duration of their illness. Factors that explain the increased car crash rate include poor judgment, impaired eye-hand-foot coordination, slowed reaction time, and diminished vision and hearing. Nevertheless, young adult men have an even higher rate. They may lack judgment and experience, but alcohol is clearly a major contributing factor.

48. Of the following, which is the greatest reason that Alzheimer's patients are placed in nursing homes?

a. Dementia
b. Incontinence
c. Hallucinations

d. Sundowning
e. Disruptive behavior

answer: e. Agitation, the interruption of the family's sleep, dangerous activities, wandering, and other disruptive behavior are the most likely precipitants of placement of Alzheimer's patients in a nursing home.

49. Which of the following statements regarding diffuse Lewy body disease are true?

a. It is possibly 15 per cent as common as Alzheimer's disease.
b. The key feature of the histology is the concentration of Lewy bodies in the substantia nigra.
c. By the time patients are 40 years old, they have all the clinical and neuropathologic features of Alzheimer's disease.
d. Lewy bodies are eosinophilic intracytoplasmic inclusions.

answer: a, d. The defining neuropathologic feature of diffuse Lewy body disease is, as its name states, Lewy bodies dispersed throughout the cerebral cortex. In Parkinson's disease, Lewy bodies are confined to the substantia nigra. By the time *Down's syndrome* patients are 40 years old, they have all the clinical and neuropathologic features of Alzheimer's disease.

50. In the search for the cause of Alzheimer's disease, to which chromosome does evidence from studies of amyloid and Down's syndrome point?

a. 14
b. 19

c. 21
d. All of the above

answer: c. Chromosomes 14, 19, and 21 have all been implicated in familial Alzheimer's disease, but a mechanism has not been established. Amyloid precursor protein and trisomy 21 (Down's syndrome) are referable to chromosome 21; however, that chromosome is not related to acetylcholine production.

51. Which of the following are reduced in Alzheimer's disease?

a. Glycine
b. Ceruloplasmin
c. Dopamine
d. Nicotine

e. Acetylcholine
f. Vasopressin
g. Norepinephrine
h. Somatostatin

answer: e, f, g, h

52. A psychiatrist is asked by the orthopedic house staff to evaluate a 55-year-old waiter who was hostile, belligerent, and uncooperative. The behavioral disturbances have occurred on two successive mornings, but have cleared completely by about 9:00 A.M. On her examination, at 2:00 P.M., the psychiatrist finds no significant abnormalities in the patient's mental, neurologic, and psychiatric status. Also, he is recovering uneventfully from hand surgery. Which conditions cause behavioral disturbances in the morning that subside within several hours?

> **answer:** The psychiatrist is faced with the opposite situation of "sundowning," in which patients with dementia become confused in the evening as environmental clues are lost in the dim light. She quite correctly deduced that the primary problem originated in a sleep disturbance, which might include hypnopompic hallucinations, sleeping medication-induced mental aberrations, and sleep rebound after sleep deprivation. Several disorders are prominent in the early morning twilight of sleep, such as seizures and cluster and migraine headaches. However, morning confusion does not indicate dementia.

53. Through which structure is CSF normally absorbed?

a. Cerebral ventricles
b. The brain parenchyma
c. Choroid plexus
d. Arachnoid villi

> **answer:** d. CSF is produced or extruded through the choroid plexus, which resides in the ventricles. It circulates through the ventricles and around the brain and spinal cord. CSF is reabsorbed through the arachnoid villi. Blocked arachnoid villi lead to communicating hydrocephalus.

54. Which of the following are common causes of communicating hydrocephalus?

a. Aqueductal stenosis
b. Chronic meningitis

c. Subarachnoid hemorrhage
d. Glioblastomas

> **answer:** b, c. Aqueductal stenosis causes obstructive hydrocephalus.

55. Which statements are true regarding the gait of the normal elderly?

a. It is characterized by a short stride.
b. Gait impairments are a frequent cause of falls.
c. Orthopedic changes are as important as most neurologic illness.
d. It is characterized by apraxia.

> **answer:** a, b, c

56. Of the following risk factors for falls in the elderly, which occurs the most frequently?

a. Use of sedatives
b. Transient ischemic attacks
c. Neuropathy
d. Normal-pressure hydrocephalus

> **answer:** a. Other risk factors are cognitive impairment, musculosketal changes, and a history of a fall.

57. Which features are typically present in Creutzfeldt-Jakob but not in Alzheimer's disease?

a. Spongiform cerebral cortex
b. Ability to transfer illness to primates by inoculation

   c.   Myoclonus
   d.   Dementia
   e.   EEG changes of burst suppression or periodic changes
   f.   Families with an autosomal dominant pattern of illness
   g.   Survival less than one year
   h.   Pyramidal or cerebellar signs
   i.   Association with trisomy 21
   j.   Association with head trauma
   k.   PrP
   l.   Inflammatory cells, indicative of infection, in brain biopsies

     answer: a, b, c, e, g, h, k

58. Which statement is *false* regarding suicide in AIDS dementia patients?

   a.   Suicide is associated with pain.
   b.   Suicide is associated with depressed mood.
   c.   The suicide rate is at least ten times greater than in control groups.
   d.   High suicide rates are found in no other neurologic illness that causes dementia.

     answer: d

59. What is the incidence of AIDS dementia in HIV positive individuals who are otherwise asymptomatic?

   a.   Less than 1 per cent   c.   About 25 per cent
   b.   About 7 per cent   d.   More than 50 per cent

     answer: a. Virtually nobody who is HIV positive but otherwise asymptomatic has cognitive impairment. AIDS dementia is rarely the first or only manifestation of HIV infection.

60. What is the incidence of dementia in HIV positive individuals at one year after developing AIDS?

   a.   Less than 1 per cent   c.   About 25 per cent
   b.   About 7 per cent   d.   More than 50 per cent

     answer: b

61. Which of the following are risk factors for AIDS dementia in HIV-positive individuals?

   a.   Anemia   c.   Late stages of AIDS
   b.   Weight loss   d.   Older age at onset of AIDS

     answer: a, b, c, d

62. What is the approximate life expectancy for AIDS patients after developing AIDS dementia?

   a.   6 months   c.   2 years
   b.   1 year   d.   Indefinite

     answer: a

63. What is the most common cause of a single discrete cerebral lesion in AIDS patients?

   a.   Cerebral lymphoma   d.   Toxoplasmosis
   b.   Kaposi's sarcoma   e.   Tuberculosis
   c.   Cryptococcal infections

     answer: a. Each of the choices could cause a cerebral lesion, but most would cause multiple lesions.

64. By those who accept the classification, which of the following illnesses would lead to cortical dementia (c) or subcortical dementia (sc)?

a. Pick's disease
b. Parkinson's disease
c. Huntington's disease
d. Normal pressure hydrocephalus
e. Alzheimer's disease
f. AIDS dementia

> *answer:* Pick's disease—c; Parkinson's disease—sc; Huntington's disease—sc; Normal pressure hydrocephalus—sc; Alzheimer's disease—c; AIDS dementia—sc

65. Which of the following statements are true concerning hepatic encephalopathy?

a. Ammonia (NH_3) crosses the blood-brain barrier more easily than ammonium (NH_4+).
b. Substances bind to benzodiazepine-GABA and increase GABA activity.
c. Ammonia (NH_3) is the primary cause of hepatic encephalopathy, and concentrations of NH_3 directly correlate with its severity.
d. Giving benzodiazepine antagonists often briefly reverses the mental aberrations of hepatic encephalopathy.

> *answer:* a, b, d

66. In which patients might brain biopsies reveal intracytoplasmic, eosinophilic inclusion bodies?

a. An 88-year-old person who had encephalitis as a child, with tremor, rigidity, and bradykinesia
b. A 70-year-old person with 1 year of dementia who develops rigidity and bradykinesia
c. A 40-year-old retired boxer with slurred speech, festinating gait, mild dementia, and resting tremor
d. A 30-year-old former intravenous drug abuser who developed tremor, rigidity, and bradykinesia

> *answer:* a, b. Intracytoplasmic, eosinophilic inclusion bodies—Lewy bodies—are found in the substantia nigra in Parkinson's disease, especially if the postencephalitic variety (a). They are also found in diffuse Lewy body disease, which causes dementia and mild parkinsonism (b). However, Lewy bodies are not found in dementia pugilistica (c) or MPTP-induced parkinsonism (d).

8 Aphasia and Related Disorders

Clinicopathologic correlations of aphasia and related disorders have long been studied to deduce how the normal brain functions. Most of these disorders are dramatic when properly demonstrated, and their identification helps localize and diagnose neurologic disease. Even when correlations are uncertain, the entire subject appeals to neurologists' desire to understand linguistics.

LANGUAGE AND DOMINANCE

Impairment in language, *aphasia*, results from damage to the *dominant hemisphere*, which is the cerebral hemisphere that governs language function. The most common cause of aphasia is a cerebrovascular accident (CVA) in the distribution of the left middle cerebral artery (see Chapter 11).

In addition to governing language function, the dominant hemisphere integrates language with intellect, emotion, and sensation (tactile, auditory, and visual). In this manner, the dominant hemisphere provides the primary avenue for the expression of thoughts, emotions, and most cognitive activity.

Language includes not only verbal language (speaking and listening) but also written language (reading and writing), sign language (American Sign Language), and languages based on ideograms, such as certain Asian dialects. All of these languages are impaired by dominant hemisphere lesions. Deficits in reading, for example, are almost always paralleled by comparable deficits in writing (but, see below, Alexia without Agraphia).

However, the dominant hemisphere does not necessarily govern languages that are learned as adults, including second languages, or the use of obscenities, i.e., cursing, which is usually a expression of strong emotions. The nondominant hemisphere probably bestows the mixture of inflection and rhythm that comprises the "tone of voice" or affective component of speech, which is called the *prosody*. Also, although musically gifted people are known to process music, as language, in the dominant hemisphere, the majority of people rely on their nondominant hemisphere for their modest musical skills.

Cerebral hemisphere dominance for normal language is accompanied by the control of fine, rapid hand movements (handedness) and, to a lesser degree, by the reception of vision and hearing. For example, right-handed people who have left cerebral hemisphere dominance not only rely on their right hand for writing and throwing a ball but they also use their right foot for kicking, right eye when peering through a telescope, and right ear for *dichotic listening*—listening to words spoken simultaneously in both ears.

These clinical observations of the dominant hemisphere are corroborated by autopsy and radiologic studies. The superior surface of its temporal lobe—the *planum temporale*—has significantly greater cortex area because it has more gyri and deeper sulci (see Fig. 20–13). This normal cortical asymmetry between the dominant and nondominant temporal lobes is lacking in many patients with autism and chronic schizophrenia—two conditions with prominent language abnormalities. Moreover, the severity of thought disorder in schizophrenia is proportional to a loss of gray matter in the left temporal lobe.

Handedness

About 90 per cent of all people are right-handed and left hemisphere dominant. In addition, the majority of left-handed people are left hemisphere dominant.

Left-handed people may have naturally occurring right hemisphere dominance, or their right hemisphere may have become dominant as a consequence of congenital injury to their left hemisphere (see Chapter 13). Left-handedness is overrepresented among children with dyslexia, other learning disabilities, stuttering, and general clumsiness, as well as among children with overt impairments—mental retardation, epilepsy, and certain major psychiatric disorders, including autism.

Left-handed people are also disproportionately represented among musicians, artists, mathematicians, and athletes. Left-handed athletes tend to be more successful than right-handed ones, at least in sports that involve direct confrontation with active defenses, such as baseball, tennis, fencing, and boxing. (In these sports, left-handed athletes benefit from certain tactical advantages, such as a left-handed batter being closer to first base. Left-handed athletes have no greater success, however, in sports without direct confrontation, such as swimming, running, and pole vaulting.)

Left-handed people, in comparison to right-handed people, become aphasic if either hemisphere is injured, but their prognosis is better. Also, the site of cerebral injury is less clearly related to the variety of aphasia (see below).

A few people are either mixed dominant or ambidextrous. Truly ambidextrous people excel in playing certain sports and performing on musical instruments. They seem to have been endowed with language, music, and motor skill function in both hemispheres.

Although the left hemisphere is dominant in almost all people (and the rest of this chapter assumes it always is), sometimes dominance must be established with certainty. For example, when the temporal lobe must be partially resected because of intractable partial complex epilepsy (see Chapter 10), only a limited resection of the dominant temporal lobe would be permissible to avoid creating aphasia. Cerebral dominance can be established with the *Wada test.* In this test, sodium amobarbital is injected directly into each carotid artery: When the dominant hemisphere is perfused, the patient becomes temporarily aphasic.

APHASIA

Components of the Perisylvian Language Arc

Impulses conveying speech, music, and uncomplicated sound travel from the ears along the acoustic (eighth cranial) nerves into the brainstem. Crossed and uncrossed brainstem tracts bring the impulses to the primary auditory cortex, *Heschl's gyri*, in each temporal lobe (see Fig. 4–15). Most music and some other auditory impulses remain in the nondominant hemisphere. Language impulses are transmitted to *Wernicke's* area, which is in the dominant (L.) temporal lobe. They circle in the *arcuate fasciculus,* back through the temporal and parietal lobes, and then forward to *Broca's area,* which is immediately anterior to the frontal lobe's motor centers for the right arm, face, larynx, and pharynx (Fig. 8–1). Broca's area receives the processed, integrated language and governs the articulation of speech. The horseshoe-shaped cerebral cortex surrounding the sylvian fissure, the *perisylvian language arc*, contains Wernicke's area, the arcuate fasciculus, and Broca's area. This region of the cerebral cortex perceives language, integrates it with other cerebral activities, and articulates its expression. Words live in the perisylvian language arc.

Using the perisylvian language arc model, normal and abnormal language patterns—the aphasias—have been established. For example, when normal people repeat aloud what they hear, impulses go to Wernicke's area, pass around the arcuate fasciculus, and land in Broca's area for speech production (Fig. 8–2A). Also, when people read aloud, impulses are initially received by the visual cortex in both the left and right occipital lobes (see Fig. 4–1). Those impulses from the left visual field are received by the right occipital cortex and must travel through the posterior corpus callosum to reach the left (dominant) cerebral hemisphere. There, the combined impulses from both the left

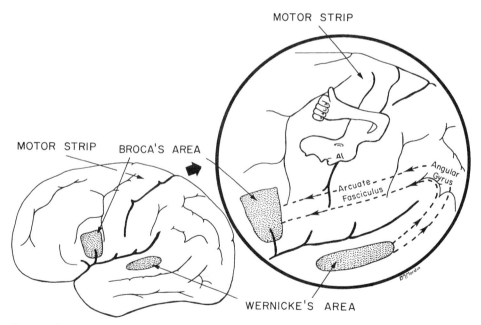

FIGURE 8–1

The left cerebral hemisphere contains *Wernicke's area* in the temporal lobe and *Broca's area* in the frontal lobe, where it is adjacent to the cerebral cortex motor area for the right hand, face, and language. The arcuate fasciculus, the "language superhighway," connects Wernicke's and Broca's areas. It curves rearward from the temporal lobe to the parietal lobe. It then passes through the angular gyrus and forward to the frontal lobe. These structures surrounding the sylvian fissure, which comprise the perisylvian language arc, form the central processing unit of the language system.

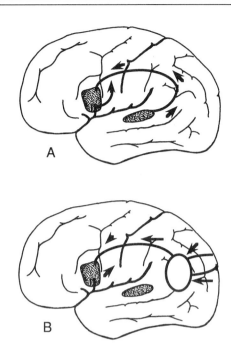

FIGURE 8–2

A, When people *repeat aloud*, language is received in Wernicke's area and transmitted through the parietal lobe by the arcuate fasciculus to Broca's area. This area innervates the adjacent cerebral cortex for the tongue, lips, larynx, and pharynx, as well as for the right face and arm. *B*, When people *read aloud*, visual impulses are received by the left and right occipital visual cortex regions. Both regions send impulses to a left parietal lobe's association region (the oval), which converts text to language. Impulses from the left visual field, which are initially received in the right cortex, must first pass through the posterior corpus callosum to reach the language centers (see Fig. 8–4).

and right visual cortex travel through the arcuate fasciculus to Broca's area for articulation (Fig. 8–2B).

Patients cannot repeat phrases if they have lesions almost anywhere in the perisylvian arc. Conversely, when the arc is isolated from the surrounding cerebral cortex, patients can repeat phrases, but they cannot initiate conversation (see below, Isolation or Transcortical Aphasia).

Several frequently occurring injuries simultaneously strike portions of the perisylvian arc and important neighboring structures to create readily recognizable neurologic deficits that include one or another variety of aphasia. The most common situation, fully predictable from the neuroanatomy, is a left middle cerebral artery occlusion that damages Broca's area and the adjacent motor cortex: This lesion produces dysarthria and right hemiparesis, as well as aphasia. Because lesions have depth—they are not two-dimensional postage stamps—they often include the underlying visual pathway, as well as the perisylvian arc. Thus, aphasia is often accompanied by a right homonymous hemianopsia.

Clinical Evaluation

Before diagnosing aphasia, the clinician must keep in mind normal language variations. Normal people may struggle and stammer when confronted with a novel experience, such as a mental status examination. People have their own style and rhythm. Some may be reticent because they are uneducated, intimidated, or hostile. Some people, before speaking, consider each word and formulate every phrase as though they were carefully considering which apple to eat from a barrel, but others just blurt things impulsively.

In diagnosing aphasia, the clinician can choose from various classifications. One of the most widely used distinguishes *receptive* (*sensory*) from *expressive* (*motor*) aphasia on the basis of the relative impairment of verbal reception or expression; however, this division is not practical because most aphasic patients have mixtures of receptive and expressive impairments. The most clinically useful classification is the *nonfluent* and *fluent* division because it is based on the patient's verbal output (Table 8–1).

Fluent and nonfluent aphasias are usually evident during conversation, history taking, or mental status examination. A standard series of simple verbal tests identify and classify these aphasias. This entire test sequence can be repeated with written requests and responses; however, with almost only one exception (described below), written deficits generally parallel verbal deficits. The standard aphasia tests evaluate *three basic language functions*: comprehension, naming, and repetition (Table 8–2).

- Comprehension is tested by asking the patient to follow simple requests, such as picking up one hand.
- Naming is tested by asking the patient to say his or her own name and that of common objects, such as a pen or key.
- Repetition is tested by asking the patient to recite several short phrases, such as, "The boy went to the store."

Nonfluent Aphasia

Characteristics.   Nonfluent aphasia is characterized by a paucity of speech. Patients are nonverbal. Whatever speech is produced consists almost exclusively of single words and short phrases, with the preferential use of highly meaningful words, such as nouns and verbs. Important modifiers—adjectives, adverbs, and conjunctions—are missing. Many utterances are only stock phrases or bytes, such as, "Get out of here."

TABLE 8–1. SALIENT FEATURES OF MAJOR APHASIAS

Feature	Nonfluent Aphasia	Fluent Aphasia
Previous descriptions	Expressive	Receptive
	Motor	Sensory
	Broca's	Wernicke's
Spontaneous speech	Nonverbal	Verbal
Content	Paucity of words, mostly nouns and verbs	Complete sentences with normal syntax
Articulation	Dysarthric, slow, stuttering	Good
Errors	Telegraphic speech	Paraphasic errors, nonspecific phrases, circumlocutions
Response on testing		
Comprehension	Preserved	Impaired
Repetition	Impaired	Impaired
Naming	Impaired	Impaired
Associated deficits	Right hemiparesis (arm, face > leg)	Hemianopsia, hemisensory loss
Localization of lesion	Frontal lobe	Temporal or parietal lobe Occasionally diffuse

TABLE 8–2.   CLINICAL EVALUATION FOR APHASIA

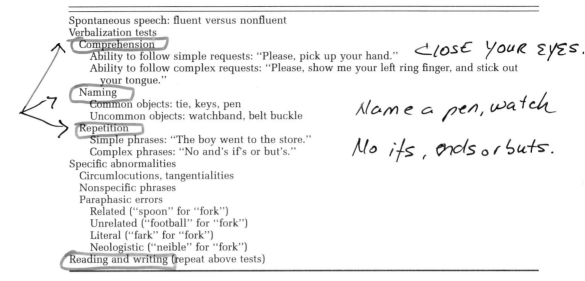

Spontaneous speech: fluent versus nonfluent
Verbalization tests
  Comprehension
    Ability to follow simple requests: "Please, pick up your hand."   *Close Your Eyes.*
    Ability to follow complex requests: "Please, show me your left ring finger, and stick out
      your tongue."
  Naming
    Common objects: tie, keys, pen   *Name a pen, watch*
    Uncommon objects: watchband, belt buckle
  Repetition   *No ifs, ands or buts.*
    Simple phrases: "The boy went to the store."
    Complex phrases: "No and's if's or but's."
  Specific abnormalities
    Circumlocutions, tangentialities
    Nonspecific phrases
    Paraphasic errors
      Related ("spoon" for "fork")
      Unrelated ("football" for "fork")
      Literal ("fark" for "fork")
      Neologistic ("neible" for "fork")
  Reading and writing (repeat above tests)

Nonfluent speech is also slow. The rate is typically less than 50 words per minute, which is much slower than normal (100 to 150 words per minute). Another hallmark is that the flow of speech is so interrupted by excessive pauses that its pattern is termed "telegraphic." For example, in response to a question about food, a patient might stammer "fork . . . steak . . . eat . . . no." A well known example of telegraphic speech might be, "In Paris . . . need money . . ."

Patients with nonfluent aphasia are unable to say either their own name or the names of common objects. They cannot repeat simple phrases. However, they have relatively normal comprehension that can be illustrated by their ability to follow verbal requests, such as "Close your eyes" or "Raise your left hand." Nonfluent aphasia was originally designated "expressive" because of this combination of speech impairment and preserved comprehension.

Localization and Etiology.   The lesions responsible for nonfluent aphasia are located in or near Broca's area (Fig. 8–3A). Their etiology is usually a middle cerebral artery CVA or other discrete structural lesion. Usually extensive, these lesions damage neighboring structures, such as the motor cortex and the posterior sensory cortex. Moreover, because they are spherical or conical, these lesions damage underlying white matter tracts, including the geniculo-calcarine (visual) pathway. Diffuse cerebral injuries, such as metabolic disturbances or Alzheimer's disease, are practically never responsible for them.

Associated Deficits.   Because the responsible lesion usually damages the motor cortex and other adjacent and underlying regions, nonfluent aphasia is characteristically associated with a right hemiparesis, with particular weakness of the arm and lower face, and with poor articulation (dysarthria). Deep lesions typically induce a right homonymous hemianopsia (visual field cut) and hemisensory loss. One of the most common syndromes in neurology is an occlusion of the left middle cerebral artery that produces the combination of nonfluent aphasia and right-sided hemiparesis with the arm much more involved than the leg, visual field cut, and hemisensory impairment. The usual

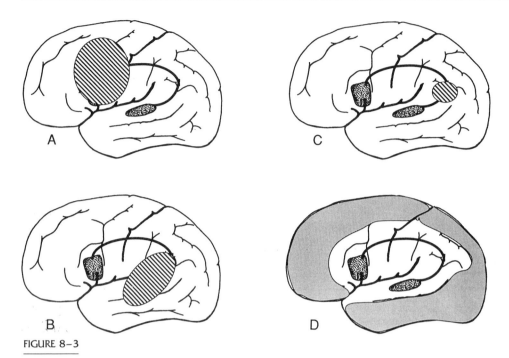

FIGURE 8–3

A, Lesions that cause *nonfluent aphasia* are typically located in the frontal lobe and encompass Broca's area and the adjacent cortex motor strip. *B*, Those causing *fluent aphasia* are in the temporoparietal region, may even be a diffuse injury, such as Alzheimer's disease, and encompass Wernicke's areas and the posterior regions. They usually spare the motor strip. *C*, Those causing *conduction aphasia*, which are relatively small, interrupt the arcuate fasciculus in the parietal or posterior temporal lobe. *D*, Those causing isolation aphasia are circumferential injuries of the watershed region that spare the perisylvian language arc.

localization and frequently occurring motor problems of this variety of aphasia have given rise to similar terms: "Broca's" and "motor" aphasia.

Regarding a related symptom, nonfluent aphasia is associated with *buccofacial apraxia*, which is also called "oral apraxia." This apraxia, like other apraxias, is not paresis, but an inability to execute normal voluntary movements. When buccofacial apraxia is associated with nonfluent aphasia, it impedes patients' facial, lip, and tongue movements. It causes poor articulation and, in severe cases, *aphemia* (mutism) or *abulia* (lack of speech).

To demonstrate buccofacial apraxia, the examiner must ask the patient to say "La . . Pa . . La . . Pa . . La . . Pa," protrude the tongue in different directions, pretend to blow out an imagined match, and pretend to suck through a straw. Patients with buccofacial apraxia will not be able to follow these abstract requests, but yet they can use the same muscles reflexively or when provided with cues. For example, patients who cannot speak might sing, and those who cannot pretend to suck through a straw might be able to drink water through an actual straw.

Nonfluent aphasia is also characteristically associated with depression. Many explanations for this association are possible. Patients with aphasia, which is usually accompanied by marked physical impairments, have suffered a major loss of bodily function and naturally feel sad and hopeless. Also, their awareness of their deficits leaves them perpetually frustrated. Nonfluent aphasia is generally caused by large frontal lobe lesions that alone lead to apathy and abulia (see Frontal Lobe Syndrome, Chapter 8). Signs of depression in aphasic patients, particularly those who have had several CVAs, may actually be manifestations of dementia or pseudobulbar palsy. In fact, although nonfluent aphasia, dementia, pseudobulbar palsy, and depression may mimic each other, all four are manifestations of frontal lobe injury and may, in various combinations, occur together.

Global Aphasia. An extreme form of nonfluent aphasia is *global aphasia*, in which complete dominant hemisphere damage abolishes language function. Aside from uttering some unintelligible sounds and following an occasional gestured request, patients with global aphasia are mute and unresponsive. They have comparably severe physical deficits: right hemiplegia, right homonymous hemianopsia, and conjugate deviation of the eyes toward the left. Frequent causes are internal carotid or middle cerebral artery occlusions, cerebral hemorrhages, and penetrating injuries that obliterate the dominant hemisphere.

Frontal lobe injury =>

1. nonfluent aphasia
2. dementia
3. Pseudobulb. palsy
4. Depress

Fluent Aphasia

Paraphasias and Other Characteristics. Fluent aphasia is characterized by the inability to comprehend language and the incessant use of *paraphasic errors* or *paraphasias*, which are incorrect or even nonsensical words. Paraphasias are included within relatively complete, well-articulated, grammatically correct sentences that are spoken at a normal rate. They can render conversation unintelligible.

Paraphasias include word substitution, such as "clock" for "watch" (a related paraphasia); "glove" for "knife" (an unrelated paraphasia); or "that" for any object (a generic substitution). Words may be altered, such as "breat" for "bread" (a literal paraphasia). Most striking are strings of nonsensical coinages (*neologisms*), such as "I want to fin gunt in the fark," and use of words that rhyme (*clang associations*).

Patients may speak in *circumlocutions*, as though they were trying to avoid dealing with their word-finding difficulty. They may also tend toward *tangential discussions*, as though once the wrong word were chosen, they pursued the idea triggered by their error.

Nevertheless, since nondominant hemisphere functions are not injured, nonverbal expressions are preserved. Patients' prosody is true to their emotions. Also, whether words are adequate or not, emotions are revealed by facial gestures, body movements, and cursing. Most patients are still able to produce a melody even though they may be unable to say the lyrics. For example, patients can hum a tune, such as "Jingle Bells," but if they attempt to sing, their lyrics are strewn with paraphasias.

Associated Deficits. In contrast to nonfluent aphasia, fluent aphasia is not associated with significant hemiparesis because the responsible lesion is distant from the cerebral cortex motor strip (Table 8–1). Only right-sided hyperactive deep tendon reflexes (DTRs) and a Babinski sign may be elicited. A right-sided sensory impairment and visual field cut may be present, however, because of interruptions of the sensory and visual cerebral pathways.

More striking, patients are strangely unaware of their paraphasias, unable to edit them, and oblivious to their listener's consternation. At the same time, patients develop anxiety, agitation, or even paranoia. Clinicians not seeing any hemiparesis and unable to capture the patient's attention for detailed testing often do not appreciate the neurologic basis of the language, thought, or behavioral abnormalities. For many psychiatric consultations, the sudden onset of fluent aphasia often turns out to be the explanation for an "acute psychosis," marked change in behavior, or management problem in a patient on a medical service.

Localization and Etiology. Usually discrete structural lesions, such as small CVAs, in the temporoparietal region cause fluent aphasia (Fig. 8–3B). They do not necessarily damage Wernicke's area, the arcuate fasciculus, or the sensory cortex, but fluent aphasia is often termed "Wernicke's" or "sensory" aphasia. Unlike nonfluent aphasia, fluent aphasia is sometimes caused by diffuse cerebral injury, including Alzheimer's disease.

Varieties of Fluent Aphasia. Varieties of fluent aphasia tend to be subtle, and their diagnosis turns on fine points. Moreover, their clinical-pathologic correlations are subject to great individual variations in anatomy, language production, and the presence of dementia.

A common variety of fluent aphasia is *anomic aphasia* or *anomia*, which is simply an inability to name objects. Anomia is often produced by a small CVA, but it can be a symptom of Alzheimer's disease.

Another variety, *transcortical aphasia* or *isolation aphasia*, results from isolation of the perisylvian arc because the surrounding cerebral cortex is damaged. Often the entire cerebral cortex, except for the perisylvian arc, is devastated, and patients have overwhelming dementia. Precisely because the language system remains intact, patients with isolation aphasia can characteristically repeat whatever they hear. In contrast, they cannot participate in a conversation, follow requests, or name objects because the language system cannot communicate with the rest of the cerebral cortex. Depending on the injury, patients may have a right hemiparesis or a tendency toward decorticate posture. The salient feature of isolation aphasia is a remarkable disparity between patients seeming to be mute, yet repeating long and complex sentences. They actually repeat readily, involuntarily, and apparently compulsively. Their parrot-like echoing of visitor's words is called *echolalia*. A cursory examination could understandably confuse their speech with irrational jargon.

The perisylvian arc cerebral cortex is well perfused by major branches of large cerebral arteries. In contrast, the surrounding cerebral cortex is a large border zone between the middle, anterior, and posterior cerebral arteries (the *watershed area*) that is tenuously perfused by thin, fragile vessels. Isolation aphasia is usually caused by a *watershed infarction*, which occurs when the cerebral cortex "at the end of the line" sustains a widespread infarction (Fig. 8–3D). Thus, isolation aphasia is usually the result of a cardiac or respiratory arrest, other hypotensive or hypoxic episodes, or showers of small emboli (see Chapter 11). It is also found among several neurologic deficits caused by suicide attempts with carbon monoxide (CO) poisoning. (CO has a predilection for damaging the globus pallidus, cerebellum, and hippocampus, as well as the cerebral cortex.) Occasionally, Alzheimer's disease causes isolation aphasia.

If varieties of aphasia are understood as damage to Broca's area, Wernicke's area, and the surrounding cerebral cortex, the clinician could predict a variety of aphasia that results from arcuate fasciculus damage. In *conduction aphasia*, a small, discrete arcuate fasciculus lesion, usually in the parietal or posterior temporal lobe (Fig. 8–3C), interrupts or *disconnects* Wernicke's and Broca's areas. (Given that both major centers are preserved but separated, conduction aphasia may be seen as one of the disconnection syndromes [see below].) Patients with conduction aphasia are fluent and have good comprehension, but they cannot repeat phrases or short sentences. They are particularly maladept at repeating strings of syllables. Their clinical deficit is the opposite of isolation aphasia.

The most frequent cause of conduction aphasia is a small, embolic CVA in the posterior temporal branch of the left middle cerebral artery, but other CVAs and structural lesions may be responsible. The responsible lesions are so small that they cause little or no physical deficits. At most, patients have right lower facial weakness.

Language TESTS:
- *comprehens.*
- *naming*
- *repetition.*

MENTAL ABNORMALITIES WITH LANGUAGE IMPAIRMENTS

Dementia and Aphasia

DSM #.

Aphasia may mimic dementia because it can impair such common tasks as saying the date and place, repeating a series of numbers, and following requests. Aphasia also clouds thinking and memory because these crucial cognitive functions are heavily dependent on language and communication.

Nevertheless, aphasia has several distinguishing features. It usually begins suddenly. Its major varieties—fluent and nonfluent—cause difficulty with one or more of the three standard language function tests: comprehension, naming, and repeating. Nonfluent aphasia, the more common variety, is usually readily recognizable because it is accompanied by dysarthria and obvious lateralized signs: right-sided hemiparesis and visual field cut. Fluent aphasia, although less common, is readily identifiable by characteristic paraphasias.

Dementia
aphasia
apraxia
agnosia

On the other hand, patients with dementia in its early stages may have anomia while being fully verbal, articulate, and able to perform reasonably well on the standard language function tests. Patients with severe dementia have a paucity of speech and a limited vocabulary, i.e., they are nonverbal. When these patients do speak, they tend to perseverate.

Occasionally, patients have both aphasia and dementia. This combination occurs with multiple infarctions or Alzheimer's disease and a superimposed CVA. These situations are notoriously difficult to clarify because aphasia invalidates many tests of intellectual function.

Distinguishing aphasia from dementia and recognizing when they coexist are more than academic exercises. A diagnosis of aphasia almost always suggests that a patient has had a discrete dominant cerebral hemisphere injury. Since a CVA or other structural lesion would be the most likely cause, the appropriate evaluation would include a CT or MRI scan (see Chapter 20). In contrast, a diagnosis of dementia suggests that the most likely cause would be Alzheimer's disease or another diffuse process, and the evaluation might include an electroencephalogram (EEG), lumbar puncture, and various blood tests, as well as a scan.

(Left).

Schizophrenia and Aphasia

#.

Although the distinction between aphasia and dementia may be difficult, the one between fluent aphasia and schizophrenic speech can be even more troublesome. These two conditions share circumlocutions, tangentialities, neologisms, and a reduced meaning of their words. As the thought disorder of schizophrenia becomes more pronounced, its language abnormalities increase in frequency and similarity to aphasia. Likewise, the sudden onset of aphasia can be so frightening and bewildering that patients become irrational, agitated, and paranoid.

Despite these similarities, many differences can be discerned. Schizophrenic speech usually develops gradually in patients who are relatively young (in their third decade) and have had long-standing illness. Their neologisms and other paraphasias are relatively infrequent and inconspicuous. Schizophrenic patients, unlike most fluent aphasia patients, can repeat multisyllabic words and complex phrases, such as "Methodist Episcopal Church."

People who develop aphasia usually do so suddenly when in their seventh or eighth decade. Except for some with fluent aphasia, aphasic patients are aware that they cannot communicate. They often request help in this regard and, possibly because of self-monitoring, keep their responses short and pointed. Although lateralized findings are often undetected because they are subtle or the patient's excitement or confusion precludes a neurologic examination, right-sided hemiparesis indicates aphasia.

Other Disorders

Language abnormalities are a prominent aspect of *childhood autism*. Autistic children begin to speak later than normal and often remain mute until they do. Their grammar is poor, incorrect pronouns are assigned (pronoun reversal), and echolalia is common. Also, they have limited prosody and generally do not use meaningful gestures. On the other hand, autistic children do not display cardinal features of aphasia: paraphasias, anomias, and impaired comprehension.

Mutism and apparent language abnormalities can also be associated with psychogenic disturbances. In these situations, the language impairment is usually inconsistent and amenable to suggestion. For example, if requested, a patient might communicate in writing and thereby reveal intact language function. If this does not work, an amobarbital interview might be appropriate.

A common aphasia-like psychogenic condition is difficulty in word finding or name recalling. It is sometimes explained by psychodynamic processes, such as "blocking." The classic example is the Freudian slip. (Freud himself was an expert on aphasia and its neurologic substrate.) Examples found in everyday conversation can be termed either paraphasias or insights into the unconscious. When a physician's former secretary is being evaluated for a neurologic disorder and says that she has been Dr. So-and-So's "medical cemetery," a clinician could interpret the comment as her feelings about the competence of the doctor, an indication of the patient's own fears of death, a sign of a dominant hemisphere lesion, or a transient anomic aphasia.

DISORDERS RELATED TO APHASIA

Alexia and Agraphia

Alexia is an inability to read, and *agraphia is* an inability to write. Both are almost always found together as part of aphasia.

The important although rare exception is *alexia without agraphia*. In this condition, patients who have little or no impairment in comprehending speech or expressing themselves by writing cannot read. For example, though they are unable to read anything, even their own writing, patients can transcribe dictation and write their thoughts. Alexia without agraphia, which should really be called "alexia with graphia," results from a destructive lesion encompassing the dominant (left) occipital lobe and adjacent posterior corpus callosum (Figs. 8–4 and 20–10B). Aside from the right homonymous hemianopsia, patients have no physical deficits.

Gerstmann's Syndrome

Agraphia may also occur in *Gerstmann's syndrome*. In this condition, which has been attributed to lesions in the *angular gyrus* of the dominant parietal lobe (Fig. 8–1), agraphia is accompanied by three other abnormalities: *acalculia* (impairment of arithmetic skills), *finger agnosia* (inability to identify fingers), and *left/right confusion*.

The status of Gerstmann's syndrome as a distinct clinical entity has been questioned because patients rarely display all four components, and those patients with many components usually also have aphasia or dementia. Nevertheless, the constellation of Gerstmann's signs, even if they do not constitute a syndrome, is useful. The signs may be sought in adults with CVAs. In evaluating children for learning disabilities, those with dyscalculia frequently also have poor handwriting (agraphia) and left/right confusion accompanied by physical signs of dominant hemisphere injury, such as right-sided hyperactive DTRs and a Babinski sign (see Chapter 13).

Agnosia and Anomia

Another disturbance referable to dominant hemisphere injury is *agnosia.* This is a perceptual disorder in which patients cannot recognize objects despite intact sensory systems, intellectual capabilities, and language function. For example, if a man with agnosia were shown a stop sign, he could name it and describe it, but he would be unable to explain its meaning. Agnosia should not be confused with either dementia or aphasia—other conditions in which patients might not be able to say the names of objects, but can recognize them.

Another perceptual disorder, *prosopagnosia,* is the inability to identify familiar faces, such as those of historical figures or family members. It is often found with an inability to identify objects out of their usual (visual) context, such as a shirt pocket cut from a shirt. Prosopagnosia is frequently the result

FIGURE 8–4

Alexia without agraphia is caused by lesions that damage the left occipital lobe and the posterior corpus callosum. Patients are unable to see anything in their right visual field because of the left occipital cortex damage. Left visual images still reach the right cortex, but they cannot be transmitted to the left cerebral language centers because the critical posterior corpus callosum is damaged. Thus, patients cannot comprehend written material presented to either visual field. In contrast, they can still write full sentences from memory, imagination, or dictation because these forms of information still reach the language centers. (See Fig. 20–10B for the corresponding CT scan.)

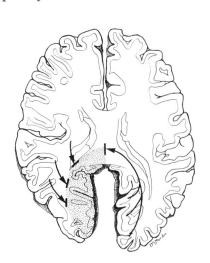

of bilateral occipitotemporal lesions. In contrast, identification of unknown faces, which probably relies more on spatial concepts than simple memory, is primarily a function of the nondominant hemisphere.

Color agnosia or *anomia* is the inability to identify color that is not a manifestation of color blindness, dementia, or aphasia. It is attributed to damage to the dominant occipitotemporal region. Patients with color agnosia are unable to name the colors of painted cards or other objects; however, in striking contrast, they are able to match cards of the same color and also recite from memory the colors of common objects, such as the sky (see Agnosia, Chapter 12).

Apraxia

Apraxia, which is roughly the motor system's equivalent of nonfluent aphasia, is the inability to execute learned actions despite normal strength, sensation, coordination, and, more important, comprehension. This disorder is attributed to the disruption of motor areas and the disconnection of motor centers from each other and from language centers.

In demonstrating apraxia, in general the examiner first tests the patient's buccofacial (lips, face, and tongue) and limb movements in making gestures or "symbolic acts." Then the examiner asks the patient to perform actions that are imagined and real (Table 8–3). The object in the "imagined" sequence is pretend, but the one in the "real" sequence is the actual object. When given the object, patients with apraxia can often perform the action because of the cue. Similarly, after seeing the examiner perform an action, they can copy it. Depending on circumstances, further testing includes performing a series of steps, copying figures, arranging match-sticks, walking, or dressing.

Although apraxia can be easily differentiated from simple paresis, it is often inseparably associated with aphasia or dementia. Also, patients are typically unaware that they have apraxia. After all, patients usually do not spontaneously attempt the various tests for apraxia, such as saluting unseen officers or using an imaginary screwdriver. Moreover, an unsophisticated staff might naturally assign motor impairments to paresis or incoordination.

Despite the complexity of the situation, several clinically useful apraxias have been described. *Ideomotor apraxia*, the most frequently occurring, is basically the impairment of converting an idea into an action. It can be pictured as a disconnection of cognitive or language regions from motor regions (Fig. 8–5). The underlying lesion is usually a left-sided frontal or parietal lobe infarction.

One of its two varieties, *buccofacial apraxia*, was discussed as a feature of nonfluent aphasia. In the other variety, *limb apraxia*, patients are not able to execute simple requests involving their arms or legs. They cannot salute or

TABLE 8–3. TESTING FOR APRAXIA			
		Action	
	Gesture[a]	Imagined	Real
Buccofacial	Kiss the air	Pretend to blow out a match	Blow out a match
	Repeat "Pa"	Suck on a straw	Drink water through a straw
Limb	Salute	Pretend to use a comb	Comb the hair
	Stop traffic	Pretend to write	Write with a pencil or pen

[a]Symbolic acts.

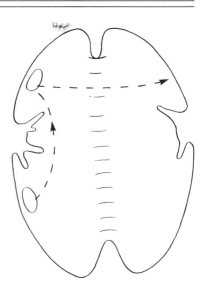

FIGURE 8–5

In a schematic transaxial view, requests for *normal movements* are received by Wernicke's area in the dominant (left) posterior temporal lobe. They are transmitted anteriorly to the motor regions and, through the anterior corpus callosum, to the contra-lateral motor strip. Interruptions of the path within the left cerebral hemisphere result in ideomotor apraxia of both arms, causing bilateral limb apraxia. Lesions in the anterior corpus callosum interrupt only those impulses destined to control the left arm and leg, which causes unilateral, left arm and leg ideomotor apraxia.

move their hands in certain abstract patterns. They cannot pretend to brush their teeth, turn a key, comb their hair, or kick a ball. When asked to pretend to *use* an object, these patients characteristically use their hands as though they *were* the actual objects. For example, they will brush their teeth with their forefingers instead of pretending to hold a toothbrush. Both varieties are associated with aphasia.   *w/Dementia.*

In *ideational apraxia*, patients cannot perform motor activities that require several sequential steps. For example, patients cannot pretend to take an imag- *eg:* inary pack of cigarettes, remove a cigarette, and then light it. Similarly, they cannot pretend to fold a letter, place it into an envelope, and then affix a stamp. Ideational apraxia is usually found in either frontal lobe injuries or diffuse cerebral disease. Whereas ideomotor apraxia is associated with nonfluent aphasia, ideational apraxia is almost inseparable from dementia. In particular, ideational apraxia is often a manifestation of Alzheimer's disease and multiple infarctions because the dementia they induce causes trouble with organization, planning, and thinking conceptually. Thus, it is sometimes called "conceptual apraxia."

Several other apraxias are not referable to dominant hemisphere or diffuse lesions and are covered in more detail elsewhere. *Construction apraxia* is associated with nondominant parietal lobe lesions (see below and Chapter 2). *Dressing apraxia* is usually manifested by an inability to clothe the left limbs and is also associated with nondominant hemisphere lesions (see below). A different but better-known condition is *gait apraxia* (see Fig. 7–7), which is a hallmark of normal pressure hydrocephalus.

NONDOMINANT HEMISPHERE SYMPTOMS

Hemi-Inattention

Although aphasia, agraphia, and apraxia are attributable to dominant hemisphere injury, several important and potentially dramatic neuropsychologic disturbances are attributable to nondominant hemisphere injury. These disturbances require considerable clinical acumen to detect because they tend to be short lived, subtle, and dependent on the patient's premorbid intelligence, personality, and defense mechanisms.

Hemi-inattention (*hemispatial neglect*) is the most prominent manifestation of nondominant hemisphere injury. It gives rise to related disorders and behavioral disturbances. Hemi-inattention usually originates in a CVA of the nondominant parietal lobe cortex and its underlying thalamus and reticular activating system, which are responsible for sensory perception, arousal, and attention.

Patients with hemi-inattention ignore visual, tactile, and other sensory stimuli that originate from their left side. They disregard, fail to perceive, or misinterpret objects in their left visual field, even though the examiner may suggest that important things reside there (Fig. 8–6). Also, when both sides of their body are touched, patients neglect the left-sided stimulation (*extinction on double simultaneous stimulation* [*DSS*]) and report that only their right side was touched. Sometimes patients even fail to shave the left side of their face and leave their left side undressed. Their failure to dress completely, however, does not constitute *dressing apraxia*, which is the inability to dress, especially if clothing is presented inside-out. For example, patients with dressing apraxia put both hands into one sleeve or persistently misalign the buttons on a shirt.

An extreme form of hemi-inattention is the alien hand syndrome. In this disorder, which typically follows a nondominant hemisphere CVA, a patient's left hand retains some rudimentary motor and sensory functions, but they can-

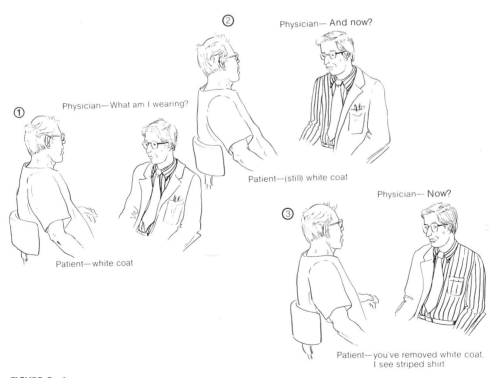

FIGURE 8–6

In a classic demonstration of left *hemi-inattention*, the patient, neglecting left-sided stimulation, perceives only what the examiner is wearing in his right visual field. Even if the patient's problem were simply a left homonymous hemianopsia, he still would have explored and discovered, with his intact right visual field, that the examiner was half-dressed.

not be appreciated by the rest of the patient's brain. Without the patient's awareness, the hand moves semipurposefully, makes its own explorations, and performs simple tasks, such as scratching and moving bedclothes. In a unique, often quoted example, a patient reported that her hand was attempting to choke her.

The alien hand syndrome rests on the patient having at least two misperceptions: (1) the patient does not possess the hand and (2) the hand's movements are independent or governed by another person (the alien). Most patients feel divorced from the hand or, at most, express a tenuous attachment to it. As for the dominant hand, sometimes it is affected by a frontal lobe injury. Several cases have been attributed to corpus callosum injury, suggesting that the alien hand syndrome is another disconnection syndrome.

Anosognosia, which is the inability to accept a physical deficit (usually a left hemiparesis), is an aspect of hemi-inattention. Patients typically cannot identify the affected part of their body (*somatotopagnosia* or *autotopagnosia*). They occasionally claim the examiner's hand and deny ownership of the paretic hand. Sometimes they attribute the weakened hand to a third person. Whatever their defense mechanism, patients fail to use the hand, which usually lies motionless.

Patients with anosognosia often refuse to accept physical therapy and other hospital routines. Some become belligerent. Patients with left hemiparesis, especially those with behavioral problems, should be evaluated for anosognosia. They should also be evaluated for depression because it can coexist with anosognosia.

Denial and confabulation, of course, are not restricted to nondominant hemisphere injury. Both are prominent signs in suddenly occurring cortical blindness (see Anton's syndrome, Chapter 12), and confabulation is found in Wernicke-Korsakoff syndrome (see Chapter 7).

Another manifestation of nondominant hemisphere injury is constructional apraxia. This disorder is characterized by *visual-spatial* perceptual impairments, in which patients are unable to organize visual information or integrate it with fine motor skills. The standard tests show that patients cannot copy simple figures or arrange match-sticks in patterns (Fig. 8–7). Constructional apraxia, however, cannot always be ascribed to a nondominant lesion. It can also be found in patients with diffuse cerebral dysfunction and those with left hemisphere damage.

Aprosody

Prosody, as mentioned previously, is the emotional or affective qualities of speech. The inability to appreciate or endow speech with these qualities is *aprosody*.

Nondominant hemisphere lesions, which cause aprosody, interfere with the ability of patients to discern emotions from others' tone of voice. For example, a patient with aprosody would be unable to appreciate the contrasting feelings in the question, "Are you going home?" asked first by a jealous hospital roommate and then by a gleeful spouse. Unable to express emotionally charged sentences, patients speak without inflection or style. They are unable to sing a song, although they can repeat the lyrics, because they cannot convey its melody.

Aprosody tends to be accompanied by the loss of nonverbal communication, popularly recognized as "body language" or technically as *paralinguistic com-*

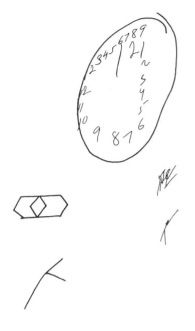

FIGURE 8–7

When asked to draw a clock, a patient with *constructional apraxia* drew an incomplete circle, repeated (perseverated) the numerals, and placed them asymmetrically. When attempting to copy the figure on the upper left, the patient repeated several lines, failing to draw any figure. The patient also misplaced and rotated the position of the lower left figure (also see Fig. 2–8).

ponents of speech, such as facial expression and limb gesture. These physical aspects of communication are similar to prosody: They lend conviction, emphasis, and affect to spoken words. Indeed, gestures seem independent and sometimes more credible than speech. Well-known examples are children crossing their fingers when promising, adults who wink while telling a joke, and people who smile while relating sad events.

To assess prosody, the examiner recreates a short version of the aphasia examination. During spontaneous speech, the examiner notes the patient's variations in volume, pitch, and emphasis. The patient is requested to ask a question, such as "May I have the ball?" in the manner of a friend and then a stern schoolteacher. The question should be asked with appropriate vocal and facial expressions. The examiner then asks a similar question, impersonating the same characters while the patient tries to identify them. An alternative but less demanding test is to ask the patient to describe pictures of people displaying extreme emotions.

Extending the concept that the nondominant hemisphere confers affect on language, several authors have suggested that the nondominant hemisphere is responsible for perception and expression of emotion, complex nonverbal processes, and a holistic approach. The dominant hemisphere, they suggest, is responsible for verbal, sequential, analytic cognitive processes, and reflection.

DISCONNECTION SYNDROMES

Virtually all human endeavors require communication pathways between several areas located within one cerebral hemisphere and often between both hemispheres. The arcuate fasciculus, for example, provides intracerebral communication. Intercerebral communication is provided by other myelin-coated axonal (white matter) bundles, *commissures*, of which the most conspicuous is the *corpus callosum*. Other intercerebral connections are the massa intermedia and the anterior, posterior, and hippocampal commissures.

Injuries that damage these pathways but spare the actual neurologic centers cause *disconnection syndromes*. Each is uncommon, but permits examination of the particular neurologic function. The existence of several was predicted before actually being demonstrated, much as certain subatomic particles were predicted and then proved to exist. Disconnection syndromes that have already been discussed are (1) alexia without agraphia, (2) conduction aphasia, and (3) ideomotor apraxias with its varieties, buccofacial and limb apraxia. Although the medial longitudinal fasciculus syndrome (MLF) or intranuclear ophthalmoplegia (INO) (see Chapters 4, 12, and 15) is strictly a brainstem disorder, it shares many disconnection syndrome characteristics.

Most disconnection syndromes result from corpus callosum damage. In addition to alexia without agraphia and some of the apraxias, the *anterior cerebral artery syndrome* is a good example. In this disorder, a CVA of the anterior cerebral arteries leads to an infarction of both frontal lobes and the anterior corpus callosum. It obstructs information passing between the left hemisphere language centers and the right hemisphere motor centers. Although the patient's left arm and leg will have normal spontaneous movement, these limbs will not respond to an examiner's verbal or written requests, i.e., the patient will have unilateral (left-sided) limb apraxia (Fig. 8–5).

In several corpus callosum disorders, disconnection signs may be present, but they are subtle and variable. The corpus callosum occasionally fails to develop in utero (*congenital absence*), and sometimes it is damaged by excessive consumption of red wine (*Marchiafava-Bignami syndrome*).

Split Brain

The most important disconnection syndrome, which also involves the corpus callosum, is the *split brain syndrome*. This disorder usually results from a longitudinal surgical division of the corpus callosum (commissurotomy) for control of intractable epilepsy (see Chapter 10). After a commissurotomy, each cerebral hemisphere is virtually isolated. Examiners may present certain information to only one hemisphere. For example, pictures, writing, and other visual information shown within one visual field will present information to only the contralateral hemisphere (Fig. 8–8). Likewise, tactile information can be presented to only one hemisphere by having a blindfolded patient touch objects with the contralateral hand. However, since auditory pathways are duplicated in the brainstem (see Fig. 4–15), sounds detected in one ear are ultimately received to a certain extent by both hemispheres.

In testing a patient's left cerebral hemisphere function, the examiner writes questions in patients' right visual field and places objects in their right hand. Patients respond correctly by speaking and writing with their right hand. To written requests for right arm and leg movements, patients respond correctly; however, left limbs are unable to follow the same requests because the left hemisphere cannot let the right hemisphere know what to do, i.e., the patient has left limb apraxia (Figs. 8–5 and 8–8).

In testing right hemisphere function, visual information is shown in patients' left visual field. Since impulses cannot travel to the language centers, patients cannot read, respond to written requests, or name objects. Nevertheless, they are able to use their left hand to copy figures and—more striking—solve mathematical problems, discriminate patterns, recognize faces, and perceive emotions.

Requests Shown In
Left Visual Field

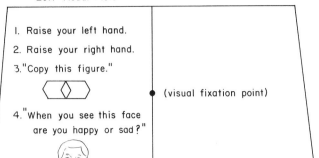

1. Raise your left hand.
2. Raise your right hand.
3. "Copy this figure."

4. "When you see this face
   are you happy or sad?"

(visual fixation point)

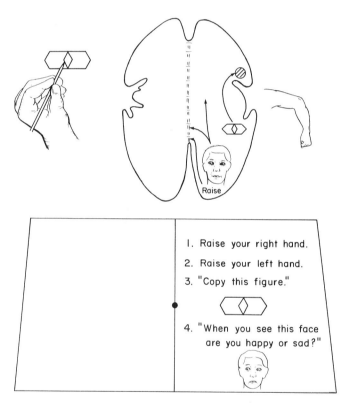

1. Raise your right hand.
2. Raise your left hand.
3. "Copy this figure."

4. "When you see this face
   are you happy or sad?"

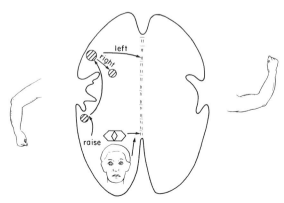

FIGURE 8–8

After a *commissurotomy*, patients often have the *split brain syndrome*. Each hemisphere can be tested individually by showing requests, objects, and pictures in the contralateral visual field. *A,* Objects and written requests shown in the left visual field are perceived by the right visual field. Since connections to the ipsilateral motor area are intact, the *left* hand can copy figures. However, since the right hemisphere is unable to transmit information through the corpus callosum to the left cerebral hemisphere, patients cannot read the requests or describe the objects. Although patients cannot speak of the feelings evoked by emotionally laden pictures shown in their left visual field, they have sympathetic, nonverbal responses. *B,* Written requests and objects shown in the right visual field are perceived by the left hemisphere. Patients can read those written requests, copy those objects with the right hand, and comply with the requests; however, since the language areas cannot send information through the corpus callosum, the left hand cannot comply. Patients can describe the emotions in a picture, but their language lacks affect.

Not only can each hemisphere detect visual, tactile, and auditory sensations, but each might perceive emotions that are different. For example, a picture that evokes humor can be shown in one visual field and simultaneously one that evokes sadness shown in the other. Moreover, each hemisphere can reason independently—by nonverbal, if not verbal, processes. However, some right hemisphere information, experience, emotion, and knowledge does not reach patients' consciousness at least to the point of verbal expression because right hemisphere functions cannot be shared with the left's language centers.

Split brain studies have suggested that normal people may have, in their two hemispheres, mental systems that are parallel, nonverbal, and operating simultaneously. Although the systems usually complement each other, they might occasionally come into conflict.

REFERENCES

Absher JR, Benson DF: Disconnection syndromes: An overview of Geschwind's contributions. Neurology *43*: 862–867, 1993

Alexander MP, Baker E, Naeser MA, et al: Neuropsychological and neuroanatomical dimensions of ideomotor apraxia. Brain *115*: 87–107, 1992

Basso A, Scarpa MT: Traumatic aphasia in children and adults: A comparison of clinical features and evolution. Cortex *26*: 501–514, 1990

Basso A, Farabola M, Grassi MP, et al: Aphasia in left-handers. Comparison of aphasia profiles and language recovery in non-right-handed and matched right-handed patients. Brain Lang *38*: 233–252, 1990

Benton AL: Gerstmann's syndrome. Arch Neurol *49*: 445–447, 1992

Critchley M, Henson RA (eds): Music and the Brain: Studies in the Neurology of Music. London, William Heinemann Medical Books Ltd, 1977

Damasio AR: Aphasia. N Engl J Med *326*: 531–539, 1992

Faber R, Abrams R, Taylor MA, et al: Comparison of schizophrenic patients with formal thought disorder and neurologically impaired patients with aphasia. Am J Psychiatry *140*: 1348–1351, 1983

Feinberg TE, Schindler RJ, Flanagan NG, et al: Two alien hand syndromes. Neurology *42*: 19–24, 1992

Heilman KM, Valenstein E (eds): Clinical Neuropsychology (3rd ed). New York, Oxford University Press, 1993

Hemenway D: Bimanual dexterity in baseball players. N Engl J Med *309*: 1587, 1983

Homan RW, Criswell E, Wada JA, et al: Hemispheric contributions to manual communication (signing and finger-spelling). Neurology *32*: 1020–1023, 1982

Klein SK, Masur D, Farber K, et al: Fluent aphasia in children: Definition and natural history. J Chid Neurol *7*: 50–59, 1992

Levine DN, Calvanio R, Rinn WE: The pathogenesis of anosognosia for hemiplegia. Neurology *41*: 1770–1781, 1991

Loonen MCB, Dongen HR: Acquired childhood aphasia: Outcome 1 year after onset. Arch Neurol *47*: 1324–1328, 1990

Mastronardi L, Ferrante L, Celli P, et al: Aphasia in polyglots. Neurosurgery *29*: 621–623, 1991

McGuire PK, Shah GMS, Murray RM: Increased blood flow in Broca's area dusing auditory hallucinations in schizophrenia. Lancet *342*: 703–706, 1993

Motley MT: Slips of the tongue. Sci Am *253*: 116–125, 1985

Portal JM, Romano PE: Patterns of eye-hand dominance in baseball players. N Engl J Med *319*: 655, 1988

Shenton ME, Kikinis R, Jolesz FA, et al: Abnormalities of the left temporal lobe and thought disorder in schizophrenia. N Engl J Med *327*: 604–612, 1992

Starkstein SE, Berthier ML, Fedoroff P, et al: Anosognosia and major depression in 2 patients with cerebrovascular lesions. Neurology *40*: 1380–1382, 1990

Starkstein SE, Federoff JP, Price TR, et al: Neuropsychological and neuroradiologic correlates of emotional prosody comprehension. Neurology *44*: 515–522, 1994

Therapeutics and Technology Subcommittee of the American Academy of Neurology: Melodic intonation therapy. Neurology *44*: 566–568, 1994

Tupper DE, Cicerone KD (eds): The Neuropsychology of Everyday Life. Norwell, MA, Kluwer Academic Publishers, 1991

Weinstein EA, Friedland RP (eds): Advances in Neurology: Hemi-Inattention and Hemisphere Specialization. New York, Raven Press, 1977

QUESTIONS and ANSWERS: CHAPTER 8

1-5.   Formulate the following cases:

Case 1

A 68-year-old man suddenly develops right hemiparesis. He only utters "Oh, Oh!" when stimulated. He makes no response to questions or requests. His right lower face is paretic, and the right arm and leg are flaccid and immobile. He is inattentive to objects in his right visual field.

Case 2

A 70-year-old man, since suffering a CVA the previous year, can only say "weak, arm," "go away," and "give . . . supper me." His speech is slurred. He can raise his left arm, protrude his tongue, and close his eyes. He can name several objects, but he cannot repeat phrases. His right arm is paretic, but he can walk.

Case 3

Over a period of 6 weeks, a previously healthy 64-year-old woman has developed headaches, progressively severe difficulty in finding words, and apparent confusion. She speaks continuously and incoherently: "Go to the warb," "I can't hear," "My heat hurts." She is unable to follow commands, name objects, or repeat phrases. On examination, there is pronation of the outstretched right arm, a right Babinski sign, and papilledema. Visual fields cannot be tested.

Case 4

A 34-year-old man with mitral stenosis has the sudden onset of aphasia after a transient left-sided headache. Although articulate and able to follow requests and repeat phrases, *OK* he has difficulty in naming objects. For example, when a pen, pin, and penny are held up in succession, which is a frequently used test, he substitutes the name of one for the other and repeats the name of the preceding object; however, he can point to the "money," "sharp object," and "writing instrument" when these objects are placed in front of him. No abnormal physical signs are present.

Case 5

A 54-year-old man complains of several months of difficulty in thinking and the inability to remember the word he desires. Although his voice quivers, he is fully conversant and articulate. He is able to write the correct responses to questions; however, he has slow and poor penmanship. He is able to name six objects, follow double requests, and repeat complex phrases. On further testing, he has difficulty recalling six digits, three objects after 3 minutes, and both recent and past events. Judgment seems intact. The remainder of the neurologic examination is normal.

answer: 1-5.

Case 1.   He has complete loss of language function, *global aphasia*, accompanied by right hemiplegia and homonymous hemianopsia. The cause is probably an occlusion of the left internal carotid artery creating an infarction of the entire left hemisphere.

Case 2.   Since he can manage only a few phrases or words in a telegraphic pattern, he has nonfluent aphasia. This variety of aphasia is typically accompanied by right hemiparesis, in which the arm is more paretic than the leg. It is usually caused by an occlusion of the left middle cerebral artery. An underlying infarction would encompass Broca's area and the adjacent cortical motor region, but spare the cortical fibers for the leg, which are supplied by the anterior cerebral artery.

Case 3.   The patient has fluent aphasia characterized by a normal quantity of speech interspersed with paraphasic errors, but only subtle right-sided corticospinal tract abnormalities. She probably has a lesion in the left parietal or posterior temporal lobe. The headaches and papilledema, given her age and the course of the illness, suggest that it is a mass lesion, such as a glioblastoma multiforme, rather than a CVA.

Case 4.   He has anomic aphasia, which is a variety of fluent aphasia in which language impairment is restricted to the improper identification of objects, i.e., a naming impairment. Its origin may be Alzheimer's disease, but in view of the history of mitral stenosis and headache, the origin was probably a small embolic CVA (see Chapter 11).

Case 5.   The patient does not have aphasia. His difficulty with memory could be either an early dementia or psychogenic inattention. Further evaluations might include neuropsychologic studies and evaluation for dementia.

6–10.   Match the lesions that are pictured schematically with those expected in cases 1–5.

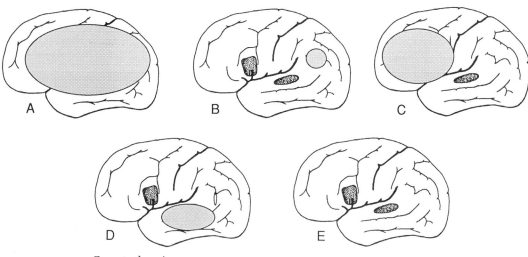

A   B   C

D   E

answer: *Case 1,* drawing a

answer: *Case 2,* drawing c

answer: *Case 3,* drawing d

answer: *Case 4,* drawing b or d

answer: *Case 5,* drawing e

11–26.   Match the lesion with the expected associated finding(s).

a. Dysarthria, including hoarseness
b. Dysphagia
c. Dementia
d. Dyscalculia
e. Fluent aphasia
f. Constructional apraxia
g. Dyslexia
h. Deafness
i. Mutism
j. Left-right disorientation

k. Finger agnosia
l. Hyperactive reflexes
m. Sixth cranial nerve palsy
n. Alexia
o. Ataxia
p. Dressing apraxia
q. Anosognosia
r. Hemi-inattention
s. Left limb apraxia

11.   Paresis of one recurrent laryngeal nerve

answer: a

12.   Pseudobulbar palsy

answer: a, b, l

13.   Bulbar palsy

answer: a, b

14. Dominant hemisphere temporal lobe lesion

    answer: e

15. Lateral medullary syndrome

    answer: a, b, o

16. Laryngitis

    answer: a

17. Dominant hemisphere angular gyrus lesion

    answer: d, j, k (Gerstmann's syndrome)

18. Dominant hemisphere parietal lobe lesion

    answer: d, e, g, j, k

19. Nondominant hemisphere parietal lobe lesion

    answer: f, p, q, r

20. Bilateral frontal lobe tumor

    answer: c, possibly also a, b, and i

21. Bilateral anterior cerebral artery infarction

    answer: s and possibly c and i

22. Streptomycin toxicity

    answer: h, o

23. Alcohol intoxication

    answer: a, d, o

24. Periaqueductal hemorrhagic necrosis (Wernicke's encephalopathy)

    answer: c, m, o

25. Phenytoin (Dilantin) toxicity

    answer: o

26. Infarction of left posterior cerebral artery

    answer: n Alexia

27. A 34-year-old man was revived after attempting suicide by sitting in a garaged car with the motor running. During the next week he only sat in bed and looked out of the window. He displayed no emotion and did not respond to requests. Although he was virtually mute, he seemed to repeat in intricate detail whatever he was asked and occasionally whatever was said on television. His deep tendon reflexes were brisk, and he had bilateral palmomental reflexes. His plantar reflexes were equivocal.

The examiner was uncertain whether the patient had depression, dementia, or other neuropsychologic abnormality. Please discuss the case and suggest further evaluation.

    answer: The patient was probably exposed to excessive carbon monoxide. As in cases of cardiac arrest and strangulation where patients survive, any form of cerebral anoxia creates cerebral cortex damage. When patients permanently lose all intellectual and voluntary motor function, they are said to be in the *persistent vegetative state* (see Chapter 11).

    In this case, the cerebral damage was incomplete. It probably isolated the perisylvian language arc of the cerebral cortex comprising Wernicke's area, the arcuate fasciculus, and Broca's area. Isolation of this crucial region from the rest of the cerebral cortex causes *transcortical* or *isolation aphasia* that permits repetition of words and phrases, no matter how complex; however, since language information cannot connect with the rest of the brain's language system, patients cannot name objects or follow requests. Since a large portion of the cerebral cortex is damaged, patients usually also have dementia, paresis, and frontal release signs.

In cases where cerebral cortex damage is superimposed on depressive illness or other psychologic aberrations, the clinical picture is unpredictable. In such patients, detailed testing of language function must be part of the mental status examination.

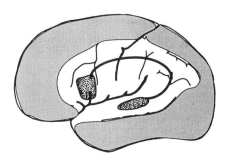

Fig. (above) In isolation aphasia, which is usually induced by hypoperfusion-induced hypoxia, the most vulnerable portions of the cerebral cortex are damaged, sparing the perisylvian language arc. Language processes may continue within this region, but they receive no input from other regions of the cerebral cortex.

28. A left-handed 64-year-old male schoolteacher sustained a cerebral thrombosis of the right middle cerebral artery. What might be predicted regarding language function?

a. He will certainly develop aphasia.
b. He will have left hemiparesis if he has aphasia.
c. If he develops aphasia, his prognosis is relatively good.
d. If he has aphasia, he will have a homonymous hemianopsia.

answer: c. Left-handed individuals who have normal intelligence are often still predominantly left-hemisphere dominant or they have mixed cerebral dominance. Moreover, language centers in the right hemisphere are not arranged consistently with respect to those on the left or to the motor and visual tracts within the hemisphere. If left-handed individuals suffer an infarction of the right cerebral hemisphere, they do not necessarily develop aphasia or the usual associated deficits. In fact, they may develop aphasia if they have an infarction in the left cerebral hemisphere. Left-handed individuals, compared to right-handed individuals, have a better prognosis for the resolution of aphasia.

29. If the patient in the previous question were discovered to have a resectable tumor in the right temporal lobe, how could language function of the right cerebral hemisphere be established before surgery?

a. An MRI scan could be performed.
b. A CT scan could show differences in the *planum temporale*.
c. Barbiturates infused into the carotid artery of the dominant hemisphere would cause aphasia.
d. A PET study would indicate cerebral dominance for language.

answer: c. Infusion of barbiturates directly into the dominant carotid artery produces aphasia (the *Wada Test*). It is the standard procedure to determine if a cerebral hemisphere is dominant before removal of cerebral neoplasms or an epilepsy scar focus. PET scans are difficult to perform because of the need for short-lived cyclotron-generated substrates and the PET scan's relatively poor resolution of metabolic function. Although the *planum temporale* (the superior surface of the temporal lobe cortex) has a greater area in the dominant than nondominant temporal lobe, the difference is not always present and, even when present, cannot be reliably visualized with CT or MRI scans.

30. In which conditions are confabulations *not* found?

a.   Anton's syndrome
b.   Gerstmann's syndrome
c.   Anosognosia
d.   Wernicke-Korsakoff syndrome

answer: b. Gerstmann's syndrome is a controversial entity that consists of the combination of right and left confusion, dyslexia, dyscalculia, and finger agnosia. It is usually attributed to lesions in the angular gyrus of the parietal lobe of the dominant hemisphere. In denial of blindness (Anton's syndrome), blind patients typically confabulate or fantasize about the appearance of objects presented to them. It occurs most often in elderly people who undergo ophthalmologic surgical procedures and cannot temporarily see out of either eye. Failure to acknowledge a left hemiparesis or similar deficit (anosognosia) is often accompanied by confabulation, denial, and other defense mechanisms. Although confabulations are described in the Wernicke-Korsakoff's syndrome, they are rare. When they do occur, the patients usually also have marked memory impairments.

31. Match the speech abnormality (dysarthria) (a–d) with the illness (1–4).

a.   Hypophonia
b.   Scanning speech
c.   Nasal speech
d.   Strained and strangled speech

1.   Myasthenia gravis
2.   Parkinsonism
3.   Multiple sclerosis
4.   Spasmodic dysphonia

answer: a-2, b-3, c-1, d-4

32. Which conditions *usually* cause aphasia?

a.   Chronic subdural hematomas
b.   Myasthenia gravis
c.   Multiple sclerosis
d.   Parkinsonism
e.   None of the above

answer: e. Subdural hematomas are located in the extra-axial space. Although chronic subdural hematomas typically cause headaches and dementia, they usually do not cause aphasia or other localized neurologic symptoms. Myasthenia gravis is a disorder of the neuromuscular junction and therefore does not cause dementia, aphasia, or other signs of a CNS dysfunction. Multiple sclerosis (MS) affects the cerebral white matter to a large extent only late in its course. Although MS may then cause dementia, it rarely causes aphasia. Parkinsonism may cause dysarthria (hypophonia and tremor) and, late in the illness, dementia; however, it rarely causes aphasia.

33.   A 45-year-old airplane pilot describes that when she awoke earlier in the morning, for approximately 5 minutes she had "expressive aphasia," by which she meant that she was unable to speak or gesture, but she understood most of the news on the radio. During that time she had no other symptoms, and she remained in bed. Which of the following conditions are reasonable explanations for her episode?

a.   Seizure
b.   TIA
c.   Migraine
d.   Sleep disorder

answer: All. She might have had a partial seizure originating in the left frontal lobe. During a postictal period, she might have had aphasia and a right hemiparesis that prevented her from gesturing. A TIA in the distribution of the left carotid artery might also have caused aphasia, with or without right hemiparesis. Hemiplegic migraines, which can cause speech impairment, can occasionally affect adults. An episode of "sleep paralysis," such as hypnopompic cataplexy, may cause virtual quadriparesis and mutism. The etiologies of transient aphasia and transient hemiparesis are similar (see Hemiplegic Migraines, Chapter 9, and Carotid Artery TIAs, Chapter 11).

34.   A 70-year-old man complains of the sudden inability to read. Although he can write his name and most sentences that are dictated to him, he cannot read aloud or copy written material. His speech is fluent and contains no paraphasic errors. On further examination, he can see objects only in his left visual field. What is this man's difficulty, and where is the responsible lesion(s)?

> ***answer:*** He clearly has alexia, as demonstrated by his inability to read, and also a right homonymous hemianopsia. He does not have agraphia because he can transcribe dictation and write words from memory, nor does he have aphasia. Thus, he has the syndrome of alexia without agraphia. This syndrome is caused by a lesion in the (left) occipital lobe and posterior corpus callosum. The left occipital lesion would explain the failure of visual information to pass from the intact right visual cortex through the corpus callosum to the left (dominant) hemisphere for integration (see Fig. 8–4). Since memory and auditory circuits, as well as the corticospinal system, are intact, he can write words that he hears or remembers. Such lesions are usually caused by infarctions of the left posterior cerebral artery or by infiltrating brain tumors, such as a glioblastoma multiforme.

35. A 68-year-old man has had a car accident as a result of drifting into oncoming traffic. He is now unaware of a weak left arm. An examination shows that he has a left homonymous hemianopsia, a mild left hemiparesis (which the patient denied), and the failure to recognize his weak left arm. Which intellectual processes are present?

> ***answer:*** He probably had the accident because a left homonymous hemianopsia prevented him from seeing oncoming traffic. More important, he has anosognosia (failure to recognize one's illness). This man displays perceptual distortions characteristic of patients with parietal lobe lesions. (R) – nondominant .

36. A 60-year-old woman with long-standing depression has agitation, a language disturbance, and dysarthria. Initially misdiagnosed as having an exacerbation of her psychiatric disorder, she was recognized as suffering from an aphasia that was characterized by a paucity of words with an impaired ability to express herself. She was also shown to have a mild right hemiparesis. An MRI scan indicated an occlusion of the left middle cerebral artery. In planning her rehabilitation management, which additional associated findings should be sought?

a.	Constructional apraxia	d.	Left homonymous hemianopsia
b.	Gait apraxia	e.	Buccofacial apraxia
c.	Limb apraxia	f.	Ideational apraxia

> ***answer:*** c, e. Limb and buccofacial apraxias, which are associated with dominant hemisphere lesions, are potentially major obstacles to speech and physical therapies.

37. Patients with nondominant hemisphere lesions are reported to have loss of the normal inflections of speech and diminished associated facial and limb gestures. What are the technical terms used to describe these findings?

> ***answer:*** Aprosody and loss of paralinguistic components of speech

38. A man who has undergone a commissurotomy for intractable seizures is shown a written request to raise both arms. What will be his response when the request is shown in his left visual field? In the right visual field?

> ***answer:*** When the request is shown in his left visual field, he will not raise either arm because the written information does not reach the left hemisphere language centers. When the request is shown in his right visual field, the information reaches the language centers and he will raise his right hand; however, the command to move his left hand may not reach the right hemisphere's motor center (Fig. 8–8).

39–44. With which conditions are the various forms of apraxia (a–h) associated?

a. Aphasia
b. Hemi-inattention
c. Dementia
d. Dysarthria
e. Incontinence

f. Left homonymous hemianopsia
g. Right homonymous hemianopsia
h. Aprosody

39. Gait *apraxia*

answer: c, e

40. Constructional *apraxia*

answer: b, f, h

NPH — confusion
— gait abn
— incontinence

41. Ideational *apraxia*

answer: c

42. Limb

answer: a, g

43. Buccofacial

answer: a, d, g

44. Ideomotor

answer: a, g

45. How does aphasia in truly left-handed people differ from aphasia in right-handed people?

a. Aphasia can result from lesions in either hemisphere.
b. The variety of aphasia is less clearly related to the site of cerebral injury.
c. The prognosis is better.
d. The etiologies are different.

answer: a, b, c

46. Which of the following are disconnection syndromes?

a. Internuclear ophthalmoplegia   d. Isolation aphasia
b. Conduction aphasia   e. Alexia without agraphia
c. Split brain syndrome   f. Global aphasia

answer: a, b, c, e. Disconnection syndromes refer to disorders in which connections between the primary neuropsychologic centers are severed. Although not generally considered a disconnection syndrome, internuclear ophthalmoplegia has the same features: centers or nuclei are normal, but interconnecting fasciculi are damaged. In contrast, isolation aphasia results from extensive cerebral cortex injury that preserves the language arc, and its elements remain connected. Global aphasia results from extensive destruction of the entire language arc.

47. Which artery supplies most of the perisylvian language arc?

a. Anterior cerebral artery   c. Posterior cerebral artery
b. Middle cerebral artery   d. Vertebrobasilar artery system

answer: b

48. What is the term applied to the area of the cerebral cortex between branches of the major cerebral arteries?

a. Watershed area   c. Cornea
b. Limbic system   d. Arcuate fasciculus

answer: a. "Watershed" technically refers to a geographic region or divide drained by a river or stream. To neurologists, the term refers to areas of the cerebral cortex that are perfused by the terminal branches of arteries. The blood supply, thus tenuous, is insufficient during hypotension or anoxia.

49. Which is/are true regarding sign language?

a. Sign language, like spoken language, is based in the dominant hemisphere.
b. Middle cerebral artery occlusions in deaf people will probably cause aphasia in sign language.
c. Sign language relies on visual rather than auditory input.
d. American Sign Language (ASL) is the proper name for the common, gesture-based sign language.

answer: all

50. In nonfluent aphasia, why is the arm typically more paretic than the leg?

a. The motor cortex for the arm is supplied by the middle cerebral artery, which is usually occluded. The motor cortex for the leg is supplied by the anterior cerebral artery, which is usually spared.
b. The arm has a larger cortical representation.
c. The infarct occurs in the internal capsule.
d. The motor cortex for the arm is supplied by the anterior cerebral artery, which is usually occluded. The motor cortex for the leg is supplied by the middle cerebral artery, which is usually spared.

answer: a

51. After a right parietal infarction, patients may develop an alien hand syndrome. Which of the following characteristics are descriptive of this phenomenon?

a. Persistent pain in an amputated hand
b. The misperception that a paralyzed hand is normal
c. Attraction to another person's hand
d. A perception that the paralyzed hand is not the patient's
e. Perception that the paralyzed hand acts independently or under another person's control

answer: d, e

52. Which two of the following varieties of apraxia are most closely associated with dementia?

a. Ideational   d. Buccofacial
b. Dressing   e. Oral
c. Ideomotor   f. Gait

answer: a, f. Ideational apraxia is a manifestation of dementia. Gait apraxia and dementia are manifestations of normal-pressure hydrocephalus.

53. In which disorders is echolalia a symptom?

a. Autism   d. Tourette's syndrome
b. Isolation aphasia   e. All
c. Dementia

answer: e. Echolalia, an involuntary repetition of visitors' or examiners' words, is a manifestation of diverse neurologic conditions.

54. Which disconnection syndromes stem from corpus callosum damage?

a. Alexia without agraphia   e. Split brain syndrome
b. Buccofacial apraxia   f. Anterior cerebral artery syndrome
c. Left limb apraxia   g. Marchiafava-Bignami syndrome
d. Isolation aphasia

answer: a, c, e, f, g

55. Which conclusions have stemmed from studies of patients who have undergone a commissurotomy?

a. The corpus callosum is vital to routine cognitive function.
b. Patients with the split brain have gross, readily identifiable physical and cognitive abnormalities.

c. Emotions generated in the right hemisphere are not as readily described as those generated in the left hemisphere.
d. Emotions generated in the left hemisphere are not as readily described as those in the right hemisphere.

answer: c

9 Headaches

Almost 90 per cent of Americans have at least occasional headaches. Most of them are beset with *tension, migraine,* or *cluster headaches* (Chronic Recurring Headache).[1] These headaches are diagnosed not by physical or laboratory tests, which are characteristically normal, but by their distinctive symptoms.

Acutely occurring or steadily progressive headaches, in contrast, are often manifestations of life-threatening diseases of the brain. These headaches include *temporal arteritis, intracranial mass lesions, pseudotumor cerebri, meningitis,* and *subarachnoid hemorrhage* (Headaches Secondary to Organic Disease). Their symptoms are less specific, and their diagnosis rests on abnormal physical findings and laboratory tests results. (*Postconcussion* syndrome headaches, which could be considered in this group, are discussed in Chapter 22, Head Trauma.)

CHRONIC RECURRING HEADACHE

Tension Headache (Tension-Type Headache)

Formerly called "muscle contraction headaches," tension headaches are the almost universal intermittent, frontal, cervical, or generalized dull pain. They plague women more than men and, probably because of psychology or environment rather than genetics, affect multiple family members. The symptom of tension headaches is exclusively pain—unaccompanied by photophobia, hyperacusis or phonophobia (sensitivity to noise); autonomic disturbances, such a nausea or vomiting; or prostration: People with tension headaches may complain, but they go about their business.

Tension headaches were attributed to contraction (tension) of the scalp, neck, and face muscles (Fig. 9–1), but recent concepts place them at the opposite end of a headache spectrum from migraine. Tension may be produced by physical factors—fatigue, cervical spondylosis, bright light, or loud noise —as well as by emotional stress (Table 9–1).

Treatment. Neurologists generally assure patients that their headaches do not represent a brain tumor or other potentially fatal illness, which are frequent unspoken fears. In conjunction with prescribing medications (Table 9–2), neurologists commonly refer these patients to formal or informal counseling about psychologic factors, general health, diet, and exercise.

---

[1]The classification within parentheses is taken from the International Headache Society (see references). Although accepted in academic neurologic circles, the terminology is often descriptive, arbitrary, and, in some areas, controversial. In particular, the term "Headaches Secondary to Organic Disease" implies that migraines and other headaches are not the result of physiologic disease.

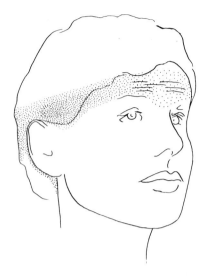

FIGURE 9–1

Tension headaches produce a band-like squeezing, symmetric pressure at the neck, temples, or forehead.

For headaches that occur less than twice a week, neurologists usually prescribe "abortive therapy"—medicine taken only at the onset of a headache. Most often they prescribe simple analgesics, such as aspirin, aspirin-caffeine compounds, acetaminophen, or, especially for menses-related headaches, nonsteroidal anti-inflammatory drugs (NSAIDs). These medicines should be kept in the car, at work, and in pocketbooks to be taken at the first inkling of a headache (or any pain) to prevent its full development. However, daily use of these and other medications may lead to daily, rebound, or withdrawal headaches (see below).

TABLE 9–1. IMPORTANT ITEMS IN A HEADACHE HISTORY

What is its nature?
  Type: throbbing[a], aching, sharp
  Location at onset: bilateral, unilateral (hemicranial)[a],
    periorbital[a,b], trigeminal distribution
  Precipitants: stress, relief of stress[a], menses[a],
    missing meals[a], too much or too little sleep[a],
    glare[a], alcohol[a], chocolate[a], medications
    (vasodilators, oral contraceptives), touching the
    face
  Relief: bed rest[a], pacing[b]
What are its temporal characteristics?
  Duration
  Pattern: random[b], during sleep[b] or early morning[a],
    end of the day, weekends[a], seasons[b]
  Do they occur in groups?[b]
  Were they present in childhood?[a]
  Is there a history of carsickness as a child?[a]
What symptoms are associated with the headache?
  Aura[a], visual, sensory disturbance, personality
    change
  Autonomic dysfunction[a]: nausea, vomiting,
    polyuria, polydipsia
  Photophobia[a], hyperacusis or phonophobia[a]
  Ptosis and tearing ipsilateral to the headache[b]
Is there a parent or sibling with similar headaches?[a]

[a]Migraine symptoms.
[b]Cluster headache symptoms.

TABLE 9–2.   HEADACHE MEDICATIONS[a]

ANALGESICS	
Acetaminophen	
Aspirin	Aspirin, (one 5-gr tablet = 325 mg)
Bufferin	Aspirin (325 mg), aluminum glycinate, magnesium carbonate
Esgic	Butalbital, acetaminophen, caffeine (40 mg)
Excedrin	Aspirin (250 mg), acetaminophen, caffeine (65 mg)
Fioricet	Butalbital, acetaminophen, caffeine (40 mg)
Fiorinal	Butalbital, caffeine (40 mg), aspirin (325 mg)
Midrin	Isometheptene, dichloraphenazone, acetaminophen
BETA-BLOCKERS[b]	
Propranolol	
CALCIUM CHANNEL BLOCKERS[b]	
Verapamil	
ANTI-INFLAMMATORY AGENTS[b]:	
Nonsteroidal Anti-Inflammatory Drugs (NSAIDs)	
Aspirin	
Ibuprofen	
Naproxen	
Steroids	
Prednisone	
Dexamethasone	
SEROTONIN-ACTIVE MEDICATIONS	
Cafergot	Ergotamine, caffeine (100 mg)
DHE	Dihydroergotamine
Sansert[b]	Methysergide
Sumatriptan	Imitrex
Wigraine	Ergotamine, caffeine (100 mg)
MISCELLANEOUS	
Amitriptyline[b]	
Lithium[b]	
Valproate[b]	

[a]Consult package insert for indications, dosage, contraindications, precautions, and side effects. Several of these medications are widely and successfully prescribed for headaches without FDA indication.
[b]Prophylactic therapy of migraines. The other medications are generally used as abortive treatment. However, the NSAIDs, including aspirin, may be used as either prophylactic or abortive treatment.

Preventive, "prophylactic" therapy—medicine taken daily—is recommended if severe headaches occur more frequently than once a week, if abortive therapy is ineffective, or if medication requirements are excessive. Neurologists usually avoid prescribing minor tranquilizers, except for limited periods. Instead, they often recommend NSAIDs or, even if patients have no history of depression, antidepressants in small nighttime doses.

Biofeedback, relaxation, physical therapy, and stress reduction may be helpful, especially for pregnant women, for whom no medications are recommended, and young adults. Insight-oriented psychotherapy and classic psychoanalysis directed toward headaches do not reduce the headaches. Of course, these techniques might provide insight, reduce anxiety, treat depression, and offer other benefits.

Migraines

Migraines are complex, variable, and accompanied by characteristic sensory, psychologic, and autonomic features that accompany, overshadow, or even replace the headache. These associated features separate migraines from other chronic recurrent headaches. Two major migraine varieties—defined by the presence or absence of an *aura*—and several variations can be discerned by their different symptoms.

Classic Migraine (Migraine with Aura). In the *classic* variety of migraine, which affects only about 15 per cent of migraine patients, the headache is preceded by an aura that can be almost any symptom of brain dysfunction. The subsequent headache is similar to migraines without an aura (see below).

Auras gradually evolve, last 20 minutes or less, and evaporate rapidly. Although auras are usually visual phenomena, they can consist of any particular transient alteration in sensory and language function; sensory distortions, misperceptions, and complex hallucinations; or overwhelming and unprovoked personality change (Table 9–3). Surprisingly, in view of the impending headache, they mesmerize patients.

When auras are not followed by a headache, which often happens, they consist of recurrent, free-standing hallucinations. Whether or not they are not followed by a headache, auras are important because they are a distinctive neurologic symptom, can mimic other neurologic disorders (transient ischemic attacks [TIAs], drug ingestion, and partial complex seizures), and are an "organic cause" of altered perception, mood, and behavior.

The most common auras are individualistic visual hallucinations (see Chapter 12). They can involve a graying of a region of the visual field (*scotoma*; Fig. 9–2A), flashing zigzag lines (*scintillating scotomata*; Fig. 9–2B), crescents of brilliant colors (Fig. 9–2C), tubular vision, or distortion of objects (*metamorphopsia*). Although olfactory hallucinations can be a migraine aura, they are more likely a manifestation of a partial complex seizure. In children, auras can be recurrent colicky or "cyclic abdominal pain" with nausea and vomiting.

Common Migraine (Migraine without Aura). The *common* variety, which affects about 75 per cent of migraine patients, has no aura preceding the head-

TABLE 9–3. VARIETIES OF MIGRAINE AURA

Sensory phenomena
   Special senses
      Visual, olfactory, auditory, gustatory
   Paresthesias, especially in lips and hand
Motor deficits
   Hemiparesis, hemiplegia
   Ophthalmoplegia
Neuropsychologic changes
   Aphasia
   Perceptual impairments, especially for size, shape, and time
Emotional and behavioral
   Anxiety, depression

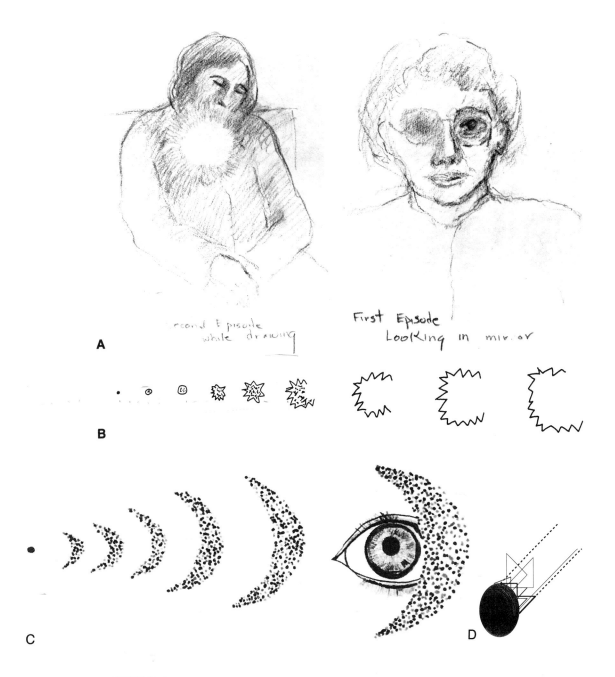

A, Second Episode while drawing

First Episode Looking in mirror

FIGURE 9–2

A, These drawings by a migraine patient show the typical visual obscurations of a *scotoma* that precedes her migraine headache. In both cases, a small circular area near the center of vision is lost entirely or reduced in clarity. Even though the aura is gray and has a relatively simple shape, she is captivated by it. *B,* The patient who drew this aura, a *scintillating scotoma,* wrote, "In the early stages, the area within the lights is somewhat shaded. Later, as the figure widens, you can sort of peer right through the area. Eventually, it gets so wide that it disappears." The scotoma is typical: It consists of an angular, brightly lit margin and an opaque interior that begins as a star and expands into a crescent. It scintillates at 8 to 12 Hz. Angular auras are sometimes called *fortification scotomas* because of their similarity to military fortresses. *C,* A 30-year-old woman artist in her first trimester of pregnancy had several classic migraine headaches that were heralded by this scotoma. It began as a blue dot and, over 20 minutes, enlarged to a crescent of brightly shimmering, multicolored dots. When the crescent's intensity was at its peak, she was so dazzled that she lost her ability to see and think clearly. *D,* Having patients draw visual hallucinations has great diagnostic value. One patient, who had no artistic talent, reconstructed this "visual hallucination" using a computer drawing program. Children might provide similar valuable diagnostic information if they are asked to draw what they "see" before a headache or before they "feel bad."

ache. The headache, which typically lasts 4 to 24 hours, is initially throbbing or pulsating, hemicranial (felt on one side of the head), and predominantly temporal, retro-orbital (located behind the eye), or periorbital (around the eye). In about 50 per cent of patients, the headache moves to the opposite side or becomes generalized (Fig. 9–3). When migraines occur frequently, the pain evolves into a dull, symmetric, and continual headache that mimics a tension headache.

Accompanying nonheadache symptoms are characteristic: sensory hypersensitivity, autonomic dysfunction, and disability. In common terms, people want to go to bed; they are nauseated if not vomiting; and they seek dark, quiet places.

In conjunction with that seclusive behavior, patients often have episodic mood changes that can mimic those produced by other neurologic disorders and possibly psychiatric disturbances (Table 9–4). Patients with migraines may become feverishly active and work excessively. Most become depressed, feel dysphoric, and try to escape from other people, light, smells, and noise. If unable to find solitude, they may become distraught. Partly because of autonomic dysfunction, they tend to drink large quantities of water and crave food or sweets, particularly chocolate. Some children become confused and overactive. When they can sleep, children may be so withdrawn as to appear stuporous. After a migraine clears, especially when it ends with sleep, people sometimes sense a remarkable tranquillity or even euphoria.

Both classic and common migraines, as well as tension headaches, occur more frequently in women than in men and tend to affect more than one family member. In contrast to tension headaches, migraines begin in the early morning, rather than the afternoon. Migraines in women tend to start at menarche, to recur premenstrually and to be aggravated by oral contraceptives. During pregnancy, about three quarters of women with migraines experience a dramatic relief; however, the others have no improvement or experience an exacerbation. Some women develop their very first migraine during their pregnancy's first trimester. In men and women, migraines may occur during REM sleep (see Chapter 17), sometimes exclusively (*nocturnal migraines*).

Another important characteristic of migraines is that they can be precipitated by certain physical factors, such as skipping meals, too little or excessive sleep, menses, psychologic stress, and alcoholic drinks. (Alcoholic drinks can also provoke cluster headaches. According to common belief, red wine and brandy are most likely to precipitate migraines and vodka and white wine, the least likely.) In contrast, alcoholic drinks tend to ameliorate tension headaches.

Contrary to old, elitist views, migraines are not particularly prevalent among people in upper-income brackets or those who are rigid and perfectionist. Nevertheless, the role of psychologic stress is interesting. On one hand, stress can precipitate migraines, as it probably does with tension headaches. On the other hand, the *relief* of stress, "letdown," also produces migraines. People with difficult weekday jobs, for example, often awaken on weekend and holiday mornings with a migraine. Likewise, at the start of a vacation, especially after examinations, students develop migraines.

Other Migraine Varieties.   Migraines in children, *childhood migraines*, are similar to those in adults. However, they affect boys as often as girls and may cause cyclic, incapacitating nausea and vomiting. Children often become confused, incoherent, or distraught. Overall, children are more susceptible to basilar artery, ophthalmoplegic, and hemiplegic migraines (see below).

In *basilar migraines*, headaches are accompanied by symptoms—ataxia, vertigo, dysarthria, and diplopia—that reflect dysfunction in the basilar artery dis-

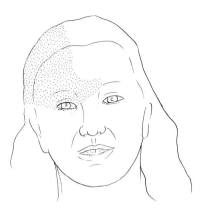

FIGURE 9-3

Patients with migraines have throbbing, hemicranial headaches that, in about 50 per cent of cases, either move to the other side of the head or become generalized.

tribution: the cerebellum, brainstem, and posterior cerebrum (see Fig. 11–2). Also, possibly because both temporal lobes may be impaired, victims may have recent memory impairments, e.g., transient global amnesia (see Chapter 11).

Hemiplegic migraines are characterized by combinations of various grades of hemiparesis, hemiparesthesia, and aphasia preceding or accompanying otherwise typical migraines. Sometimes the hemiparesis may even develop without an associated headache. Thus, in evaluating a patient who has had transient hemiparesis, the physician must consider hemiplegic migraines along with transient ischemic attacks (TIAs), postictal (Todd's) hemiparesis, and psychogenic disorders. In *complicated migraine* or *migrainous stroke*, hemiplegic migraine deficits become permanent in a situation that is virtually identical to a stroke. In view of the association of oral contraceptives, migraines, and stroke, women who have migraines with aura are usually advised not to take oral contraceptives.

Migraine-Like Conditions: Food-Induced Headaches. Certain foods and medications can cause nonspecific headaches, and in susceptible individuals, they precipitate a typical migraine. However, other than alcohol, the role of foods is overemphasized: Food precipitates migraines in only about 15 to 20 per cent of patients.

The clearest examples of foods precipitating a headache are the *Chinese restaurant syndrome*, where the offending agent is monosodium glutamate

TABLE 9-4. CAUSES OF TRANSIENT OR RECURRENT ALTERED MENTAL STATUS IN COMMON NEUROLOGIC CONDITIONS

Drugs
  Illicit
  Medicinal
Metabolic aberrations, e.g., hypoglycemia
Migraines
Seizures (see Chapter 10)
  Absence
  Partial complex
  Frontal lobe
Sleep attacks, e.g., narcolepsy, sleep apnea naps (see Chapter 17)
Transient global amnesia (see Chapter 11)
Transient ischemic attacks (TIAs; see Chapter 11)

(MSG), and the *hot dog headache*, where the offending agent is the nitrites in processed meats. Another example is the *ice cream headache*, which is precipitated by any very cold food that overstimulates the pharynx. Some people develop migraine-like headaches after eating tyramine-containing foods, such as ripened cheese, or phenylethylamine-containing foods, especially chocolate.

In the opposite situation, people deprived of their regular coffee develop a *caffeine-withdrawal syndrome* that consists of moderate to severe headache possibly accompanied by anxiety, depression, and lethargy. Although this syndrome is almost synonymous with coffee deprivation, it can be precipitated by withdrawal of other caffeine-containing beverages or medications (see Table 9–2 and Chapter 17). In fact, daily headaches may be caused partly by withdrawal of caffeine-containing medications (see below). Caffeine-withdrawal headaches pose a dilemma for heavy coffee drinkers: Excessive coffee leads to irritability, palpitations, and gastric burning, but foregoing it results in headaches, anxiety, and other symptoms.

Medication-Induced Headaches. Anti-anginal medicines, such as nitroglycerin or isosorbide (Isordil), probably because they contain toxic nitrites or dilate cerebral as well as cardiac arteries, cause headaches. Elderly patients who have cerebrovascular atherosclerosis are particularly vulnerable. Curiously, whereas some calcium channel blockers, such as nifedipine (Procardia), precipitate headaches, others, such as verapamil (Calan), may prevent them. For the psychiatrist, the most notorious iatrogenic headache, which is often complicated by cerebral hemorrhage, is caused by the interaction of monoamine oxidase inhibitor (MAOI) antidepressants with other agents (see below).

Sex-Related Headaches. Migraine-like headaches often occur after strenuous physical activity. In particular, sexual activity, whether intercourse or masturbation, may precipitate migraine-like headaches, *orgasmic headaches* or *coital cephalgia*. This condition is benign and relatively common, especially in people with migraines. Nevertheless, before dismissing severe headaches occurring during athletic or sexual activity, physicians might consider intracerebral or subarachnoid hemorrhage (see below).

Proposed Causes of Migraines. A long-standing, but probably outdated, theory is that the aura of migraines is caused by constriction of cerebral arteries in the carotid system (see Fig. 11–1), followed by dilation that allows unsuppressed pulsations to stretch the arteries and cause headaches. The current theory is that the aura of migraines is caused by "neuronal depression,"—that is, the impaired metabolism of cerebral neurons—that spreads in an orderly fashion over the cerebral cortex. According to this theory, decreased cerebral metabolic requirements, rather than vasoconstriction, reduce cerebral blood flow.

Modern theories suggest that the trigeminal nerve, which supplies the meninges and large blood vessels in the head, releases neuropeptides and other chemicals, such as substance P and neurokinin A. They incite painful perivascular inflammation and vasodilation.

"Central theories" are based on faulty serotonin (5-hydroxytryptamine [5HT]) neurotransmission. Although no single mechanism has been proven, several observations are important. Most brain serotonin neurons are in the brainstem's dorsal raphe nuclei. Serotonin plasma concentration falls at the onset of a migraine, and reserpine, which depletes serotonin, induces migraines. Several dramatically effective acute migraine medications act primarily on certain serotonin receptors ($5HT_1$); dihydroergotamine (DHE), ergotamine (Cafergot, Wigraine), and sumatriptan (Imitrex). Similarly, prophylactic migraine medications act on other serotonin receptors ($5HT_2$); for example, methysergide (Sansert).

There is undoubtedly a genetic predisposition to migraines because 70 per cent of migraine patients have a close relative with migraines. Moreover, strong laboratory evidence indicates that a hemiplegic variety results from an abnormal gene.

Treatment. In trying to discover migraine precipitants, neurologists usually suggest that patients create a "headache diary" to record headache days, medications, diet, menses, school examinations, and other potentially significant events. If precipitants cannot be avoided, at least they can be anticipated.

Simple analgesics useful for tension headaches often abort mild to moderate migraines. More potent migraine-abortive medications usually act on serotonin receptors in trigeminal nerve endings and cerebral vessels. Ergotamine preparations can be administered by pill, suppository, inhaler (Cafergot, Wigraine), or injection (DHE,). They are very effective, but tricky to use. They should be administered at the onset of the headache, and they routinely cause nausea and vomiting that may require phenothiazine-containing antiemetic medications, such as metoclopramide (Reglan). After taking ergotamines, many patients remain at rest in a darkened room and, if possible, sleep. Excessive ergotamine use can lead to chronic daily headache and *ergotism*, with spasm of coronary or limb arteries that might be severe enough to cause angina or gangrene.

Sumatriptan (Imitrex), a specific serotonin receptor agonist, is self-injected or taken by pill. Unlike conventional orally or rectally administered medications, sumatriptan injections act within minutes, are effective at any time during the migraine, and ameliorate nausea. Although expensive, sumatriptan can obviate emergency room visits or hospital admissions. Because it is metabolized by monoamine oxidase (MAO), sumatriptan should be given in reduced doses or not at all to patients receiving MAO inhibitors.

Prophylactic therapy is appropriate if headaches occur more than three or four times a month, abortive medicines are ineffective, or acute medications are taken excessively. Propranolol (Inderal) and other beta-adrenergic blockers are widely used for migraine prophylaxis, as well as for the treatment of angina, hypertension, and essential tremor (see Chapter 18). Physicians and their patients must both be aware that some side effects of this medicine, regardless of its indication, may be mental changes akin to depression.

Methysergide (Sansert), which is a congener of LSD that blocks certain serotonin receptors, is an effective prophylactic medicine; however, it too may induce mood and mental changes. Most worrisome, if methysergide is taken for longer than 6 months, it may cause retroperitoneal, pleural, and endocardial fibrosis.

Tricyclic antidepressants, such as amitriptyline, are clearly effective in migraine prophylaxis. They reduce the severity, frequency, and duration of migraines. Apart from any elevation of mood, antidepressants may be useful because they decrease or alter REM sleep during which some migraine headaches develop and they possess analgesic activity (see Chapter 14). New antidepressants that specifically affect serotonin metabolism have not been completely compared to the standard tricyclic antidepressants, but early studies have been disappointing.

Calcium channel blockers, such as verapamil (Calan), and NSAIDs are also widely used and effective in migraine prophylaxis. Although their benefit cannot be reliably predicted, they have a relatively low incidence of serious side effects.

As in tension headaches, neither insight-oriented psychotherapy nor classic psychoanalysis has been shown in adequately controlled studies to be effective. However, biofeedback and relaxation therapy have helped migraine patients.

Other Strategies. Whether tension headaches and migraines are actually separate illnesses or not, physicians should estimate what portion of their patients' headaches are migraines. If the headaches are at some time unilateral, throbbing, accompanied by nausea, precipitated by menses, or preceded by the other known migraine precipitants, the diagnosis of migraine is appropriate. Physicians should institute migraine treatments without requiring an aura, severe pain, or prostration.

Patients with chronic daily headache (see below) who have been overmedicated—for one reason or another—might be considered to have drug addiction. The offending medications will determine the rapidity of the withdrawal and the need for alternate analgesics, vasoconstrictors, NSAIDs, or antidepressants during and afterward.

Under certain circumstances, headache patients should be hospitalized. Those with migraines lasting for more than 3 days (*status migrainosus*), prostration, or nausea and vomiting that has led to dehydration would benefit from hospitalization for parenteral medication, intravenous fluids, antiemetics, and a quiet, dark refuge. Also, abuse of over-the-counter medications as well as narcotics may require hospitalization for withdrawal. Ergotism often requires hospitalization.

Chronic Daily Headaches

''Chronic daily headaches'' (CDH), while not yet officially recognized as a distinct condition, are encountered in numerous people who have had migraines and medication abuse. They are often accompanied by symptoms of depression. The headaches have most of the characteristics of tension headaches. Only a minority of headaches have any other characteristic, such as a throbbing sensation, nausea, or hypersensitivity to light or sound. The diagnosis of CDH is precluded by underlying organic disease, head trauma, or overt psychologic illness.

Most cases of CDH are attributable to dependence on over-the-counter or physician-prescribed medications, especially acetaminophen, aspirin-butabarbital-caffeine compounds, benzodiazepines, barbiturates, ergotamine, and caffeine. Thus, CDH may be a complication of antimigraine medications.

CDH may result from years of migraine or represent a combination of migraine-tension headaches. Although those conditions are usually portrayed as separate entities (Table 9–5), they too possibly represent points on a spectrum. In practice, many patients clearly have a combination that seems to blend, vary, and recur.

Cluster Headaches

As their name implies, cluster headaches occur in groups (clusters) of one to eight times daily for a period of several weeks to months. Many patients have a cyclic pattern that occurs most often in the spring. Cluster-free intervals range from a few months to several years.

TABLE 9–5.   COMPARISON OF TENSION AND COMMON MIGRAINE HEADACHES

	Tension	Migraine
Location of headache	Bilateral	Hemicranial[a]
Nature of headache	Dull ache	Throbbing[a]
Severity	Slight to moderate	Moderate to severe
Associated symptoms	None	Nausea, hyperacusis, photophobia
Activity	Continues working	Seeks bed rest
Effect of alcohol	Reduces headache	Worsens headache

[a]In approximately one half of patients, at least at onset.

Each headache is sharp, nonthrobbing pain that seems to bore into one eye and adjacent areas for one half to 3 hours. Suffering from repetitive bouts of agitating and excruciating pain, patients speak of wanting to kill themselves. The pain is accompanied by ipsilateral eye tearing, conjunctival injection, nasal congestion, and a partial Horner's syndrome (Figs. 9–4 and 12–15).

During a cluster period, headaches can occur randomly throughout the day and can be precipitated by alcoholic drinks, but they often occur with stereotyped regularity, especially during REM sleep. Compared to the symptoms of a migraine, a cluster headache is extraordinary pain devoid of frills. Cluster headaches are not preceded by an aura or other warning, are unaccompanied by nausea, are not alleviated by bedrest or seclusion, and are not associated with mental changes.

The demography is also unique. Cluster headaches affect men six to eight times more commonly than women. In fact, they are the only form of chronic headache that develops more frequently in men than women. In addition, unlike migraines, cluster headaches typically have no familial tendency. They typically begin between age 20 and 40 years. More than 80 per cent of patients smoke, and 50 per cent drink alcohol excessively.

Cause and Treatment.   Cluster headaches are probably caused by a different form of cerebrovascular dysfunction than migraines. Nevertheless, since cluster and migraine headaches probably result from cerebrovascular dysfunction and have several common clinical features (episodic, unilateral pain), both are called "vascular headaches."

Abortive medicines are relatively ineffective for cluster headaches because of their abrupt, unexpected onset and relatively short duration. However, oxygen inhalation at 8 to 10 L/min, vasoconstrictors, and sumatriptan may interrupt them. Prophylactic medicines include lithium, as well as those useful for migraines. (Lithium was introduced because cluster headaches, like manic-depressive episodes, are cyclic and afflict middle-aged people.) Medications

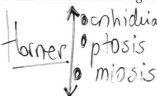

FIGURE 9–4

Patients with cluster headaches usually have unilateral periorbital pain accompanied by ipsilateral tearing and nasal discharge, along with ptosis and miosis (a partial Horner's syndrome).

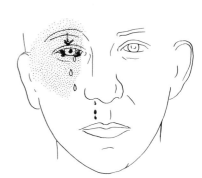

of choice are verapamil, methysergide, and ergotamine after a short course of prednisone. Psychotherapy and biofeedback do not help.

TRIGEMINAL NEURALGIA

Trigeminal neuralgia, also called *tic douloureux,* is a recurring condition that is classified as a "cranial neuralgia," rather than a "chronic recurring headache." Patients, for whom that distinction is of no importance, suffer from dozens of brief, 20- to 30-second jabs of excruciatingly sharp pain that extend along one of the three divisions of the trigeminal nerve. The division most often affected is V_2 (see Fig. 4–11). Unlike all other headaches, stimulating the affected area can provoke the pain. These regions, *trigger zones,* when stimulated by eating, even light touch, brushing teeth, or drinking cold water, evoke a dreadful shock. The pain usually ceases at night, allowing the patient a full night's sleep.

Trigeminal neuralgia typically develops after age 60 years, making it one of the most important causes of headache in the elderly (Table 9–6). As in most other chronic headaches and illnesses that affect the elderly, the male to female ratio is 3:2.

Cause and Treatment

In most cases, the cause is an aberrant superior cerebellar artery or other cerebral blood vessel compressing the trigeminal nerve root as it emerges from the brainstem. Tumors of the cerebellopontine angle may have the same effect. When trigeminal neuralgia develops in young adults, a multiple sclerosis plaque that irritates the trigeminal nerve nucleus may be responsible.

Whatever the cause, treatment is usually begun with carbamazepine (Tegretol). In the majority of patients, in whom an aberrant vessel is responsible for the neuralgia, the most effective procedure is a craniotomy that places a barrier between the vessel and trigeminal nerve (Fig. 9–5). Less risky procedures are percutaneous glycerol injections and placing radiofrequency lesions in the root of the trigeminal nerve.

HEADACHES SECONDARY TO ORGANIC DISEASE

Temporal Arteritis

Temporal arteritis is a disease of unknown etiology in which the temporal and other cranial arteries become inflamed. Since histologic examination of

TABLE 9–6. COMMON NEUROLOGIC CONDITIONS THAT CAUSE HEADACHES IN THE ELDERLY

Brain tumors: glioblastoma, metastases
Cerebrovascular insufficiency
Cervical spondylosis
Medication-induced migraines
Subdural hematomas after little or no trauma
Temporal arteritis
Trigeminal neuralgia

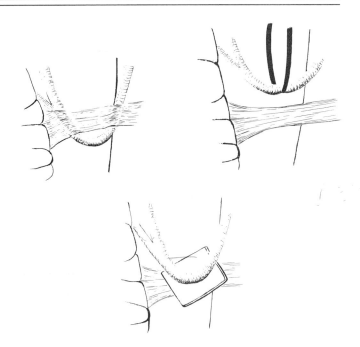

FIGURE 9–5

Top left, Microscopic vascular decompression to alleviate trigeminal neuralgia is a major neurosurgical advance. As pictured through an operating microscope, the brainstem is on the left side of the field, and the trigeminal nerve lies horizontally to the right. The nerve is compressed from below by a large, aberrant artery. *Top right*, A surgical loop plucks the artery out from beneath the nerve. *Bottom*, The artery is then placed over a barrier that protects the trigeminal nerve.

affected arteries reveals giant cells, the condition is properly called *giant cell arteritis*.

Patients are almost always older than 55 years. They usually have a dull, continual headache in one or both temples. Almost pathognomic, but rare, is increasing jaw pain on chewing ("jaw claudication"). In advanced cases, the temporal arteries are red and tender. Temporal arteritis is often accompanied by signs of systemic illness, such as malaise, low-grade fever, and weight loss. It may be only one aspect of polymyalgia rheumatica or other rheumatologic disorder.

Since untreated arterial inflammation leads to arterial occlusion, serious complications may develop when the diagnosis is delayed. Most importantly, ophthalmic artery occlusion will cause blindness, and cerebral artery occlusion will cause cerebral infarctions. In over 90 per cent of cases, an erythrocyte sedimentation rate (ESR) above 40 mm supports the diagnosis. A temporal artery biopsy is the definitive test, but it is often unnecessary, hazardous, or impractical. Timely treatment with high dose steroids will relieve the headaches and prevent complications.

Intracranial Mass Lesions

Brain tumors and subdural hematomas often induce persistent or progressively severe headaches as their first or most bothersome symptom (see Chapters 19 and 20). Headaches that result from brain tumor headaches most often mimic tension because they are bilateral, dull, and less intense than vascular headaches. They worsen when intracranial pressure is raised, as when people bend over, cough, or strain at stool, and during early morning REM sleep. Although brain tumors notoriously wake patients up, that pattern is present in less than half the patients, and moreover, numerous other headache conditions begin during sleep: migraines, cluster headaches, carbon dioxide retention, sleep apnea, and caffeine withdrawal.

Brain tumor-induced headaches are usually accompanied by at least subtle cognitive and personality changes. If they are not present initially, lateralized signs usually develop within 8 weeks. However, evidence of increased intracranial pressure—papilledema and stupor—may be late or absent. Neurologists tend to order CT or MRI scans in almost all patients with unexplained progressive headaches and, in those with the onset of headaches after 55 years, an ESR.

Chronic Meningitis

CSF:
Lymphocyt ↑
glue ↓
prot ↑

Chronic meningitis, most often from *Cryptococcus*, causes continual, dull headaches that are accompanied by signs of systemic illness and dementia (see Chapter 7). Patients who have impaired immune systems, including the elderly, those taking steroids, and those with AIDS, are particularly susceptible. A CT or MRI scan, which should be performed before a lumbar puncture (LP), may show communicating hydrocephalus. The LP will yield cerebrospinal fluid (CSF) that has a lymphocytic pleocytosis, low glucose concentration, elevated protein concentration, and often specific antigens. Since fungi and tubercle bacilli may take weeks to culture (see Chapter 20), the diagnosis is usually based on the clinical evaluation and preliminary CSF results.

Pseudotumor Cerebri   *benign i. e. HTN.*

Pseudotumor cerebri (benign intracranial hypertension), which stems from idiopathic cerebral edema, occurs predominantly in young obese women who have menstrual irregularities. The intracranial hypertension gives rise to papilledema and a dull, generalized headache. Many patients have a surprising discrepancy between florid papilledema and an otherwise unremarkable examination. In particular, despite marked, generalized cerebral edema, patients have no alteration in their intellect or mood.

CSF pressure can reach levels over 400 mm H_2O. Papilledema may lead to blindness from optic atrophy (see Chapter 12). Treatment usually consists of diuretics, dieting, repeated LPs to drain CSF, and sometimes steroids. In refractory cases, surgeons decompress the system by installing CSF shunts or performing an optic nerve sheath fenestration.

Bacterial Meningitis and Subarachnoid Hemorrhage

Commonly occurring, life-threatening, headache-producing illnesses are bacterial meningitis and subarachnoid hemorrhage. Bacterial meningitis is usually caused by *meningococcus* or *pneumococcus* that often spreads in epidemic fashion among young adults in confined areas, such as dormitories or military training camps. It causes a rapidly developing, severe headache accompanied by photophobia, malaise, fever, and nuchal rigidity. When bacterial meningitis is suspected, the CSF must be examined and treatment started with penicillin or another antibiotic.

Viral infections of the brain, *encephalitis*, or meninges, *meningitis*, cause headaches. These conditions are usually nonspecific clinically and more benign than bacterial infections. They are diagnosed by an LP, CT or MRI, and sometimes EEG.

In contrast to almost all other forms of encephalitis, *Herpes simplex* encephalitis has distinct clinical findings. This virus, which is the most frequent cause of serious, nonepidemic encephalitis, has a predilection for the inferior surface of the frontal and temporal lobes. It causes fever, somnolence, and delirium and, because the temporal lobe is infected, partial complex seizures and memory impairment (amnesia). Bilateral temporal lobe damage in some patients has led to the human variety of the Klüver-Bucy syndrome (see Chapter 16).

The other important, acutely occurring headache is the *subarachnoid hemorrhage* from a ruptured cerebral *berry aneurysm*. Cerebral artery aneurysms —shaped like "berries"—usually develop in the arteries that comprise the circle of Willis (see Fig. 11–2 and Chapter 20). If the arteries are incompletely fused in utero, the weak junctions eventually form an aneurysm. If an aneurysm ruptures, blood spurts into the brain and subarachnoid space, which normally contains clear CSF. After a subarachnoid hemorrhage, blood can be seen on a CT or MRI and in the CSF.

A subarachnoid hemorrhage typically causes a severe headache, prostration, and nuchal rigidity—symptoms similar to those in bacterial meningitis. However, sentinel bleeds ("leaks") or otherwise atypical subarachnoid hemorrhages are not as dramatic. Subarachnoid hemorrhages often occur during exertion, including exercise, straining at stool, and sexual intercourse. They are sometimes misdiagnosed as a common migraine or tension headache. If the CSF is examined several days after a subarachnoid hemorrhage, it will be xanthochromic (yellow) from blood breakdown products.

Although the LP provides important diagnostic information, it frequently leads to a severe headache called the "post-LP headache." As though withdrawal of excessive CSF lets the brain "bounce" unprotected against the inside of the skull, the patient's headache is exacerbated by sitting upright or even rapidly turning the head and neck. The pain often radiates to the back of the neck and is accompanied by nausea. Recommended treatments have included intravenous fluid infusions, bed rest, caffeine, and, to stop CSF leaks from the LP site, instillation of a blood patch.

Monoamine Oxidase Inhibitor (MAOI) and Hemorrhage. A variation of the ruptured congenital aneurysm—almost peculiar to psychiatric practice—is the striking, iatrogenic intracerebral or subarachnoid hemorrhage induced by a hypertensive reaction to MAOI antidepressants. If patients taking these medicines eat tyramine-containing foods or receive particular medications, the interaction can precipitate severe hypertension, excruciating headache, and hemorrhage. High-tyramine foods that must be avoided are aged cheese, pickled herring, Chianti wine, beer with and without alcohol, and numerous other spicy, delectable, and seemingly innocuous staples and appetizers. The medicines that must not be administered with MAOI antidepressants are ones often used by neurologists and psychiatrists. The list includes sumatriptan, meperidine (Demerol), L-dopa (as in Sinemet), sympathomimetics, such as amphetamines, and the entire class of dibenzepin derivatives, which includes carbamazepine (Tegretol) and the tricyclic antidepressants.

Commonly used MAOI antidepressants—isocarboxazid (Marplan), pargyline (Eutron), phenelzine (Nardil), and tranylcypromine (Parnate)—normally cause an accumulation of epinephrine, norepinephrine, and serotonin. Although MAOIs used to treat depression place patients at risk of hypertensive reactions, those used in Parkinson's disease, such as selegiline or deprenyl (Eldepryl), do not hold the same danger. A hypertensive reaction should be treated by intravenous phentolamine (Regitine), which is an alpha-adrenergic blocking agent. Substitutes, which are possibly more readily available, are chlorpromazine and propranolol.

REFERENCES

Abramowicz M (ed): Sumatriptan for migraine. Med Lett *34*: 91–93, 1992

Akpunonu BE, Ahrens J: Sexual headaches: Case report, review, and treatment with calcium blocker. Headache *31*: 141–145, 1991

Breslau N: Migraine, suicide ideation, and suicide attempts. Neurology *42*: 392–395, 1992

Dalessio DJ, Silberstein SD (eds): Wolff's Headache and Other Head Pain (6th ed). New York, Oxford University Press, 1993

Davidoff RA: Migraine: Manifestations, Pathogenesis, and Management. Philadelphia, F.A. Davis, 1994

Finelli PF: Coital cerebral hemorrhage. Neurology *43*: 2683–2685, 1993

Forsyth PA, Posner JB: Headaches in patients with brain tumors: A study of 111 patients. Neurology *43*: 1678–1683, 1993

Headache Classification Committee of the International Headache Society: Classification and diagnostic criteria for headache disorders, cranial neuralgias and facial pain. Cephalalgia *8* (Suppl 7): 1–96, 1988

Jensen R, Brink T, Olesen J: Sodium valproate has a prophylactic effect in migraine without aura. Neurology *44*: 647–651, 1994

Kaufman DM, Solomon S: Migraine visual auras: A medical update for the psychiatrist. Gen Hosp Psychiatry *14*: 162–170, 1992

Kumar KL, Reuler JB: Uncommon headaches: Diagnosis and treatment. J Gen Intern Med *8*: 333–341, 1993

Leibold RA, Yealy DM, Coppola M, et al: Post dural puncture headache: Characteristics, management, and prevention. Ann Emerg Med *22*: 1863–1870, 1993

Lipton RB, Stewart WF: Migraine in the United States: A review of epidemiology and health care use. Neurology *43* (Suppl 3): S6–S10, 1993

Littlewood JT, Glover V, Davies PTG, et al: Red wine as a cause of migraine. Lancet *1*: 558–559, 1988

Mathew NT: Chronic refractory headache. Neurology *43* (Suppl 3): S26–S33, 1993

Ostergaard JR, Kraft M: Benign coital headache. Cephalalgia *12*: 353–355, 1992

Raskin NH: Acute and prophylactic treatment of migraine: Practical approaches and pharmacologic rationale. Neurology *43* (Suppl 3): S39–S42, 1993

Rasmussen BK: Migraine and tension-type headache in a general population: Precipitating factors, female hormones, sleep pattern and relation to lifestyle. Pain *53*: 65–72, 1993

Richards W: The fortification illusions of migraines. Sci Am *224*: 89–96, 1971

Sacks OW: Migraine: Revised and Expanded. Berkeley, University of California Press, 1992

Silberstein SD: The role of sex hormones in headache. Neurology *42* (Suppl 2): 37–42, 1992

Silberstein SD: Tension-type and chronic daily headache. Neurology *43*: 1644–1649, 1993

Silverman K, Evans SM, Strain EC, et al: Withdrawal syndrome after the double-blind cessation of caffeine consumption. N Engl J Med *327*: 1109–1114, 1992

Solomon S, Lipton RB, Newman LC: Clinical features of chronic daily headache. Headache *32*: 325–329, 1992

The Subcutaneous Sumatriptan International Study Group: Treatment of migraine attacks with sumatriptan. N Engl J Med *325*: 316–321, 1991

The Subcutaneous Sumatriptan International Study Group: Treatment of acute cluster headache with sumatriptan. N Engl J Med *325*: 322–326, 1991

Welch KMA: Drug therapy of migraine. N Engl J Med *329*: 1476–1483, 1993

Ziegler DK, Hurwitz A, Preskorn S, et al: Propranolol and amitriptyline in prophylaxis of migraine. Arch Neurol *50*: 825–830, 1993

QUESTIONS and ANSWERS: CHAPTER 9

1–4. A 17-year-old Marine recruit has developed a severe generalized headache, lethargy, and nuchal rigidity.

1. What disease must be considered first?

2. What diagnostic procedure must be performed first?

3. What would the typical result be?

4. What is the therapy?

> ***answer:*** Acute bacterial meningitis, particularly meningococcal meningitis, is a common, often fatal disease in military recruits, schoolchildren, and other young people brought into confined areas. The possibility of bacterial meningitis

merits immediate investigation with a lumbar puncture (LP) for cerebrospinal fluid (CSF) analysis. With bacterial meningitis, the CSF reveals a low glucose concentration (0–40 mg/100 ml), high protein concentration (greater than 100 mg/100 ml), and a polymorphonuclear pleocytosis (over 1000/ml). Although alternatives have been suggested, penicillin, 20 million U/day intravenously, remains the standard treatment.

5–9. A 45-year-old man has had moderate bitemporal headaches and then the gradual onset of stupor over 5 days. He has episodes of unusual, repetitive behavior, complaints of unusual smells, and photophobia. He has fever, delirium, mild nuchal rigidity, and bilateral Babinski signs.

5. What might the episodic behavioral disturbances indicate?

6. What do the delirium and Babinski signs suggest?

7. What is the most common cause of sporadic (nonepidemic) encephalitis?

8. What areas of the brain are particularly susceptible?

9. What are the major sequelae of this infection?

> *answer:* He is having partial complex seizures that usually originate in the temporal lobes. He probably has cerebral as well as meningeal involvement. *Herpes simplex* encephalitis is the most common, nonepidemic encephalitis. *Herpes simplex* encephalitis has a predilection for the temporal lobes, which include portions of the limbic system. Temporal lobe inflammation may cause partial complex seizures and, because of the limbic system involvement, profound memory impairment (amnesia) and in rare cases a human form of the Klüver-Bucy syndrome (see Chapter 16).

10. A young hypertensive woman suddenly develops severe right retro-orbital pain, prostration, and a right third cranial nerve palsy. What is the most likely cause?

> *answer:* Although there are many causes of severe retro-orbital pain, a third nerve palsy indicates that a posterior communicating artery aneurysm has ruptured and caused a subarachnoid hemorrhage.

11. A middle-aged hypertensive man has the sudden onset of the worst headache of his life while watching television. Although he has nausea and vomiting, he is able to speak coherently. What are the likely possible causes?

> *answer:* The symptom, "the worst headache of my life," suggests a cerebral or subarachnoid hemorrhage. Migraine or cluster headaches, which may appear in middle age, might be the correct diagnosis; however, they should be considered only when headaches have become a chronic illness (often requiring months of observation) and when potentially fatal conditions have been excluded.

12. An elderly, depressed man has a moderately severe generalized headache and decreased attention span, but no "hard" findings. What entities should be given special consideration?

> *answer:* Although elderly people are subject to most forms of headaches, they are prone to develop a variety of conditions (see Table 9–6) that probably reflect a depressed immune system; atherosclerotic, inflamed, or fragile cerebral vessels; falls leading to head trauma and thus subdural hematomas; and overmedication. Of course, headaches may be a symptom of depression.

13. What medicines are known to cause headaches?

> *answer:* Nitroglycerin, long-acting vasodilators (e.g., Isordil), and several other anti-anginal medications cause headaches. Reserpine and hydrazaline cause a dull frontal pain and nasal stuffiness. The monamine oxidase (MAO) inhibitors cause hypertensive headaches when foods containing tyramine are eaten. Birth control pills can precipitate or exacerbate migraines.

14–25. Match the disease (Q14–25) with the characteristic symptoms (a–l):

a. Severe ocular pain, "red eye," decreased vision
b. Papilledema, generalized headache, obesity, and menstrual irregularity
c. Mastoid pain followed by facial palsy
d. Lancinating pain in the jaw
e. Moderate headache, focal seizures, fever
f. Mild headache and hemiparesis after a fortification scotoma
g. Chronic pain, depressed sensorium
h. Temporal pain, malaise, jaw claudication, high sedimentation rate
i. Daily dull headaches, inattention, and insomnia
j. Generalized headache, nuchal rigidity
k. Horner's syndrome
l. Headache, nausea, vomiting, diplopia, and ataxia

14. Tic douloureux

    answer: d (Nevralg. Vigemen)

15. Bell's palsy

    answer: c

16. Pseudotumor cerebri

    answer: b

17. Basilar migraine

    answer: l

18. Subarachnoid hemorrhage

    answer: j

19. Temporal arteritis

    answer: h

20. Angle-closure glaucoma

    answer: a

21. Subdural hematoma

    answer: f, g, i, or l

22. Postconcussion headache

    answer: i

23. Medulloblastoma

    answer: l

24. Viral meningitis

    answer: j

25. Hemiplegic migraine

    answer: f

26. What features of a headache suggest that it is a migraine?

    answer: Typically, a migraine is unilateral (in 50 per cent), pulsating, and accompanied by autonomic nervous system dysfunction, e.g., nausea, vomiting, fatigue, and diaphoresis. Migraine with aura (classic migraine), which is relatively infrequent (only 15 per cent of migraine sufferers have this variety) is preceded by visual scotoma or other hallucinations.

27. What are common precipitants of migraine headaches?

answer: Menses, glare, alcohol, missing meals, REM sleep, too much as well as too little sleep, and relief of stress may precipitate migraines. REM sleep, however, is more closely associated with the development of cluster headaches.

28. How do migraine headaches in children differ from those in adults?

answer: Although patients of all ages may have autonomic dysfunction, these symptoms may be the primary or exclusive manifestation of migraines in children. Children are also more prone than adults to develop ophthalmoplegic and basilar artery migraine. They are also more likely to have behavioral disturbances, such as agitation, withdrawal, or stupor. They are particularly prone to have cyclic vomiting and abdominal pain as a manifestation of migraine.

29. Which neurologic disorders cause visual hallucinations?

answer: Migraines with auras (classic migraines), seizures originating in the temporal or occipital lobes, narcolepsy, hallucinogens (PCP and LSD), and alcohol withdrawal (DTs) all may precipitate visual hallucinations.

30. In which parts of the brain are serotonin-containing neurons concentrated?

a. Limbic system
b. Frontal lobes
c. Dorsal raphe nucleus
d. Cerebellum

answer: c

31. In regard to migraine, to which process does "cortical depression" refer?

a. The organically based changes in affect that accompany migraines
b. The wave of neuron hypometabolism that, according to one theory, causes the migraine
c. The inability of the cortex to respond to stimulate during the migraine

answer: b

32. What does "xanthochromic" CSF indicate?

a. The CSF is yellow.
b. Subarachnoid bleeding probably occurred within the previous several days.
c. The serum bilirubin concentration or CSF protein concentration may be highly elevated.

answer: a, b, c

33. What are signs of *Herpes simplex* encephalitis?

a. Partial complex seizures
b. Amnesia
c. Klüver-Bucy syndrome
d. Hemorrhagic lesions in the temporal lobes

answer: a–d. The *Herpes simplex* virus, which is the most common cause of nonepidemic encephalitis, invades the undersurface of the brain where it invades the temporal and frontal lobes. Damage to those regions, which is hemorrhagic, causes seizures, limbic system impairment, and rarely changes in sexuality, oral behavior, and aggressiveness.

34–37. Do these headaches (34–37) respond to sleep?

34. Classical migraine

answer: Yes. Sleep typically relieves migraines, but it may precipitate them.

35. Trigeminal neuralgia

answer: Yes. Trigeminal neuralgia does not disturb sleep.

36. Cluster

answer: No. In fact, REM sleep typically precipitates cluster headaches.

37.   Temporal arteritis

answer: No. Temporal arteritis is independent of sleep.

38–44.   Which of these headaches typically awaken the patient from sleep?

38.   Migraine

answer: Yes

39.   Sleep apnea

answer: Yes

40.   Brain tumor

answer: Yes

41.   Subdural hematoma

answer: Yes

42.   Tension

answer: No

43.   Cluster headaches

answer: Yes

44.   Chronic obstructive pulmonary disease

answer: Yes

45.   In what stage of sleep do migraine and cluster headaches begin?

answer: REM

46.   What common laboratory tests are abnormal with migraine headaches?

answer: None.

47.   A group of many severe periorbital headaches occurs every winter when the patient goes to Miami. Of which kind of headache is this pattern typical?

answer: A cluster headache. The grouping of the headaches is most important.

48.   What diseases or conditions cost industry the largest number of man-hours?

answer: Low back pain and headache

49–51.   Which of the following headaches follow family patterns?

49.   Migraine headaches

answer: Yes

50.   Cluster headaches

answer: No

51.   Tension headaches

answer: Yes

52–56.   Which medicines (a–h) are useful for the following headaches?

a.   Methysergide (Sansert)
b.   Propranolol (Inderal)
c.   Cafergot
d.   Carbamazepine
e.   Aspirin, acetaminophen, caffeine, barbiturate compounds

f. Lithium
g. Sumatriptan
h. None of the above

52. Tension headaches
answer: e

53. Infrequently occurring migraine with aura (classic migraine)
answer: c, g, and, for infrequent headaches, e

54. Frequent, severe migraine without aura (common migraine)
answer: a, b, g

55. Temporal arteritis
answer: h

56. Trigeminal neuralgia
answer: d

57–60. What are the prominent adverse effects of the following medications?

57. Methysergide (Sansert)
answer: Retroperitoneal, pleural, and cardiac fibrosis

58. Propranolol (Inderal)
answer: Bradycardia, asthma, cardiac failure, and fatigue

59. Cafergot
answer: Nausea and vomiting in acute stage; vascular spasm, claudication, and muscle cramps with prolonged use, i.e., ergotism

60. Aspirin
answer: Painful gastric distress, gastroduodenal bleeding, and easy bruisability

61. Which headache variety is cyclic or periodic, develops only in men, and responds to lithium treatment?
answer: Cluster headaches were initially treated with lithium because of their periodicity similar to manic-depressive illness.

62. Which variety of headache is partly or entirely genetically transmitted?
a. Cluster
b. Trigeminal neuralgia
c. Giant cell arteritis
d. Migraine
e. Pseudotumor cerebri
f. Hemiplegic migraines
answer: d (partly), f (definitely)

63. Which headaches are associated with mood changes?
a. Cluster
b. Trigeminal neuralgia
c. Giant cell arteritis
d. Migraine
e. Pseudotumor cerebri
answer: d

64. Which headache variety occurs more often in men than women?
a. Classic migraine
b. Common migraine
c. Pseudotumor cerebri
d. Trigeminal neuralgia
e. Tension headaches
f. Cluster headaches
answer: f

65. Which are CNS pain-sensitive structures?

a. Optic nerves
b. Meninges

c. Cerebral neurons
d. Ventricles

answer: a, b

66–73. Match the headache (Q66–73) with its most likely cause (a–l):

a. Giant cell inflammation of extra- and intracranial arteries
b. Autonomic nervous system dysfunction
c. Vascular compression of the trigeminal nerve
d. Nitrites
e. Monosodium glutamate (MSG)
f. Cerebral edema
g. Nightmares
h. REM sleep
i. NREM sleep
j. Night terrors
k. Cerebral artery as well as coronary artery effects
l. Spread of infection to cause meningitis or a brain abscess

66. Tic douloureux

answer: c

67. Hot-dog headache

answer: d

68. Sinusitis with seizures

answer: l

69. Pseudotumor cerebri

answer: f

70. Temporal arteritis

answer: a

71. Chinese restaurant syndrome

answer: e

72. Nocturnal migraine

answer: h

73. Anti-anginal medication-induced headaches

answer: k

74. Which of the following are valid reasons why tricyclic antidepressants (TCA) are helpful in migraine headaches in people without overt depression?

a. TCA may improve sleep patterns.
b. TCA may increase the concentration of serotonin, which is analgesic.
c. TCA are analgesic themselves.
d. TCA are endorphins.
e. These patients may have occult depression.

answer: a, b, c, e

75. In the treatment of migraines, why is rectal or parenteral administration preferable to oral administration of vasoconstrictors, such as ergotamine?

answer: Parenteral or rectal vasoconstrictor medication administration produces effective blood levels much faster than oral administration. Early treatment is essential because once vasodilation is established, migraines are relatively refractory to vasoconstriction medications. In addition, when a patient has a migraine, autonomic gastrointestinal disturbances impair the absorption of orally administered medications.

76. Which of the following are indications for changing the emphasis from abortive to prophylactic migraine therapy?

a. More than four migraines monthly
b. Tinnitus from aspirin-containing medications
c. Ergotism
d. Habitual narcotic use
e. Once monthly migraine with aura (classic migraine)

answer: a, b, c, d

77. Which conditions are apt to occur in several family members, although not necessarily on a genetic basis?

a. Temporal arteritis
b. Tuberous sclerosis
c. Multiple sclerosis
d. Migraines
e. Absence (petit mal) seizures
f. Cluster headaches
g. Pick's disease
h. Tension headaches
i. Tourette's syndrome

answer: b, c, d, e, g, h, i

78. When are women's migraines exacerbated?

a. Premenstrual days
b. Menopause
c. Taking oral contraceptives
d. Menarche

answer: all

79. Which type of headache do brain tumors most often cause?

a. Tension
b. Migraine
c. Cluster
d. Subarachnoid hemorrhage
e. Trigeminal neuralgia

answer: a

80. A 35-year-old man, who suffers several migraines a year, developed a uniquely severe headache during sexual intercourse. He described it as "the worst headache of his life." Two evenings later, this headache recurred during masturbation. What advice should be given to the patient?

answer: The patient probably has developed a sexually induced benign headache (coital migraine); however, the development of a uniquely severe headache in any patient, especially when it occurs during vigorous activity, requires further evaluation. In particular, a subarachnoid or intracerebral hemorrhage must be considered. A CT or MRI scan or lumbar puncture, depending upon the circumstances, is usually performed because the possibility of a potentially fatal subarachnoid hemorrhage should always be borne in mind when confronted with a patient with the "worse headache" of his or her life.

81. What are the advantages of sumatriptan over ergotamine in the treatment of acute migraines?

a. Sumatriptan is self-injectable.
b. Sumatriptan does not cause nausea.
c. Sumatriptan is inexpensive.
d. Sumatriptan can be effective after the headache is established.

answer: a, b, d

82. Which are causes of the entity called "chronic daily headache" (CDH)?

a. Post-trauma headaches
b. Analgesic abuse
c. Ergotism
d. Depression

e. Narcotic abuse
f. Cluster headaches
g. Trigeminal neuralgia

answer: a−e

83. Which cranial nerves innervate the meninges?

a. Olfactory
b. Oculomotor

c. Trigeminal
d. Facial

answer: c

84. Which of the following statements concerning the role of serotonin in migraine are true?

a. Serotonin (5HT) is metabolized to 5-hydroxyindolacteic acid (5HIAA).
b. 5HT concentration falls at the onset of the attack.
c. Sumatriptan, dihydroergotamine, and ergotamine act on serotonin receptors.
d. Serotonin-containing neurons are concentrated in the dorsal raphe.

answer: all

10 Seizures

Seizures are characterized by specific clinical features and electroencephalographic (EEG) patterns and are associated with distinctive etiologies, age at onset, and medical treatment (anticonvulsants). A tendency to have recurrent seizures, *epilepsy*, affects about 6 of every 1000 people.

Seizures can mimic psychiatric disturbances, have prominent cognitive and affective components, and be precipitated by psychotropic medicines. The EEG, which is the most specific laboratory test for seizures, is also helpful in the diagnosis of many other neurologic conditions. This chapter concentrates on partial complex seizures and their neuropsychologic traits within a review of the clinical, EEG, and treatment aspects of the major varieties of seizures.

THE ELECTROENCEPHALOGRAM (EEG)

Normal and Abnormal

The routine EEG records cerebral electrical activity detected by "surface" or "scalp" electrodes (Fig. 10–1). Four frequency bands of cerebral activity, represented by Greek letters, are detectable over certain parts of the brain and under particular conditions (Table 10–1).

EEG readers first determine the display of the electrodes (the EEG *montage*). They also note the time scale, which is determined by vertical lines on the EEG paper or displayed as a 1-second horizontal bar (Fig. 10–1). Although approaches vary, readers then determine its *dominant* or *background rhythm* (see below), organization, and symmetry. Abnormal patterns, especially if they occur in paroxysms, are noted and given special attention. All of these features are judged in the context of the patient being awake, unresponsive, or asleep.

The normal dominant or background EEG activity is in the *alpha* range of 8 to 13 cycles-per-second, or Hertz (Hz), and occurs over the occipital region (Fig. 10–2). Alpha activity is prominent when individuals are relaxed with their eyes closed, but it disappears if they open their eyes, concentrate, or become anxious. Thus, alpha activity reflects an anxiety-free state and is a guideline in biofeedback, "alpha training," and other behavior modification techniques. Alpha activity is also lost when people fall asleep or take any medicine that affects mental function. It typically slows in the elderly and in almost every neurologic illness that affects the brain. However, in the early stages of Alzheimer's disease, alpha activity, although slower than average, may remain at or above 8 Hz.

Beta activity, frequencies faster than 13 Hz, usually has relatively low voltage and overlies the frontal lobes. Although present in normal persons, beta activity is prominent when people are concentrating, anxious, or taking minor tranquilizers.

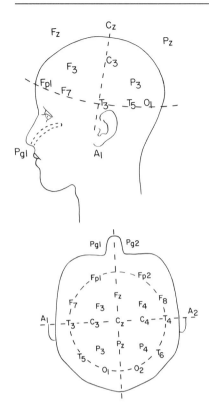

FIGURE 10-1

In the standard array of scalp electrodes, most are named for the underlying cerebral lobe. Odd-numbered ones are on the left and even-numbered ones on the right. The P_g electrodes are from the nasopharyngeal leads; the C electrodes, the center of the skull; and the A electrodes, the ears.

Theta (4- to 7-Hz) and *delta* (1- to 3-Hz) frequencies are normally detected in children, in all people as they enter deep sleep, and in many people with trivial disturbances; however, these slow frequencies are usually absent in healthy, alert adults. When present diffusely over the entire brain, theta or delta activity may indicate a degenerative illness or metabolic derangement. When found continuously over a particular area with *phase reversal* (Fig. 10–3), these slow activities suggest a cerebral lesion, but their absence certainly does not exclude one.

Whatever their frequency, unusually pointed waves—"sharp waves" or "spikes"—may suggest a cerebral lesion and a predisposition to seizures. When they are "phase reversed," spikes or sharp waves indicate an irritative focus that has the potential to produce a seizure. However, this EEG abnormality alone does not prove that a patient has epilepsy.

Seizures

The EEG is most useful in diagnosing and categorizing seizures. During a seizure (*ictus*), the EEG reveals *paroxysmal* EEG activity that usually consists

TABLE 10-1.   COMMON EEG RHYTHMS

Activity	Hz (cycles/sec)	Usual Location
Alpha	8–13	Posterior
Beta	>13	Anterior
Theta	4–7	Generalized[a]
Delta	1–3	Generalized[a]

[a]May be focal.

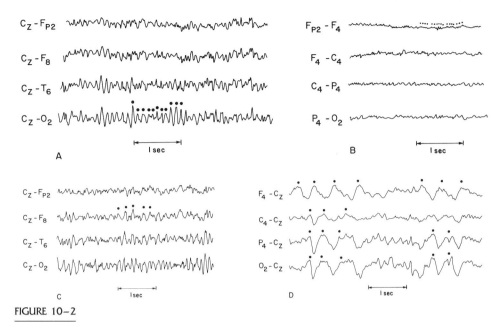

FIGURE 10–2

A, Alpha activity is the regular 11-Hz activity overlying the occipital lobe. *B, Beta* activity is the low-voltage, irregular 17-Hz activity overlying the frontal lobe. *C, Theta* activity is the 5-Hz activity overlying the right frontal lobe. *D, Delta* activity is the high-voltage 2- to 3-Hz activity present over the entire hemisphere.

of bursts of spikes, slow waves, or complexes of spike-and-wave or polyspike-and-waves. Unfortunately, ictal EEGs may be obscured by muscle or movement artifacts. After the seizure, in the *postictal period*, EEGs usually show only low-voltage activity, *postictal depression*, often followed by diffuse high-voltage slowing.

EEGs obtained between seizures, in the *interictal period*, contain specific abnormalities that support a diagnosis in up to 80 per cent of epilepsy patients. However, about 20 per cent of epilepsy patients have normal interictal EEGs. Thus, normal interictal EEGs do not exclude a diagnosis of seizures. Moreover, their value is further confused by the finding that about 15 per cent of the normal population has nonspecific EEG changes, such as an occasional slow wave or spike. These same EEG changes also confound EEG studies of patients having various neurologic, psychiatric, or medication-induced disorders.

In patients suspected of having epilepsy, several maneuvers are used to evoke characteristic EEG abnormalities. Such patients are usually asked to hyperventilate for 3 minutes or to look toward a stroboscopic light while an EEG is obtained. If these maneuvers do not yield diagnostic information and a strong suspicion of seizures persists, an EEG is performed after sleep deprivation. In about 15 per cent of epileptic patients, a *sleep-deprived EEG* reveals abnormalities not apparent in routine studies.

In some epilepsy patients, specially placed electrodes will reveal abnormalities undetectable by ordinary scalp electrodes. For example, anterior temporal scalp, nasopharyngeal, or sphenoidal electrodes can detect discharges from the inferior-medial (mesial or medial) surface of the temporal lobe (Fig. 10–4). Electrodes surgically implanted in the subdural space or within the cerebral cortex can pinpoint an epileptic focus. They can also demonstrate

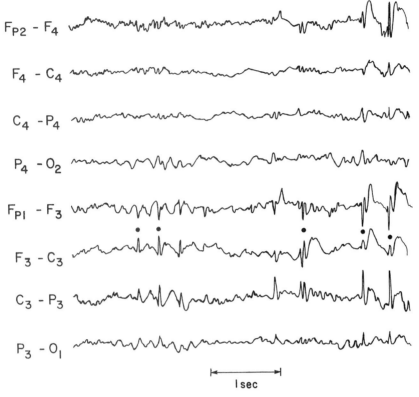

FIGURE 10-3

This montage shows four channels from the right side above four from the left. Each side progresses from the frontal to the occipital region. On at least six occasions (marked by dots), sharp waves and spikes, in *phase reversal*, appear to point toward each other. They originate from the F_3 electrode, which is over the left frontal lobe. A finding of such isolated, phase-reversed sharp waves is associated with seizures; however, without additional clinical or EEG evidence, it is insufficient for diagnostic purposes.

that areas of the brain that appear to be a seizure focus only reflect ("mirror") the actual focus.

Intensive EEG-video monitoring consists of several days of continuous, split-screen videotaped clinical and EEG recordings of seizures, changes in behavior, and effects of sleep (or sleep deprivation). Serum anticonvulsant concentrations and various physiologic data can be monitored and correlated with seizures. EEG-video monitoring is extremely useful in diagnosing, classifying, and determining the frequency of seizures; evaluating patients for epilepsy surgery; treating patients who seem to suffer from *refractory seizures* (frequent seizures that seem unaffected by anticonvulsants); and identifying disorders that mimic seizures.

Routine, office-based *EEG brain mapping,* with surface or scalp electrodes, consists of topographic displays and automatic comparisons to normal EEG data. This technique has serious, inherent problems. It cannot diagnose epilepsy because the prolonged tracings "average out" important transient abnormalities, such as spikes. They also tend to misinterpret normal variants. In contrast, EEG data mapped from electrodes implanted in the dura, subdural, or brain itself are valuable in locating a seizure focus.

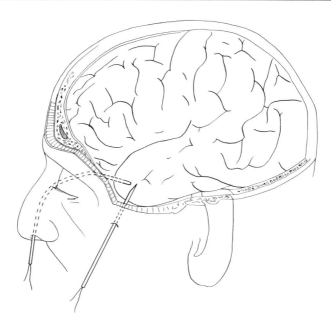

FIGURE 10-4

Nasopharyngeal electrodes, which are inserted through the nostrils, reach the posterior pharynx. There, separated by the thin sphenoid bone, they are adjacent to the medial surface of the temporal lobe, which is the focus or origin of about 80 per cent of partial complex seizures. (Refer to figures in Chapter 20 to see the relatively great distance between the medial surface of the temporal lobe and the scalp, and also the close relationship between the temporal lobe and the sphenoid bone). *Sphenoidal* electrodes are inserted through the skin to reach the lateral, external surface of the sphenoid wing. Electrodes in this location are near the inferior surface of the temporal lobe. (However, specially placed scalp electrodes, new arrays, and critical reading of the EEG may be just as accurate.)

Toxic-Metabolic Encephalopathy

The EEG is useful in detecting toxic-metabolic encephalopathy or "delirium" produced by hepatic or renal failure, medicines, illicit drugs, or systemic illnesses. During the initial phase of these conditions, when patients have only subtle behavioral or cognitive disturbances, the EEG loses alpha activity and shows generalized theta and delta activity. In addition, hepatic and uremic encephalopathy are characteristically associated with *triphasic waves* (Fig. 10-5), which, in hepatic failure, may appear before the bilirubin levels rise. Equally important, a normal EEG virtually excludes a toxic-metabolic encephalopathy.

Dementia

In early Alzheimer's disease, the background alpha activity characteristically slows from about 10 to 12 Hz down to 8 Hz. This slowing is subtle and, especially for people older than 65 years, remains within the normal range. In moderately advanced Alzheimer's disease, however, the background EEG is unequivocally slow. Eventually, the EEG becomes disorganized.

Multi-infarct dementia also induces EEG abnormalities. Although multi-infarct EEG changes may be unilateral or asymmetric if the underlying infarctions are asymmetric (see Chapters 7 and 11), the EEG cannot reliably differentiate between multi-infarct dementia and Alzheimer's disease.

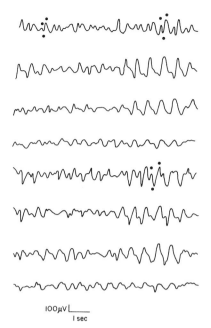

100μV └──
    I sec

FIGURE 10–5

This EEG obtained from a patient with hepatic encephalopathy reveals typical *triphasic waves,* which can be seen in the first and fifth channel. There is also a lack of organized background activity—ordinarily seen clearly in the lowermost channels—consisting of medium-voltage alpha frequency over the occipital lobes.

In contrast, the EEG is almost definitive in diagnosing subacute sclerosing panencephalitis (SSPE) and Creutzfeldt-Jakob disease (see Chapter 7). In these conditions in which dementia is accompanied by myoclonic jerks, the EEG shows *periodic complexes* (Fig. 10–6).

The EEG is also effective in distinguishing *pseudodementia* from dementia (see Chapter 7). In pseudodementia, the EEG is normal or shows only slightly slowed background activity, but in advanced dementia from almost any cause, it shows theta and delta activity. Of course, in the many patients who have a mixture of depression and mild dementia, the EEG cannot measure the relative contribution of each condition.

Altered States of Awareness

The EEG shows distinctive changes during normal sleep's progressively deeper stages and dreaming. Coupled with monitors of ocular movement and muscle activity in the polysomnogram (PSG), the EEG is critical in diagnosing sleep disturbances (see Chapter 17).

The EEG is useful in diagnosing the *locked-in syndrome,* a condition in which a patient might appear to be comatose, but is fully alert and cognizant (see Chapters 2 and 11). People in the locked-in syndrome usually have sustained infarctions in their pons or medulla. Thus, they cannot speak or move their trunk or limbs. However, since their cerebral hemispheres and upper brainstem are normal, these otherwise devastated people are alert, have normal cerebral activity including cognitive function, and have a normal EEG.

The locked-in syndrome must be differentiated from the *persistent vegetative state.* This condition typically follows marked cerebral cortex anoxia from cardiac arrest, drug overdose, or carbon monoxide poisoning. Because these insults lead to extensive cerebral cortex injury, patients have profound dementia accompanied by an inability to speak or move. Their "vegetative functions," such as digesting food and breathing, continue, and their eyes open

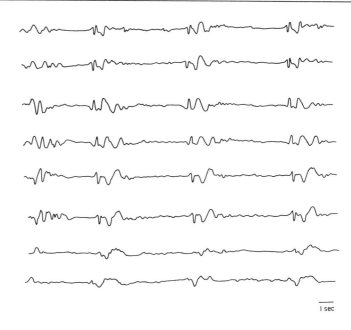

1 sec

FIGURE 10-6

Periodic complexes are seen in all channels as four fairly regular bursts of electrical activity followed by minimal activity, which is termed "burst suppression." Periodic complexes are associated with myoclonic jerks, and together they are cardinal features of two illnesses characterized by dementia: subacute sclerosing panencephalitis (SSPE), which occurs in children, and Creutzfeldt-Jakob disease, which occurs in the elderly (see Chapter 7).

and close. As would be expected after extensive cerebral cortical damage, the EEG is usually slow and disorganized, i.e., markedly abnormal.

Finally, if the EEG detects no electrical activity—that is, shows *electrocerebral silence*—in the absence of extenuating conditions, such as hypothermia and barbiturate overdose, it can be instrumental in declaring death. Making the determination before the heart stops beating is important for harvesting organs, deciding medical-legal situations, and for management of severely brain injured patients.

Structural Lesions

The EEG does not reliably detect or exclude structural lesions that cause seizures, such as brain tumors, abscesses, strokes, or subdural hematomas. It is normal in many of these conditions. When abnormal, it cannot distinguish among them. Computed tomography (CT) and especially magnetic resonance imaging (MRI) are the standard tests that, despite their expense, are cost effective in detecting structural lesions that cause seizures. The CT is usually satisfactory. However, mesial temporal sclerosis, which underlies many partial complex seizures, is a special situation where the MRI is superior to the CT (see below).

Psychiatric Disturbances

Although the EEG is useful for diagnosing toxic-metabolic encephalopathy, some of the dementias, and the persistent vegetative state, it is inadequate for diagnosing most other illnesses characterized by impaired mentation. There is no consensus on the nature or frequency of various EEG abnormalities in psychiatric illnesses. Furthermore, the EEGs in psychiatric illnesses with virtually any neurologic component show at least minor, nonspecific EEG abnormalities.

Antipsychotic, antidepressant, anticonvulsant, and other psychotropic medications induce EEG abnormalities that may be prominent and persist for up to 2 months after medications are withdrawn. Benzodiazepines and barbiturates typically produce beta activity. Otherwise, psychotropic medications give rise to EEG changes that vary with the dose and are nonspecific, such as background slowing, intermittent theta and delta activity, increased beta activity, and sharp waves.

Sometimes antidepressant and antipsychotic agents do more than produce EEG changes. Many precipitate seizures or, at least, increase a patient's tendency to have seizures (see below).

Electroconvulsive therapy (ECT) also induces EEG changes. During and immediately after ECT, EEG changes resemble those of a generalized tonic-clonic seizure and its aftermath. With increasing numbers of ECT treatments, EEG slow-wave activity over the frontal lobes or the entire cerebrum lasts up to 3 months. Although ECT-induced EEG slowing is associated with memory impairment, it is also associated with a more effective treatment of depression. When ECT is unilateral, EEG slowing is less pronounced and more restricted to the treated side.

VARIETIES OF SEIZURES

The two major categories of seizures are *partial seizures* and *primary generalized seizures (generalized seizures)*. Most partial seizures are classified either as *partial with elementary symptoms* or *partial with complex symptoms*. Most generalized seizures are classified as either *absences* or *tonic-clonic seizures* (Table 10–2).

Partial seizures are said to have *elementary* symptoms when their clinical manifestation is only a particular movement or sensation. Impaired consciousness, with or without psychologic abnormalities, constitutes a *complex* symptom. Both varieties of partial seizures originate from paroxysmal electrical discharges in a discrete region of the cerebral cortex—the *focus*. For example, partial seizures with motor symptoms are attributed to a focus in the contralateral frontal lobe.

TABLE 10–2. A MODIFIED VERSION OF THE INTERNATIONAL CLASSIFICATION OF EPILEPSIES

Partial (or focal) epilepsies
  Partial seizures with elementary symptomatology:
    Without impairment of consciousness
  Partial seizures with complex symptomatology: *With*
    impairment of consciousness
  Partial seizures with secondary generalization
Generalized epilepsies
  Primary generalized epilepsies
    Absences (petit mal)
    Tonic-clonic (grand mal)

Partial and other seizures consist of similar, *stereotyped* symptoms for the patient in almost every episode. Thus, variable symptoms suggest a nonseizure disorder.

The EEG during and between partial seizures shows abnormalities in electrodes overlying the focus. Because neither the entire cortex nor the deep structures are incorporated into a partial seizure, consciousness is preserved.

Although most partial seizures last between several seconds and several minutes, in a condition known as *epilepsia partialis continua* or *focal status epilepticus*, these seizures continue for many hours or days. While the discharge remains confined to its focus, the original symptoms persist. The symptoms may interfere with complex mental and physical activity, but routine tasks can continue *despite* the seizure.

More often, the cerebral cortex discharges spread in a slow, brush-fire-like manner to include adjacent areas of the cortex and create additional symptoms. Discharges can spread over the entire cortex, sometimes traveling through the corpus callosum to the other cerebral hemisphere. If the entire cerebral cortex is engulfed, *secondary generalization*, patients lose consciousness, develop bilateral motor activity, and have generalized EEG abnormalities.

In primary generalized seizures, in contrast to partial seizures with secondary generalization, discharges are propagated diffusely from the thalamus or other subcortical structures. They immediately spread upward to excite the entire cerebral cortex. Primary generalized seizures are bilateral, symmetric, and without focal clinical or EEG findings.

Usually caused by a genetic propensity or metabolic aberration, primary generalized seizures are characterized by unconsciousness and generalized EEG abnormalities; however, they do not necessarily generate gross motor activity. Generalized seizures can persist for many hours, in which case they become a life-threatening condition, *generalized status epilepticus.*

Partial Elementary Seizures

Partial seizures with elementary *motor* symptoms, formerly called "focal motor seizures," usually consist of rhythmic jerking (clonic movement) of a body part that may be as limited as one finger or as extensive as an entire side (Fig. 10–7). These seizures can develop into focal status epilepticus or undergo secondary generalization. Sometimes, in a "Jacksonian march," a seizure discharge spreads along the motor cortex, and movements that began in a finger extend to the entire arm and then to the face. After any partial motor seizure, affected muscles may be weakened. A postictal (Todd's) monoparesis or hemiparesis may persist for up to 24 hours. Thus, the differential diagnosis of transient hemiparesis includes transient ischemic attacks (TIAs), hemiplegic migraines, psychogenic disturbances, and Todd's hemiparesis.

Seizures with elementary *sensory* symptoms, which usually are attributed to a focus in the parietal lobe's sensory cortex, typically consist of tingling or burning paresthesias in regions of the body that have extensive cortical representation, such as the face. Sometimes sensory loss, which is a "negative symptom," might be a seizure's only manifestation.

Partial elementary seizures with "special sensory" symptoms consist of specific, simple auditory, visual, or olfactory sensations. Although these symptoms are so vivid that they can be described as "hallucinations," patients readily recognize them as manifestations of cerebral dysfunction, rather than actual events.

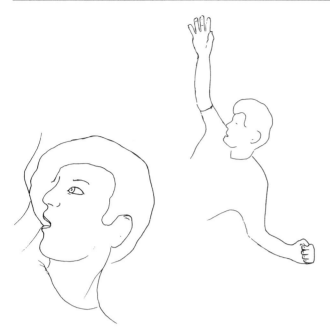

FIGURE 10–7

A patient having a partial seizure with motor symptoms has his head, neck, and eyes deviated toward the right, his right arm extended, and his left flexed. This "adversive posture" suggests that a seizure originated in the left frontal lobe, i.e., in the cerebrum contralateral to the body's direction.

Auditory symptoms are usually repetitive noises, musical notes, or single words that have no meaning. They are attributable to temporal lobe lesions. Visual symptoms, which are attributable to occipital lesions, usually are perceived as relatively simple or elementary bright lines, spots, or splotches of color that move slowly across the visual field or, like a view through a kaleidoscope, stars rotating around the center of vision. In contrast, elaborate visual phenomena, alone or combined with other sensory symptoms or emotional changes, are "complex" symptoms that must be differentiated from elementary symptoms and other visual hallucinations (see Table 9–3 and Chapter 12).

Olfactory symptoms usually consist of smelling vaguely recognizable odors, such as the most frequent one, burning rubber. Since olfactory hallucinations usually result from discharges in the anterior inferior tip of the temporal lobe, the *uncus*, partial seizures with olfactory symptoms are often called *uncinate seizures* or *fits*. If discharges spread from the uncus to engulf a larger area of the temporal lobe, partial complex seizures ensue.

EEG and Etiology.   During partial elementary seizures, EEGs show spikes, slow waves, or spike-wave complexes overlying the seizure focus. For example, during seizures with motor symptoms, EEG abnormalities may be prominent in channels over the frontal lobe (Fig. 10–8), and during the interictal period, EEGs may still show occasional spikes in the same channels.

Depending mostly on the patient's age at the seizures' onset, particular lesions may be suspected. When young children develop these seizures, frequent causes are congenital cerebral injuries, neonatal meningitis, and neurocutaneous disorders, such as tuberous sclerosis and Sturge-Weber syndrome (see Chapter 13). Thus, many children have combinations of epilepsy, mental retardation, and "cerebral palsy."

In young adults, common causes of partial elementary seizures are head trauma, arteriovenous malformations (AVMs), and previously asymptomatic congenital injuries. Post-traumatic seizures are not associated with trivial head injuries, but with trauma that has caused a loss of consciousness for more than 30 minutes, a skull fracture that is depressed (not just linear), or a penetrating

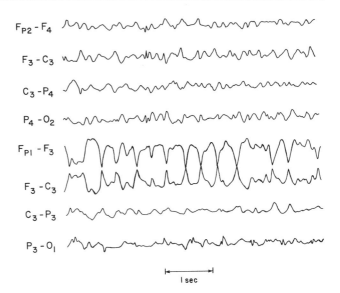

FIGURE 10-8

This EEG obtained during a partial seizure with motor symptoms contains a paroxysm of 4-Hz sharp wave activity with phase reversals referable to the F_3 electrode. Since this electrode overlies the left frontal region, the seizure probably consists of right face or arm motor activity and, in 50 per cent of cases, a deviation of the head and eyes to the right.

wound. Young adults with major psychiatric disturbances, particularly autism, are prone to have seizures.

Drug and alcohol abuse—which carries numerous, ominous, neurologic ramifications—should be considered in young adults presenting with a seizure. Often in the setting of psychotic or otherwise abnormal behavior, cocaine, phencyclidine (PCP), and amphetamines cause focal or generalized seizures within an hour of their administration. Cocaine induces seizures regardless of the route of administration: injecting, inhaling, smoking, sucking, or swallowing. Rather than occurring immediately after the use of illicit substances, seizures follow—by several days—withdrawal from benzodiazepines (especially alprazolam) and alcohol when taken in daily, high doses. Once they begin, withdrawal seizures also often evolve into status epilepticus. Also, a profound overdose of benzodiazepines or alcohol can produce a seizure. (Most cases of benzodiazepine-withdrawal seizures are associated with prescription medications, rather than "street" drugs.)

Although seizures associated with drug or alcohol abuse do not necessarily constitute epilepsy, they reveal dependency or addiction. Moreover, a drug-related seizure may have been caused by an acute, life-threatening neurologic problem, rather than the drug itself. Cocaine, for example, routinely causes cerebral hemorrhages that cause seizures. Similarly, heroin and other drugs, which themselves usually do not cause seizures, can lead to bacterial endocarditis, acquired immune deficiency syndrome (AIDS), hepatitis, and vasculitis.

Adults aged 40 to 60 years develop seizures most often because of a structural lesion, typically a primary or metastatic brain tumor. Older people are more likely to have sustained a stroke than a tumor. In South and Central Americans, cysticercosis is the most common structural lesion that induces seizures. In young adults with AIDS, it is cerebral toxoplasmosis.

Partial Complex Seizures

Partial complex seizures usually begin between patients' late childhood and their early thirties. Affecting about 65 per cent of epilepsy patients, they are the most frequent variety of seizure. EEG-video monitoring studies have defined ictal and postictal seizure manifestations and separated them from non-seizure disturbances. Nevertheless, several important aspects of partial complex seizures remain unclear. One is the genuineness of the broad range of purported ictal symptoms, including violence. Another is the relationship of epilepsy to several interictal neuropsychologic disorders, including certain personality traits, violence, and cognitive impairment.

Before discussing partial complex seizures, however, a preliminary note on nomenclature must be inserted. In the past, less cumbersome but less accurate titles, *psychomotor seizures* and *temporal lobe seizures* or *epilepsy* (*TLE*), have been used. The term "psychomotor seizures" is properly applied only to the rare variety of partial complex seizures with exclusively behavioral abnormalities. Likewise, TLE is inappropriate because the seizure focus in about 10 per cent of cases is not located in the temporal lobe. TLE is also inconsistent with the current classification of seizures based on symptoms, rather than anatomic origin.

Using current nomenclature, the symptoms of partial complex seizures in about 10 per cent of patients include a characteristic premonitory sensation, an *aura*. Not merely a warning, this symptom is actually the first part of the seizure.

During most of a partial complex seizure, patients usually display only a blank stare, and they are inattentive and uncommunicative. They always (by definition) have impaired consciousness. In most cases, they also have partial or complete memory loss, *amnesia*, presumably because the limbic system in the temporal lobe is beset with seizure discharges. Since the amnesia is so striking, it may seem to be a patient's only symptom. (Therefore, partial complex seizures must be strongly considered among the neurologic causes of the acute amnestic syndrome [Table 7–1].)

The only physical signs of partial complex seizures are usually *automatisms*, which are simple, repetitive, and purposeless movements. Automatisms of the face and hands are most common. They include swallowing, kissing, and lip-smacking, or fumbling with clothing, scratching, and rubbing the abdomen (Fig. 10–9). Automatisms are present in more than 80 per cent of complex seizures and are induced more frequently than mental aberrations.

Other physical manifestations are adversive postures (see Fig. 10–7) and performing simple activities, such as standing, walking, and pacing, or even driving; however, these actions may be naturally occurring rote activities that persist despite a seizure. Likewise, about 25 per cent of patients utter brief phrases or unintelligible sounds.

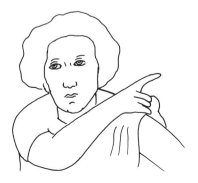

FIGURE 10–9

During partial complex seizures, patients are typically dazed. They perform rudimentary, purposeless actions, such as pulling on their clothing. Repetitive, simple body movements, *automatisms*, such as lip smacking, are present in 80 per cent of cases.

Partial complex seizures that originate or spread to the frontal lobe, *frontal lobe seizures*, produce complex verbal and physical behavior. The manifestations of frontal lobe seizures may be bizarre and consist of movements suggestive of *pseudoseizures* (psychogenic seizures, see below), such as pelvic thrusting and flailing movements.

Regardless of the site of the focus of partial complex seizures, many times actions and words are cued by the environment. For example, a child may clutch and continually stroke a nearby stuffed animal while repeating an endearing phrase. What would distinguish this activity from normal would be the child's impaired consciousness, apparent self-absorption, and subsequent failure to recall the event.

Symptoms might occasionally be elaborate visual or auditory hallucinations accompanied by emotions appropriate to the hallucination. Although these symptoms are notorious, they are rare.

In addition, a wide variety of symptoms could be considered manifestations of seizures; however, certain ones cannot be accepted in isolation. In particular, the various "experiential phenomena," such as *déjà vu, jamais vu*, dreamlike states, mind-body dissociations, and floating feelings, cannot automatically be accepted as seizure symptoms because they are rarely associated with other clinical or any EEG evidence of seizures. Experiential phenomena are too nonspecific and have been so romanticized and popularized that they have virtually no diagnostic value.

Another frequently encountered symptom that has a dubious association with partial complex seizures is the *rising epigastric sensation*. This symptom consists of a perception of a swelling in the abdomen that, as if progressing upward within the body, turns into tightness in the throat and then suffocation. Although it could be an aura, the rising epigastric sensation has a striking similarity to a panic attack, claustrophobia, and *globus hystericus*, a common psychogenic disturbance in which people also feel tightening of the throat and an inability to breathe.

After a partial complex seizure, which usually has a duration of 2 to 3 minutes, patients characteristically experience postictal confusion, clouding of their sensorium, disorientation, a flat affect, and a tendency to sleep. Postictal confusion may be intensified if a seizure involves the brain's language centers, in which case patients may have transient aphasia. Also depending on the focus of the seizure, patients may have a Todd's hemiparesis. For 15 to 30 minutes after the seizure, at least 40 per cent of patients have a markedly elevated serum prolactin concentration. They may also have focal postictal EEG depression.

Whatever their ictal manifestations, most partial complex seizures sooner or later undergo secondary generalization. Thus, a guideline for differentiating them from a recurring psychogenic event is that at least every 1 to 2 years partial complex seizures are complicated by their exploding into generalized seizures.

Another important but rare complication of partial complex seizures is *partial complex status epilepticus*. Despite its prevalence in popular literature as a cause of bizarre behavior, only about two dozen cases have been described in neurologic journals. In this disorder, patients experience up to 24 hours of confusion that is sometimes accompanied by thought and language disorders, automatisms, and other purposeless motor activity. Attacks may mimic schizophrenia and occasionally merit their description, *ictal psychosis*.

Otherwise, partial complex seizures and psychotic episodes are unlikely to be mistaken for each other. Partial complex seizures are not triggered by the environment, last only a few minutes, are stereotyped, necessarily include impaired consciousness, have a postictal period characterized by sleepiness and amnesia, and are followed by a gradual return to the interictal personality, which admittedly might be abnormal. Psychotic episodes, in contrast, often are responsive to the environment, have a duration of at least several days, vary greatly in their manifestations, which often include hypervigilance, and are not followed by sleepiness and amnesia.

Ictal Sex. In many people with or without epilepsy, seizure-like symptoms, including hyperventilation, that occur during sexual activity are simply manifestations of anxiety. During a seizure, patients commonly fumble with buttons or tug at their clothing and thus may seem to partially undress, but they are not exhibitionists or attempting to engage in sex.

Other activity that might be considered sexual is only rudimentary or nonspecific, such as masturbatory movements, scratching of the perineum, and pelvic thrusting. Except for rare instances, seizures are unaccompanied by erotic or interactive sexual behavior. For the most part, partial complex epilepsy patients are hyposexual.

Ictal Violence. EEG-video monitoring has demonstrated that *ictal violence*, which usually consists only of random shoving, pushing, kicking, or verbal abuse, such as screaming, occurs during less than 0.1 per cent of seizures. This behavior is fragmented, unsustained, and unaccompanied by rage or anger. When patients whose consciousness is always impaired naturally combat restraints, they have "resistive violence." Ictal violence is not considered "aggression" because it is neither directed nor purposefully destructive.

During seizures with or without violent manifestations, patients cannot perform sequential activities or interactions with other people or mechanical devices, such as cars or guns. They are unable to commit premeditated violent acts. Few neurologists accept violence, aggression, or criminal activity as the sole manifestation of a partial complex or any other variety of seizure.

Partial Complex Interictal Mental Abnormalities

Personality Changes. Classic studies by Bear, Fedio, and others described distinctive personality traits in patients with "temporal lobe epilepsy." These patients were found to be circumstantial, hyposexual, humorless, "sticky" in interpersonal relations, and overly concerned with general philosophic and religious questions, such as the order of the universe. They characteristically displayed *hypergraphia*, a tendency to write excessively and compulsively, which is typical in mania and schizophrenia.

Related older studies also suggested that different emotional traits depended upon whether the seizure focus was in the right or left temporal lobe. Right-sided foci supposedly predisposed a patient to anger, sadness, and elation and left-sided ones to ruminative and intellectual tendencies.

Recent studies, based on EEG-video monitoring and strict methodology, have either not corroborated those personality traits or found them in as little as 7 per cent of patients. In fact, these same traits were found in patients without epilepsy. The studies also found no difference in personality traits when foci are in different temporal lobes or even other brain areas, and no difference in personality traits between patients with different varieties of epilepsy.

As a general rule, personality disturbances and cognitive impairments (see below)—to the extent that they exist—are associated with a variety of factors that indicate extensive brain damage: the onset of seizures in childhood, episodes of status epilepticus, multiple seizure types, need for two or more anticonvulsants, and signs of brain damage on the neurologic examination, CT, or MRI.

"Schizophreniform Psychosis."   Partial complex seizures are associated in up to 10 per cent of patients with schizophrenia-related symptoms, such as hallucinations, paranoia, and social isolation; however, unlike typical schizophrenic patients, seizure patients' affect is relatively normal, they do not deteriorate, and their families do not have an increased incidence of schizophrenia. These symptoms, subsumed in Slater and Beard's term "schizophreniform psychosis," arise, on the average, when patients are 30 years old and when epilepsy began in childhood, especially between ages 5 and 10 years. Therefore, the schizophreniform psychosis develops more than 10 years after the onset of epilepsy. Patients are likely to have their seizure focus in the left temporal lobe. Pathologic studies show that epilepsy patients with psychosis, compared to those without psychosis, have larger cerebral ventricles, greater periventricular gliosis, and increased focal damage. In contrast, despite having extensive cerebral damage, multiple sclerosis (MS) patients rarely have schizophrenic symptoms.

Although most studies have reported that psychosis is more likely to occur when seizures are poorly controlled, some report that it is precipitated by vigorous anticonvulsant suppression of seizures ("forced normalization," see below). Other studies found that schizophrenic symptoms are associated with seizures that have auras.

In treating acute schizophreniform psychosis or other psychoses in epileptic patients, routine psychiatric treatments should be added to the anticonvulsants regimen, keeping in mind that anticonvulsants interact with haloperidol, chlorpromazine, and other antipsychotic agents. More important, patients with or without epilepsy can have seizures precipitated by antipsychotic agents.

Seizures occur in approximately 1 per cent of patients who receive antipsychotic medications and are associated with high-dose or parenteral administration, brain injury, and, in the majority of cases, a pre-existing seizure disorder. Of those individuals with a pre-existing seizure disorder, seizures that developed with psychotropic medications followed noncompliance with anticonvulsant medications and polypharmacy.

Clozapine (Clozaril) has induced seizures, which were mostly generalized tonic-clonic seizures, in 4 per cent of patients at high doses ($\geq$600 mg/day), but in only 1 per cent at low doses (<300 mg/day). Likewise, in routine doses, risperidone (Risperdal) has not been associated with seizures. Of the standard antipsychotic agents, chlorpromazine carries the highest seizure risk according to some studies; haloperidol, a moderate risk; and thioridazine and fluphenazine, the lowest risk. Lobectomy and similar surgical procedures that reduce the frequency of seizures or even eliminate them do not relieve the schizophreniform disorder.

Cognitive Impairment.   Although most epilepsy patients have normal intelligence, many have either static or progressively severe intellectual impairments. When epilepsy begins in early childhood, 10 to 25 per cent of the children are found to have mental retardation. Children with congenital cerebral injuries often have the well-known triad of motor impairments (cerebral palsy), mental retardation, and seizures (see Chapter 13). In addition, many epileptic children, with or without mental retardation, have been uneducated.

Except for those with absences, epilepsy patients are liable to develop progressive cognitive impairment. Of several factors responsible for their deterioration, the most common ones are frequent seizures and multiple seizure types. Seizures lead to cognitive impairment because, in addition to their biochemical and physiological disruption, they lead to head trauma, cerebral anoxia, and treatment with one or more anticonvulsants. Epileptogenic mesial temporal sclerosis, in particular, progressively damages the surrounding limbic system, which is one of the bases of the memory circuit.

Seizures also reflect underlying brain injury that may be progressive. In certain degenerative illnesses, such as in tuberous sclerosis and the storage diseases, refractory seizures are naturally accompanied by increasingly greater cognitive and motor impairments.

Cognitive decline must also be distinguished from the development of personality disturbances, depression, and other psychiatric complications. These traits could develop singly or together and result from various neurologic problems.

Crime and Violence. Another established, but potentially misleading, interictal trait of epilepsy patients is their high incidence of criminality. For example, among men in prison, the incidence of epilepsy is at least four times as great as in the general population. However, taking the association of crime and epilepsy at face value is liable to be misleading: Crimes of adult epileptic prisoners are no more violent than those of nonepileptic ones, and the prevalence of epilepsy is the same in violent as nonviolent criminals. Also, violent behavior is no more prevalent among patients with partial complex seizures than with other seizures. The consensus is that having epilepsy does not cause crime. However, epilepsy, head trauma, and other brain injuries lead to conditions, such as poor impulse control and lower socioeconomic status, that lead people to crime.

Another aspect of interictal violence is that it tends to occur in epileptic patients who are schizophrenic or mentally retarded. Otherwise, patients' violent and nonviolent seizures have a similar seizure type, frequency, EEG changes, and anticonvulsants. Overall, underlying neurologic, psychiatric, and social disorders—without invoking an additional effect of epilepsy—are sufficient to account for interictal violence, as well as aggressive personality traits.

Depression. Depression is more prevalent in epilepsy patients than in persons with comparable conditions. It occurs particularly in epilepsy patients who have partial complex seizures, are male, or require multiple anticonvulsants. However, the severity of the depression is not related to the duration of epilepsy, seizure frequency, or a family history of depression. Also, epilepsy-associated depression is rarely bipolar. Although depression in epilepsy has been correlated with left-sided temporal lobe foci, the finding is inconsistent, the left hemisphere cannot be assumed to be dominant in epilepsy patients, and any association's practical significance has been exaggerated.

Suicide occurs four to five times more frequently in epilepsy patients, especially those with partial complex seizures, than in the general population. Suicide associated with epilepsy is more likely to be a manifestation of psychotic behavior or borderline personality disorders than depression, psychosocial burdens, or anticonvulsant medications. (Other neurologic illnesses associated with an increased incidence of suicide are MS, Huntington's disease, spinal cord lesions, and AIDS dementia.)

Depression is one of several psychiatric disturbances that may contribute to refractory seizures. Other potential explanations are that epilepsy patients are sometimes surreptitiously noncompliant with their anticonvulsant regimen. They may consciously or unconsciously superimpose pseudoseizures on epileptic seizures. In these situations, valuable diagnostic tests are EEG-video monitoring and frequent determinations of serum anticonvulsant levels. Also, sleep deprivation, whatever its cause, and the use of or withdrawal from drugs or alcohol—depression-associated behavior—may precipitate seizures.

Treatment of depression in epileptic patients is based on medication (antidepressants) more than psychotherapy. Successful medical treatment often produces better control of epilepsy, as well as improvement in mood.

Although the physician can expect success, antidepressants must be given cautiously in epilepsy patients because they can interact with anticonvulsants. Moreover, both the new and old antidepressants, even at therapeutic concentrations, can cause seizures.

Risk factors for seizures in nonepilepsy patients taking antidepressants are a personal or family history of seizures, abnormalities on a pretreatment EEG, underlying brain damage, prior ECT, drug or alcohol use or withdrawal, and concomitant use of other medications. Antidepressant-induced seizures usually occur in the first week of treatment and are related to excessive or sudden elevations in serum concentrations. Physicians must guard against the emergence of structural lesions, such as a brain tumor, that cause both a depressed affect and a seizure. They must also keep in mind that some seizures may result from a deliberate drug overdose and others are actually pseudoseizures.

Clomipramine (Anafranil) has led to seizures in 1.5 percent of patients taking 300 mg/day or less. Seizures are clomipramine's most significant adverse reaction, and the risk does not diminish over time as with most other antidepressants. Until suggested doses were reduced, maprotiline (Ludiomil) and bupropion (Wellbutrin) would also frequently induce seizures. Depending on the dose, imipramine has a seizure rate of 0.1 to 1.1 per cent, and amitriptyline has a lower rate.

The use of serotonin-based antidepressants is rarely complicated by seizures. For example, use of therapeutic doses of Fluoxetine (Prozac) has been complicated by seizures in only 0.2 per cent of cases. Venlafaxine (Effexor) is not associated with seizures.

Alprazolam, lithium, and monamine oxidase inhibitors carry a low incidence of seizures. However, withdrawal from alprazolam and other benzodiazepines can lead to seizures and even status epilepticus.

Although ECT in epilepsy patients may be complicated by prolonged seizures, that complication is rare and readily treated. ECT is not contraindicated in depressed epilepsy patients.

Confusion. Epilepsy patients may develop confusion, which might also be called "delirium" or toxic-metabolic encephalopathy. Confusion has several neurologic and potentially life-threatening causes. In addition, it must be distinguished from both cognitive decline and depression.

Confusion frequently develops in patients with pre-existing cognitive and physical impairments. Its immediate cause is usually anticonvulsant intoxication that is inadvertently induced by changes in the medication regimen or by adding new medications, including psychotropics. However, occasionally patients deliberately induce anticonvulsant intoxications by taking them in excessive quantities or mixing them with alcohol or illicit drugs.

Other causes of confusion include prolonged seizures—partial complex or absence status epilepticus ("nonconvulsive status epilepticus"). They may cause mental changes, but little or no physical manifestations. Seizures also lead to head trauma that can be further complicated by intracranial bleeding.

The postictal period has great diagnostic importance. This period's duration is usually longer than the seizure. Physicians often observe patients only in the postictal state because the seizures occur at home. More important, postictal mental aberrations can mimic serious neurologic or psychiatry illness. Patients are disoriented, amnestic, and possibly aphasic. They are sometimes irrational, agitated, and combative. Their affect is typically flat, and they may have paranoid delusions and hallucinations.

A rare and controversial cause of confusion and other mental impairments is *forced normalization*. In this condition, after anticonvulsants have controlled an epileptic patient's seizures and "forced" the EEG to be normal, the patient develops psychotic behavior. The usual explanation is that seizures had suppressed abnormal behavior.

At the other extreme, abruptly stopping anticonvulsants is unequivocally risky. A flurry of seizures or even status epilepticus may develop after abruptly withdrawing anticonvulsants. The risk is especially great after the withdrawal of benzodiazepines and phenobarbital. Moreover, in *anticonvulsant withdrawal-emergent psychopathology*, anxiety, depression, and other mental aberrations appear in about a third of patients after the withdrawal of anticonvulsants. These conditions are, of course, analogous to *withdrawal emergent dyskinesia*, in which tardive dyskinesia-like movements appear after the withdrawal of antipsychotic agents (see Chapter 18).

The EEG During and After Partial Complex Seizures.   During a partial complex seizure, the EEG typically shows paroxysms of spikes, slow waves, or other abnormalities in channels overlying the temporal or frontotemporal region. Even though the seizure focus may be unilateral, EEG abnormalities may be found bilaterally because of additional foci, interhemispheric projections, or "reflections."

In the interictal period, the routine EEG reveals spikes or spike and slow-wave complexes over the temporal lobes in about 40 per cent of cases. Accompanied by an appropriate history, these EEG abnormalities are specific enough to corroborate the diagnosis. Looking at the situation in reverse, about 90 per cent of persons with anterior temporal spikes on the EEG will have partial complex seizures. Nevertheless, the diagnosis of seizures should not be based on EEG spikes without an appropriate history.

If nasopharyngeal leads, specially placed scalp leads, and sleep recordings are used, EEG abnormalities will be found in as many as 80 per cent of cases (Fig. 10–10). If the diagnosis remains a problem, especially where episodic behavioral abnormalities are believed to result from seizures, EEG-video monitoring should be used. In short, the EEG diagnosis of partial complex seizures should be approached with a routine EEG, which has a 40 per cent yield; an EEG with nasopharyngeal leads during sleep for an 80 per cent yield; and then EEG-video monitoring, with virtually a 100 per cent yield.

Other Tests.   Before embarking on costly tests, the physician should review the clinical situation by looking for cognitive impairments, lateralized signs,

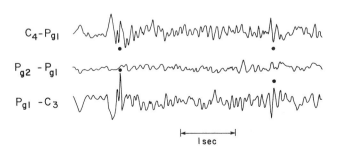

FIGURE 10–10

An interictal EEG with nasopharyngeal electrodes (Pg_1 and Pg_2) shows phase-reversed spikes that routine scalp electrodes may not detect.

and stigmata of the neurocutaneous syndromes. Screening tests, depending on the circumstances, might include alcohol levels, drugs screens, HIV screening, and anticonvulsant levels.

Since partial elementary and partial complex seizures usually originate from structural lesions, CT or MRI scans (see Chapter 20) are routinely performed. Even when the neurologic evaluation is normal, these scans may reveal structural lesions, including temporal lobe atrophy, tuberous sclerosis nodules, strokes, and AVMs. In partial complex epilepsy, where the etiology is often mesial temporal sclerosis, minute vascular malformations, or other cryptic lesions, the MRI with gadolinium is superior to the CT because of its greater resolution and freedom from artifacts produced by the bones surrounding the middle fossa.

A CT or MRI scan is also performed for tonic-clonic seizures because clinical and EEG data may not be able to distinguish between primary generalized seizures and partial seizures with secondary generalization. With drug- or alcohol-withdrawal seizures and absences (see below), these scans may be unnecessary.

Positron emission tomography (PET) has been used to study cerebral metabolism in epilepsy and to plan surgery in epilepsy patients with partial complex seizures. With those seizures, PET studies in the interictal period show that the affected temporal lobe—a region usually far larger than the focus—is hypometabolic. However, PET metabolic alterations are unrelated to the seizure's clinical or EEG manifestations. Moreover, PET's relatively low resolution does not permit precise anatomic correlations.

Magnetoencephalography (MEG) is the plot of magnetic fields that are comparable to the EEG of electric fields. The equipment, which is as expensive as MRI equipment, can be coupled with the EEG. Nevertheless, MEG cannot yet be used reliably for epilepsy or any other illness.

Etiology. Lesions that cause partial complex seizures include not only those that cause partial elementary seizures but also temporal lobe hamartomas, astrocytomas, and especially mesial temporal sclerosis. Probably the most common cause of partial complex seizures, mesial temporal sclerosis is thought to lead to sclerosis of the hippocampus and temporal lobe atrophy. Except for about 10 per cent of cases, as noted previously, the lesion is within the temporal lobe. Like other seizures, partial complex seizures may be precipitated by menses, intercurrent illness, and low anticonvulsant serum concentration.

Anticonvulsants

Although surgery is often indicated (see below), anticonvulsants are the primary treatment for partial, secondarily generalized, and all primary generalized seizures (Table 10–3). Although some controversy remains regarding anticonvulsants' mechanism of action and their specific indications, several guidelines are applicable.

Using a single anticonvulsant, *monotherapy*, is preferable to using two or more anticonvulsants, *polypharmacy*, because this strategy minimizes side effects, noncompliance, and, in most cases, cost. Except in an emergency, anticonvulsants must be introduced slowly. Since anticonvulsants are most often metabolized primarily in the liver, the addition of other medications that undergo hepatic metabolism alters the serum concentration of each. In particular, anticonvulsants interfere with the metabolism of antidepressants, antipsy-

TABLE 10–3.   COMMONLY USED ANTICONVULSANTS[a]

Anticonvulsant	Usual Daily Dose (mg)	Therapeutic Serum Concentration[b] (mg/ml)
Carbamazepine (Tegretol)[c]	600–1200	5–12
Ethosuximide (Zarontin)	2000	40–100
Gabapentin (Neurontin)	900–1800	
Phenytoin (Dilantin)	300–400	10–20
Valproate (Depakote)	1500–2000	50–100

[a]These anticonvulsants have mostly replaced phenobarbital and its closely related anticonvulsant, primidone (Mysoline), which both cause inordinate sedation and cognitive impairments. Also, barbiturates, particularly when used in children and adults with brain damage, may, in a "paradoxical reaction", induce excitement and hyperactivity, rather than sedation.

[b]Recommended concentrations vary and should be altered by the clinical situation. Often a "subtherapeutic level" is sufficient, and increasing the dose will create side effects without improving seizure control.

[c]To reach a steady state, five "half-lives" are required: carbamazepine 4–6 days; phenytoin 5–10 days; and valproate 3–6 days.

chotics, antibacterials, narcotics including methadone, contraceptives, and, with polypharmacy, each other. Anticonvulsants may be safely discontinued in many patients, especially children, but careful planning, slow withdrawal, and subsequent monitoring are necessary.

Side Effects.   Most anticonvulsant side effects are common to the entire class and are apt to complicate their use for psychiatric as well as for neurologic indications. Excessive concentrations cause lethargy, confusion, and, in extreme cases, coma. In particular, phenytoin (hydantoin or diphenylhydantoin [Dilantin]) intoxication causes a well-known combination of nystagmus, ataxia, and dysarthria. Most anticonvulsants, even in therapeutic levels, can cause liver and bone marrow toxicity that is frequent but self-limited and harmless. Similarly, anticonvulsants induce a benign rash shortly after they are initiated. On the other hand, anticonvulsants rarely and unpredictably cause a frequently fatal, fulminant mucocutaneous allergic reaction, the *Stevens-Johnson syndrome* (erythema multiforme), which consists of weeping, often confluent blisters on the mouth, eyes, and skin.

Epilepsy, whether the father or the mother has the disorder, has teratogenic effects. Taking anticonvulsants in pregnancy, especially during the first trimester when the fetus is most vulnerable, further increases the incidence of fetal malformations. Anticonvulsant teratogenicity is widespread, but not specific. Although phenobarbital may be the most dangerous of the commonly used anticonvulsants, none is risk free, and none induces a particular malformation. For example, the *fetal hydantoin syndrome*, which includes craniofacial abnormalities and limb defects, is not peculiar to hydantoin (phenytoin [Dilantin]). The more serious fetal malformations of meningomyelocele and other neural tube defects (see Chapter 13) have been associated with both carbamazepine and valproate. Anticonvulsants can also induce abnormalities later in life. For example, hydantoin therapy begun before puberty may retard normal cerebellar growth.

Anticonvulsants can superimpose cognitive impairments on those originating from the underlying brain damage. Most often, anticonvulsant-induced cognitive impairment results from polypharmacy, excessive anticonvulsant concentration, use of phenobarbital or primidone, or too rapid introduction of the medication.

The cognitive impairments may consist of memory difficulties, intellectual dulling, and inattention. However, in most cases the impairments are nonspecific and mild. When related to phenytoin, the cognitive deficits are partly attributable to slowed motor activity that impairs performance on timed psychologic tests. On the other hand, carbamazepine has a beneficial effect that probably results from its structural similarity to the tricyclic antidepressants. Phenytoin, carbamazepine, and valproate otherwise do not create significantly different incidences or types of cognitive impairment.

Surgery

When partial complex seizures are refractory to anticonvulsants, surgical removal of a seizure focus may be greatly beneficial. Surgical candidates ought to have a single frontal or temporal lobe lesion that is clearly identifiable on clinical, EEG, and radiographic testing. They must often undergo a Wada test to avoid postoperative aphasia and amnesia.

In epilepsy that originates in the temporal lobe, patients typically undergo a partial or complete lobectomy. This surgery has been a major medical advance. Almost 50 per cent of patients enjoy a complete cessation of seizures. Another 25 per cent have a major reduction in frequency. In addition, if only by reducing the need for multiple or high doses of anticonvulsants, surgery often improves mental function. Unfortunately, surgery does not relieve interictal psychosis, and postoperatively a small proportion (less than 8 per cent) of patients develop behavioral and cognitive deterioration. These complications occurs in spite (or possibly because of) greater seizure control.

Patients with multiple foci causing seizures that undergo secondary generalization may benefit from a *commissurotomy*. This procedure is a sectioning of the corpus callosum to interrupt the spread of discharges between cerebral hemispheres. Despite the extent of the surgery, postoperative deficits are so subtle that special neuropsychologic tests are required to demonstrate its major consequence, the *split brain syndrome* (see Fig. 8–8).

Rolandic Epilepsy

Another variety of partial seizures is *rolandic epilepsy* (*benign childhood epilepsy with centrotemporal spikes*). Virtually always beginning between ages 5 and 9 years, remitting by puberty, and occurring predominantly in boys, rolandic epilepsy is the most common partial epilepsy of childhood. Unlike other varieties of partial epilepsy, this condition is restricted to childhood, not associated with an underlying structural lesion, and inherited (in an autosomal dominant pattern). Also, children with this epilepsy are not at risk of developing other varieties of epilepsy as adults.

The seizures consist of unilateral paresthesias and movements of the face accompanied by speech arrest and are associated with tonic-clonic seizures that occur mostly at night. Rolandic epilepsy is infrequent and easily suppressed with anticonvulsants. Interictal EEG changes—high-voltage spikes in the central temporal region (rolandic spikes)—are readily detectable in sleep.

GENERALIZED SEIZURES

Generalized seizures are characterized by an immediate loss of consciousness accompanied by bilateral, symmetric, synchronous, paroxysmal EEG discharges. These seizures are usually the result of either an autosomal dominant genetic disorder, a physiologic disturbance, or a metabolic aberration, including drug and alcohol withdrawal. In contrast to partial seizures, generalized seizures lack an aura, lateralized motor or sensory disturbances, and focal EEG abnormalities. Also, they practically never result from brain tumors, cerebral infarctions, or other structural lesions. Most generalized seizures are of either the absence (*petit mal*) or tonic-clonic (*grand mal*) variety.

Absences

Absence (petit mal) seizures usually begin between ages 4 and 10 years and usually disappear in early adulthood. However, for about 40 per cent of children, tonic-clonic seizures replace the absences.

Absences, which can occur many times daily, are 1- to 10-second lapses in attention accompanied in almost all cases by automatisms, subtle clonic limb movements, or blinking (Fig. 10–11). Notably, the blinking occurs rhythmically at 3 Hz, which is the frequency of the associated EEG abnormality. Although children do not have retrograde amnesia and they maintain muscle tone and bladder control, their mental and physical activity is interrupted. After the ictus, as though it had never occurred, children have no confusion, agitation, or sleepiness.

Children with unrecognized absences may be misdiagnosed as being inattentive, dull, or even mentally retarded. Their seizures may be mislabeled as partial complex seizures, but the two conditions can be differentiated (Table 10–4). The distinction is especially important because treatment requires different anticonvulsants and, on occasion, absence status epilepticus leads to a several-hour episode of apathy, psychomotor retardation, and confusion. The attack can be diagnosed only with an EEG, and it can usually be terminated by intravenous administration of a benzodiazepine. This condition usually develops virtually only in children and young adults with a history of absences or other seizures who have suddenly stopped taking their anticonvulsants. As noted previously, it is a cause of acute confusion.

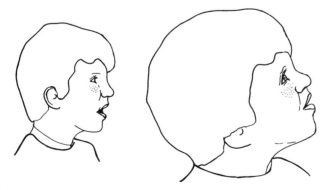

FIGURE 10–11

During a typical absence, this 8-year-old boy has brief, 1- to 3-second staring spells during which he becomes glassy-eyed and mute. Typically he rolls his eyes upward and blinks at 3 Hz. Although he loses consciousness, he maintains bodily tone and does not become incontinent. Absence seizures and the accompanying EEG abnormality (see Fig. 10–12) may be demonstrated by having the child count numbers slowly while hyperventilating. Seizures occur when the counting slows or pauses. At the end of the seizure, the child will resume counting at the appropriate number, which indicates that there is no retrograde amnesia.

TABLE 10–4. COMPARISON OF PARTIAL COMPLEX AND ABSENCE SEIZURES

Feature	Partial Complex	Absence
Aura	Often	Never
Consciousness	Impaired	Lost at onset
Movements	Usually simple, repetitive, but may include complex activity	Blinking and facial and finger automatisms
Postictal behavior	Amnesia, confusion, and tendency to sleep	No abnormality, but amnesia for ictus
Frequency	One to two per week	Several daily
Duration	2 to 3 minutes	1 to 10 seconds
Precipitants		Hyperventilation, photic stimulation
EEG	Spikes and polyspike and waves, usually over both temporal regions	Generalized 3-Hz spike-and-wave complexes
Anticonvulsants	Carbamazepine, phenytoin	Ethosuximide, valproate

EEG, Etiology, and Treatment. During an absence, the EEG shows synchronous 3-Hz spike and slow-wave complexes in all channels (Fig. 10–12). Even in the interictal period, occasional asymptomatic bursts of 3-Hz spike and slow-wave complexes lasting 1 to 1.5 seconds may be observed. In patients with absences, either hyperventilation or photic stimulation can precipitate the characteristic clinical and EEG abnormalities. Just as the EEG abnormality

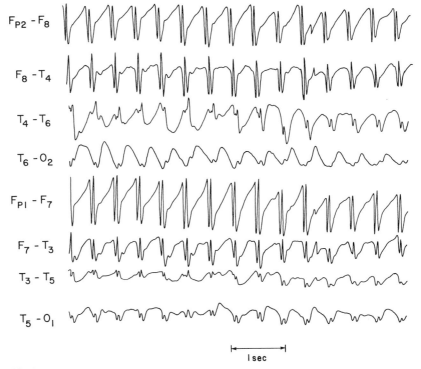

FIGURE 10–12

During an absence, the EEG characteristically shows regular, symmetric, and synchronous 3-Hz spike-and-wave complexes. The discharge arises from and returns to a normal EEG background.

is generalized, PET scans performed during absences show increased metabolism in the thalamus and entire cerebral cortex.

Patients' relatives, when young, also often have absences or 3-Hz spike and slow-wave complexes that can be precipitated by hyperventilation. This finding supports the hypothesis that absences are inherited in an autosomal dominant pattern. In contrast to tonic-clonic seizures, absences are not associated with drug withdrawal, metabolic aberrations, or structural lesions. Therefore, CT and MRI scans are usually not performed.

Absences are treated with ethosuximide, valproate, or occasionally clonazepam. Most children readily respond to one or another of these anticonvulsants. After adolescence, anticonvulsants often can be withdrawn without precipitating recurrence of the absences.

Tonic-Clonic Seizures

Tonic-clonic seizures, unlike absences, begin at any age after infancy, persist into adult life, and cause massive motor activity and profound postictal residua. Although patients may have a prodrome of malaise or mood change, tonic-clonic seizures are usually unheralded, explosive events. In the initial tonic phase, patients lose consciousness, roll their eyes upward, and extend their neck, trunk, and limbs as if to form an arch. Subsequently, they undergo a dramatic clonic phase in which their limbs, neck, and trunk are wracked by violent jerks (Fig. 10–13).

A potential diagnostic problem is that during this terrible episode of tonic-clonic activity, the primary generalized seizure appears similar to a partial seizure that has undergone secondary generalization. Often, only a detailed history, a trained observer, or an intraictal EEG can distinguish between them.

During the tonic phase, if the superimposed muscle EEG artifact can be eliminated by administering muscle relaxants, the EEG shows repetitive, increasingly higher amplitude spikes occurring with increasing frequency in all channels. In the clonic phase, the spikes, which become less frequent but greater in amplitude, are interrupted by slow waves (Fig. 10–14).

Afterward, the EEG shows postictal depression. The postictal EEG is often the only one available, but it can confirm the diagnosis. Similarly, the EEG is also slow after ECT. After either a tonic-clonic seizure or ECT-induced seizure, the serum prolactin level rises for 15 to 30 minutes in most cases. After a pseudoseizure, in contrast, the EEG is relatively normal, and the prolactin level remains at baseline.

About 20 to 30 per cent of patients with tonic-clonic seizures have interictal asymptomatic, brief bursts of spikes, polyspikes, or slow waves. Seizures and accompanying EEG abnormalities may be precipitated by photic stimulation or hyperventilation.

Etiology.   Many tonic-clonic seizures are the result of an autosomal dominant trait expressed between the ages of 5 and 30 years. In many cases, patients have a history of childhood absences.

Sleep deprivation is one of the most common precipitants. In particular, medical house officers who have worked all night are susceptible to tonic-clonic seizures early the following morning. Also, stage 1 and stage 2 NREM sleep precipitate tonic-clonic seizures in epileptic patients (see Chapter 17). Many epileptic patients have these seizures predominantly or exclusively while asleep, and some patients have them virtually only on awakening. Oc-

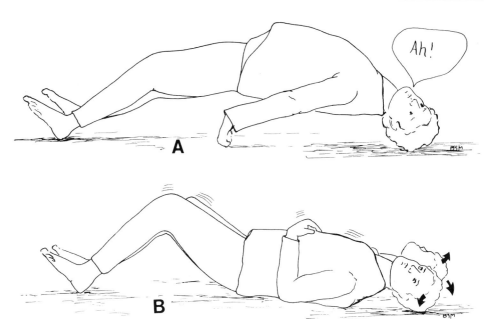

FIGURE 10–13

A, This patient in the tonic phase of a tonic-clonic seizure arches his torso and extends his arms and legs. He assumes this position because of the relatively greater strength of the extensor muscles over the flexor muscles. Simultaneous diaphragm, chest wall, and laryngeal muscle contractions force air through a tightened larynx and cause the shrill, epileptic cry. During this phase, patients often bite their tongue and involuntarily force urine out of their bladder. *B*, In the clonic phase, the patient's head, neck, and legs have symmetric and forceful contractions for about 10 to 20 seconds. Saliva, which becomes aerated and often blood-tinged from tongue lacerations, appears as a froth at the mouth. The pupils dilate, and the patient sweats profusely. Finally, muscular contractions become progressively less frequent and weaker. The seizure usually ends with a sigh, followed by stertorous breathing. In the immediate postictal period, patients are unresponsive. Before regaining consciousness, they may pass through a state of confusion and agitation, loosely called "postictal psychosis."

casionally, seizures are precipitated exclusively by stroboscopic light (photo-convulsive epilepsy).

Alcohol can precipitate seizures in cases of profound intoxication, alcohol-induced hypoglycemia, or sleep deprivation. Abrupt withdrawal from chronic, excessive alcohol consumption produces "alcohol-withdrawal seizures," which usually occur after 1 to 3 days of abstinence. Although the clinical and EEG manifestations of these seizures are similar to those in genetically determined seizures, the interictal EEG is normal.

A small but noteworthy group of children, adolescents, and some adults have absences or tonic-clonic seizures in response to particular sensory stimulation, *reflex epilepsy*. In its most common variety, *photosensitive epilepsy*, seizures are triggered by specific visual stimuli, such as flickering lights, disco stroboscopic lights, television pictures that have lost their vertical stability, or video games. Even certain patterns of letters, words, or figures may trigger seizures in some individuals. Likewise, musical stimuli, such as musical passages, may trigger seizures.

Treatment. Anticonvulsants commonly used for tonic-clonic seizures are valproate, phenytoin, and carbamazepine. As in the treatment of partial seizures, neurologists usually attempt to control these seizures with monother-

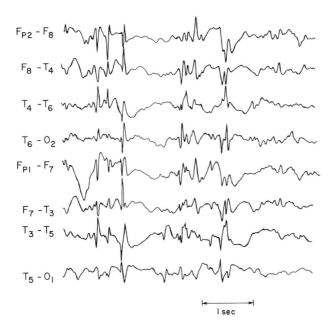

FIGURE 10-14

During a tonic-clonic seizure, the EEG would ideally show paroxysms of spikes, polyspikes, and occasional slow waves in all channels; however, unless a muscle relaxant is administered, muscle artifact obscures this pattern. The interictal background EEG activity usually contains multiple bursts of generalized spikes. In contrast to occasional temporal lobe spikes, this is a pattern that confirms a diagnosis of epilepsy.

apy. Anticonvulsants are usually given for at least 6 to 12 months, except in cases of a single seizure or those in which a precipitating factor, such as sleep deprivation or alcohol withdrawal, can be identified and avoided.

Febrile Seizures

The most common variety of seizure to occur in childhood is febrile seizures. They occur in 2 to 4 per cent of all children and recur in one third of them. A small fraction of children with recurrent febrile seizures subsequently develop partial complex epilepsy. However, febrile seizures do not increase the risk of cerebral palsy, mental retardation, or death.

Daily phenobarbital had been given as a prophylactic anticonvulsant or administered at the onset of fever; however, phenobarbital impairs cognitive function, produces hyperactivity, and provides little protection. To prevent recurrent febrile seizures, neurologists recommend oral diazepam only when fevers develop.

OTHER ISSUES

Driving

Patients with epilepsy have increased rates of traffic violations, including driving under the influence of alcohol or drugs, and traffic accidents. Traffic problems are strongly associated with a driver who is male, younger than 25 years old, and with underlying neurologic or psychiatric illness.

Almost all states require a "waiting period" for driving after having a seizure, but modifications are sometimes allowed for seizures that arose from an isolated medical illness, such as hypoglycemia, and for seizures with a prolonged aura. Most states set a waiting period of 3 to 6 months, but several, including New York, California, and New Jersey, require 12 months. Patients are usually required to reveal any history of seizures to a state's motor vehicle department. In addition, several states require physicians to report drivers with seizures.

DISORDERS THAT MIMIC SEIZURES

Pseudoseizures

Psychogenic episodes mimicking seizures, *pseudoseizures*, are more prevalent in women, children, and adolescents. Not necessarily representing a conversion disorder, as was originally suggested, pseudoseizures are associated with a wide range of psychiatric disturbances, including childhood sexual abuse.

About 50 per cent of patients with pseudoseizures also have epileptic seizures. Thus, in some epileptic patients, pseudoseizures occur together with epileptic seizures and can be responsible for "refractory epilepsy." Partial complex seizures that originate in the frontal lobe are uncommon, but are notoriously apt to be misdiagnosed as psychogenic seizures. Therefore, although patients may seem to have only pseudoseizures, they should undergo an investigation for seizures, as well as a psychiatric evaluation.

Like epileptic seizures, pseudoseizures tend to be stereotyped for each individual. However, in most cases, pseudoseizures begin slowly with gradually developing flailing, struggling, alternating limb movements (asymmetric or out-of-phase clonic movements), and similar side-to-side head movements. They are also identifiable by sexually suggestive pelvic thrusting. As fatigue ensues, the movements decline in intensity and regularity, but their duration is often longer than 2 minutes, which is much longer than an epileptic seizure. Also, the movements usually have no tonic phase, tongue biting, or incontinence. Despite the apparent generalized nature of the pseudoseizure, consciousness during the episode is preserved, patients have no postictal symptoms, and retrograde amnesia is absent.

If a routine EEG were obtained during a pseudoseizure and muscle artifact were eliminated, it would be normal. An EEG performed afterward, which is more feasible, would not show postictal depression. In addition, the serum prolactin concentration, which is usually transiently elevated after a generalized or partial complex seizure, would not rise.

EEG-video monitoring is invaluable in determining the presence of pseudo- and epileptic seizures. Preliminary information might be gathered in children with episodic behavioral disturbances, including temper tantrums, breath-holding spells, as well as seizures, by having parents videotape their child during the episodes. The psychiatrist and other physicians could then review the videotape. (Home videos are also helpful in diagnosing sleep disorders, movement disorders, and behavioral disturbances.)

While pseudoseizures with a tonic-clonic appearance are usually theatrical, those mimicking partial seizures are often subtle. Patients who mimic partial elementary seizures usually have apparent memory lapses, episodes of inattention, visual aberrations, other subjective phenomena, or nonspecific sensations, such as dizziness or epigastric sensations. When these symptoms result from pseudoseizures, they are variable, last longer than the usual limit of several minutes, and are not accompanied by dulling of the sensorium. Also, these pseudoseizures rarely seem to include automatisms or undergo progression to a generalized seizure.

Nevertheless, since partial complex seizures may induce bizarre thoughts and behavior, the clinical distinction in most studies is no more reliable than 85 to 90 per cent. Misdiagnosing seizures that originate in the frontal lobe and not appreciating the combination of epileptic and pseudoseizures are two of the most common pitfalls. In difficult cases, long-term (many day) EEG-video monitoring is usually required to make a reliable diagnosis of these disorders.

Episodic Dyscontrol Syndrome

The episodic dyscontrol syndrome, which is roughly equivalent to recurrent rage attacks, consists of violent, aggressive, primitive, destructive outbursts provoked by minor stimuli, such as verbal threats, anger, or frustration. The outbursts, which are variable, *nonstereotyped*, are typically associated with consuming alcohol—even minor amounts.

In contrast to violent partial complex seizures, episodic dyscontrol is at least momentarily purposeful, directed, and accompanied by a highly charged affect. Also, these patients may barbarically scream, punch, wrestle, and throw glasses or bottles and then claim either repentance or amnesia.

Episodic dyscontrol attacks occur almost exclusively in young men who have either congenital cerebral injury or traumatic brain injury. The patients often have borderline intelligence, specific cognitive impairments, or minor physical neurologic abnormalities. Moreover, many have epilepsy and interictal EEG abnormalities that have undoubtedly been responsible for some reports of aggression in seizures. Suggested medical treatments for episodic dyscontrol syndrome, in addition to prohibiting alcoholic beverages, have included stimulants, beta-blockers, and anticonvulsants—most recently carbamazepine. However, no particular treatment has been proved effective.

Cerebrovascular Disturbances

TIAs resemble partial seizures in that both may involve momentarily impaired consciousness and physical deficits (see Chapter 11). In general, however, TIAs have a slower onset, rarely cause loss of consciousness, and tend to begin only when the patient is standing upright.

Of the various cerebrovascular disturbances that can mimic partial complex seizures, the most important is *transient global amnesia* (*TGA*; see Chapter 11). During an episode of TGA, which is a frequent cause of transient amnesia (see Table 7–1), patients cannot memorize new information, such as the date, location, and examining physicians, for several hours. The EEG may show spikes, but not epileptic bursts. TGA is probably caused by vascular insufficiency of the temporal lobes that leads to ischemia of the limbic system. It may be diagnosed, although with some difficulty, by relying on the clinical features.

Migraines, another vascular disturbance, may induce episodes of confusion and personality change followed by a tendency to sleep (see Chapter 9). They also mimic seizures because they can cause hemiparesis for several hours and abnormal EEGs. In fact, the incidence of seizures in migraine patients is greater than in the general population. Correct diagnosis, which is frequently difficult, relies on the patient's history and response to medications.

Sleep Disorders

Some unresponsive patients who might be suspected of having seizures are actually undergoing sleep attacks associated with hallucinations or the momentary loss of body tone, i.e., the *narcolepsy-cataplexy syndrome* (see Chapter 17). Unlike seizures, narcolepsy has no aura, motor activity, incontinence, or subsequent symptoms. Moreover, an EEG during narcolepsy displays rapid eye movement (REM) activity.

Metabolic Aberrations

Of the various metabolic aberrations that mimic seizures, reactions to medicines are probably the most common. Many medicines, including some eye drops, produce transient mental and physical alterations. However, they practically never induce movements or stereotyped thoughts.

Hyperventilation, another common metabolic alteration, induces giddiness, confusion, and other psychologic symptoms that can be confused with seizures (see Chapter 3). Severe hyperventilation can precipitate seizures, although probably only in epileptic individuals.

Hypoglycemia, which can result from excessive insulin, alcohol intoxication, and prediabetic states, can induce symptoms of panic attacks, as well as of seizures. Also, similar symptoms occur with excessive coffee intake or skipping meals. Although the severity and frequency of symptomatic hypoglycemia are probably overestimated, small frequent meals along with reduction of caffeine intake should remedy most cases.

REFERENCES

Anticonvulsants and Surgical Treatment

Abramowicz M (ed): Drugs for epilepsy. Med Lett *31*: 1–3, 1989
Abramowicz M (ed): Gabapentin—A new anticonvulsant. Med Lett *36*: 39–40, 1994
Abramowicz M (ed): Valproate for bipolar disorder. Med Lett *36*: 74–75, 1994
Dodrill CB, Troupin AS: Neuropsychological effects of carbamazepine and phenytoin: A reanalysis. Neurology *41*: 141–143, 1991
Engel J: Update on surgical treatment of the epilepsies. Neurology *43*: 1612–1617, 1993
Gallassi R, Morreale A, DiSarro R, et al: Cognitive effects of antiepileptic drug discontinuation. Epilepsia *33* (Suppl 6): S41–44, 1992
Harden CL: New antiepileptic drugs. Neurology *44*: 787–795, 1994
Ketter TA, Malow BA, Flamini R, et al: Anticonvulsant withdrawal-emergent psychopathology. Neurology *44*: 55–61, 1994
Mattson RH, Cramer JA, Collins JF, et al: A comparison of valproate with carbamazepine for the treatment of complex partial seizures and secondarily generalized tonic-clonic seizures in adults. N Engl J Med *327*: 765–771, 1992
Meador KJ, Loring DW, Allen ME, et al: Comparative cognitive effects of carbamazepine and phenytoin in healthy adults. Neurology *41*: 1537–1540, 1991
Pellock JM, Willmore LJ: A rational guide to routine blood monitoring in patients receiving antiepileptic drugs. Neurology *41*: 961–964, 1991
Rosman NP, Colton T, Labazzo J, et al: A controlled trial of diazepam administration during febrile illnesses to prevent recurrence of febrile seizures. N Engl J Med: *329*: 79–84, 1993
Shinnar S, Berg AT, Moshe SL, et al: Discontinuing antiepileptic drugs in children with epilepsy: A prospective study. Ann Neurol *35*: 534–545, 1994

Spencer SS, Spencer DD, Williamson PD, et al: Corpus callosotomy for epilepsy. Neurology *38*: 19–24, 1988

Trimble MR: Antiepileptic drugs, cognitive function, and behavior in children: Evidence from recent studies. Epilepsia *31* (Suppl 4): S30–S34, 1990

Trimbel MR: Neurobehavioral effects of anticonvulsants. JAMA *265*: 1307–1308, 1991

Waters CH, Belai Y, Gott PS, et al: Outcomes of pregnancy associated with antiepileptic drugs. Arch Neurol *51*: 250–253, 1994

Interictal Disorders

Bear DM, Fedio P: Quantitative analysis of interictal behavior in temporal lobe epilepsy. Arch Neurol *34*: 454–467, 1977

Bruton CJ, Stevens JR, Frith CD: Epilepsy, psychosis, and schizophrenia. Neurology *44*: 34–42, 1994

Devinsky O, Kelly K, Yacubian EMT, et al: Postictal behavior: A clinical and subdural electroencephalographic study. Arch Neurol *51*: 254–259, 1994

Flor-Henry P: Psychosis and temporal lobe epilepsy. Epilepsia *10*: 363–395, 1969

Hansotia P, Broste SK: The effect of epilepsy or diabetes mellitus on the risk of automobile accidents. N Engl J Med *324*: 22–26, 1991

Indaco A, Carrieri PB, Nappi C, et al: Interictal depression in epilepsy. Epilepsy Res *12*: 45–50, 1992

Mendez MF, Doss RC, Taylor JL, et al: Depression in epilepsy: Relationship to seizures and anticonvulsant therapy. J Nerv Ment Dis *181*: 444–447, 1993

Mendez MF, Doss RC, Taylor JL, et al: Interictal violence in epilepsy: Relationship to behavior and seizure variables. J Nerv Ment Dis *181*: 566–569, 1993

Mendez MF, Grau R, Doss RC, et al: Schizophrenia in epilepsy: Seizure and psychosis variables. Neurology *43*: 1073–1077, 1993

Morrell MJ, Sperling MR, Stecker M, et al: Sexual dysfunction in partial epilepsy: A deficit in physiologic arousal. Neurology *44*: 243–247, 1994

Pincus JH: Violence: The neurologic contribution. Arch Neurol *49*: 595–603, 1992

Rodin E, Schmaltz S: The Bear-Fedio personality inventory and temporal lobe epilepsy. Neurology *34*: 591–596, 1984

Slater E, Beard AW: The schizophrenic-like psychosis of epilepsy. Br J Psychiatry *109*: 109: 95–150, 1963

Stenager EN, Stenager E: Suicide and patients with neurologic diseases. Arch Neurol *49*: 1296–1303, 1992

Trimble MR: The Psychoses of Epilepsy. New York, Raven Press, 1991

Whitman S, Coleman TE, Patmon C, et al: Epilepsy in prison: Elevated prevalence and no relationship to violence. Neurology *34*: 775–782, 1984

Seizures and Epilepsy

Alldredge B, Lowenstein DH, Simon RP: Seizures associated with recreational drug abuse. Neurology *39*: 1037–1039, 1989

Alper K, Devinsky O, Perrine K: Nonepileptic seizures and childhood sexual and physical abuse. Neurology *43*: 1950–1953, 1993

Berg AT, Shinnar S, Hauser WA, et al: A prospective study of recurrent febrile seizures. N Engl J Med *327*: 1122–1127, 1992

Devinsky O, Honigfeld G, Patin J: Clozapine-related seizures. Neurology *41*: 369–371, 1991

Fagan KJ, Lee SI: Prolonged confusion following convulsions due to generalized nonconvulsive status epilepticus. Neurology *40*: 1689–1694: 1990

French JA, Williamson PD, Thadani VM, et al: Characteristics of medial temporal lobe epilepsy. Ann Neurol *34*: 774–780, 1993

Gates JR, Ramani V, Whalen S, et al: Ictal characteristics of pseudoseizures. Arch Neurol *42*: 1183–1187, 1985

Goossens LAZ, Andermann F, Andermann E, et al: Reflex seizures induced by calculation, card or board games, and spatial tasks: A review of 25 patients and delineation of the epileptic syndrome. Neurology *40*: 1171–1176, 1990

Hsiao JK, Messenheimer JA, Evans DL: ECT and neurologic disorders. Movement Disorders *3*: 121–136, 1987

Meierkord H, Will B, Fish D, et al: The clinical features and prognosis of pseudoseizures diagnosed using video-EEG telemetry. Neurology *41*: 1643–1646, 1991

Pacia SV, Devinsky O: Clozapine-related seizures: Experience with 5,629 patients. Nuerology *44*: 2247–2249, 1994

Pascual-Leone A, Dhuna A, Altafullah I, et al: Cocaine-induced seizures. Neurology *40*: 404–407, 1990

Rosenstein D, Nelson JC, Jacobs SC: Seizures associated with antidepressants: A review. J Clin Psychiatry *54*: 289–299, 1993

Sackheim HA, Prudic J, Devanand DP, et al: Effects of stimulus intensity and electrode placement on the efficacy and cognitive effects of electroconvulsive therapy. N Engl J Med *328*: 839–846, 1993

Saygi S, Katz A, Marks DA, et al: Frontal lobe partial seizures and psychogenic seizures. Neurology *42*: 1274–1277, 1992

Scheuer ML, Pedley TA: The evaluation and treatment of seizures. N Engl J Med *323*: 1468–1474, 1990

Shen W, Bowman ES, Markland ON: Presenting the diagnosis of pseudoseizure. Neurology *40*: 756–759, 1990

Simon RP: Alcohol and seizures. N Engl J Med *319*: 715–716 1988

Spencer SS, Spencer DD, Williamson PD, et al: Sexual automatisms in complex partial seizures. Neurology *33*: 527–533, 1983

Williamson PD, Thadani VM, Darcy TM, et al: Occipital lobe epilepsy: Clinical characteristics, seizure spread patterns, and results of surgery. Ann Neurol *31*: 3–13, 1992

Testing

Therapeutics and Technology Assessment Subcommittee of the American Academy of Neurology: Assessment: EEG brain mapping. Neurology *39*: 1100–1101, 1989

Therapeutics and Technology Assessment Subcommittee of the American Academy of Neurology: Assessment: Intensive EEG/video monitoring for epilepsy. Neurology *39*: 1101–1102, 1989

Therapeutics and Technology Assessment Subcommittee of the American Academy of Neurology: Assessment: Magnetoencephalography (MEG). Neurology *42*: 1–4, 1992

QUESTIONS and ANSWERS: CHAPTER 10

1–4. Match the EEG with the interpretation (see pages 252–253).

a. Spike and polyspike and wave
b. 3-Hz spike and wave
c. Normal
d. Temporal spike focus

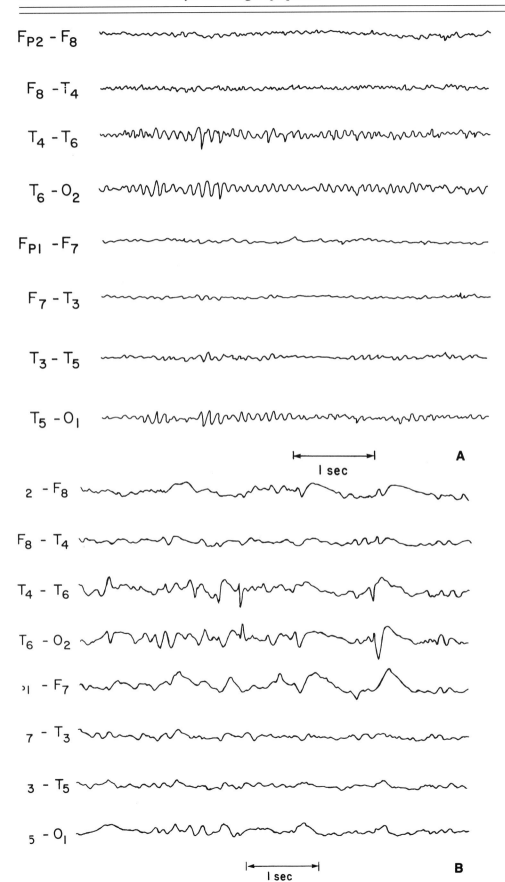

F$_{P2}$ - F$_8$

F$_8$ - T$_4$

T$_4$ - T$_6$

T$_6$ - O$_2$

F$_{P1}$ - F$_7$

F$_7$ - T$_3$

T$_3$ - T$_5$

T$_5$ - O$_1$

I sec

A

2 - F$_8$

F$_8$ - T$_4$

T$_4$ - T$_6$

T$_6$ - O$_2$

$_1$ - F$_7$

7 - T$_3$

3 - T$_5$

5 - O$_1$

I sec

B

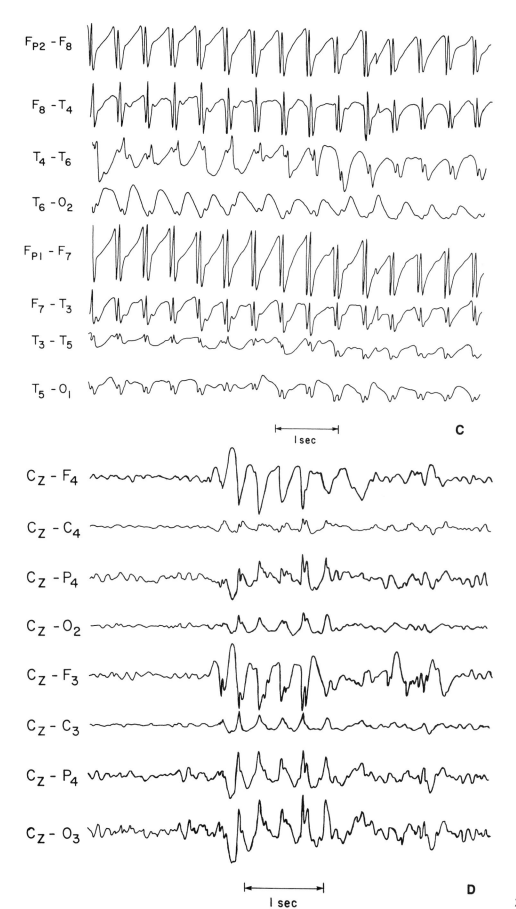

F_{P2} - F_8

F_8 - T_4

T_4 - T_6

T_6 - O_2

F_{P1} - F_7

F_7 - T_3

T_3 - T_5

T_5 - O_1

|← 1 sec →|

C

C_Z - F_4

C_Z - C_4

C_Z - P_4

C_Z - O_2

C_Z - F_3

C_Z - C_3

C_Z - P_4

C_Z - O_3

|← 1 sec →|

D

253

1. Fig. EEG-A

   answer: c

2. Fig. EEG-B

   answer: d

3. Fig. EEG-C

   answer: b

4. Fig. EEG-D

   answer: a

5–8. Match the EEG with the associated seizures.

a. Tonic-clonic (grand mal)
b. Partial elementary
c. Partial complex
d. Absence (petit mal)

5. Interictal temporal lobe spikes

   answer: c

6. Generalized 3-Hz spike and wave

   answer: d

7. Generalized spike and polyspike and wave

   answer: a

8. Occipital spike and wave

   answer: b

9–16. Match the EEG pattern with its most likely cause (a–j).

a   Normal relaxation
b.   Hepatic encephalopathy
c.   Use of minor tranquilizers
d.   Brain tumor
e.   Cerebral death
f.   REM sleep; dreaming
g.   Unilateral ECT
h.   Psychoses
i.   Creutzfeldt-Jakob disease
j.   Barbiturate overdose

9. Delta activity, phase reversed over left occiput

   answer: d

10. Bifrontal beta activity

    answer: c

11. Alpha rhythm

    answer: a

12. Triphasic waves

    answer: b

13. Rapid extraocular movement artifact

    answer: f

14. Periodic complexes

answer: i

15. Right cerebral theta and delta activity

answer: g

16. Electrocerebral silence

answer: e, j

17. In which conditions will an EEG be helpful in making a specific diagnosis?

a. Cerebral tumor
b. Hepatic encephalopathy
c. Neurosis
d. Huntington's disease
e. Cerebral abscess
f. Creutzfeldt-Jakob disease
g. Psychogenic seizures

h. Manic-depressive illness
i. Cerebellar tumor
j. SSPE
k. Psychoses
l. Multiple sclerosis
m. Early Alzheimer's disease
n. Pseudodementia

answer: b, f, g, j, n

18–20. Match the rare but serious complication of anticonvulsant treatment with its definition.

a. Conversion to a normal EEG and suppression of seizure activity that purportedly may trigger a psychosis
b. Frequently fatal allergic reaction that primarily involves the gastrointestinal mucosa
c. Psychosis as an allergic reaction
d. Excitement instead of sedation, especially with phenobarbital in children and brain-damaged adults

18. Stevens-Johnson syndrome

answer: b

19. Forced normalization

answer: a

20. Paradoxical hyperactivity

answer: d

21–24. Identify the following statements as true or false.

21. Use of the EEG in the diagnosis of psychologic disturbance is complicated by drug-induced EEG changes.

answer: True

22. Diazepam (Valium), meprobamate (Miltown), and barbiturates induce rapid (beta) EEG activity.

answer: True

23. Tricyclic antidepressants and phenothiazines may induce nonfocal sharp wave EEG activity.

answer: True

24. The major tranquilizers, antidepressants, and lithium may cause slowing of EEG background activity.

answer: True

25. Carbamazepine (Tegretol) is often used in the treatment of epilepsy patients who are depressed. Which of the following medications has the chemical structure that is the closest to carbamazepine?

a. Lithium
b. Phenytoin
c. Imipramine

d. Haloperidol
e. Phenelzine
f. Tranylcypromine

answer: c

26–33. Match the visual disturbance with the probable cause.

a. Amaurosis fugax
b. Partial complex seizure of temporal lobe origin
c. Partial elementary seizure of occipital lobe origin
d. Petit mal seizure
e. Hysteria
f. Tension headache
g. Migraine with aura
h. Delirium tremens
i. Partial elementary seizures of occipital origin with secondary generalization

26. A red blotch of color in the left homonymous field followed by clonic movements of the left arm and leg, then the entire body

answer: i

27. Loss of central vision in both eyes followed by a throbbing, unilateral headache

answer: g

28. Fortification scotomata

answer: g

29. Visualization of the American flag, accompanied by hearing drumbeats

answer: b

30. Seeing and smelling garbage

answer: b

31. A kaleidoscopic movement of bright lights in the right visual field

answer: c

32. A "shade of gray" covering one eye for 3 minutes

answer: a

33. Tremor, sweating, tachycardia, and seeing rodents

answer: h

34–43. The patient's age when partial (elementary or complex) seizures begin often suggests the cause. Match the seizure cause with the age when it is likely to first appear.

a. Childhood, e.g., 3–8 years
b. Adolescence, e.g., 13–21 years
c. Middle age, e.g., 45–65 years

34. Head injury

answer: a, b, c

35. Congenital cerebral malformation

answer: a

36. Arteriovenous malformation

answer: a, b

37. Glioblastoma multiforme

answer: c

38. Metastatic brain tumor

> *answer:* c

39. Cocaine use

> *answer:* b

40. Cerebrovascular accident

> *answer:* c

41. Pseudoseizure

> *answer:* b

42. Medial temporal sclerosis

> *answer:* a, b

43. Perinatal cerebral hypoxia

> *answer:* a

44–46. A 60-year-old man, who has been previously healthy, is brought to the Emergency Room in a state of apparent confusion and excitement. Careful evaluation reveals that he has poor memory for recent and past events, but he can recall his own and his wife's name. His judgment, language, and other cognitive processes are intact. There are no physical abnormalities. He gradually improves during 2 hours.

44. What is the name of this condition?

a. Delirium
b. Fugue state

c. Acute amnestic syndrome
d. Acute confusional state

> *answer:* c

45. Which one of the following is *not* a frequent cause?

a. Partial complex seizures
b. Wernicke-Korsakoff syndrome
c. Psychogenic disturbances

d. Medications
e. Transient global amnesia
f. Anticonvulsant intoxication

> *answer:* f

46. When a neurologic cause is responsible, which area of the brain is most often affected?

a. Temporal lobe
b. Entire cerebrum

c. Thalamus
d. Frontal lobe

> *answer:* a

47. Is it true, in general, that partial elementary and partial complex seizures are all treated with the same anticonvulsants, but absences are treated with different ones?

> *answer:* Yes. Absences are treated with ethosuximide (Zarontin) as a first-line anticonvulsant and valproic acid (Depakote) as a second-line anticonvulsant. Partial seizures are usually first treated with phenytoin (Dilantin), carbamazepine (Tegretol), and sometimes valproic acid (Depakote).

48. A 23-year-old medical student was experimenting with smoking marijuana. Its effect, which was completely different than anticipated, was anxiety and fear. The student was brought to the Emergency Room with hallucinations, agitation, fever, and nystagmus. Increasing mental and physical agitation culminated in a seizure. Of the following, which is the most likely culprit?

a. Marijuana
b. Phencyclidine (PCP)

c. Cocaine
d. A cerebral hemorrhage

> *answer:* PCP, even in minute amounts, can cause hallucinations and seizures. Higher doses of cocaine are required to produce these effects. When cocaine is

taken in higher amounts, it often causes cerebral hemorrhage, stroke, or vasculitis. Although PCP use among medical students is rare, when health care personnel develop seizures, strongly consider drug abuse.

49. A 30-year-old woman, who has a history of partial complex seizures, is brought to the Emergency Room because she developed lethargy and confusion. Which of the following conditions should be considered in the differential diagnosis?

a. Expansion of a temporal lobe tumor
b. Development of a subdural hematoma from head trauma
c. Partial complex status epilepticus
d. Anticonvulsant intoxication
e. Development of a systemic disorder, such as renal failure

> *answer:* All these causes must be considered; however, in the majority of such cases, the cause is anticonvulsant intoxication (d). If the intoxication is profound or represents one of several episodes, the physician should consider the possibility that the episode was a suicide attempt.

50. Which of the following physical signs may indicate anticonvulsant intoxication?

a. Hemiparesis
b. Ataxia of gait
c. Nystagmus
d. Aphasia
e. Dysarthria
f. Lethargy or stupor
g. Dysmetria on heel-shin testing
h. Tremor on finger-nose testing
i. Papilledema

> *answer:* b, c, e, f, g, h

51. In which part of the skull is the temporal lobe located?

a. Sella
b. Anterior fossa
c. Posterior fossa
d. Middle fossa

> *answer:* d

52. What is the duration of the serum prolactin level elevation after a generalized tonic-clonic or partial complex seizure?

a. 24 hours
b. 12 hours
c. 2 hours
d. Less than 1 hour

> *answer:* d

53. Which of the following statements are true?

(1) Epileptic people are more likely than nonepileptic people to be convicted of a crime and sent to prison.
(2) Epileptic criminals are no more likely than other criminals to have committed a violent crime.

> *answer:* 1-True, 2-True

54. Which of the following statements concerning neural tube defects are true?

a. Meningomyeloceles may be induced by anticonvulsant treatment of pregnant women.
b. The incidence of neural tube defects is reduced by folic acid treatment.
c. The neural tube forms from the endoderm.
d. The neural tube forms the brain, as well as the spinal cord.

> *answer:* a, b, d. The neural tube is derived from invagination of the ectodermal layer of the embryo in the first trimester.

55. A patient's head and eyes deviate to the left, and the left arm extends immediately before a generalized tonic-clonic seizure develops. Where did the seizure probably originate?

a. Cerebellum
b. Right cerebral hemisphere
c. Diencephalon
d. Left cerebral hemisphere

> *answer:* b

56. What is the frequency with which eyelids blink during an absence?

a. 8–12/sec
b. 3/sec
c. Highly variable
d. None of the above

answer: b

57. Which statements correctly complete the sentence? The EEG . . .

a. has abnormalities in 15 per cent of the general population.
b. may be abnormal in psychiatric patients if they are given psychotropics.
c. usually has a posterior background activity in the alpha (8–13 Hz) range.
d. in patients with attention deficit disorder shows frequent but no diagnostic abnormalities.
e. in patients with Gilles de la Tourette's syndrome shows frequent but no diagnostic abnormalities.

answer: a, b, c

58. Which three statements correctly complete the sentence? Partial complex seizures (e.g., psychomotor seizures), compared with absences (petit mal seizures), are . . .

a. longer in duration.
b. more apt to begin in childhood.
c. associated with an aura and postictal confusion.
d. more likely to induce retrograde amnesia.
e. likely to disappear in young adult life.

answer: a, c, d

59. Which are causes of electrocerebral silence despite a regular sinus rhythm on the electrocardiogram?

a. Psychogenic unresponsiveness
b. Depression
c. Brain death
d. Barbiturate overdose
e. Hypothermia

answer: c, d, e

60. Which is the best test for demonstrating mesial temporal sclerosis?

a. MRI of the head
b. SPECT of the head
c. CT of the head
d. CT of the head with contrast
e. EEG
f. EEG with nasopharyngeal leads

answer: a

61. What are the relationships between the EEG and ECT treatment?

a. When unilateral ECT is administered, the EEG changes are found predominantly over the right, nondominant hemisphere.
b. Generalized EEG changes after ECT are associated with more successful treatment of depression.
c. Generalized EEG changes after ECT are associated with greater amnesia.
d. ECT can precipitate status epilepticus in patients with epilepsy or a structural lesion.

answer: a, b, c, d

62. A patient taking carbamazepine is given erythromycin. What will happen to the carbamazepine level?

a. Rise
b. Fall
c. Show no change

answer: a. Most anticonvulsants are metabolized in the liver. Numerous medications, which also undergo hepatic metabolism, compete for the enzyme sites. One or both medications will be metabolized more slowly, and their concentration will increase. Subsequently, as hepatic enzymes are induced, both medications will probably be metabolized more rapidly.

63. An alcoholic man who has epilepsy treated with phenytoin presents with confusion, nystagmus, and ataxia. He has alcohol on his breath. After a routine medical and neurologic evaluation, what should be the two first steps?

a. Determine the blood alcohol concentration.
b. Obtain an EEG.
c. Administer more phenytoin.
d. Administer thiamine.

answer: a, d. Many alcoholics have epilepsy. When inebriated, they pose several dilemmas. Wernicke-Korsakoff syndrome, hypoglycemia from liver disease, or head trauma could cause confusion and obtundation. Although he has the signs, phenytoin intoxication is unlikely because alcoholics during binges usually do not take their medications, which might include insulin and antihypertensive medications, as well as anticonvulsants.

64–65. A 32-year-old left-handed woman has had partial complex seizures since she was 14 years old. Her seizures have been refractory to anticonvulsants, except when two or more were given or intoxicating doses were used. EEG-video monitoring documented that her seizures were partial complex, they occurred when appropriate anticonvulsant concentrations were therapeutic, and the focus was in the left anterior temporal lobe.

64. In contemplating surgery, what test should be performed next?

a. Amobarbital interview   c. PET scan
b. Withdrawal of anticonvulsants d. Wada test

answer: d. The patient will undoubtedly be advised to undergo a partial or complete left temporal lobectomy. If that temporal lobe is dominant, she would be able to undergo only a limited resection.

65. What is the likelihood of her achieving a complete or near-complete remission in her seizures from a temporal lobectomy?

a. 25 per cent   c. 75 per cent
b. 50 per cent   d. Almost 100 per cent

answer: c

66. Which of the following statements is/are true regarding rolandic epilepsy?

a. It is also called "benign childhood epilepsy with centrotemporal spikes."
b. The most common cause is mesial temporal sclerosis.
c. When children with the condition become adults, they are prone to develop other varieties of seizures.
d. Rolandic epilepsy often requires EEG-video monitoring, and if a single focus is identified, a partial lobectomy would be indicated.

answer: a. Rolandic epilepsy is peculiar to children, an inherited condition, and readily responsive to anticonvulsants. EEGs performed during sleep may be necessary for diagnosis, but elaborate monitoring is rarely necessary.

67–71. Match the condition with its description.

a. Psychiatric disturbances, including psychotic behavior, after control of seizures
b. Psychiatric disturbances, especially anxiety and depression, after the complete withdrawal of anticonvulsants
c. Pseudoseizures
d. Repetitive or prolonged seizures that cause mental impairment as the primary or exclusive symptom

67. Nonconvulsive status epilepticus

answer: d

68. Activity under conscious control that mimics a seizure

answer: c

69. Activity not under conscious control that mimics a seizure

answer: c

70. Withdrawal emergent psychopathology

answer: b

71. Forced normalization

answer: a

72. Which statements are true regarding the relationship of interictal violence to epilepsy?
a. Violence is associated with epileptic patients using two or more anticonvulsants.
b. Violence tends to occur in epileptic patients who are schizophrenic or mentally retarded.
c. Crimes of adult epileptic incarcerated criminals (prisoners) are no more violent than those of nonepileptic ones.
d. The prevalence of epilepsy is no greater in prisoners than in the general population.

answer: b, c

73. Which variety of seizure is most apt to be misdiagnosed as a pseudoseizure?
a. Partial complex seizure that originates in the temporal lobe
b. Partial complex seizure that originates in the frontal lobe
c. Febrile seizure
d. Absence
e. Drug withdrawal seizure

answer: b. A partial complex seizure that originates in the frontal lobe can induce behavior that is characteristic of pseudoseizures, such as pelvic thrusting, flailing limb movements, and alternating head movements.

74. Which findings are associated with postictal depression?
a. Vegetative symptoms   c. Sleep-wake disturbances
b. Tendency toward suicide   d. Slow, low voltage activity

answer: d. "Postictal depression" is a term applied to the slow, low-voltage EEG patterns detected after seizures, including those induced by ECT. This pattern is not detectable after many focal seizures or, of course, after a pseudoseizure. It is associated with a transient rise in the serum prolactin concentration.

75. A commercial airliner from South America crashed in New York after exhausting its fuel supply. A young man with blunt abdominal trauma, but no head injury, was initially coherent. However, 30 minutes after arriving in the hospital he became agitated, incoherent, diaphoretic, and hypertensive. During an evaluation, which showed no signs of abdominal or head injuries, he developed a series of seizures and unstable respiration, pulse, and blood pressure. During one seizure, he passed through his rectum several condoms filled with white powder. What is the cause of his seizures?
a. An epidural hematoma   d. Cocaine overdose
b. Cysticercosis   e. Hypoxia
c. An isodense subdural hematoma

answer: d. Smuggling cocaine and other contraband into the United States by swallowing numerous substance-filled condoms is a common, but hazardous practice. If one breaks, enough cocaine, heroin, or other illicit drug is absorbed by the intestines to cause an overdose. In this case, a cocaine overdose caused psychosis, cardiac instability, and seizures. In addition to stabilizing vital functions, treatment would have included intravenous benzodiazepine or phenytoin for control of seizures.

11 Cerebrovascular Disease

Cerebrovascular disease most commonly causes *transient ischemic attacks* (*TIAs*), *cerebrovascular accidents* (*CVAs or strokes*), and *multi-infarct dementia*, conditions that result in temporary or permanent neuropsychologic and physical deficits. The complexity of cerebrovascular disease belies the adage, "A stroke is a stroke is a stroke." Well-informed psychiatrists can recognize common TIAs and strokes, localize the lesion, and predict associated mental disturbances, such as aphasia, dementia, and amnesia.

TRANSIENT ISCHEMIC ATTACKS (TIAs)

As the name suggests, transient ischemic attacks (TIAs) are temporary interruptions in cerebral circulation that cause physical and mental impairments. TIAs typically last from 5 seconds to 15 minutes, but occasionally for as long as 12 to 24 hours. Most TIAs result from platelet emboli that arise from the inner surface of atherosclerotic, stenotic, and ulcerated plaques in the *extracranial arteries*: the carotid and vertebral arteries. When an embolus courses through a cerebral artery, it interrupts the circulation and induces ischemia. The resulting constellation of symptoms and signs usually implicates either the carotid or vertebral artery.

Mental and physical deficits from TIAs mimic other transient neurologic disturbances, particularly partial seizures, postictal confusion and (Todd's) hemiparesis, migraine, and metabolic aberrations. In occasional cases, suddenly occurring, transient neuropsychologic deficits, such as aphasia, occur without any associated physical deficits. These cases mimic psychogenic episodes.

TIAs not only cause neurologic deficits but they also indicate underlying atherosclerotic cerebrovascular disease and a tendency toward sustaining a CVA. TIAs lead to CVAs when atherosclerotic plaques give rise to large emboli that permanently block a cerebral artery, or the plaques grow large enough to occlude the extracerebral vessel. Without treatment, about 5 to 25 per cent of individuals with TIAs develop a CVA within 1 year.

Carotid Artery TIAs

Platelet emboli that form on plaques at the bifurcation of the common carotid artery (Fig. 11–1) lead to cerebral hemisphere TIAs. These carotid artery TIAs are characterized by (contralateral) hemiparesis, hemisensory loss, paresthesias, or hemianopsia. Also, since the ophthalmic artery is the first branch

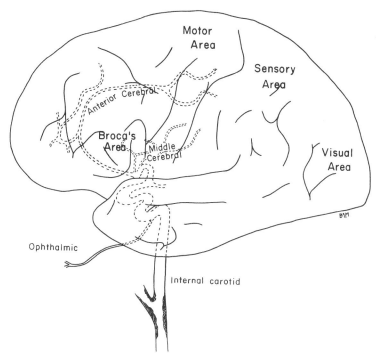

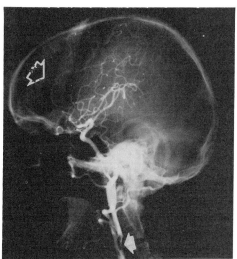

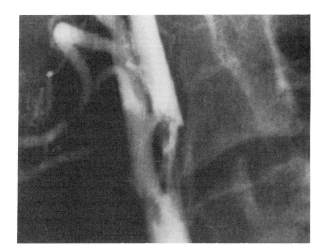

FIGURE 11–1

Top, At its bifurcation in the neck, the common carotid artery divides to form the external and internal carotid arteries. Within the skull, the internal carotid artery gives rise to the ophthalmic artery, and then it branches into the anterior and middle cerebral arteries. It also gives a branch to the posterior cerebral arteries. Thus, each internal carotid artery perfuses the ipsilateral eye and most of the ipsilateral cerebral hemisphere.

Each *middle cerebral artery* supplies the deep and midsection of the hemisphere that contain most of the motor cortex, sensory cortex, and, in the dominant hemisphere, the language arc (see Fig. 8–1). Each *anterior cerebral artery* supplies the frontal lobe, including the medial surface of the motor cortex, which contains the motor innervation for the leg (see Fig. 7–6). Each *posterior communicating artery* joins with a terminal branch of the basilar artery to form the posterior cerebral artery, which supplies the occipital and most of the temporal lobes. Anterior and posterior communicating arteries form collateral circulation with the contralateral hemisphere via the circle of Willis (see Fig. 11–2).

Left, An arteriogram of the carotid artery and its branches prominently displays the bifurcation (*closed arrowhead*), the typical "candelabra" of branches of the middle cerebral artery rather than a single vessel, and a faint anterior cerebral artery that sweeps from anterior to posterior (*open arrowhead*).

Right, A magnification of the bifurcation shows that the internal carotid artery is constricted by an extensive circumferential plaque. The remaining blood flow appears as an "apple core." The rough interior surface of the artery gives rise to retinal and cerebral emboli.

of the internal carotid artery, emboli that flow into this artery cause several minutes of visual obscuration or blindness in the eye. Patients with the distinctive symptom, *amaurosis fugax*, typically describe a "blanket of gray" descending slowly in front of one eye (Table 11–1).

Dominant hemisphere TIAs may cause suddenly occurring but transient aphasia. Similarly, nondominant hemisphere TIAs may cause a brief period of hemi-inattention and related neuropsychologic deficits (see Chapter 8). In both situations, the deficits, which may not be accompanied by hemiparesis, may induce or mimic amnesia, confusion, or agitation.

TIAs in patients with Alzheimer's disease or multi-infarct dementia may convert a mild, compensated intellectual impairment into a marked confusional state. A similar deterioration may develop when both cerebral hemispheres derive their blood supply from one carotid artery through the circle of Willis (Fig. 11–2) because the other carotid artery is occluded. In this case, emboli from the patent artery lead to generalized cerebral ischemia.

Between TIAs, patients may be normal and have no signs of cerebrovascular disease. Although a harsh systolic sound, *bruit*, over the carotid artery bifurcation suggests atherosclerotic cerebrovascular disease, it does not necessarily mean that the patient has carotid stenosis. Retinal emboli (Hollenhorst plaques), which are atheromatous material detectable on funduscopy, may indicate carotid artery stenosis.

Laboratory Tests.   Since TIAs are precursors of strokes and might be confused with other conditions, neurologists attempt to confirm that diagnosis and search for highly stenotic atherosclerotic plaques that might be amenable to surgery (see below). Ultrasound (Doppler and duplex studies), which can measure blood flow and portray artery structure, is a generally reliable technique for revealing or excluding carotid artery stenosis. The traditional, definitive diagnostic procedure has been arteriography; however, since it requires an intra-arterial insertion of a catheter and injection of a "contrast agent," this procedure may cause a CVA or other serious complications. Magnetic resonance imaging arteriography (MRI-A), which will supplant traditional arteriography (angiography) when its resolution improves, readily permits the noninvasive observation of extracerebral and intracerebral vessels (see Chapter 20).

TABLE 11–1.   CAROTID ARTERY TIAs

Symptoms
   Contralateral hemiparesis, hemianopsia, hemisensory loss
   Aphasia
   Ipsilateral amaurosis fugax
Associated findings
   Carotid bruit
   Retinal artery emboli
Tests
   Ultrasonography (carotid duplex studies)
   Magnetic resonance imaging angiography (MRI-A)
   Cerebral arteriography
Therapy
   Medical: platelet inhibitors, e.g., aspirin, ticlopidine (Ticlid); warfarin
   Surgical: carotid endarterectomy, if stenosis >70% and symptomatic

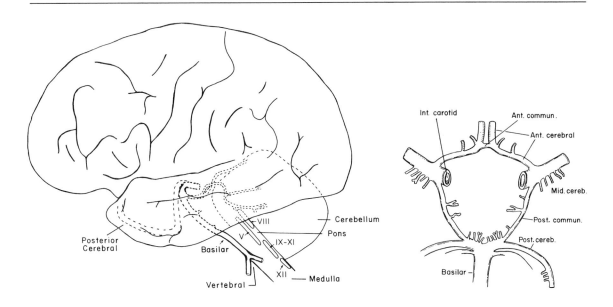

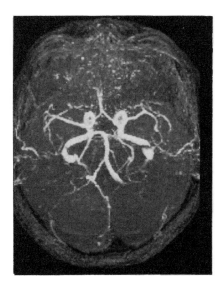

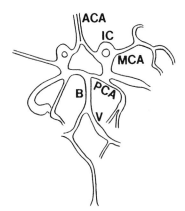

FIGURE 11-2

Top left, After ascending encased in the cervical vertebrae, the two vertebral arteries enter the skull and join to form the basilar artery at the base of the brain. Small, delicate branches from the basilar artery supply the brainstem. (The Roman numerals refer to cranial nerve nuclei.) Large branches, as if wrapping their arms around the brainstem, supply the cerebellum and posterior portion of the cerebrum, i.e., the occipital lobes and infero-medial portions of the temporal lobes.

Top right, The circle of Willis, the "great anastomoses," is circular and completely patent only in textbooks. In fact, only about 20 per cent of people have a completely patent circle. It is formed by connections between the basilar and internal carotid arteries. It gives off the anterior, middle, and posterior cerebral arteries. The circle also potentially provides anastomoses between anterior-posterior and right-left cerebral circulations. Although the circle confers advantages, junctions of the arteries are weak spots. Their defects may balloon outward, form berry aneurysms, rupture, and produce subarachnoid hemorrhages.

Bottom left, An MRI-A-generated axial view of the vertebral arteries shows them merging to form the basilar artery. The basilar artery terminates by dividing into the posterior cerebral arteries, which form the posterior segment of the circle of Willis.

Bottom right, This sketch of the MRI-A to the left shows the basilar (B) and internal carotid (IC) arteries fusing. The circle gives rise to the anterior (ACA), middle (MCA), and posterior (PCA) cerebral arteries. (Communicating arteries are not labeled.)

Other tests help determine if a TIA has led to a CVA and exclude other diagnoses. A CT or MRI scan is almost always performed to exclude CVAs and cerebral mass lesions. A routine evaluation for briefly occurring neurologic deficits includes an electrocardiogram (ECG) and sometimes a 24-hour study of the cardiac rhythm (a Holter monitor). An electroencephalogram (EEG) is ordered if the patient is likely to be having seizures. On the other hand, lumbar punctures and skull x-ray films have no diagnostic value.

Therapy. Nonsurgical (medical) therapy, basically an attempt to inhibit platelet aggregation, is effective for most patients. Common aspirin (one tablet daily) is a potent platelet inhibitor and the most widely prescribed medicine to reduce the incidence of TIAs and also possibly of CVAs. Other effective medicines, such as ticlopidine (Ticlid), also primarily inhibit platelet aggregation. Warfarin (Coumadin), an anticoagulant that has effects on clotting factors, is given to patients with atrial fibrillation, mitral stenosis, and certain other conditions.

Carotid endarterectomy is a delicate surgical procedure in which the carotid artery is briefly opened for the removal of atheromatous plaque. During the procedure, the cerebral blood supply may be briefly interrupted, or atheromatous material may fly off from the surgical site to lodge in the brain. Nevertheless, a major cooperative study has established that, in skilled hands, this surgery is usually the best treatment for patients with carotid artery TIAs whose arteriograms show at least 70 per cent carotid artery stenosis. Comparable studies have not established the best treatment for asymptomatic individuals with ipsilateral carotid stenosis. Surgery is not feasible for complete occlusion of the artery.

Basilar Artery TIAs

The two vertebral arteries join to form the basilar artery at the undersurface of the brain. This group of vessels, which is usually called the *vertebrobasilar system* or simply the *basilar artery*, supplies the brainstem, cerebellum, and the posterior-inferior portion of cerebrum (the occipital and medial-inferior portion of the temporal lobes [Fig. 11–2]). The emboli-generating plaques are located at the origin of the vertebral arteries (in the chest) and at their junction. In both of these locations, plaques are inaccessible to surgeons.

Symptoms and signs of basilar artery TIAs, distinctly different from those of carotid artery TIAs, usually result from patchy ischemia of the brainstem cranial nerve nuclei and cerebellar tracts (Table 11–2). Typical symptoms are tingling around the mouth (circumoral paresthesias), dysarthria, nystagmus, ataxia, and vertigo. On rare occasions, when all blood flow through the basilar artery is momentarily interrupted and the entire brainstem becomes ischemic, a patient will have a *drop attack*, which consists of a brief loss of consciousness and body tone that causes patients to collapse. (Drop attacks appear similar to cataplexy [see Chapter 17].)

Vertigo, one of the most characteristic symptoms of basilar artery TIAs, is the sensation of either revolving in space or feeling one's surroundings revolve. No other descriptions should be accepted by the thoughtful physician. In particular, the common complaint of "dizziness" has no clinical value because it can also mean lightheadedness, giddiness, anxiety, confusion, or imbalance.

Though useful in carotid artery evaluation, ultrasound testing is inapplicable to vertebrobasilar system evaluation because those arteries are shielded

TABLE 11–2.   VERTEBROBASILAR ARTERY TIAs

Symptoms
    Vertigo, vomiting, tinnitus
    Circumoral paresthesias or numbness
    Dysarthria, dysphagia
    Transient global amnesia
    Drop attacks
Associated findings
    Nystagmus
    Ataxia
    Cranial nerve abnormalities
Tests
    Ultrasonography (transcranial Doppler studies)
    Magnetic resonance imaging angiography (MRI-A)
    Cerebral arteriography
Therapy
    Medical: platelet inhibitors, e.g., aspirin, ticlopidine
      (Ticlid); warfarin
    Surgical: none

by the chest, vertebrae, and skull. A transcranial Doppler examination, which can penetrate the skull, may portray the vertebrobasilar system architecture and blood flow. MRI-A and conventional arteriography are applicable. Since vertebrobasilar stenosis is ultimately not surgically correctable, whatever the results of these studies, standard treatment remains similar to medical therapy for carotid artery TIAs.

Transient Global Amnesia

Although seizures, migraines, and other conditions have been suggested as etiologies, basilar artery TIAs are most likely the cause of the fascinating and mysterious condition, *transient global amnesia (TGA)*. In the scenario involving ischemia, basilar artery TIAs impair circulation in this artery's terminal branches, the posterior cerebral arteries, which supply the temporal lobes (see Fig. 11–2). Since the temporal lobes contain portions of the limbic system (see Fig. 16–5), ischemia induces temporary memory impairment (amnesia) and personality change.

During the attack, which starts abruptly, patients characteristically have profound amnesia. They cannot memorize or learn new information, such as a sequence of digits, and they cannot recall recently acquired information, such as the events of the last several hours or days. Typically, patients do not know how they came to the physician's office or the Emergency Room, and their recall of other recent events is filled with gaps. Patients lose track of their responses during an interview by a physician who may have to be reintroduced several times during the evaluation. As a secondary aspect, some patients become perplexed or even agitated, but others, as if recoiling, become apathetic and immobile. Nevertheless, patients' general knowledge remains intact, and given the circumstances, their affect is usually explainable. Despite their amnesia, they do not confabulate in the manner of Wernicke-Korsakoff patients. They may be able to perform complex tasks that were learned before the TGA. Since the motor system is completely spared, patients walk and talk normally—making TGA a prime example of a transient mental deficit unaccompanied by physical deficits.

Often precipitated by exertion, particularly sexual activity, TGAs last for 3 to 24 hours and have a recurrence rate of about 10 per cent. TGAs are a frequently cited cause of the *acute amnestic syndrome* (see Chapter 7) and a *transient altered mental status* (see Table 9–3). Unlike the other conditions, TGA is diagnosed predominantly in older people who are apt to have cerebrovascular disease. Partial complex seizures, which most closely mimic TGA, are characterized by a diffuse cognitive impairment of the sensorium, simple repetitive actions, and epileptiform EEG changes (see Chapter 10). Psychogenic amnesia, unlike TGA, usually consists of people seeming to forget their name, occupation, and other basic information.

CEREBROVASCULAR ACCIDENTS (CVAs)

CVAs cause permanent neuropsychologic and physical deficits from infarctions, hematomas, or related forms of brain damage. Most CVAs result from arterial thrombosis, embolus, or hemorrhage that disrupt cerebral blood flow. Predisposing conditions, *risk factors*, are numerous and sometimes avoidable.

The greatest risk factor is age. The incidence of CVAs rises almost exponentially after the age of 65 years, but still about 20 per cent of CVA victims are under the age of 65 years. Hypertension, the other major risk factor, leads to CVAs in middle-aged as well as older individuals, and it is probably the cause of most cases of multi-infarct dementia (see below). Antihypertensive medications can reduce the incidence of CVAs, but they may have bothersome side effects. In various cardiac conditions—valvular disease, acute myocardial infarction, atrial fibrillation, and possibly mitral valve prolapse—thromboses tend to form on the endocardial surface and embolize to the brain. Diabetes mellitus and cigarette smoking are also risk factors. Although oral contraceptives have been implicated, their danger may be restricted to women who have migraines, smoke, or use relatively high-dose preparations. Migraines themselves are a risk factor for CVA, but probably only in young women. Curiously, although the lack of exercise, Type A personality, heavy alcohol consumption, and cholesterol-rich diets may be risk factors for coronary artery disease, they carry little risk for CVAs.

Narcotic abuse is in its own category. It causes CVAs frequently and through a variety of mechanisms: intravenous injection of particulate material, episodes of anoxia and hypotension, and cerebral vasculitis. In particular, cocaine alkaloid ("crack") causes cerebral hemorrhage.

Thrombosis and Embolus

The majority of CVAs are caused by a thrombosis that propagates within an atherosclerotic extracranial or intracerebral (cerebral) artery and simply occludes it. This type of CVA, which comprises the vast majority of CVAs, is frequently called a *stroke* in the neurologic literature, as well as in the lay press; however, that designation is too all encompassing because it includes hemorrhages and CVAs caused by entirely different mechanisms.

Another cause is emboli, which originate in a carotid artery, lodging in a cerebral artery, i.e., an *arterial-arterial embolus*. Likewise, a cerebral artery embolus may have originated on the endocardial surface. Other causes of thrombosis and embolism are vasculitis, sickle-cell disease, drug abuse, and other blood dyscrasias. In short, the causes of CVAs are usually abnormalities of the heart, blood vessels, or blood.

The exact cause of cell death in CVAs may be an accumulation of excitatory, neurotoxic neurotransmitters, such as *glutamate*. For example, during a CVA, the N-methyl-D-aspartate (*NMDA*) receptors, which normally bind glutamate to open calcium channels, are overstimulated and flood cells with fatal concentrations of calcium.

Infarctions in the Carotid Artery Distribution. Cerebral artery thrombosis and embolism cause infarction in the distribution of the artery and characteristic deficits (Fig. 11–1 and Table 11–3). As in TIAs, anatomy is destiny.

- *Middle* cerebral artery infarction, which is the most common, results in contralateral hemiparesis, hemisensory loss, aphasia with dominant hemisphere lesions, and hemi-inattention with nondominant hemisphere CVAs (see Fig. 20–8).

- *Anterior* cerebral artery infarction causes paresis and apraxia of the contralateral leg because of damage to the anterior and medial aspects of the frontal lobe. With bilateral anterior cerebral artery infarctions, extensive frontal lobe damage causes pseudobulbar palsy, apathy, mutism, and the other signs of the "frontal lobe syndrome" (see Chapter 7), as well as impairments of both legs.

- *Posterior* cerebral artery infarction causes a contralateral homonymous hemianopsia and possibly alexia without agraphia because of occipital lobe damage (see Chapters 8 and 12).

Cerebral emboli-induced infarctions develop suddenly and painfully as the embolus lodges in a cerebral vessel. Cerebral thromboses generally develop slowly or intermittently, begin during sleep, and are relatively painless. In both cases, the region surrounding the infarction becomes edematous. When edema is most severe, during the third to fifth days, the deficits are most pronounced.

TABLE 11–3.   CEREBROVASCULAR ACCIDENTS (CVAs)

Carotid artery
  Anterior cerebral
    Contralateral lower extremity paresis
    Mutism, apathy, pseudobulbar palsy[a]
  Middle cerebral
    Contralateral hemiparesis
    Hemisensory loss
    Aphasia
    Hemi-inattention
  Posterior cerebral
    Contralateral homonymous hemianopsia
    Alexia without agraphia
Vertebrobasilar system
  Basilar artery
    Total occlusion
      Coma
      Locked-in syndrome[b]
    Occlusion of branch
      Cranial nerve palsy with contralateral hemiparesis[b]
      Internuclear ophthalmoplegia[b]
  Vertebral artery
    Lateral medullary (Wallenberg's) syndrome[b]

[a]With bilateral infarctions.
[b]No cognitive impairments.

Some clinical recovery occurs as the edema resolves; however, the infarction remains a functionless scar that can produce seizures (see Chapter 10).

Infarctions in the Basilar Artery Distribution.   Infarctions in the distribution of the basilar artery cause brainstem, cerebellar, or posterior cerebral injuries. In contrast to cerebral hemisphere infarctions, brainstem infarctions generally do not cause language or intellectual impairment. They typically cause constellations of cranial nerve injuries and hemiparesis. Large brainstem infarctions usually cause coma if not immediate death.

Precise localization of brainstem infarctions is often desirable for practical as well as academic reasons. Lesions of the midbrain cause ipsilateral oculomotor nerve and contralateral paresis (see Fig. 4–8). Pontine lesions cause ipsilateral abducens nerve and contralateral paresis (see Fig. 4–10). Midline pons or midbrain infarctions cause the MLF syndrome (see Chapters 12 and 15). Finally, lateral medullary infarctions, which are the most common, cause ipsilateral limb ataxia, palatal paresis, Horner's syndrome, and alternating hypalgesia (see Wallenberg's syndrome, Fig. 2–10).

Most important, once the lesion is localized to the brainstem, the physician can usually conclude that the patient's mental function is intact. For example, a patient with right hemiparesis and a left sixth cranial nerve palsy is unlikely to have aphasia.

Hemorrhages

Cerebral hemorrhages most often result from hypertension and develop in the basal ganglia, thalamus, pons, and cerebellum (see Figs. 18–1 and 20–8). As would be expected with an exploding blood vessel, cerebral hemorrhages occur abruptly and are often accompanied by headaches, nausea, and vomiting, i.e., signs of abruptly increased intracranial pressure. Patients usually lose consciousness and have profound neurologic deficits.

Although most patients with cerebral hemorrhage are sent to neurologists, psychiatrists should be able to identify several varieties of cerebral hemorrhage. They should recognize the potentially devastating cerebral hemorrhage induced by certain monamine oxidase inhibitors, especially since it can be attenuated with antihypertensive medications (see Chapter 9). The *cerebellar hemorrhage*, which can be readily evacuated in a life-saving step, should be diagnosed by its characteristic occipital headache, gait ataxia, dysarthria, and lethargy. *Subarachnoid hemorrhage (SAH)*, usually the result of a ruptured berry aneurysm (a balloon-like arterial dilation), most often causes a prostrating headache and nuchal rigidity, but not necessarily any physical deficits. Sometimes a SAH mimics a migraine or muscle tension headache (see Chapter 9); however, when it occurs, the CT or MRI will usually reveal blood in the subarachnoid space at the base of the brain or within the ventricles, and the lumbar puncture will yield bloody or xanthochromic CSF.

CEREBROVASCULAR ACCIDENTS AND COGNITIVE CHANGES

Dementia

CVA-induced dementia—*multi-infarct dementia* to neurologists—usually results from one massive cerebral infarction, bilateral frontal lobe infarctions, or many small subcortical infarctions. It is more closely associated with left-

sided than right-sided lesions, even allowing for aphasia. Multi-infarct dementia is the second most common cause of dementia—Alzheimer's disease
is the first—and the most common cause in people older than 85 years. Multi-
infarct dementia is roughly similar to *état lacunaire* and *Binswanger's disease*,
conditions in which hypertensive cerebrovascular disease causes multiple
small (0.5 to 1.5 cm) cerebral scars or *lacunes*, particularly in the cerebral
white matter.

Multi-infarct dementia is included in DSM-IV as a *vascular dementia*,
which is a term with a limitation. Although it leads to TIAs and CVAs through
cerebral insults, atherosclerotic cerebrovascular disease itself does not directly
cause cognitive, emotional, or neuropsychologic abnormalities.

The clinical hallmark of multi-infarct dementia is the presence of *focal neurologic deficits*, which are typically hemiparesis, dysarthria, and clumsiness
that probably results from apraxia, rigidity, or spasticity. Another important
although not pathognomonic feature is a stepwise deterioration in neurologic
function that presumably results from an irregular succession of CVAs. In addition, signs of frontal lobe injury—apathy, emotional instability, incontinence, and difficulty walking—often predominate.

The focal neurologic physical deficits, certainly more than the quality of the
cognitive changes, distinguish multi-infarct from Alzheimer's disease dementia. The distinction between cortical and subcortical dementia, even if it has
some validity, is not applicable to these two illnesses. Both produce signs of
cortical injury, such as aphasia, and usually in the middle stages, both may
cause gait impairment and other signs that are "subcortical." Early in both
conditions, the EEG is either normal or contains only some nonspecific slowing. CT and MRI scans usually show atrophy in both conditions, although in
multi-infarct dementia high-resolution MRI scans show small infarctions. Positron emission tomography (PET) scans show multiple hypometabolic regions.

Other Mental Changes

The most common situation is that discrete CVAs cause constellations of
neuropsychologic disturbances and physical signs. Well-known examples are
aphasia, Gerstmann's syndrome, apraxia, and hemi-inattention.

Discrete CVAs may also cause partial complex and other seizures because
about 5 per cent of cerebral infarctions become irritative, i.e., these scars have
epileptogenic potential. Therefore, in patients with cerebrovascular disease,
brief, generalized confusion may result from TIAs, transient global amnesia,
or partial complex seizures.

The opposite situation occurs when virtually the entire cerebral cortex suffers an infarction from severe hypotension or anoxia. The cortex is vulnerable
because its blood supply depends on delicate terminal branches of the cerebral
arteries. The cortex at the periphery of the arterial supply, the *watershed areas*,
is the most vulnerable. When people survive an episode of cardiac arrest,
strangulation, carbon monoxide poisoning, or similar insult, they may suffer
a *watershed infarction*. Depending on the origin, extent, and severity of the
cerebral cortex damage, patients surviving those insults may develop dementia, persistent vegetative state, cortical blindness, or, because the perisylvian
language arc is relatively well perfused, isolation aphasia (see Chapter 8).

An entirely different situation is depression, which is said to occur in about
30 per cent of CVA patients. Those patients with depression in most studies
have greater functional disability, aphasia, cognitive impairment, and subse-

quent mortality. Depression should be considered not only in CVA patients who have a change in their affect, sleep disturbances, and poor appetite, but in those who are recovering slower than expected and those who are "underachievers" in rehabilitation programs. However, before diagnosing depression in CVA patients, physicians must bear in mind CVA-induced conditions that can mimic, induce, or coexist with depression: nonfluent aphasia, frontal lobe syndromes, dementia, pseudobulbar palsy, and aprosody.

CVAs affecting the left frontal lobe have been associated most closely with depression; however, some studies have been unable to confirm the association. In any case, antidepressant medications are often helpful and have minimal side effects in depressed CVA patients. Possibly because these patients have lost cerebral tissue, they usually require small doses.

Alternatively, some mood changes can be induced by medications that stroke patients are apt to be taking. For example, many antihypertension medications, such as methyldopa (Aldomet) and propranolol (Inderal), impair mental function by reducing cerebral blood flow, acting as false neurotransmitters, or otherwise interfering with neuronal function. Diuretics can also cause confusion and seizures when they reduce serum sodium concentration below 125 mEq/ml. Antihypertensive medications also lead to orthostatic hypotension, lightheadedness, and vertigo when patients suddenly stand upright. They can even lose consciousness.

Locked-In Syndrome

Among the innumerable patients who have sustained multiple CVAs and appear demented, mute, and quadriplegic, physicians should search for the patient who has the *locked-in syndrome*. In this rare but important condition, mute and quadriplegic patients have *intact cognitive capacity* and, if only through moving their eyes, some ability to communicate.

The locked-in syndrome usually results from infarction of the inferior portion (base or ventral surface) of the pons or medulla (bulb) when a branch of the basilar artery is occluded (Fig. 11–3). Patients are mute because of complete bulbar palsy and are quadriplegic because of interruption of the corticospinal tract. They usually require a tracheostomy and ventilator support because of the bulbar palsy. The locked-in syndrome also develops as a result of peripheral nervous system diseases in which the cranial nerves as well as the peripheral nerves are affected, such as myasthenia gravis, botulism, amyotrophic lateral sclerosis, and the Guillain-Barré syndrome (see Chapters 5 and 6).

Whatever the particular cause, the upper brainstem, dorsal surface of the bulb, and their interconnections with the cerebral cortex are all intact. Thus, patients are alert and have normal cognition and affective capacity. They can purposefully move their eyes and eyelids. Then, by closing their eyes in a "yes-no" pattern, they can answer questions. Given appropriate clues, they will maintain a normal sleep-wake schedule. Their EEGs are relatively normal because the physiologic connections between the thalamus and cerebral cortex are preserved.

The medical, social, and legal management of locked-in syndrome patients should be based on their being cognizant individuals. They can understand people talking and reading to them, and they can accurately convey their wishes, including decisions regarding their care. Although patients who have suffered a brainstem infarction occasionally partially recover, their overall

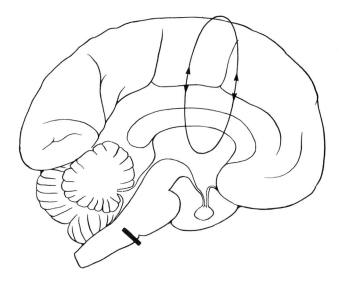

FIGURE 11–3

The locked-in syndrome usually results from an infarction of the ventral surface of the lower brainstem. A lesion in this area (indicated by the bar) would sever the corticospinal tracts and directly injure cranial nerves IX through XII, but it would not damage the reticular activating system, which governs attention.

    More importantly, the cerebral cortex and upper brainstem are still intact and able to maintain normal interactions. This lesion, which is nowhere near the cortex, obviously does not affect the brain's cognitive, language, or visual centers. It also spares the cerebral centers governing eye movement and their connections to the upper brainstem (see Fig. 12–12). The EEG is relatively normal because the reverberating circuits between the thalamus and the cerebral cortex (indicated by the loop), which generate the organized relatively regular background EEG activity, are also unharmed.

prognosis is poor. On the other hand, those debilitated from peripheral nervous system illnesses often totally recover.

    An examination for the locked-in syndrome might be undertaken in patients who are unable to speak or move their limbs, but can voluntarily look from side to side. The physician should ask these patients to blink a certain number of times. If they respond, a system of communication can be developed. (One patient communicated freely using eyelid blinks in Morse code.) If patients can blink meaningfully, the physician should test their ability to see and calculate. Afterward, detailed status testing can be undertaken.

Persistent Vegetative State

    Extensive cerebral damage resulting in *permanent mental incapacity* causes the *persistent vegetative state* (Fig. 11–4). This condition, which has previously been known as "akinetic mutism" or "coma vigil," is much more common than the locked-in syndrome. Patients in the persistent vegetative state are devoid of cognitive capacity, unaware of their surroundings, and unable to communicate in any manner—although they are seemingly awake or arousable, able to open their eyes to strong stimulation, breathe without respirators, and move from noxious stimulation (Fig. 11–5). Vegetative patients have only spontaneous, random eye movements and reflex eyelid blinks. Their eyes may momentarily fix on a face or, as the result of reflex activity, turn toward sounds, including voices. Unfortunately, this activity may be misinterpreted by rela-

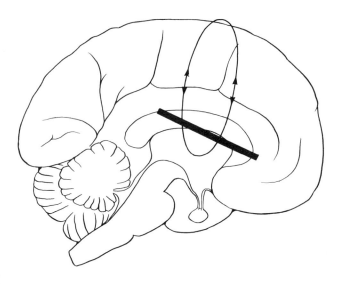

FIGURE 11–4

The persistent vegetative state, which can be caused by cerebral anoxia or numerous other conditions, results from extensive damage to the cerebral cortex or the cerebral tissue immediately underlying it (indicated by the bar). These injuries impair all cerebral functions, including cognitive ability, purposeful motor activity, vision, and speech. The brainstem, being relatively unaffected by these conditions, becomes independent of cerebral control. It then operates by reflex to regulate the body's vegetative functions: swallowing, digestion, breathing, metabolism, and temperature regulation. The EEG is abnormal because the cerebral hemispheres and the interactions with the brainstem (indicated by the loop) are damaged.

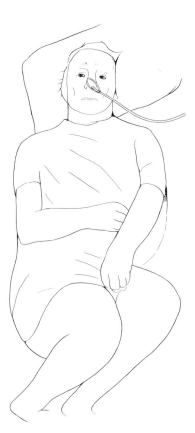

FIGURE 11–5

Patients in the persistent vegetative state tend to assume a decorticate (flexed or fetal) posture because of extensive cerebral damage. Although they are awake, have roving eye movements, and usually do not require a respirator, they are mute, virtually motionless, and unable to respond to visitors or examiners. Patients are often dependent on nasogastric tubes, intravenous lines, urinary catheters, and tracheostomies or endotracheal tubes for respirators. Since they are immobile, they are vulnerable to aspiration pneumonia, urinary tract infections, and pressure sores.

tives as appreciating their presence or understanding their words. Once patients have been in the persistent vegetative state for 1 month, there is no chance of recovery.

Patients are not in suspended animation, and they are not like "Sleeping Beauty." Moreover, their eye movements and continued vegetative functions are so rudimentary that they are found in animals with a very low level of neurologic function.

Most patients are comatose for days or weeks before they enter a vegetative state. The conditions that most often cause coma leading to the persistent vegetative state are cerebral anoxia from cardiac arrest, profound hypoglycemia, major head trauma, and massive CVAs. Alternatively, some patients slip into the vegetative state, without first being comatose, from an accumulation of small cerebral infarctions or the progression of Alzheimer's disease or other degenerative illness. School-aged children and teenagers also may sustain cerebral injuries—usually from motor vehicle and other accidents, drug overdoses, or suicide attempts—that produce this hopeless state.

Beyond its heart-wrenching neurologic aspects, this problem has important legal considerations. Many patients, while in better health, had directed that they "not live like a vegetable," and their relatives have sought to discontinue nutrition, as well as artificial supports. Several ethical and legal contests, starting with the case of Karen Ann Quinlan, have explored the limits of maintaining vegetative patients according to or against their wishes, or when it is futile. Without having to enter those debates, the role of the psychiatrist in this grim situation might be to asses the patient's cognitive function; ascertain that the patient does not have a toxic-metabolic encephalopathy, the locked-in syndrome, or a correctable cause of dementia; and discuss the prognosis with colleagues and family members.

Laboratory Tests in CVAs

The diagnosis of a CVA is based, in most cases, on the clinical evaluation and is confirmed with a CT or MRI scan. The most common alternative diagnoses are structural lesions, such as a brain tumor, abscess, or subdural hematoma, and systemic illnesses with neurologic complications, such as vasculitis and temporal arteritis. Either type of scan will indicate the presence and location of almost all CVAs, except those that are fresh or small, and at the same time exclude other structural lesions. Skull x-rays and EEGs are superfluous. Arteriography is done only in selected cases to diagnose carotid stenosis, cerebral aneurysms, and vascular malformations.

Examination of the cerebrospinal fluid through a lumbar puncture (LP) is used to diagnose a subarachnoid hemorrhage and cerebral infections, such as meningitis and encephalitis, that might mimic a CVA. However, an LP is usually unnecessary for a routine CVA and should be avoided when an intracranial mass lesion is present (see Transtentorial Herniation, Chapter 19).

Therapy of CVAs

During the initial phase of a patient's CVA, neurologists maintain a patent airway and support vital functions. Anticoagulants and other treatments have been introduced to abort thromboses or lyse those that have just been formed, but these medicines can be dangerous and their usefulness has not been established. Other treatments are aimed at promoting cerebral blood flow to ischemic areas. Steroids, oxygen, and vasoactive medicines have no proven benefit.

Medical and nursing care are directed at preventing complications: aspiration pneumonia, decubitus ulcers (bed sores), and urinary tract infections. If the patient is not alert or the gag reflex is diminished, medications and nutrition are given intravenously or by a nasogastric tube. To prevent decubiti, which are unsightly, malodorous, and can lead to sepsis, physicians usually order air mattresses, sweat-absorbent bed surfaces (e.g., artificial sheepskins), and elbow and heel cushions for paretic limbs. Since urinary incontinence adds to the likelihood of developing a bed sore, makes patients cold and wet, and creates odors repugnant to family and staff, physicians generally order catheters.

The patient's bed should be placed against the wall so that all visitors and staff must approach the patient from the side without perceptual impairment. For example, a patient with a left hemiparesis and a *left* homonymous hemianopsia should be placed with his or her *left* side against the wall so that people approach from the *right*, and important objects (e.g., call-buttons, television, clock, and pictures) can be seen and grasped.

In the initial phase, relatives who act as caregivers of CVA patients can be helpful by orienting the patient and bringing a luminous dial clock, a calendar, and pictures; repositioning the patient and moving paretic limbs to avoid contractures; and locating appropriate rehabilitation facilities. Eventually they may have greater difficulty in coping with the patient's mental than physical impairments. Such caregivers are subject to depression at about three times the expected rate.

Traditional physical therapy will often maintain the patient's muscle tone, forestall bed sores, and prevent contractures. It will usually help patients with simple hemiparesis to regain their ability to walk, circumvent some impediments, and avoid maladaptive but expeditious physical compensations. Speech therapy may help with dysarthria and offer patients encouragement. "Cognitive and perceptual skill training" for impaired mentation, sensory impairment, and visual loss remains unproven.

Hemi-inattention and anosognosia resolve over a period of 1 to 3 weeks. However, aphasias usually improve to almost their fullest extent in 4 to 6 weeks, after which deficits are usually permanent. Poor prognostic factors for recovery—as any physician might intuit—are advanced age, dementia, persistent hemi-inattention, incontinence, bilateral brain damage, and prior CVAs.

Depression and pathologic crying, which are often manifestations of pseudobulbar palsy, can be treated with antidepressants. Likewise, agitation, overwhelming anxiety, and hallucinations can be treated with neuroleptics. Control of these aberrations helps patients accept deficits, restraints, and therapies. When a patient's sleeping schedule is disrupted, mild hypnotics are appropriate, but phenobarbital and other barbiturates should be avoided because they may create agitation in brain-injured patients, i.e., a paradoxical reaction.

Attempting to prevent new or recurrent strokes, neurologists recommend aspirin, one tablet (325 mg) daily, to adults in addition to antihypertensive medications and general medical care. They often advise people who are unable to tolerate aspirin and those in whom it fails to take ticlopidine. They recommend warfarin to most people with atrial fibrillation, prosthetic valves, and rheumatic valvular disease.

REFERENCES

Abramowicz M (ed.): Ticlopidine for prevention of stroke. Med Lett *34*: 65–66, 1992

ANA Committee of Ethical Affairs. Persistent vegetative state: Report of the American Neurologic Association Committee on Ethical Affairs. Ann Neurol *33*: 386–390, 1993

Astrom M, Adolfsson R, Asplund K: Major depression in stroke patients. Stroke *24*: 976–982, 1993

Chui HC, Victoroff JI, Margolin D, et al: Criteria for the diagnosis of ischemic vascular dementia proposed by the State of California Alzheimer's disease diagnostic and treatment centers. Neurology *42*: 473–480, 1992

Gilman S: Advances in neurology. N Engl J Med *326*: 1608–1616 and 1671–1976, 1992.

Hale G: The Source Book for the Disabled. Philadelphia, The Saunders Press, 1979

Kaufman D, Lipton R: The persistent vegetative state: An analysis of clinical correlates and costs. NY State J Med *92*: 381–387, 1992

Kritchevsky M, Squire LR, Zouzounis JA: Transient global amnesia: Characterization of anterograde and retrograde amnesia. Neurology *38*: 213–219, 1988

Levine SR, Burst JCM, Futrell N, et al: A comparative study of the cerebrovascular complications of cocaine: Alkaloidal versus hydrochloride—a review. Neurology *41*: 1173–1177, 1991

Melo TP, Ferro JM, Ferro H: Transient global amnesia. A case study. Brain *115*: 261–270, 1992

North American Symptomatic Carotid Endarterectomy Trial Collaborators: Beneficial effect of carotid endarterectomy in symptomatic patients with high-grade carotid stenosis. N Engl J Med *325*: 445–453, 1991

Robinson RG, Parikh RM, Lipsey JR, et al: Pathological laughing and crying following stroke: Validation of a measurement scale and a double-blind treatment study. *Am J Psychiatry 150*: 286–293, 1993

Stern RA, Bachman DL: Depressive symptoms following stroke. Am J Psychiatry *148*: 351–356, 1991

Tatemichi TK, Desmond DW, Paik M, et al: Clinical determinants of dementia related to stroke. Ann Neurol *33*: 568–575, 1993

The Multi-Society Task Force on PVS: Medical aspects of the persistent vegetative state. N Engl J Med *330*: 1499–1508, 1572–1579, 1994

Zivin JA, Choi DW: Stroke therapy. Sci Amer *July*, 56–63, 1991

QUESTIONS and ANSWERS: CHAPTER 11

1–10. Match the neurologic deficit with the most likely artery of infarction.

Artery

a. Right posterior cerebral
b. Left posterior cerebral
c. Anterior cerebral
d. Middle cerebral
e. Right middle cerebral
f. Left middle cerebral
g. Ophthalmic
h. Vertebral or posterior inferior cerebellar
i. Perforating branch of basilar
j. Anterior spinal
k. Basilar

Deficit

1. Hemiparesis with relative sparing of the leg

   answer: d

2. Lower extremity monoparesis

   answer: c

3. Monocular blindness from optic nerve ischemia

   answer: g

4. Left homonymous hemianopsia

   answer: a

5. Left palate paresis, left limb ataxia

answer: h

6. Right third cranial nerve palsy with left hemiparesis

answer: i

7. Right hemiparesis with aphasia

answer: f

8. Quadriplegia and mutism with intact mentation

answer: i

9. Left sixth and seventh cranial nerve palsy with right hemiparesis

answer: i

10. Coma, quadriparesis

answer: k

11–20. Match the type of transient neurologic deficit with the artery involved (carotid [a], basilar [b], both, or neither).

Artery

a.   Carotid
b.   Basilar

Deficit

11. Transient global amnesia

answer: b

12. Amaurosis fugax

answer: a (ophthalmic arteries)

13. Paresthesias of right arm and aphasia

answer: a

14. Vertigo, nausea, nystagmus, and ataxia

answer: b

15. Migraines

answer: a usually, but sometimes b

16. Locked-in syndrome

answer: b

17. Diplopia

answer: b

18. Dysarthria

answer: Both

19. Transient hemiparesis

answer: Both

20. Quadriparesis and anesthesia below the chest, but preserved position and vibration sensation

answer: Neither. Occlusions of the anterior spinal artery, as occasionally complicate surgery involving the aorta, injure the entire spinal cord except for the posterior columns.

21–30. A 74-year-old man has had a steadily worsening left-sided headache for 7 days, a nonfluent aphasia, right hemiparesis with hyperreflexia, a Babinski sign, and right homonymous hemianopsia. Which of the following should be considered as likely possibilities?

21. Cerebral hemorrhage

    answer: No. Cerebral hemorrhages usually are suddenly occurring catastrophic processes.

22. Subarachnoid hemorrhage

    answer: No. The headaches would also be sudden and incapacitating. Nuchal rigidity would be present.

23. Brain tumor

    answer: A good choice. With the relatively short history and extensive deficits, only a rapidly growing brain tumor, such as a metastasis or glioblastoma, would be possible.

24. Subdural hematoma

    answer: Unlikely. Although the headache and hemiparesis are consistent, the aphasia and hemianopsia are rare with masses outside the brain substance, i.e., extra-axial lesions.

25. Basilar artery occlusion

    answer: No. He would be comatose.

26. Carotid artery occlusion

    answer: Good choice. This is a typical story of progressive carotid stenosis leading to occlusion.

27. Brain abscess

    answer: Another good choice.

28. Toxoplasmosis

    answer: Unlikely. Toxoplasmosis is found virtually only as a complications of AIDS, but it typically causes such lateralized symptoms.

29. Cerebral embolus

    answer: No. Although the deficits are compatible, emboli occur suddenly.

30. Multiple sclerosis

    answer: No. The headache, extent of the lesion, and his age are inconsistent.

31–36. After a CVA, a 65-year-old man is alert but mute and unable to move his palate, arms, or legs. He has bilateral hyperreflexia and Babinski signs. He responds to verbal and written questions by blinking his eyelids.

31. Does this man have a fluent, nonfluent, or global aphasia?

    answer: No. There is no evidence of aphasia. He can understand spoken language and respond appropriately.

32. Is his vision impaired?

    answer: No. He can read written questions.

33. Is there evidence of cerebral damage?

    answer: No. The palatal and other motor pareses may be the result of brainstem damage. Cortical functions seem to be intact.

34. How would the EEG appear?

answer: The EEG might appear normal since cortical functions are intact.

35. What is this syndrome called?

answer: It is called the locked-in syndrome.

36. Where is the lesion?

answer: The lesion is in the ventral surface of the lower brainstem, i.e., the base of the pons.

37–41. A 64-year-old man, who had sustained a right cerebral infarction the previous year, is admitted after the sudden, painless onset of right hemiparesis and mutism. He now has bilateral paresis and no verbal output. Although his eyes are frequently open, he fails to respond to either voice or gesture.

37. Where is the probable site of the recent injury?

answer: The new lesion is in the left (dominant) hemisphere. With the history of a prior right cerebral infarction, he now has bilateral infarctions.

38. What is the probable cause?

answer: The sudden, painless onset suggests a thrombotic or embolic CVA.

39. Would the EEG be normal?

answer: The EEG will be abnormal because of extensive cerebral damage.

40. If he were not paralyzed, would he be able to write?

answer: No. Aphasic patients generally have difficulty in all modes of communication. Moreover, as the result of extensive cerebral cortex damage, he probably has dementia, i.e., multi-infarct dementia.

41. Would he have bulbar or pseudobulbar palsy?

answer: He would probably have pseudobulbar palsy because of bilateral cerebral infarctions. Moreover, since he has evidence of no cognitive function and the EEG is abnormal, if he makes no improvement in 1 month, he will probably evolve into a persistent vegetative state.

42–52. A 20-year-old woman awakens from sleep and finds that she has a mild left hemiparesis. Which are the possible causes of her deficit?

42. Cerebral thrombosis associated with oral contraceptives

43. Cerebral vasculitis from lupus, drug abuse, etc.

44. Cerebral embolus from mitral stenosis

45. Cerebral embolus from drug abuse

46. Septic cerebral embolus from bacterial endocarditis

47. Cerebral embolus from an atrial myxoma

48. Cerebral toxoplasmosis from a previously undiagnosed HIV infection

49. Infarction from sickle-cell disease

50. Migraine-induced transient paresis, i.e., hemiplegic migraine

51. A prolonged postictal (Todd's) paresis

52. Multiple sclerosis

answer: 42–49. All yes. CVAs in young people are the result of diseases of the heart, blood, or blood vessels.

answer: 50–52. All yes. These other processes, although not strictly CVAs, may mimic strokes.

53–56. A 20-year-old woman is brought to the Emergency Room by her family because she is suddenly unable to speak or move her right side. She looks directly forward, but does not follow commands. On inspection of her fundi, her eyes constantly evert. She seems to respond to visual images in all fields. The right arm and leg are flaccid and immobile, but her face is symmetric. Deep tendon reflexes are symmetric, and no pathologic reflexes are elicited. She does not react to noxious stimuli on the right side of her face or body.

53. Where is the apparent lesion?

answer: A patient who seems to have global aphasia and a right hemiparesis would usually have a left hemisphere lesion.

54. (a) What pathologic features usually found with such a lesion are not present in the patient? (b) What nonpathologic features are present?

answer: (a) She does not have the usual paresis of the lower (right) face, asymmetric deep tendon reflexes, Babinski signs, or a right homonymous hemianopsia. (b) Eversion of the eyes during inspection is almost always a voluntary act. Inability to perceive noxious stimuli is rare in cerebral lesions. Likewise, a sharply demarcated sensory loss (splitting the midline) is not neurologic.

55. What is the most likely origin?

answer: A psychogenic disturbance is the most likely origin.

56. What readily available laboratory tests would lend great support to the diagnosis?

answer: A normal EEG, CT, or MRI scan would support the diagnosis.

57–61. A 70-year-old man has the sudden onset of an occipital headache, nausea, vomiting, and an inability to walk. He has no paresis, but a downward drift of the right arm and symmetrically active deep tendon reflexes with normal plantar response. He has dysmetria on right finger-nose and heel-shin movements. His gait is so ataxic that he must be supported when he attempts to walk.

57. Where is the lesion?

answer: The lesion is in the cerebellum.

58. Which side?

answer: Abnormal cerebellar findings are referable to the ipsilateral hemisphere, which is the right in this case.

59. What is its origin?

answer: In view of the patient's age and the sudden onset, a CVA is most likely. Since it is painful, a cerebellar hemorrhage, especially because it is potentially lethal, must be given first consideration.

60. Why is there a "drift" of the right arm?

answer: The right arm drifts downward probably not on the basis of a mild paresis (because strength is normal and no corticospinal tract findings were elicited), but because damage to the cerebellar system disturbs coordination.

61. What is the consequence of increased size of the lesion?

answer: If the hemorrhage were to expand, the fourth ventricle would be compressed and hydrocephalus would result. With further compression, the brainstem would be compressed, and coma and then death would follow.

62–65. A 75-year-old man has had 5 days of moderately severe, unremitting left-sided headaches and then right-sided hemiparesis with hyperreflexia and a Babinski sign. On admission, he has neither aphasia nor visual field loss. During the initial 3 days in the hospital, however, he develops stupor with a dilated, unreactive left pupil and bilateral Babinski signs.

62. Where is the lesion?

answer: In view of the left-sided headaches and contralateral hemiparesis, the lesion would be on the "left side" of the CNS, but the physician cannot initially be certain that the deficit is referrable to the cerebral hemisphere rather than the brainstem because the patient has no language or visual disturbance. The development of transtentorial herniation, however, makes it clear that the lesion had been in the left supratentorial (cerebral) compartment.

63. What are the possible causes?

answer: The rapid demise with transtentorial herniation suggests that a mass lesion continued to expand. An occlusion of the internal carotid artery with subsequent cerebral swelling and herniation is possible, but a subdural hematoma is more likely. Tumors, arteriovenous malformations, and abscesses are less common causes (see Chapter 19).

64. Which would be the most appropriate diagnostic test?

answer: The most appropriate diagnostic test would be a CT or MRI scan. Presumably, a routine history, physical examination, and initial hematologic and chemistry tests would have been done on admission. By the time he "herniates," however, emergency measures must be instituted and those preliminary studies postponed.

65. What is the origin of the pupillary abnormality?

answer: The dilation and unreactivity of the left pupil are caused by compression of the third cranial nerve as the subdural hematoma squeezes the temporal lobe through the tentorial notch.

66–67. Found wandering about in a confused manner, a 45-year-old woman is brought to the Emergency Room. She is lethargic, inattentive, and confused, but not aphasic. Her pupils are equal and reactive, and her fundi are normal. Extraocular movements are full. All her extremities move well. She has hyperactive deep tendon reflexes and bilateral Babinski signs.

66. Where is the lesion?

answer: The woman has delirium. Since she has no lateralizing signs or indications of increased intracranial pressure, one cannot say that she has a "lesion."

67. What is the most likely cause?

answer: Causes of diffuse neurologic dysfunction are usually metabolic alterations (uremia, hypoglycemia), postictal confusion, infectious processes (encephalitis), or intoxications (alcohol, drugs, barbiturates).

68. Which of the following varieties of CVAs most often appears as patients awaken in the morning?

a. Cerebral hemorrhage
b. Cerebral thrombosis

c. Cerebral embolus
d. Subarachnoid hemorrhage

answer: b

69. Which of the varieties of CVAs described in question 68 most often develops during sexual intercourse?

answer: d

70. Which of the following CVA risk factors is the most important and correctable?

a. Advanced age
b. High cholesterol diet
c. Obesity
d. Cigarette smoking
e. Hypertension
f. Lack of exercise

    answer: e

71. Which of the following is the standard therapy for vertebrobasilar artery TIAs?

a. Endarterectomy
b. Surgical anastomosis
c. Coumadin
d. Aspirin

    answer: d

72. Which of the following is thought to be the most important cause of multi-infarct dementia?

a. Carotid bifurcation atherosclerosis
b. Cerebral emboli
c. Generalized atherosclerosis
d. Hypertension

    answer: d

73. Which of the following is the greatest difference between Alzheimer's disease and multi-infarct dementia?

a. Quality of dementia
b. CT findings
c. EEG findings
d. Clinical course
e. Focal physical findings

    answer: e. Focal physical findings are the most reliable feature, but the clinical course of a stepwise deterioration is also reliable and important.

74. A 28-year-old man has had a 3-day history of increasing left arm weakness and clumsiness and also a mild generalized headache. Examination reveals only hyperactive deep tendon reflexes in the mildly paretic left arm. Routine medical evaluation reveals no abnormalities. Both CT and MRI scans show a large right ring-enhancing cerebral lesion. Of the following, which is the most likely cause of the patient's neurologic difficulties?

a. Cerebral infarction
b. Cerebral hemorrhage
c. Toxoplasmosis
d. Glioblastoma
e. Meningioma

    answer: c. Further inquiry revealed that the patient was a homosexual, and laboratory testing revealed that he had acquired immune deficiency syndrome (AIDS). This condition is typically complicated by the development of cerebral toxoplasmosis, which is the most common cause of a ring-enhancing cerebral lesion in young adults. Cerebral infarction in a 28-year-old man is unlikely. Also, the scans in cerebral infarctions usually have a "pie-shaped" pattern. Cerebral hemorrhage is typically a suddenly occurring event, associated with blood-density on CT and MRI scans. A glioblastoma would be rare in a 28-year-old individual, and the scans would have indicated an infiltrating tumor. A meningioma is likewise rare in young adults, and when it does occur, it is extra-axial and slowly growing.

75–86. Match the sign (75–86) with the condition (a–b).

a. Locked-in syndrome
b. Persistent vegetative state

75. Mutism

    answer: Both

76. Quadriparesis

    answer: Both

77. Voluntary eye movement

    answer: a

78. Results from cerebral hypoxia

answer: b

79. Results from lower brainstem infarction or embolus

answer: a

80. Relatively normal EEG

answer: a

81. Cognitive capacity intact

answer: a

82. Cognitive capacity lost

answer: b

83. Due to lesion in base of pons that spares reticular activating system

answer: a

84. Due to lesion that damages virtually all of cerebral cortex or underlying cerebrum

answer: b

85. Usually caused by an extensive brainstem infarction, but may be caused by Guillain-Barré syndrome or myasthenia gravis

answer: a

86. Can be caused by insulin injections, as in attempted murder

answer: b

87. Which of the following characteristics most reliably distinguishes multi-infarct dementia (MID) from Alzheimer's dementia?

a. Stepwise onset
b. MRI scans that show atrophy
c. Aphasia
d. Focal physical findings
e. Greatest cognitive deficit is loss of memory

answer: d. The stepwise onset of multi-infarct dementia (MID) is a good but not the most characteristic aspect of the illness. Not only are histories of patients with dementia unreliable, but sometimes Alzheimer's disease seems to follow such a pattern. Atrophy is seen in both conditions, and in MID infarctions are often not visible. Aphasia is a characteristic finding of MID, but anomic aphasia and sometimes other varieties of aphasia are found in Alzheimer's disease. The particular neuropsychologic deficits cannot reliably distinguish the two conditions.

88. In patients with symptoms of carotid stenosis, what degree of stenosis has been found to justify surgery?

a. 50 per cent
b. 60 per cent
c. 70 per cent
d. 80 per cent
e. 90 per cent

answer: c

89. Several weeks after cardiac surgery that had been complicated by prolonged hypotension, a 70-year-old man had marked impairment of naming objects, following requests, disorientation, and other cognitive functions. Although he had little spontaneous speech, he seemed to repeat everything that was said to him or that he heard on television. He had generalized weakness, apraxia, and, as best as could be determined, visual impairment. Which of the following is the best diagnosis?

a. Locked-in syndrome
b. Persistent vegetative state
c. Multi-infarct dementia
d. Isolation aphasia, cortical blindness, and other watershed infarctions
f. None of the above

> ***answer:*** d. His ability to converse, albeit nonsensical, excludes the diagnoses of locked-in syndrome and persistent vegetative state. His tendency to repeat is the hallmark of isolation aphasia, which is typically accompanied by other signs of cerebral cortical hypotension injury. Multi-infarct dementia, which almost requires a history of several stroke episodes, does not cause isolation aphasia.

90. Which are the following characteristics of the N-methyl-D-aspartate receptor?

a. It is usually called the "NMDA" receptor.
b. It regulates calcium channels.
c. Excitatory neurotransmitters, such as glutamate, bind onto this receptor.
d. Overstimulation of the receptor leads to cell death by calcium flooding.

> ***answer:*** All

91. A 73-year-old woman arises from a vigorous hair washing at her local beauty parlor and finds that she is vertiginous and nauseated. A physician detects nystagmus and ataxia of her limbs and trunk. Her symptoms and signs resolve over 1 hour. What is the most likely cause of her disturbance?

a. Carotid artery TIA
b. Vertebrobasilar artery TIA
c. A chemical in the hair wash
d. Ordinary lightheadedness

> ***answer:*** b. She probably has had hyperextension (excessive backward bending) of her neck that crimped her vertebral arteries and caused a vertebrobasilar artery TIA. This condition is most common in elderly people who have osteophytes that press against the vertebral arteries as they pass upward through the cervical spine. This disorder is sometimes called by the double entendre, the *vanity syndrome*, because it was first described in (vain) patrons of beauty parlors who had their hair washed in basins (vanities).

12 Visual Disturbances

Because visual disturbances are so frequent, this chapter discusses several common neuroophthalmologic problems likely to occur in psychiatric patients, including decreased visual acuity, visual field loss, glaucoma, and certain psychologic aberrations affecting vision. The physician should determine the specific nature of visual symptoms (Table 12–1). The initial examination (Table 12–2) includes inspecting the globe or "eyeball" (Fig. 12–1); assessing visual acuity, visual fields, and optic fundi; and testing pupil reflexes and ocular movement. Examinations for special cases, such as psychogenic blindness and visual agnosia, are discussed later in the chapter.

DECREASE IN VISUAL ACUITY

Visual acuity is routinely determined by having the patient read from either a Snellen wall chart or a hand-held card (Fig. 12–2). A person with "normal" visual acuity can read 3/8-inch letters at a distance of 20 feet. This acuity, which is the reference point of the system, is designated 20/20. People with 20/40 acuity must be as close as 20 feet to see what a normal person can see from a distance of 40 feet.

Optical Disturbances

In *myopia*, usually because of either too "thick" a lens, too "long" a globe, or abnormal corneal optics, people have increasingly blurred vision at increasingly greater distances (Fig. 12–3). Myopia first becomes troublesome during adolescence when it causes difficulty with seeing blackboards, watching movies, and driving. Since reading and other close activities are unimpaired, people with myopia are said to be "near-sighted."

In its counterpart, *hyperopia* or hypermetropia (far-sightedness), the lens is usually too "thin" or the globe too "short." People with hyperopia have increasing visual difficulty at increasingly shorter distances. In *presbyopia*, a related optical condition that begins in middle age, the lenses are not able to focus on closely held objects. Patients with hyperopia and those with presbyopia have difficulty reading and sewing, and they tend to hold newspapers and needles away from themselves. "Reading glasses" correct the problem.

In addition to these naturally occurring conditions, use of certain medications can lead to important optical disturbances. The foremost is *drug-induced accommodation paresis*, in which patients have visual acuity impairment for closely held objects (Fig. 12–4). Normally, when a person looks at a closely held object, a parasympathetic-mediated *accommodation reflex* contracts the ciliary body muscles, which thickens the lens to focus the image on the retina. However, psychotropic medications with anticholinergic properties blur vi-

TABLE 12–1.   SALIENT FEATURES OF A PATIENT'S HISTORY

Is the symptom in one or both eyes? one visual field?
What is the primary symptom?
  Decreased visual acuity
  Visual field loss (one or both eyes)
  Diplopia: direction(s)
  Visual distortions or hallucinations, including halos around lights
What associated symptoms are present?
  Ocular: pain, scintillations
  Neurologic: headache, paresis, ataxia, impotence
  Systemic: fever, malaise, nausea, excessive thirst
Is there is a history of any of the following conditions?
  Diabetes, hypertension, syphilis
  Use of psychotropic, anticholinergic, antituberculous, or other medications
  Abuse of tobacco, alcohol, or methanol
  Exposure to hallucinogens or industrial toxins
Is there a family history of visual disturbances, especially glaucoma?

sion largely because they impair accommodation. Blurred vision is also a relatively common side effect of the serotonin reuptake inhibitors and clozapine, as well as the tricyclic antidepressants, which have well-known anticholinergic properties. For example, venlafaxine (Effexor) causes paresis of accommodation in 9 per cent of patients taking 75 mg daily, and sertraline (Zoloft) causes blurred vision for unspecified reasons in 4.2 per cent of patients. In fact, these medicines can impair accommodation without producing other anticholinergic effects, such as dry mouth, constipation, and urinary hesitancy.

Abnormalities of the Lens, Retina, and Optic Nerve

Cataracts (loss of lens transparency) result from complications of old age (senile cataract), trauma, diabetes, and myotonic dystrophy (see Chapter 6). In

TABLE 12–2.   SALIENT FEATURES OF A PATIENT'S EXAMINATION

Gross evaluation of the globe (eyeball)
  Injection of conjunctival vessels[a]
  Clarity of cornea and lens
  Inspection for Kayser-Fleischer rings (see Chapter 18)[a]
  Corneal reflex
Determination of visual acuity
  Naked eye
  Corrected with eyeglasses or lens
Determination of visual fields
  Confrontation (see Fig. 4–2)
Inspection of fundi
  Optic disk: color, clarity of margins
  Retina: color, hemorrhages[a], exudates[a], pigment deposit[a]
  Vessels: arterial pulsations[a], venous pulsations
Testing of pupils
  Size, shape, and equality
  Light reflex
  Accommodation
Measurement of extraocular movement
  Position at rest
  Position when looking horizontally or vertically (diplopia[a], nystagmus[a])
  Strength of orbicularis oculi (eyelids)
  Paresis with fatigue

[a]Abnormalities.

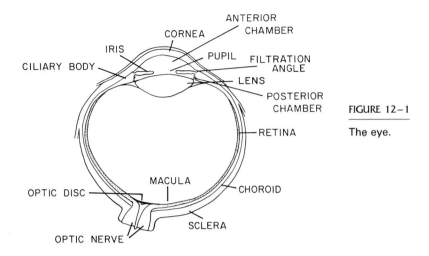

FIGURE 12–1

The eye.

prolonged, high doses, phenothiazines induce minute lens opacities that rarely impair vision.

Pigmentary changes in the retina that do interfere with vision can be manifestations of congenital injuries, degenerative diseases, diabetes, or the use of massive doses of phenothiazines (Fig. 12–5). In addition, acquired immune deficiency syndrome (AIDS) is associated with opportunistic infections of the retinas and other layers of the eye.

In contrast, optic nerve injuries almost always produce marked visual loss. Sometimes they also produce psychiatric symptoms. One example is olfactory groove or sphenoid wing *meningiomas*, which compress the adjacent optic nerve (see Chapters 19 and 20). When they grow into the frontal or temporal lobe, these tumors can trigger partial complex seizures and induce intellectual

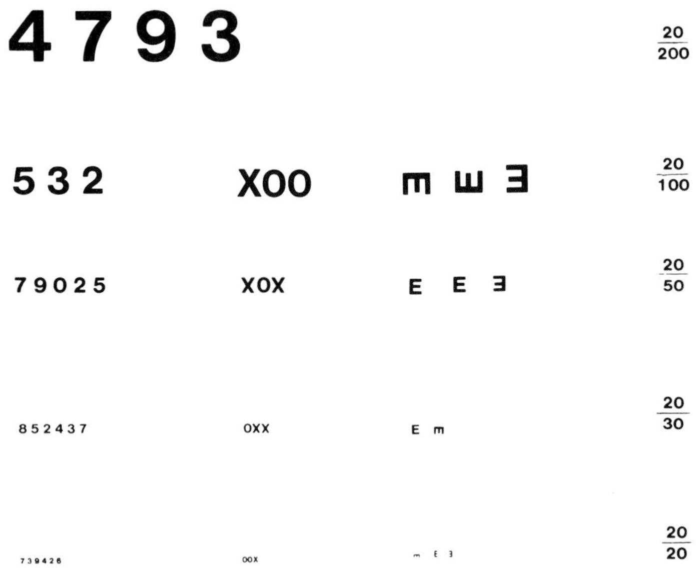

FIGURE 12–2

This hand-held visual acuity chart should be held 14 inches from the patient. The acuity is that line that can be read without a mistake. Each eye should be tested individually, and for neurologic evaluations, glasses or contact lenses should be worn.

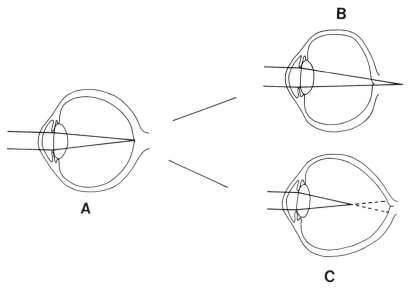

FIGURE 12-3

Image focusing in myopic and hyperopic eyes. *A,* In normal eyes, the lens focuses the image on to the retina. *B,* In hyperopic eyes, the shorter globe or improperly focusing lens causes the image to fall behind the retina. *C,* In myopic eyes, the longer globe or improperly focusing lens causes the image to fall in front of the retina. Traditionally, glasses or contact lenses have corrected hyperopia. In addition, surgical "flattening" of the lens corrects myopia in many individuals.

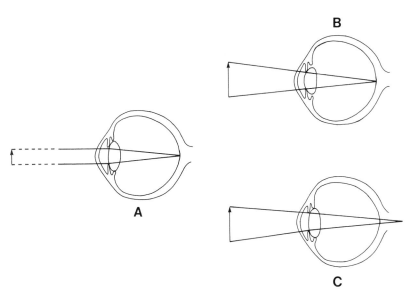

FIGURE 12-4

Accommodation and accommodation paresis. *A,* When looking at a distant object, parallel light rays are refracted little by a relatively flat lens onto the retina. *B,* Accommodation: When looking at a closely held object, ciliary muscle contraction increases the curvature of the lens, greatly refracting the light rays. *C,* Accommodation paresis: If the ciliary muscles are paretic, the lens cannot form a rounded shape. Its weakened refractive power can only focus the light rays from closely held objects behind the retina; however, parallel light rays from distant objects are still focused on the retina. Therefore, with accommodation paralysis, closely held objects will be blurred, but distant ones will be distinct.

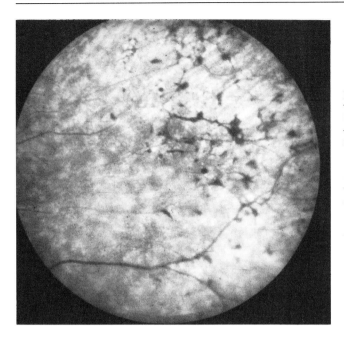

FIGURE 12–5

Retinal hyperpigmentation —described as "black bone spicules" or "salt and pepper"—can be induced by massive doses of thioridazine (Mellaril). Before these retinal pigmentary changes are visible, patients may complain of blurred vision or impaired night-time vision.

and personality changes. Another example is pituitary tumors, such as *adenomas* or *craniopharyngiomas*, which can grow upward to compress the optic chiasm and hypothalamus and downward to damage the pituitary gland (see Fig. 19–4). Compression of the optic chiasm causes optic atrophy and bitemporal hemianopsia, and compression of the hypothalamus and pituitary causes headache, decreased libido, diabetes insipidus, and loss of secondary sexual characteristics.

Inflammation of the optic nerve, *optic* or *retrobulbar neuritis,* causes sudden, painful visual loss in one eye (Fig. 12–6). The pupil usually has a preserved but diminished reaction to light (reactivity) during the initial attack. Since patients are usually otherwise in good health, the optic disk appears normal, and the pupil is still reactive, patients might be misdiagnosed as suffering from a psychogenic disturbance (see Chapter 3). In fact, at least one third of optic neuritis patients ultimately develop multiple sclerosis (MS) (see Chapter 15). With recurrent optic neuritis attacks, whatever their origin, the optic nerve becomes atrophic, the pupil unreactive, and the eye blind.

Another inflammatory condition of the optic nerve is *temporal,* or *giant cell, arteritis.* Typically affecting old people, temporal arteritis causes headaches, malaise, weight loss, and sometimes the appearance of depression. Worse, if it is not promptly treated with steroids, temporal arteritis leads to optic nerve and cerebral infarctions (see Chapter 9). Optic atrophy, blindness, and some-

FIGURE 12–6

Optic Nerve

Optic Disk

Retrobulbar Portion

The long segment of the optic nerve behind the eye, the *retrobulbar* portion, is subject to multiple sclerosis and other inflammatory conditions. The resulting condition, called *optic* or *retrobulbar neuritis,* causes pain and loss of vision (see Fig. 15–2). However, in the early stages, optic neuritis does not cause any observable change in the optic disk, which is the *bulbar* portion of the nerve.

times mental aberrations also result from methanol intoxication, which occasionally occurs in alcoholics. Brain tumors (see Chapter 19) and pseudotumor cerebri (Chapter 9), if untreated, cause optic atrophy.

GLAUCOMA

Glaucoma, in most cases, is elevated intraocular pressure that results from the obstructed outflow of aqueous humor through the *filtration angle* of the anterior chamber of the eye (Fig. 12–7). Two common varieties—*open-angle* and *angle-closure*—are recognized, and the angle-closure variety occasionally results from psychotropic medications. If glaucoma remains untreated, it damages the optic nerve head, causes visual field impairments, and eventually leads to blindness.

Open-Angle Glaucoma

Open-angle or *wide-angle glaucoma* occurs seven times more frequently than closed-angle glaucoma. People at greatest risk are older than 40 years, diabetic, myopic, and relatives of glaucoma patients. Since symptoms are usually absent at the onset, glaucoma might be diagnosed only by an ophthalmologist detecting either elevated intraocular pressure or certain visual field losses. Later, when central vision or acuity is impaired, the optic cup is abnormally deep and permanently damaged. The lack of symptoms in the initial phase of open-angle glaucoma is the best reason for a yearly ophthalmologic examination.

Open-angle glaucoma usually responds to topical medications (eye drops), laser therapy, or surgery. Psychotropic medications do not precipitate open-angle glaucoma. Patients with open-angle glaucoma may be given antidepressants and other psychotropic medications provided that their glaucoma treatment is continued.

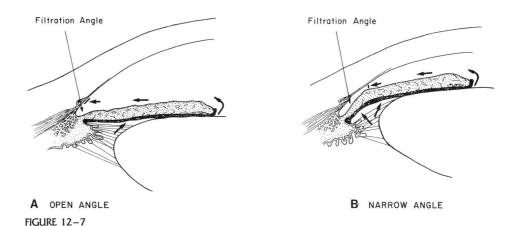

A OPEN ANGLE   **B** NARROW ANGLE

FIGURE 12–7

A, Open-angle glaucoma: The aqueous humor is not drained despite access to the absorptive surface of the angle. Impaired flow from the eye leads to gradually increased intraocular pressure (glaucoma). *B,* Narrow-angle glaucoma: When the iris is pushed forward, as may occur during pupil dilation, the angle is narrowed or even closed. Obstruction of aqueous humor flow, which usually occurs suddenly, leads to angle-closure glaucoma.

Angle-Closure Glaucoma

In *angle-closure glaucoma*, which is also called *closed-angle* or *narrow-angle glaucoma,* intraocular pressure is usually raised by the iris blocking aqueous humor outflow at the filtration angle. The fluid becomes trapped behind the iris. Patients with narrow-angle glaucoma, like those with open-angle glaucoma, usually are older than 40 years and often have a family history, but they also have had long-standing narrow angles. Few have had symptoms, such as seeing halos around lights, preceding an attack of angle-closure glaucoma. In contrast to the relatively normal appearance of the eye in open-angle glaucoma, in acute angle-closure glaucoma, the eye is red, the pupil dilated, and the cornea hazy. Moreover, the eye and forehead are painful, and vision is impaired.

Angle-closure glaucoma is sometimes iatrogenic. When the pupils are dilated for ocular examinations, the "bunched-up" iris can block the angle. Likewise, angle-closure glaucoma can be precipitated by medications with anticholinergic properties probably because they dilate the pupil. However, the incidence of glaucoma complicating antidepressant use is remarkably low (less than 0.1 per cent).

Whatever the cause, prompt treatment of angle-closure glaucoma is mandatory. Topical and systemic medications open the angle (by constricting the pupil) and also reduce aqueous humor production. Laser iridectomy immediately and painlessly creates a passage directly through the iris to drain aqueous humor.

Since measuring the intraocular pressure does not predict who will develop angle-closure glaucoma, few rules concerning prescribing medicines are practical. Everyone older than 40 years should have intraocular pressure measured every 2 years, and those older than 65 years, every year. Patients who are under treatment for either form of glaucoma may receive psychotropic medications. Glaucoma medications, such as pilocarpine, and ophthalmic beta-blockers, such as timolol (Timoptic), may be absorbed through the nasal mucosa and create systemic and psychologic side effects. Children are particularly susceptible; when they receive scopolamine and other atropine-like eye drops for ocular examination, they can develop agitation. On the other hand, marijuana, despite the claims of its enthusiasts, is no more effective than standard topical medications.

CORTICAL BLINDNESS AND ASSOCIATED PSYCHOLOGIC PHENOMENA

Bilateral occipital cortex damage causes visual impairment, *cortical blindness*. It usually results from posterior cerebral injuries, such as bilateral posterior cerebral artery occlusion and occipital head trauma, but it can result from extensive brain injury from anoxia, multiple infarctions, or MS. Whether the cortical blindness results from limited or generalized cortex injury, since the optic nerves and brainstem remain intact, the pupils are normal in size and reactivity to light.

Anton's Syndrome

A dramatic neuropsychologic complication of cortical blindness is *Anton's syndrome*. In this disorder, patients persist in believing that their vision is intact, i.e., they deny blindness. With little prompting, they "describe" their room, clothing, and various other objects. In addition to denying and confabulating, they sometimes behave as though they have normal vision and proceed to stumble about their room.

Many cases of Anton's syndrome are accompanied by other signs of generalized cerebral cortex injury, especially delirium and dementia. With posterior cerebral injuries as the cause of the problem, Anton's syndrome may accompany anosognosia for other deficits (from right-sided parietal lobe injury) or amnesia (from bilateral temporal lobe injury). For example, a 76-year-old man, who had just sustained a right-sided posterior cerebral infarction and had a left posterior cerebral infarction the previous year, ascribed his inability to see the examiner's blouse first to poor lighting and then to his disinterest in it. When pressed, still denying his blindness, he confabulated by calmly describing the blouse as "lovely" and "becoming," at times elaborating that it was "obviously made from good material."

Although cortical blindness and Anton's syndrome refer to the complete loss of vision, sometimes disturbances relate to a visual field cut, i.e., a hemianopsia (see below). *Palinopsia*, which may be likened to "visual perseveration," consists of images that reappear, especially in an hemianopic area. Patients recall images of family, friends, and familiar places; however, unfamiliar scenes may also recur.

Agnosia

Another neuropsychologic phenomenon, *visual agnosia*, is a perceptual inability to identify an object by sight, despite an intact visual system and the absence of aphasia and dementia. Patients with visual agnosia cannot comprehend what they see. For example, patients are unable to write or say the word "key" when a key is shown to them, but they are able to make a drawing of it, describe its use, and say "key" when one is placed in their hand. Visual agnosia differs from aphasia in that, when vision is bypassed (when patients touch objects), language function is normal. Another difference is that the lesion causing visual agnosia is not established—certainly not as well as in aphasia (see Fig. 8–1).

Visual agnosia is a major aspect of the infamous *Klüver-Bucy syndrome*. This syndrome is a behavioral disorder that is produced in monkeys by resection of both temporal lobes, which contain the amygdalae and their associated structures (see Chapter 16). The loss of a good portion of the limbic system results in visual agnosia so severe that the monkeys not only touch all objects but they also identify objects by putting them into their mouth ("psychic blindness"). Their behavior is repetitive, compulsive, and indiscriminate.

When the Klüver-Bucy syndrome occurs in people, it includes a muted version of psychic blindness, *oral exploration*. Patients only place inedible objects into their mouth partly, briefly, and absentmindedly.

Color agnosia, a variety of visual agnosia, is a particular inability to identify an object's color. It is not common color blindness, which is a sex-linked inherited retinal abnormality. Patients with color agnosia cannot say or write an object's color despite a normal ability to match colored cards, read Ishihara plates (pseudoisochromatic numbered cards), and recite the colors of well-known objects, such as the sky.

In another variety, *prosopagnosia*, patients cannot recognize *familiar faces*, although they can identify friends and relatives by voice, dress, mannerisms, and other nonfacial characteristics (see Chapter 8). Prosopagnosia is usually attributed to bilateral occipitotemporal injury. In a variation, patients with right cerebral lesions are unable to match pairs of pictures of *unfamiliar* faces. Their impairment probably reflects visual-spatial impairments from nondominant parietal lobe lesions. Although these agnosias are neatly and individually defined, patients' deficits are usually incomplete and are combined with other perceptual impairments, alexia, aphasia, dementia, and physical deficits.

Psychogenic Blindness

A completely different situation is *psychogenic blindness*. Cases of psychogenic blindness that convincingly mimic true blindness are rare because people do not have an intuitive knowledge of the visual pathways, "blindness" is too incapacitating to burden oneself, and bedside testing can easily reveal the nonanatomic origin of the problem.

An uninhibited examiner simply might make childlike facial contortions or ask the patient to read some four-letter words. The patient's reaction to these provocations would reveal an ability to see. When only one eye is affected by psychogenic blindness, fogged, colored, or polarized lenses will often confuse (or fatigue) a patient into revealing that vision is present.

Another technique is to spin a vertically striped cylinder (drum) in front of a person with questionable visual loss. The drum will elicit *opticokinetic* nystagmus in individuals with normal vision, even those too young to speak. Likewise, looking at a large, moving mirror forces almost everyone with normal vision to follow their own image. Visual evoked response (VER) testing can show diagnostically helpful electrical potentials (see Chapter 15). Alternatively, having patients wear lenses with negligible optical value may also reveal normal vision. Furthermore, it permits patients to extract themselves without embarrassment from psychogenic blindness.

A special disturbance is *tubular* or *tunnel vision* (Fig. 12–8). This pattern is inconsistent with the laws of optics that dictate that the visual area expands with increasing distance. An important exception to this law, however, is migraine with aura (see Chapter 9), in which patients have peripheral vision constriction.

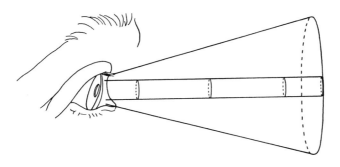

FIGURE 12–8

The area seen by a person normally increases conically in proportion to the distance from the object. In *tubular* or *tunnel vision*, which defies the laws of optics, the visual area is constant despite increasing distance.

Visual Hallucinations

Unlike auditory hallucinations, visual hallucinations almost always indicate neurologic dysfunction. They can originate in the frontal lobe, temporal lobe, or cerebral peduncles, as well as the occipital cortex. They can be manifestations of various difficulties, including intoxications, metabolic aberrations, structural lesions, and physiologic disturbances (Table 12–3). Moreover, with the exception of migraine auras, the contents of visual hallucinations do not indicate a particular origin. Diagnostic clues regarding visual hallucinations are if they are repetitive (stereotyped) or associated with headache, convulsive activity, delirium, or sleep disturbance.

With seizures, visual hallucinations tend to be stereotyped. Tumors, strokes, and other structural lesions can produce partial elementary, frontal lobe, or complex seizures with visual symptoms (see Chapter 10). These hallucinations are "seen" in both eyes and can even appear in an hemianopic area. They range from simple geometric forms in partial simple seizures to detailed visions accompanied by sounds, thoughts, emotions, and, characteristically, impairment of consciousness in partial complex seizures.

As an element of narcolepsy-cataplexy (see Chapter 17) or an occasional independent event, dreams may intrude into a patient's partial consciousness. Like dreams, these hallucinations are composed of intricate visions accompanied by rich thoughts and strong emotions. They occur while patients fall asleep (hypnagogic hallucinations) or awake (hypnopompic hallucinations). As with normal dreams during rapid eye movement (REM) sleep, these hallucinations are associated with flaccid, areflexic paresis.

A different sleep-related visual hallucination is peduncular hallucinosis. This condition is caused by infectious or vascular injuries of the midbrain and pons. (This portion of the brainstem contains the cerebral peduncles [Fig. 4–4], connections to the limbic system, and pathways involved in REM). Peduncular hallucinations are typically accompanied by somnolence and oculomotor nerve palsies.

Migraines with aura (classic migraine) include stereotyped and characteristic—virtually diagnostic—visual hallucinations (see Fig. 9–2). Distinctive crescent scotomata or scintillating fortification spectra usually move slowly across the visual field for 1 to 20 minutes before yielding to a

TABLE 12–3. COMMON NEUROLOGIC CAUSES OF VISUAL HALLUCINATION

Alzheimer's disease (see Chapter 7)
Delirium tremens (DTs)
Intoxications
    Alcoholic hallucinosis
    Hallucinogens: Phencyclidine (PCP, angel dust), lysergic acid diethylamide (LSD), mescaline, amphetamines
    Medicines: L-dopa, scopolamine, atropine, penicillin, psychotropics
Migraines: Migraine with aura (classic migraine)
Narcolepsy: Hypnopompic (awakening) and hypnagogic (falling asleep) hallucinations (see Chapter 17)
Peduncular hallucinosis
Sensory deprivation
    Sudden blindness, e.g., Anton's syndrome (see Chapter 12)
Seizures (see Chapter 10)
    Frontal lobe
    Elementary (visual)
    Complex partial

hemicranial headache. However, visual auras sometimes are the sole manifestation of a migraine.

Visual hallucinations may be caused by intoxications with medications, including psychotropics, as well as with illicit drugs. They may also result from withdrawal from alcohol and other addictive substances. The best-known example is *delirium tremens* (*DTs*). In most patients, varied hallucinations often stem from the environment and are accompanied by agitation, confusion, sweating, and tachycardia. Sometimes patients, petrified by the hallucinations, become reticent and immobile.

Finally, visual hallucinations can be produced by any sudden visual loss. Palinopsia and cortical blindness (see above) induce hallucinations that, with palinopsia, may be stereotyped. Suddenly occurring blindness from eye injury may have the same effect. Soldiers with blinding eye wounds have periods of "seeing" brightly colored forms and even entire scenes. Similarly, eye surgery in the elderly is occasionally followed by visual hallucinations along with disorientation and agitation. Visual hallucinations in all these circumstances may result from spontaneously discharging unstimulated cortical neurons, but in many cases they result from sensory deprivation superimposed on dementia. Whatever the explanation, bilateral ophthalmologic surgical procedures should be avoided in the elderly.

Visual Field Loss.   The patterns of visual loss (Fig. 12–9) are a reliable guide to localization and diagnosis. In general, the following guidelines apply.

Monocular quadrantanopias, hemianopsias, scotomata, and blindness are usually the result of optic nerve injury.

Homonymous quadrantanopias and hemianopsias almost always result from visual tract injuries between the optic chiasm and the occipital cortex (see Fig. 4–1). The most common situation is a middle cerebral artery infarction that results in a contralateral homonymous hemianopsia accompanied by hemiparesis and hemisensory loss. An homonymous superior quadrantanopia (Fig. 12–10), although rare, is noteworthy because it may be the only physical man-

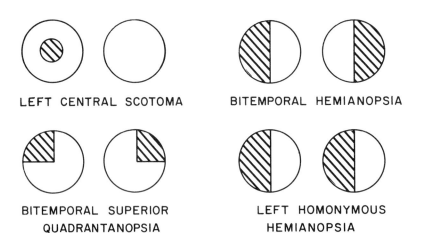

LEFT CENTRAL SCOTOMA   BITEMPORAL HEMIANOPSIA

BITEMPORAL SUPERIOR   LEFT HOMONYMOUS
QUADRANTANOPSIA   HEMIANOPSIA

FIGURE 12–9

Uniocular *central scotomata* may be caused by migraine attacks, optic neuritis, or other ipsilateral optic nerve injuries. *Bitemporal superior quadrantanopia* is usually caused by lesions of the optic chiasm, such as pituitary adenomas or craniopharyngiomas. *Bitemporal hemianopsias* are caused by more advanced compression of the optic chiasm by the same lesions. *Homonymous hemianopsias*, with or without macular sparing, are most often caused by contralateral cerebral lesions, such as infarctions.

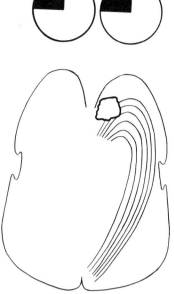

FIGURE 12-10

Large anterior temporal lobe lesions may interfere with forward sweeping optic tract fibers. Thus, these lesions, which are rare, may cause a contralateral superior quadrantanopia, as well as partial complex seizures.

ifestation of a contralateral temporal lobe lesion that produces partial complex seizures. Another noteworthy loss is an homonymous hemianopsia that excludes the center of vision (macular sparing) because it may indicate an occipital lobe lesion.

The visual field loss most commonly associated with mental aberrations is the left homonymous hemianopsia. It is often accompanied by left sensory inattention, visual-spatial impairments, and anosognosia (see Fig. 2–8 and Chapter 8).

Bitemporal quadrantanopias and hemianopsias indicate a lesion at the optic chiasm. The vast majority are pituitary adenomas, which, as discussed previously, compress the optic chiasm, cause optic atrophy, and lead to hypopituitarism with an elevated serum prolactin level.

CONJUGATE OCULAR MOVEMENT

Both eyes normally move together in a paired, coordinated (*conjugate*) manner so that people can look (*gaze*) laterally and follow (*pursue*) moving objects. Conjugate movement is generated by a succession of cerebral and brainstem *gaze centers* that receive cerebellar influence and visual feedback. Since these centers innervate pairs of oculomotor, trochlear, and abducens cranial nerve *nuclei,* conjugate movements are *supranuclear.*

Conjugate movement originates in each frontal lobe's *cerebral conjugate gaze center.* When a person is at rest, each cerebral center continuously emits impulses that go through a complicated pathway to "push" the eyes contralaterally. With the counterbalancing effect of each center, the eyes remain midline (Fig. 12–11). When a person wants to look to one side, the contralateral cerebral gaze center increases activity. For example, when someone wants to look toward a water glass on the right, the left cerebral gaze center activity increases, and as if pushing the eyes away, the eyes turn to the right. Also, if

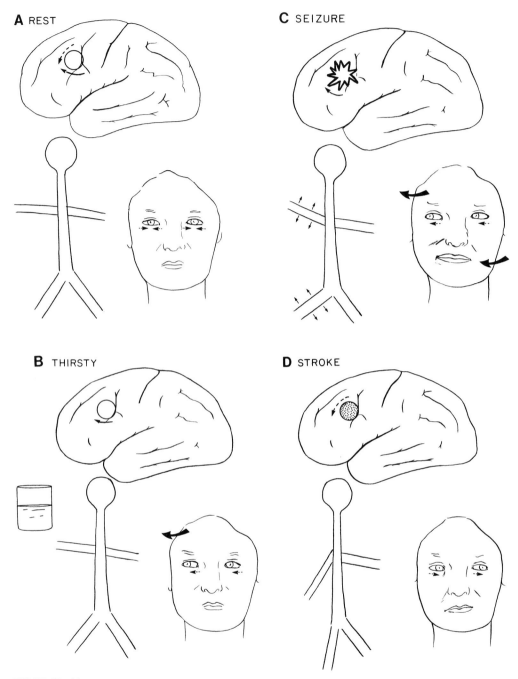

FIGURE 12–11

A, At rest, the eyes are midline because the impulses of each frontal lobe conjugate gaze center are balanced, each ''pushing'' the eyes contralaterally. *B,* Voluntarily increased activity of the left cerebral gaze center drives the eyes to the right (contralaterally). *C,* Involuntarily increased cerebral activity also drives the eyes contralaterally. Also, with left cerebral seizure activity, the right arm and leg develop tonic-clonic activity. *D,* A CVA destroys the left cerebral gaze center, permitting the right center to push the eyes toward the lesion. It also destroys the cerebral motor strip, causing contralateral paresis. This common CVA is characterized by the eyes ''looking'' away from the hemiparesis.

this person wanted to reach for the glass, the left cerebral corticospinal center, which is adjacent to that gaze center, would mobilize the right arm.

Partial seizures also increase the activity of the conjugate gaze center. They push the eyes contralaterally and, because they usually envelop the adjacent corticospinal tract, they push the head and neck contralaterally and produce tonic-clonic activity of the contralateral arm and leg. In contrast, when patients have unilateral destructive cerebral injuries, such as large cerebrovascular accidents (CVAs or strokes), the activity of the gaze center on that side is abolished. The activity of the other center, being unopposed, pushes the eyes toward the injured side. For example, with a left cerebral infarction, the eyes deviate toward the left. Also, since the corticospinal tract is generally involved, the right side of the body is paralyzed. This example illustrates the sayings, "When the eyes look away from the paralysis, the stroke is cerebral," and "The eyes look toward the stroke."

Each cerebral gaze center produces conjugate eye movements by stimulating a contralateral *pontine gaze center*, which is also called the *pontine paramedian reticular formation (PPRF)*. In contrast to the cerebral center, each pontine center *pulls* the eyes toward its own side (Fig. 12–12). A unilateral pontine infarction allows the eyes to be pulled toward the opposite side. For example, if the right pontine gaze center were damaged, the eyes would deviate to the left. Also, because the right pontine corticospinal tract would be damaged, the left arm and leg would be paralyzed. Thus, with a pontine lesion, the eyes "look toward the paralysis."

After the pontine gaze centers receive impulses from the contralateral cerebral conjugate gaze center, each pontine gaze center stimulates the adjacent abducens (sixth cranial nerve) nucleus and, through the *medial longitudinal fasciculus* (*MLF*), the contralateral oculomotor (third cranial nerve) nucleus (see Figs. 15–3 and 15–4). Innervation of one abducens nucleus and the other oculomotor nucleus is necessary for conjugate lateral eye movement. If both abducens nuclei were stimulated simultaneously, both eyes would turn outward. If both oculomotor nuclei were stimulated simultaneously, both eyes would turn inward. When the MLF is injured, as often occurs in MS and brainstem CVAs, the *MLF syndrome* (*internuclear ophthalmoplegia*) develops. In this condition, the cranial nuclei and nerves are normal, but the eyes cannot move conjugately (see Chapter 15).

Another important ocular movement is *nystagmus* (rhythmic horizontal, vertical, or rotatory eyeball oscillation). Although often a sign of CNS injury, nystagmus may be a normal variant. When people look to the extreme of lateral

FIGURE 12–12

When looking to the right, the left frontal conjugate gaze center stimulates the right (contralateral) pontine gaze center, which, in turn, stimulates the right (adjacent) abducens nerve nucleus and, through the left medial longitudinal fasciculus, the left (contralateral) oculomotor nerve nucleus.

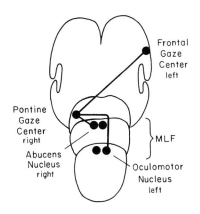

gaze, they may have horizontal nystagmus (end-point nystagmus). Some people have congenital nystagmus, which may be disconcerting to people looking at them, but it does not interfere with their vision. In these people, the nystagmus is pendular, direction changing, and absent when they look toward a particular point (the null point).

On the other hand, jerky, predominantly horizontal nystagmus is most often caused by labyrinthitis, in which case it is associated with vertigo, nausea, and vomiting. Nystagmus is also caused by various neurologic injuries, including MS, brainstem infarctions, and Wernicke-Korsakoff syndrome. It may be the most prominent physical finding in the abuse of diazepam, barbiturates, or alcohol and with excessive concentrations of antipsychotic and antidepressant medications. However, nystagmus is routinely found in seizure patients who take therapeutic doses of phenytoin (Dilantin) or phenobarbital: its absence even suggests noncompliance with an anticonvulsant regimen.

Saccades and Pursuit Movement

When anything enters the periphery of the visual field, the eyes dart toward it. They rotate conjugately, rapidly, smoothly, and without disturbing the eyelids or head. These movements, called *saccades*, are characterized by their rapidity, which may exceed 700 degrees/sec. Saccades or "saccadic eye movements" are examined in patients by asking them to stare at an object 45 degrees to one side and suddenly to shift their gaze to a different object 45 degrees to the other. Laboratory measurements are detailed, but at the "bedside," slowness is the primary abnormality. Other abnormalities are over- or undershooting (hyper- and hypometria), irregular or jerky movements, and—a subtle one—initiating the saccade by head movement or blinking.

The counterpart of saccades is *pursuit*, which is relatively slow ocular tracking of moving objects. The bedside test is to ask the patient to gaze at the examiner's finger as it moves horizontally at about 30 degrees/sec. The eye should remain on the target and smoothly follow it. The primary abnormality would be irregular or jerky movements.

Since saccadic and pursuit movements are generated by the supranuclear gaze centers, extensive structural cerebral lesions impair both movements. When lesion are relatively small, frontal lobe lesions impair saccades, and parietal, occipital, and brainstem lesions impair pursuit. Slowed or otherwise abnormal saccades may be detected early and characteristically in Huntington's disease. They are also found in other conditions that involve the basal ganglia and cerebrum and cause dementia (see Chapter 18). Abnormalities in pursuit are present in drug intoxication and the diseases that cause impaired saccades. Although various saccade and pursuit abnormalities are found in many people with schizophrenia or, less so, with affective disorders compared to controls, they only indicate an underlying biologic dysfunction and are not specific or common enough to be diagnostic.

DIPLOPIA

Diplopia ("double vision") seen with one eye is usually the result of either ocular abnormalities, such as a dislocated lens or retinal tear, or psychogenic factors. Individuals with such "monocular" diplopia will have diplopia when covering the unaffected eye. Also, their diplopia will usually persist in all directions of gaze.

Individuals who have diplopia from neurologic injuries will usually have diplopia only in certain directions of gaze, and the diplopia will be abolished by covering either eye. It is almost always caused by—in descending order— brainstem (but not cerebral) infarction, oculomotor or abducens cranial nerve injury, or extraocular muscle paresis. Supranuclear lesions cause conjugate gaze palsies, not diplopia.

Oculomotor (third cranial) nerve injury results in ptosis, lateral deviation of the eye, diplopia that is greatest when the patient looks away from the midline, and, most importantly, pupil dilation (Fig. 12–13). However, one important exception is that, in third nerve infarctions from diabetes, the pupil is spared and remains reactive to light and equal to its counterpart. Abducens (sixth cranial) nerve injury results in medial deviation of the eye and diplopia when looking laterally, but neither in ptosis nor pupil abnormality (Fig. 12– 14).

Although diplopia is frequently the result of cranial nerve injury, several conditions are important variations. When myopic adults read or drive while fatigued, they develop momentary diplopia because of ocular muscle fatigue. Also, myasthenia gravis causes diplopia and ptosis, which are initially transient and are never associated with pupil abnormalities (see Chapter 6).

On the other hand, although congenital ocular muscle weakness, *strabismus*, causes dysconjugate gaze, children do not have diplopia because the brain suppresses the image from the weaker eye. With continuous suppression of the vision of that eye, however, it will actually become blind *(amblyopic)*. Thus, babies and children with a "crossed" or "lazy eye" often have the "good" eye patched several hours each day to force them to use the visual and muscle systems of the weak eye.

Before diagnosing psychogenic diplopia, zealous physicians must not overlook subtle neurologic conditions, especially myasthenia gravis and the MLF syndrome. Psychogenic diplopia is usually intermittent, inconsistent, and

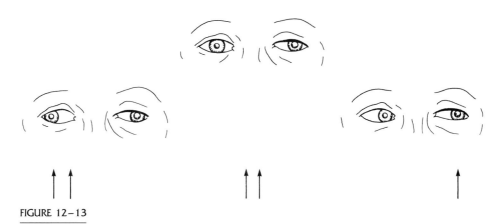

FIGURE 12–13

Left oculomotor (third cranial) nerve palsy. In the center picture, a patient looks ahead. The left upper lid is lower, the pupil larger, and the eye deviated slightly laterally. Since the eyes are dysconjugate, the patient sees two arrows (diplopia) when looking ahead. In the picture on the left, the patient looks to the right. Since the paretic left eye fails to cross medially beyond the midline (i.e., it fails to adduct), the eyes are more dysconjugate and there is greater diplopia. In the picture on the right, the patient looks to the left. The eyes are almost conjugate, and there is little or no diplopia.

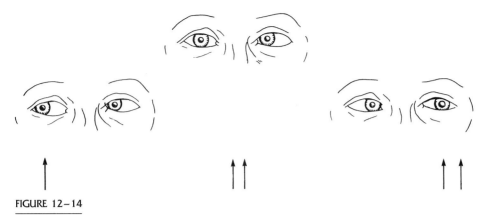

FIGURE 12–14

A left abducens (sixth cranial) nerve palsy. In the center picture, a patient looks ahead. The patient's left eye is deviated medially. The eyes are dysconjugate, and the patient sees two arrows when looking ahead. In the picture on the left, the patient looks to the right. The eyes are conjugate, and the patient sees only a single arrow. In the picture on the right, the patient looks to the left. The paretic left eye fails to cross the midline laterally, i.e., it fails to abduct. The exaggeration of the dysconjugate gaze increases the diplopia.

present in all directions of gaze. Patients with this condition have no observable abnormality. A common set of tests consists of the patient reading colored or polarized charts utilizing colored or polarized lenses. In another psychogenic disturbance, children or young adults, as if looking at the tip of their nose, fix their eyes in a downward and inward position. This position is a burlesque that can be overcome by inducing opticokinetic nystagmus.

HORNER'S SYNDROME and ARGYLL-ROBERTSON PUPILS

Contrary to a reasonable expectation that the brain would innervate the eye entirely through a short and direct pathway, the sympathetic tract follows a remarkably circuitous route (Fig. 12–15A). Injury to the sympathetic tract leads to *Horner's syndrome*: ptosis, miosis (a small pupil), and anhidrosis (lack of sweating) (Fig. 12–15B). Given the roundabout course of the sympathetic tract, Horner's syndrome can be found in several geographically diverse injuries: lateral medullary infarctions (Wallenberg's syndrome [see Fig. 2–10]); cervical spinal cord injuries; apical lung (Pancoast) tumors; and, because of a carotid artery abnormality, cluster headaches (see Fig. 9–4).

Horner's syndrome might be confused with an oculomotor nerve injury because ptosis is a prominent, common sign. However, the miosis serves as the distinguishing feature of Horner's syndrome.

When confronting a small pupil, the astute physician must also bear in mind that the real problem is that the contralateral one is abnormally large. Causes of a dilated pupil include, in addition to an oculomotor nerve injury, a congenital variation (Adie's pupil), accidentally rubbing atropine-like substances into one eye, and its notorious variant: people—usually medical personnel—purposely, surreptitiously installing such substances.

Argyll-Robertson pupils also must be differentiated from oculomotor nerve injury. They are irregular, asymmetric, and small (1 to 2 mm). Moreover, they are characteristically unreactive to light, but do constrict normally when patients look at closely held objects, i.e., during accommodation. The impaired

FIGURE 12-15

A, The sympathetic nervous system originates in the brainstem, passes through the medulla, and descends into the cervical and then the thoracic spinal cord. Some sympathetic system neurons leave the thoracic spinal cord and, after making a hairpin turn, ascend to form ganglia adjacent to the cervical vertebrae. Postsynaptic neurons ascend further. They are wrapped successively around the common carotid, internal carotid, and then the ophthalmic artery. These neurons, seeming to rise higher than their starting point, innervate the pupil dilator muscles, levator palpebrae (upper eyelid) muscles, and facial sweat glands. *B, Top,* Stimulation of the sympathetic nervous system retracts the eyelid, dilates the pupil, and prevents sweating (anhidrosis). These cardinal signs of the "flight or fright" response may also be induced by states of excitement, including amphetamine use. *Bottom,* Injury to the sympathetic tract causes Horner's syndrome—miosis, ptosis, and anhidrosis—on this patient's left side. The important clue to Horner's syndrome is the eyebrow elevation, which is an unconscious maneuver that uncovers the pupil.

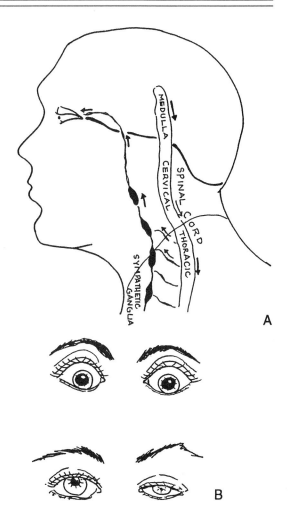

light reflex with intact accommodation has given rise to the saying, "Argyll-Robertson pupils are like prostitutes: they accommodate but do not react." Although Argyll-Robertson pupils have historically been a manifestation of syphilis, the majority of cases today result from diabetic autonomic neuropathy.

REFERENCES

Abramowicz M (ed.): Reading machines for the blind. Med Lett *34*: 13–14, 1992

Aldrich MS, Alessi AG, Beck RW, et al: Cortical blindness: Etiology, diagnosis, and prognosis. Ann Neurol *21*: 149–158, 1987

Asaad G: Hallucinations in Clinical Psychiatry, New York, Brunner/Mazel 1990.

Cummings JL, Miller BL: Visual hallucinations: Clinical occurrence and use in differential diagnosis. West J Med *146*: 46–51, 1987

Damasio AR, Damasio H, Hoesen GWV: Prosopagnosia: Anatomic basis and behavioral mechanisms. Neurology *32*:331–341, 1982

Friedman L, Abel LA, Jesberger JA, et al: Saccadic intrusions into smooth pursuit in patients with schizophrenia or affective disorder and normal controls. Biol Psychiatry *31*: 1110–1118, 1992

Gittinger JW: Functional hemianopsia: A historical perspective. Surv Ophthalmol *32*: 427–432, 1988

Grove WM, Clementz BA, Iacono WG, et al: Smooth pursuit ocular dysfunction in schizophrenia. Am J Psychiatry *149*: 1362–1368, 1992

Hamilton JD: Thioridazine retinopathy within upper dosage limit. Psychosomatics *26*:823–824, 1985

Heilman KM, Valenstein E (eds): Clinical Neuropsychology (3rd ed) New York, Oxford University Press, 1993

Keane JR: Neuro-ophthalmologic signs of AIDS. Neurology *41*: 841–845, 1991

Lieberman E, Stoudemire A: Use of tricyclic antidepressants in patients with glaucoma. Psychosomatics *28*: 145–148, 1987

McDaniel KD, McDaniel LD: Anton's syndrome in a patient with posttraumatic optic neuropathy and bifrontal contusions. Arch Neurol *48*: 101–105, 1991

Newman NM: Neuro-Ophthalmology: A Practical Text. Norwalk, CT, Appleton & Lange, 1992

McKee AC, Levine DN, Kowall NW, et al: Peduncular hallucinosis associated with isolated infarction of the substantia nigra par reticulata. Ann Neurol *27*: 500–504, 1990

Quigley HA: Open-angle glaucoma. N Engl J Med *328*: 1097–1106, 1993

QUESTIONS and ANSWERS: CHAPTER 12

1. Which findings characterize Argyll-Robertson pupils?

a. Miosis
b. Ptosis
c. Irregular shape
d. Unresponsiveness to light
e. Unresponsiveness to accommodation

> *answer:* a, c, d

2. Which medications are associated with transient visual impairment because of accommodation paresis?

a. Butyrophenones
b. Amitriptyline
c. Imipramine
d. Phenobarbital
e. Phenytoin

> *answer:* b, c

3. Which of the following cause cataracts that interfere with vision?

a. Myotonic dystrophy
b. Diabetes mellitus
c. Ocular trauma
d. Chlorpromazine

> *answer:* a, b, c

4. A 20-year-old soldier develops loss of vision in the right eye. The eye is painful, especially when he looks about. No ocular or neurologic abnormalities are found, except for a decreased light reaction in the right pupil. After 1 week, vision returns, except for a small central scotoma. What illness is he likely to have had?

> *answer:* He probably had an episode of optic neuritis.

5. What is the prognosis in the case presented in question 4?

> *answer:* About one third of male patients and three quarters of female patients later develop multiple sclerosis.

6. Which laboratory procedure will identify dysfunction of the optic nerve in patients with clinical symptoms and signs indicative of multiple sclerosis and also help distinguish patients with visual impairments from those with psychogenic impairments?

> *answer:* Visual evoked responses (VER), which are essentially analyses of the EEG when flashing light is shown into the subject's eyes, will indicate the presence and location of impairment of the visual system. It is a sensitive procedure that permits detection of asymptomatic optic nerve lesions, as might occur in multiple sclerosis. It requires little or no patient cooperation. An MRI can detect only large plaques in the optic nerves.

7. What are the characteristics of open-angle glaucoma?

a. Chronicity
b. Acute onset

c. Hereditary predisposition
d. Onset after age 40
e. Raised intraocular pressure
f. Precipitated by tricyclic antidepressant medications
g. Absolute contraindication to the use of tricyclic antidepressant medications
h. Response to ocular or systemic medical therapy

answer: a, c, d, e, h

8. What are the characteristics of angle-closure glaucoma?

a. Chronicity
b. Acute onset
c. Hereditary predisposition
d. Onset after age 40
e. Painful eye
f. "Steamy" cornea
g. Headache
h. Precipitated by tricyclic antidepressant medications
i. Surgical treatment

answer: b, c, d, e, f, g, h, i

9. Should patients with angle-closure glaucoma be given tricyclic antidepressants?

answer: They may take tricyclic antidepressants after therapy for glaucoma has been instituted. In particular, patients may undergo laser iridotomy and then take the medication with impunity.

10-15. Match the usual field loss (10-15) with the underlying illness (a-f) [answers may be used more than once]

a. A 25-year-old woman has paraparesis and ataxia.
b. A 35-year-old woman has insidious onset of loss of peripheral daytime vision and all nighttime vision. Her mother has a similar illness.
c. A 30-year-old man has episodes of seeing the American flag and hearing the first five bars of "America the Beautiful."
d. A 21-year-old man has loss of bodily hair, gynecomastia, and diabetes insipidus.
e. A 70-year-old man has global aphasia, right hemiplegia, and right hemisensory loss.
f. A 75-year-old man has fluent aphasia.

10.

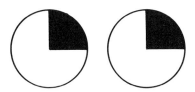

answer: c. The patient may have partial complex (e.g., psychomotor) seizures and a right superior quadrantanopia as the result of a left temporal lobe lesion. *or* f. The patient may have a left temporal lobe lesion giving him aphasia and a contralateral superior quadrantanopia.

11.

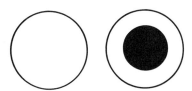

answer: a. The patient has spinal cord, cerebellar, and right optic nerve injury, probably as the result of multiple sclerosis.

12.

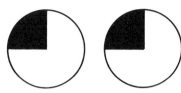

answer: c. The patient may have partial complex seizures and a left superior quadrantanopia as the result of a right temporal lobe lesion.

13.

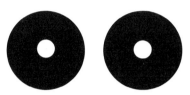

answer: b. The patient and her mother have preservation only of the central vision during daytime. If examination of her fundi showed clumping of retinal pigment, the diagnosis of retinitis pigmentosa would be certain. These visual fields might also be obtained from someone having tunnel vision.

14.

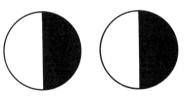

answer: e. The patient probably has a dominant hemisphere lesion, such as a cerebrovascular accident or tumor, giving a right homonymous hemianopsia.

15.

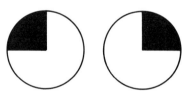

answer: d. The patient has a large pituitary tumor causing panhypopituitarism and bitemporal hemianopsia.

16–26. Match the characteristics of the visual hallucination with the source (a-c).

a.   Seizures that originate in the occipital lobe
b.   Seizures that originate in the temporal lobe
c.   Migraine with aura (classical migraine)

16. Associated musical hallucinations

answer: b

17. Flashes of bright lights in the contralateral visual field

answer: a, c

18. Associated olfactory hallucinations

answer: b, rarely c

19. Rotating blotches of color

answer: a

20. Formed hallucinations with impaired consciousness

answer: b

21. Postictal aphasia

  answer: b, rarely c

22. Throbbing unilateral headache

  answer: c

23. Nausea and vomiting

  answer: c

24. Simple blocks and stars of color

  answer: a, c

25. Twisting, complicated multicolored lights

  answer: b, c

26. Faces with distorted features or coloring

  answer: b, c

27–28. Match the symptom (27-28) with the possible origins (a-d).

a. Left third nerve palsy   c. Right third nerve palsy
b. Left sixth nerve palsy   d. Right sixth nerve palsy

27. Diplopia when looking to the right

  answer: a, d

28. Diplopia when looking to the left

  answer: b, c

29–30. Match the actions that cause blindness with the outcome.

a. Methanol-induced optic nerve injury
b. Pigmentary retinal degeneration
c. Retinal burns

29. Staring directly into the sun

  answer: c

30. Drinking nonethanol alcohols

  answer: a

31. What are common causes of ptosis?

a. Third nerve palsy   e. Myasthenia gravis
b. Sixth nerve palsy   f. Hysteria
c. Pancoast tumor   g. Blepharospasm
d. Multiple sclerosis

  answer: a, c, e

32. Which illnesses cause internuclear ophthalmoplegia?

a. Multiple sclerosis   d. Hysteria
b. Poliomyelitis   e. Heroin overdose
c. Muscular dystrophy   f. Brainstem cerebrovascular
                                    infarctions

  answer: a, f

33. Which abnormality is reported to occur in patients with schizophrenia?

a. Internuclear ophthalmoplegia   d. Conjugate gaze paresis
b. Nystagmus   e. Pursuit abnormalities
c. Ptosis

answer: e. Schizophrenic patients have irregular pursuit movement. Also, when medicated with phenothiazines, they may have oculogyric crises.

34. A 70-year-old man awakens with a right hemiparesis, vertigo, and his eyes deviated to the right. Which of the following conditions will also be found?

a. Aphasia
b. Right homonymous hemianopsia

c. Dementia
d. Nystagmus

answer: d. This patient has an infarction in the left brainstem in the pons. Thus, he would not have signs of cerebral injury, such as aphasia, hemianopsia, or cognitive impairment. He would have nystagmus because the vestibular nuclei would certainly be injured. Also, he might have injury to the left facial and abducens nerve nuclei that would cause left upper and lower facial paresis and medial deviation of the left eye.

35. Which conditions indicate that the dopamine system is involved in conjugate eye movement?

a. Internuclear ophthalmoplegia
b. Nystagmus

c. Pontine gaze center movement
d. Oculogyric crisis

answer: d. Oculogyric crises are precipitated by phenothiazines, including those used for nonpsychotic conditions, such as nausea and vomiting.

36. Which conditions have a predilection for people older than 65 years?

a. Myopia
b. Presbyopia
c. Macular degeneration
d. Classic migraines

e. Temporal or giant cell arteritis
f. Glaucoma
g. Cataracts
h. Optic neuritis

answer: b, c, e, f, g. Moreover, combinations of these conditions may occur together in the same older person. Whatever the cause of a visual impairment, it is a major threat to the mental well-being of people, especially those with other sensory deprivations, such as hearing loss, or cognitive or emotional impairment.

37. A 70-year-old man sustains a cerebral infarction. Afterward, he has a right homonymous hemianopsia, right hemisensory loss, and a mild right hemiparesis. Although he can both say and write the names of objects that he feels, he has a peculiar inability to name objects that he only sees, even when they are presented to his left visual field. What is the name of this condition and where is the lesion located?

answer: The lesion is probably in the left parietal and occipital region. The patient has visual agnosia, a condition in which patients cannot process visually acquired information. Additional testing might reveal Gerstmann's syndrome or alexia without agraphia (see Chapter 7)—conditions also resulting from posterior dominant hemisphere lesions. His problem is not aphasia because language function is normal as evidenced, once vision is circumvented, by his normal writing and speaking.

38. Match the visual disturbance (1-4) with the etiology (a-e).

1. Psychic blindness
2. Night blindness
3. Cortical blindness
4. Transient monocular blindness

a. Carotid stenosis
b. Occipital infarction (bilateral)
c. Conversion reaction
d. Bilateral temporal lobe injury
e. Vitamin A deficiency

answer: 1-d (Klüver-Bucy syndrome), 2-e, 3-b, 4-a (amaurosis fugax). (Night blindness is also a symptom of retinitis pigmentosa.)

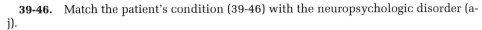

39-46. Match the patient's condition (39-46) with the neuropsychologic disorder (a-j).

a. Cortical blindness
b. Visual agnosia
c. Color agnosia
d. Color blindness
e. Prosopagnosia

f. Anton's syndrome
g. Wernicke-Korsakoff syndrome
h. Alexia without agraphia
i. Congenital cerebral injury
j. Aphasia

39. Cannot recognize familiar faces

answer: e

40. Despite visual loss, willfully but erroneously describes hospital room and physician

answer: f

41. Following cardiac arrest, blindness with intact pupil light reflex. In addition, although alert, mental impairment is prominent

answer: a

42. Cannot identify a red card, although able to match it to another red card and read a red-colored number on the Ishihara plates

answer: c

43. Despite only a right homonymous hemianopsia, inability to read. Writing ability is normal

answer: h

44. Congenital inability to read Ishihara plates

answer: d

45. Inability to name common objects under any circumstances

answer: j

46. Cannot name objects when seen, but can name objects when described or felt

answer: b

47. In which conditions are visual hallucinations stereotyped?

a. Partial complex seizures
b. Tonic-clonic seizures
c. LSD ingestions
d. Occipital lobe seizures

e. Migraine with aura
f. Migraine without aura
g. Hypnagogic hallucinations
h. Alcohol withdrawal

answer: a, d, e. In primary generalized seizures—petit mal (absences) and tonic-clonic—patients have no aura or visual symptoms. Intoxications and withdrawal cause varied symptoms and, in general, delirium. Hypnagogic and hypnopompic hallucinations are dreams that are highly variable. When migraines have an aura, it is stereotyped.

48. Which visions appear predominantly or exclusively in hemianopic areas?

a. Palinopsia
b. Partial seizures
c. Migraines

d. REM-associated dreams
e. LSD intoxication

answer: a, b. In palinopsia and partial (elementary and complex) seizures, visual hallucinations are often described exclusively within hemianopsia. Those hallucinations often result from occipital or temporal lobe lesions. Hallucinations related to migraines, dreams, and intoxications occur randomly and do not respect visual fields.

49. A patient claims to have developed a visual acuity of 20/200 in both eyes after a minimally traumatic event. Visual fields were full. The visual acuity was also measured to be 10/200 and 30/200. Where is the site of the lesion?

a. In both eyes (ocular)
b. At the chiasm
c. In the geniculocalcarine pathways
d. At the occipital cortex
e. None of the above

answer: e. The visual impairment is probably psychogenic because people's acuity should remain constant, i.e., 10/100, 20/200, 30/300.

50. Which of the following statements are true regarding saccades?

a. They are the smooth, steady tracking movements used to follow moving objects.
b. They are the quick, conjugate movements that bring objects from the periphery to the center of vision.
c. They are governed by supranuclear centers.
d. Unlike pursuit movements, they are resistant to structural lesions and degenerative illnesses.

answer: b, c. Saccades, the high-velocity conjugate gaze movements, are generated by cerebral conjugate gaze centers. They are susceptible to cerebrovascular accidents and other cerebral lesions. Moreover, abnormal saccades are one of the first findings in Huntington's disease.

51. Which of the following statements are true regarding pursuit?

a. They are the smooth, steady tracking movements used to follow moving objects.
b. They are the quick, conjugate movements that bring objects from the periphery to the center of vision.
c. They are governed by supranuclear centers.
d. Unlike saccades, they are resistant to structural lesions and degenerative illnesses.

answer: a, c. Pursuits, the relatively slow, smooth conjugate gaze movements, are generated mostly by the pontine conjugate gaze centers. They are susceptible to various illnesses and, along with saccades, are abnormal in schizophrenia and, to a lesser extent, affective disorders.

52. Which are the constituents of Horner's syndrome?

a. Mitosis
b. Miosis
c. Anhidrosis
d. Tearing
e. Third nerve palsy

answer: b, c. In addition to miosis (small pupil) and anhidrosis (lack of sweating), Horner's syndrome includes ptosis. It results from injury to the sympathetic supply of the face and eye.

53. In which conditions are Horner's syndrome found?

a. Migraine without aura
b. Migraine with aura
c. Cluster headache
d. Trigeminal neuralgia
e. Cervical spinal cord injury
f. Apical lung tumor
g. Pontine CVAs
h. Midbrain CVAs
i. Lateral medullary CVAs

answer: c, e, f, i

54. Which cerebral artery supplies the occipital lobes?

a. Anterior cerebral
b. Middle cerebral
c. Posterior cerebral
d. None of the above

answer: c. The posterior cerebral arteries, which are the final branches of the basilar artery, perfuse the occipital lobes. The occipital lobes contain the visual cortex. Occlusion of both posterior cerebral arteries leads to cortical blindness.

55. A 33-year-old man claims to have double vision in his right eye after a motor vehicle accident (MVA). When he covers the right eye the diplopia disappears, but when he covers the left eye he has persistent diplopia. The visual acuity in the left eye is 20/20 and in the right eye 20/400. Visual fields are normal in the left eye, but cannot be determined in the right eye because of the diplopia. Which of the following statements regarding this situation are true?

a. His symptom is monocular diplopia.
b. With the available information, conclusions cannot be drawn concerning the presence of central nervous system (CNS) injury causing the diplopia.
c. Monocular diplopia is virtually always the result of an ocular injury, such as a dislocated lens or retinal disruption, or psychogenic factors.
d. The first step in determining the cause of diplopia is to establish whether it arises from a single eye. In other words, ask the patient if covering one eye abolishes the diplopia.

> *answer:* a, c, d. When the brainstem or cranial nerves III, IV, or VI are injured, patients have diplopia only if both eyes are open. As a general rule, cerebral lesions do not cause diplopia. When diplopia originates from one eye, the patient is said to have monocular diplopia.

56. In which structure is the third cranial nerve located?

a. Midbrain
b. Pons
c. Medulla
d. Cerebrum

> *answer:* a

57. In which structure is the fourth cranial nerve located?

a. Midbrain
b. Pons
c. Medulla
d. Cerebrum

> *answer:* a

58. In which structure is the sixth cranial nerve located?

a. Midbrain
b. Pons
c. Medulla
d. Cerebrum

> *answer:* b

13 Congenital Cerebral Injuries

CEREBRAL PALSY

Cerebral palsy (CP) is a nonscientific, but generally accepted term. It describes the permanent neurologic *motor system* impairments that result from central nervous system (CNS) injuries sustained *in utero*, around the delivery (perinatal), during infancy, or in early childhood. In cases where the cause can be established, CP is most commonly associated with prematurity and low birth weight, particularly birth weights less than 2 Kg. Despite legal claims, less than 15 per cent of cases result from a birth injury, such as anoxia.

The two CP varieties that occur most frequently and have the greatest descriptive value are *spastic paresis* and *extrapyramidal CP* (*choreoathetosis*). Each has a characteristic motor impairment and a predictable association with seizures and mental retardation—the major consequences of cerebral injury. Each may also be associated with pseudobulbar palsy, hyperactivity, learning disabilities, hearing impairments, dysarthria, and strabismus.

Neurologists diagnose CP in children who have a "static" or "nonprogressive" motor impairment that has followed a perinatal cerebral injury (Table 13–1). The particular handicaps change little as children grow into adults. Computed tomography (CT), magnetic resonance imaging (MRI), and electroencephalography (EEG) are somewhat helpful in identifying an etiology and estimating the extent of brain damage. More important than identifying a particular congenital injury, physicians should concentrate on the problem at hand by evaluating the patient's mental and physical abilities and disabilities (Table 13–2). Since many children with CP have normal intelligence despite major motor deficits, movement disorders, dysarthria, and hearing impairments, physicians should not conclude that any child has mental retardation without a complete mental status evaluation customized for the patient.

Spastic CP

The major clinical feature of patients with spastic CP is a combination of paresis and spasticity. The spasticity, which is actually more of an impediment than the paresis, causes slow, clumsy movements that cannot be performed in isolation. Spastic CP also induces hyperactive DTRs, clonus, and Babinski signs. In addition, since the cerebral injury occurs before childhood growth, affected limbs can have *growth arrest*, i.e., the arm, leg, or both are characteristically foreshortened.

The varieties of spastic CP, which account for approximately 70 per cent of all CP cases (Fig. 13–1), are based on the clinical situation: diplegic (paresis

TABLE 13–1.   HISTORICAL FEATURES OF CEREBRAL PALSY

Description of deficit
  Motor impairment
    Paresis: extent, degree
    Movement disorder: nature, age of onset
  Delayed acquisition of motor skills
  Associated conditions
    Mental retardation
    Seizures
Search for cause
  Maternal health
    Personal or familial neurologic illness
    Prenatal illness or abnormalities
  Delivery
    Prematurity
    Low weight for date
    Prolonged labor, fetal distress
    Obstetric complications
  Neonatal period
    Low Apgar score
    Cyanosis, unresponsiveness
    Seizures
    Jaundice

TABLE 13–2.   PHYSICAL FINDINGS OF CEREBRAL PALSY

Motor Deficits
  Signs of spastic CP
    Gross impairment: paresis/spasticity, growth arrest, pseudobulbar palsy
    Subtle impairment: unequal size of hands or feet, toe walking (from shortened heel cords),
      premature hand preference, e.g., right-handedness before the age of 18 months
  Signs of extrapyramidal CP
    Choreoathetosis
Associated conditions
  Mental retardation
  Seizures
  Pseudobulbar palsy
  Impairment of special senses
    Visual: strabismus, myopia, blindness
    Auditory: deafness
    Vocal: dysarthria

FIGURE 13–1

Most cases of CP are varieties of spastic CP: hemiplegic, diplegic, and quadriplegic. The percentages are approximations because studies vary.

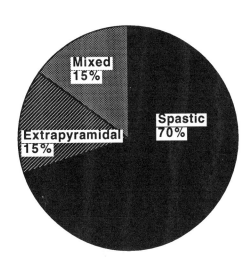

Proportion of CP Patients with Mental Retardation and Seizures

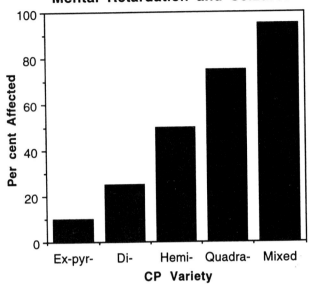

FIGURE 13–2

With more extensive *cerebral* disease, the incidence of mental retardation and seizures increases. The incidence in choreoathetosis or extrapyramidal (Ex-pyr-) CP is only approximately 10 per cent; however, the incidence in diplegic CP (Di-) is 25 per cent; hemiplegic CP (Hemi-) 50 per cent; quadriplegic CP (Quadra-) 75 per cent; and mixed CP 95 per cent.

of both legs), hemiplegic (arm and leg), and quadriplegic (all limbs). With each variety, progressively more extensive cerebral injury causes more extensive paresis, a greater incidence of seizures, and mental retardation (Fig. 13–2).

Spastic CP is associated with necrotic areas in the white matter around the ventricles, *periventricular leukomalacia*. It is detectable by ultrasound examination of an infant's head.

Diplegic CP (spastic diplegia) is symmetric paresis, primarily of the legs (Fig. 13–3). An early sign of this variety of CP is infants' legs appearing straight with the feet pointed downward (extended), drawn together (adducted), and

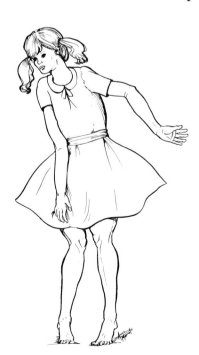

FIGURE 13–3

Spastic diplegia in this 10-year-old girl with low-normal intelligence causes straightening and inturning of the legs, a tiptoe stance, and scissors-like gait. Uncoordinated, awkward movements of her arms (posturings) are another, but subtler manifestation.

crossed over each other ("scissored"). Without surgical correction, the leg muscles' tendons shorten and hold the knees, ankles, and toes straight, adducted, and extended. When children begin to walk, the spastic diplegia forces them to stand on their toes.

Spastic diplegia is the CP variety most closely related to prematurity. The underlying pathology is *periventricular leukomalacia* that preferentially damages the corticospinal tract fibers of the legs (see Fig. 7–7). Since cerebral damage is relatively confined, both seizures and mental retardation occur less frequently (approximately 25 per cent) than in the other forms of spastic CP.

Hemiplegic CP is spastic hemiparesis that affects the face and arm more than the leg (Fig. 13–4). Hemiplegic cerebral palsy patients resemble adults with middle cerebral artery occlusions, but they have growth arrest of the affected limbs. In particular, their thumb and great-toe nail beds are smaller on the paretic side, and a short Achilles tendon forces them to walk on the toes of the affected foot. Another feature is premature hand preference. Whereas hand preference, (e.g., right-handedness) normally is apparent only after 18 months, earlier use exclusively of one hand suggests palsy of the other.

More importantly, since the right hemisphere can become dominant when the left is injured in infancy, people who have had congenital left hemisphere damage tend to develop right hemisphere dominance (see Chapter 8). They become left-handed with normal language function, albeit with right hemiparesis. In contrast, adults who sustain left cerebral hemisphere injuries almost always have aphasia in conjunction with right hemiparesis.

Since the cerebral damage in spastic hemiparesis is generally more extensive than in spastic cerebral diplegia, seizures and mental retardation develop more frequently (50 per cent of cases) in hemiplegia. However, when the damage that causes cerebral diplegia is extensive, children have profound impairments.

Quadriplegic CP is paresis of all four limbs that is usually accompanied by pseudobulbar palsy. Since it results from extensive cerebral damage, which is often caused by anoxia during delivery, a large proportion (75 per cent) of

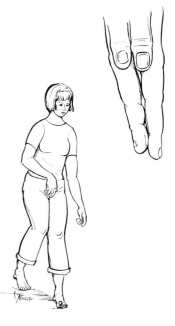

FIGURE 13–4

Spastic hemiparesis since birth in this 28-year-old woman, who has normal intelligence, causes weakness of her right arm and leg. She holds the arm, wrist, and fingers in a flexed posture. Growth arrest of her right hand has led to foreshortened fingers and, a characteristic finding, a less broad thumb nail bed. The right leg, especially the heel (Achilles) tendon, is also short, causing her to walk on her right toes and circumduct that leg. Her posture and gait are similar to that of adults after a left middle cerebral artery infarction (see Figs. 2–3 to 2–5).

these individuals suffer from seizures and mental retardation. In contrast, cervical spinal cord birth injury causes quadriplegia without cerebral damage.

Physical therapy is helpful, and surgery that transposes or lengthens tendons ameliorates spasticity. Surgical procedures in which most of the lumbosacral dorsal nerve roots are severed, *dorsal rhizotomy*, can also reduce spasticity. Although popular, oral antispastic medications are probably ineffective.

Control of seizures is difficult, especially in children with mental retardation. It often requires two or more anticonvulsants that cause sedation, hyperactivity, and behavioral disturbances.

Extrapyramidal CP

Extrapyramidal or "dyskinetic" CP is characterized by choreoathetosis, which is involuntary writhing (athetosis) of the face, tongue, hands, and feet that is punctuated and overridden by jerking movements (chorea) of the trunk, arms, and legs (Fig. 13–5; see Chapter 18). Hearing impairments often complicate the disorder. The choreoathetosis interferes with all common activities, including fine hand movements, walking, and even sitting still. Involvement of the larynx, pharynx, and diaphragm leads to incomprehensible dysarthria.

Choreoathetosis is usually caused by combinations of low birth weight, anoxia, and neonatal hyperbilirubinemia (*kernicterus*) that damage the basal ganglia and the auditory pathways. Even though the basal ganglia damage usually occurs at birth, choreoathetosis might not be apparent until children are 2 years old by which time they should have developed steady walking and fine motor movements.

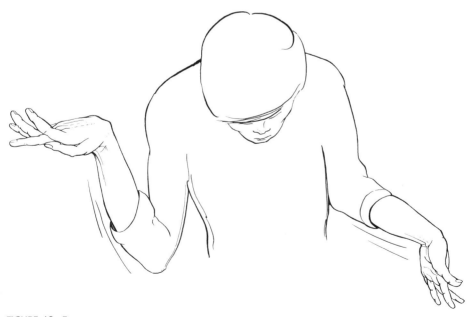

FIGURE 13–5

Choreoathetosis in a 13-year-old girl, obvious only since she was 3 years old, is manifest by slow sinuous movements (athetosis) of the wrists, hands, and fingers. It forces her hands into flexion at the wrist and her fingers into extension with overlapping positions. Intermittent, quick movements (chorea) are superimposed.

Most importantly, probably because the cerebral cortex can be relatively or entirely spared in kernicterus, this variety of CP is associated with the lowest incidence (10 per cent) of seizures and mental retardation. Many patients have been able to overcome barriers and complete college. Nevertheless, all of them are liable to be underrated by a superficial academic or medical evaluation.

Although choreoathetosis is difficult to treat, neuroleptics and sedatives may suppress some movement. Experimental, risky surgical procedures involving ablation of deep cerebral structures reportedly reduce athetosis.

Finally, *mixed forms* of CP—combinations of spastic paraparesis and choreoathetosis—account for about 15 per cent of CP cases. They reflect the most extensive CNS injury, which is naturally associated with the highest incidence of seizures and mental retardation—95 per cent.

NEURAL TUBE CLOSURE DEFECTS

This group of congenital neurologic problems results from defective embryologic development of the CNS. Normally, during the third and fourth weeks of gestation, the dorsal ectoderm invaginates to form a closed, midline neural tube that eventually gives rise to the CNS (Fig. 13–6). The ectoderm thus forms the CNS, as well as the skin. The mesoderm forms the coverings of the CNS—the meninges, vertebrae, and skull. Defects in neural tube closure, which may induce a mesodermal component, are magnified throughout gestation.

Beyond the neurologic issues, neural tube defects create some of the most public controversies in medicine: harvesting organs in cases of anencephaly

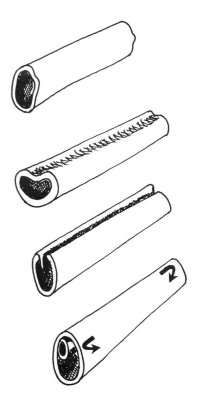

FIGURE 13–6

The neural tube's formation takes place during the third and fourth weeks when the embryo's external layer, the ectoderm, invaginates. It forms a distinct, midline neural tube that must close at both ends. Then the embryo begins to bend into a curved, fetal shape with the tube on the convex surface. Failure to complete this process results in "neural tube" or "midline closure defects" that are most common at the upper and lower ends of the spinal cord.

(see below), the problem of parents not consenting to treatment, and the burden of health care costs for infants with a dismal prognosis.

Upper Neural Tube Closure Defects

In an extreme example of a neural tube defect, in which the entire upper end of the neural tube seems not to have formed, the fetus fails to develop a skull and brain. This rare but well-publicized condition, *anencephaly*, is invariably fatal within days of birth. The organs are ideal for transplantation.

In an *encephalocele*, a skin-covered brain, meninges, or merely the CSF protrudes through a skull defect. This malformation results from incomplete closure of the mesodermal layers (bone and skin) over the upper neural tube and usually involves the occipital portion of the skull. A related malformation is the *Dandy-Walker syndrome*. In this condition, which is not evident when looking at the infant, the posterior portion of the upper neural tube fails to develop. Infants are born with only rudimentary posterior brain structures: the cerebellum, medulla, and fourth ventricle. As with many other neural tube defects, encephalocele and Dandy-Walker syndrome lead to hydrocephalus and mental retardation.

A variation of upper neural tube closure defects is a group of disorders collectively termed the *Arnold-Chiari malformation*. Usually not obvious by external appearances, they involve combinations of the medulla and cerebellum being displaced downward through the foramen magnum, aqueductal stenosis, and overlying skull and cervical spine defects. In addition, Arnold-Chiari malformations are associated with comparable defects in lower neural tube structures, such as a *meningomyelocele* (see below).

In older children and adults who may previously have had an undetected abnormality, Arnold-Chiari malformations produce headaches when bending, bulbar palsy, and neck pain. Aqueductal stenosis or blockage by the posterior brain structures of the foramen magnum causes hydrocephalus. Patients typically require neurosurgical insertion of ventricular shunts or "unroofing" of the upper cervical spine and occipital skull.

Lower Neural Tube Closure Defects

In the simplest case, *spina bifida occulta*, the spine of the lumbar vertebrae simply fails to fuse. Since both the underlying spinal cord and cauda equina and the overlying skin are intact, this disorder is usually asymptomatic.

In *meningocele*, a more serious problem, the meninges and skin protrude through a lumbosacral spine defect to form a large bulge that is filled with cerebrospinal fluid (CSF). Although this condition is usually asymptomatic, it may cause gait impairment, bladder emptying problems, and loss of the normal multiple tissue barriers that protect the CNS. To prevent bacteria from entering the CSF and causing meningitis, infants with meningoceles must undergo neurosurgery to repair the defect.

Meningomyelocele or *myelomeningocele*, the worst case, occurs far more frequently than meningocele. This defect consists of a tangle of a rudimentary spinal cord, lumbar and sacral nerve roots, and meninges protruding into a sac-like structure overlying the lumbosacral spine (Fig. 13–7). The nervous system malformation causes areflexia, paraparesis, and incontinence in infants. In addition, the defective meninges immediately subject neonates to

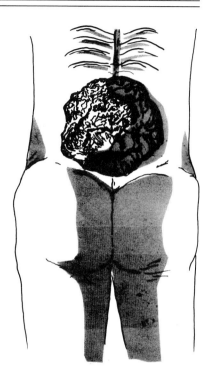

FIGURE 13–7

A newborn infant with a meningomyelocele has a broad-based, loose, translucent sac of thin, friable skin arising from the upper lumbar area that weeps a mixture of serum and CSF. The meningomyelocele contains rudiments of a spinal cord and lumbar and sacral nerves. The infant's legs are weak, flaccid, and areflexic, and the bladder is distended.

meningitis. Although hydrocephalus is present at birth in only about 25 per cent of babies with meningomyeloceles, it develops in almost all who survive.

Meningomyeloceles are repaired in the child's first week, but the clinical deficits usually worsen in childhood and again during adolescent growth spurts. Although high-technology surgery may protect infants from meningitis and reduce the impact of hydrocephalus, almost all survivors are mentally retarded and paraplegic. As children get older, they typically require urinary- and fecal-diversion procedures; revisions of shunts for hydrocephalus; further surgery on the spine; a full array of social, psychologic, and educational support services; and various appliances, ramps, and elevators.

Cause

Because a woman who has delivered a baby with meningomyelocele will have a 4 to 10 per cent chance of bearing another with a similar abnormality, a tendency toward meningomyeloceles has been attributed to an autosomal recessive genetic abnormality. Meningomyeloceles and other neural tube defects have also been attributed to radiation, vitamin deficiency, and a variety of toxins, including potato blight, vitamin A, and, most importantly, carbamazepine (Tegretol) and valproate (Depakote). Meningomyeloceles have also been attributed to folic acid deficiency. Notably, anticonvulsants lower the serum folate level.

A meningomyelocele in a fetus is suggested by excessive levels of alpha-fetoprotein in amniotic fluid and maternal serum. Fetal ultrasound examination is a complementary test. Folic acid supplements before conception and during the first trimester of pregnancy reduce the incidence of neural tube defects. Thus, the supplements are recommended for women attempting to conceive who must take anticonvulsants.

NEUROCUTANEOUS DISORDERS

Neurocutaneous disorders—paired abnormalities in the brain and skin—also stem from embryologic defects in the ectoderm. Sometimes along with abnormalities in other ectoderm and nonectoderm organs, the neurocutaneous disorders are inherited largely in an autosomal dominant pattern. Since the educated physician can deduce the cerebral pathology from a careful observation, the neurocutaneous disorders offer the optimal occasion for a *diagnosis by inspection.*

Although the neurocutaneous disorders usually remain stable through adult life, the cerebral lesions sometimes undergo malignant transformation. Of the many varieties and their numerous findings, this book presents only the main features of the most relevant disorders.

Tuberous Sclerosis

Tuberous sclerosis is usually immediately identified by smooth and firm nodules, *adenoma sebaceum,* on the malar surface of the face (Fig. 13–8). Further examination of the skin might also reveal hypopigmented areas (ash-leaf spots); leathery, scaly lesions on the trunk (shagreen patches); and periungual fibromas of the fingers.

In a classic triad, which actually occurs in the minority of children, adenoma sebaceum are accompanied by epilepsy that is intractable and cognitive decline that begins in childhood and progresses slowly, i.e., dementia. These manifestations, however, are highly variable, with many affected individuals having only skin or CNS manifestations. The variability is partly attributable to transmission by at least two different chromosomes, 9 and 16 (see Appendix 3 for a compilation of genetic disorders).

The epilepsy and dementia result from the growth of cerebral tubers, which are potato-like brain nodules, 1 to 3 cm in diameter, that compress brain tissue and irritate the surrounding cortex. Although usually benign, the tubers sometimes undergo malignant transformation. Moreover, retinal, renal, and cardiac as well as brain tumors develop. Since the cerebral tubers are relatively large and tend to calcify, they are readily detected by CT and MRI scans. In most cases, tubers cannot be removed because they are too numerous and too deep.

The combination of dementia, epilepsy, and poor prognosis forces many patients into institutions. However, the majority of patients have a relatively benign, stable course with few seizures and little or no mental retardation.

Neurofibromatosis

Commonly occurring, classic neurofibromatosis is called *neurofibromatosis type 1 (NF1),* von Recklinghausen's disease, or the "peripheral type" of neu-

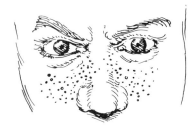

FIGURE 13–8

Adenoma sebaceum, the cutaneous component of tuberous sclerosis, is prominent on the malar surface of the face and consists of nodules that are several millimeters in diameter, firm, and uniformly pale. They may resemble acne; however, acne "pimples" have a liquid (pus) center, are surrounded by inflammation, and are present on the trunk, as well as the face.

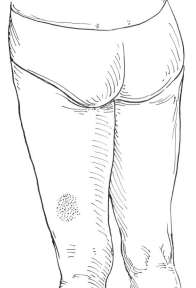

FIGURE 13–9

Café au lait spots are flat, light brown skin lesions. Six or more, each measuring at least 1.5 cm, indicate neurofibromatosis.

rofibromatosis. It is inherited on chromosome 17 in an autosomal dominant pattern, but in only 50 per cent of patients. In the others, it seems to arise sporadically as the result of a mutation.

NF1 is identified by a triad of readily identifiable manifestations: multiple *café au lait* spots, *neurofibromas*, and Lisch nodules. Café au lait spots are flat and light brown (Fig. 13–9). They are found in at least 10 per cent of normal people, but neurofibromatosis in adults is indicated by more than six café au lait spots that are each larger than 1.5 cm.

Neurofibromas are soft, palpable, subcutaneous growths, a few millimeters to several centimeters in size, that generally emerge along peripheral nerves (Figs. 13–10 and 13–11). Sometimes plexiform neuromas induce extraordinary growth of a limb. Neurofibromas can grow large enough to compress the spinal cord, nerve roots, or cauda equina and occasionally reach grotesque proportions. However, the famous 19th-century "Elephant Man," Joseph Merrick, who was thought to be an example of neurofibromatosis, actually suffered from a related condition, Proteus syndrome.

Lisch nodules, which are melanocytic hamartomas, are multiple, asymptomatic, macroscopic, yellow to brown nodules on the iris (Fig. 13–12). Al-

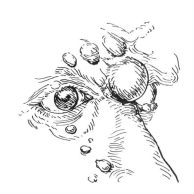

FIGURE 13–10

Neurofibromas often grow to several centimeters of disfiguring protuberances on the face.

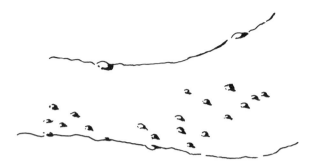

FIGURE 13–11

Neurofibromas are often subtle, multiple, subcutaneous, soft, and typically less than 0.5 cm in size.

though a slit-lamp examination may be required to distinguish Lisch nodules from inconsequential pigment collections, they are pathognomonic and the most common manifestation of NF1 in adults.

Excision of neurofibromas, except for ones compressing the spinal cord or other key structures, is impractical because the NF1 involves innumerable peripheral nerves. Café au lait spots can be blanched with laser treatment.

Most importantly, NF1 is not entirely peripheral. It induces intracerebral tumors, such as astrocytomas and optic nerve gliomas. Although mental retardation is present in only 2 to 5 per cent of patients, as many as 40 per cent may have some cognitive impairment.

Neurofibromatosis type 2 (NF2)—almost a completely different disorder—is characterized by the development of bilateral acoustic neuromas that produce steadily increasing deafness. Inherited on chromosome 22 in an autosomal dominant pattern, NF2 is also called familial acoustic neuroma or the "central type" of neurofibromatosis. NF2 may induce a few neurofibromas and large, pale café au lait spots, but the hallmark is the acoustic neuromas. In fact, the disorder is usually not diagnosed until acoustic neuromas are discovered.

Another manifestation of NF2 is meningiomas. Unless a meningioma compresses a critical area of the brain, this NF2 does not cause mental impairments. The two neoplastic complications, acoustic neuromas and meningiomas, which are "benign" tumors, can be readily detected with an gadolinium-enhanced MRI. Although the meningiomas can be removed surgically, affected nerves are usually sacrificed.

Sturge-Weber Syndrome

Sturge-Weber syndrome, or *encephalo-trigeminal angiomatosis*, consists of vascular malformations of the face, *nevus flammeus*, and underlying cerebral

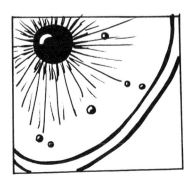

FIGURE 13–12

Lisch nodules, virtually a pathognomonic sign of NF1, are aggregations on the iris that can often be seen with the unaided eye, but a slit-lamp examination may be necessary.

hemisphere. This disorder results from a genetic abnormality, but its nature is not understood. Most cases are sporadic, and few patients have an affected sibling. The vascular malformations of the skin of the face cause a deep red discoloration (port-wine stain) in the region of one or more divisions of the trigeminal nerve (Fig. 13–13). By contrast, most people with small, patchy port-wine stains and infants with small forehead or facial angiomas, such as strawberry nevi, do not have Sturge-Weber syndrome. The facial nevus flammeus can also be bleached by laser treatment.

The cerebral component of the Sturge-Weber syndrome is a calcified vascular abnormality that is accompanied by cerebral atrophy. The calcifications can be seen on skull x-rays and CTs, but not on MRIs. Patients often have mental retardation, learning disabilities, behavioral disturbances, and refractory epilepsy. Depending on the site of the lesion, they also have focal physical deficits, such as homonymous hemianopsia and spastic hemiparesis. Recurrent seizures and progressively severe sclerosis surrounding the cerebral lesion intensify the cognitive and physical impairments.

Ataxia-Telangiectasia

Ataxia-telangiectasia is inherited, unlike most other neurocutaneous disorders, as a recessive disorder. It is associated with a genetic abnormality on chromosome 11 and is attributed to defective DNA repair.

Ataxia-telangiectasia becomes evident in children 3 to 5 years old when the neurologic component, degeneration of the cerebellar vermis, gives them a steadily progressively ataxic gait. Subsequently, they develop cognitive impairment. The cutaneous component is readily recognizable as aggregations of small, dilated vessels (telangiectasia) on the conjunctiva, bridge of the nose, and cheeks.

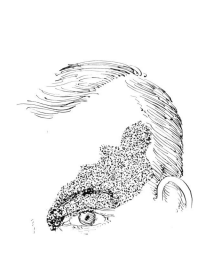 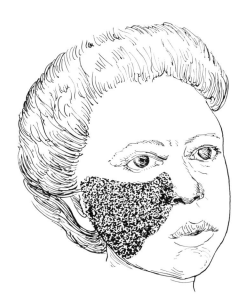

FIGURE 13–13

The cutaneous angiomatosis of Sturge-Weber syndrome involves one or more divisions of the distribution of the trigeminal nerve (see Fig. 4–11). Since the first division is the one most often affected, the most common site includes the anterior scalp, forehead, and upper eyelid. One third of patients have bilateral involvement.

As in few other neurologic diseases, ataxia-telangiectasia is consistently associated with immunodeficiency. Patients have both cellular immunity impairments and little or no IgA or IgE. The immunodeficiency leads to severe sinus and respiratory tract infections and the development of lymphomas and other neoplasms. (The association of immunodeficiency and lymphoma is well recognized in AIDS and immunosuppression for organ transplantation.)

NEURODEGENERATIVE DISORDERS

Childhood neurodegenerative diseases differ from CP in at least two ways: They are inherited conditions, and they cause progressively severe cognitive impairments as part of a generalized deterioration. Although they usually lead to death in infancy or early childhood, these diseases can present in adolescence or persist into the young adult years with personality changes, thought disorders, or dementia. They also induce seizures, myoclonus, ataxia, spastic or flaccid quadriparesis, and blindness.

Although these diseases are rare, the general category might be considered when evaluating a young person who develops dementia or an atypical psychosis, especially if there is a family history of a similar disorder. Any suspicion should be heightened when patients have signs of a systemic disorder, such as organomegaly, short stature, or other skeletal abnormalities. Most of these diseases are transmitted in an autosomal recessive genetic pattern; however, some are transmitted in a sex-linked pattern, and the mitochondrial disorders are transmitted entirely from the mother. None can be cured, and the only treatable ones are Wilson's disease and possibly adrenoleukodystrophy.

To appreciate the scope of these diseases—in keeping with the practical approach of this book—one may arbitrarily put them into a classification scheme that is admittedly overlapping: enzyme deficiencies that lead to systemic and neuronal abnormalities (storage diseases), "white matter" or myelin abnormalities (leukodystrophies), impaired energy production from mitochondria abnormalities, and chromosomal abnormalities (Table 13–3). Most conditions are discussed in chapters related to their primary symptom. This sec-

TABLE 13–3.   CHILDHOOD NEURODEGENERATIVE DISEASES[a]

Storage Diseases
  Ceroid lipofucinosis (Kuf's disease)
  Gangliosidoses
    GM1 beta-galactosidase deficiency ("gargoylism")
    GM2 hexosaminidase deficiency (Tay-Sachs disease)
  Gaucher's disease (beta glucocerebrosidase deficiency)
Leukodystrophies (see Chapters 6 and 15)
  Adrenoleukodystrophy (lignoceroyl deficiency)
  Metachromatic leukodystrophy (arylsulfatase deficiency)
  Globoid cell leukodystrophy (Krabbe's disease)
Mitochondrial disorders (see Chapter 6)
  Mitochondrial encephalopathy with ragged red fibers (MERRF)
  Mitochondrial encephalopathy, lactic acidosis, and stroke-like episodes (MELAS)
Chromosomal disorders
  Trisomy 21 (Down's syndrome; see Chapter 7)
  Rett syndrome
  Fragile X syndrome
  Lesch Nyhan (see Chapter 18)
  Wilson's disease (see Chapter 18)

[a]Commonly cited examples that may be encountered in older children, adolescents, or young adults.

tion considers several genetic illnesses that produce progressive cognitive impairment and behavioral disturbances. Their physical stigmata allow an astute clinician to make a diagnosis by inspection.

Down's Syndrome

Down's syndrome is the most widely known and, at 1 in 600 births, the most frequently occurring disorder in this group and the most readily recognizable (Fig. 13–14). It usually causes mild to moderate degrees of mental retardation, with a median IQ of 40 to 50. An unfortunate but extraordinarily important complication of Down's syndrome is that, by patients' fourth or fifth decade, Down's syndrome uniformly leads to an Alzheimer-like dementia (see Chapter 7). In fact, one theory holds that Down's syndrome and Alzheimer's disease stem from a common genetic abnormality (on chromosome 21, see below).

Down's syndrome children also have delayed motor development. Even allowing for mental retardation, they occasionally have inattention, hyperactivity, or other behavioral disturbances.

In most children, the cause is chromosome 21 trisomy; however, in some children, whose phenotype is identical, the cause is a translocation of that chromosome. The incidence of Down's syndrome infants is correlated with increasing maternal age (especially older than 40 years). Because a fetus with Down's syndrome can be identified in most cases by a chromosome analysis of amniotic fluid cells, women older than 40 years are urged to undergo amniocentesis. Nevertheless, since Down's syndrome is not transmitted through generations, it is not classified as an inherited disorder of mental retardation.

Fragile X Syndrome

The *fragile X syndrome* occurs less frequently than Down's syndrome, but is still responsible for as many as 10 per cent of cases of mental retardation. As in other genetically determined disorders of mental retardation, non-neurologic physical abnormalities are prominent and characteristic (Fig 13–15).

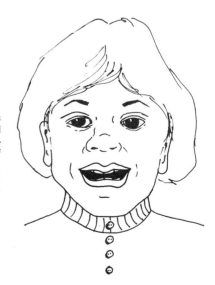

FIGURE 13–14

Children with Down's syndrome are short. Their ears are low-set with small lobes. Their eyes' epicanthal folds are wide, and the lids appear to slant upward—thus, the outdated term "Mongolism." The bridge of the nose is depressed. The tongue, which is large, tends to protrude over a slack jaw. Their palms are broad with a single midline crease, and their fingers are short and stubby.

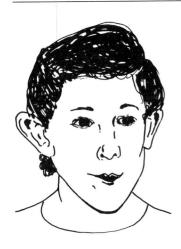

FIGURE 13-15

Boys with the fragile X syndrome tend to have a long thin face but a prominent forehead and jaw, large low-set "seashell-shaped" ears, and, after puberty, testicles that are disproportionately larger (*macro-orchidism*) than the penis.

The faulty gene consists of excessive repetitions of a trinucleotide in the X chromosome. (Similar defects in autosomal chromosomes produce myotonic dystrophy and Huntington's disease). Analysis of amniotic fluid cells can identify the abnormal gene. Unlike Down's syndrome, the fragile X syndrome is regularly and predictably transmitted from a parent to one or more children. Thus, it is the most common form of inherited mental retardation, occurring in about 1 in 1500 males and half as frequently in females.

Having one normal gene affords partial protection to females who are presumably heterozygote. (If the gene did not act in a mostly recessive manner, twice as many females would have the disorder.) Nevertheless, the abnormal gene is not completely recessive, and many females have mild mental retardation.

Children's manifestations can be limited to learning disabilities, but most children with the disorder have moderate to profound mental retardation. In particular, they usually have slowly acquired and ultimately defective language skills, hyperactivity, and other behavior disturbances that have been termed "autistic features."

Rett Syndrome

Rett syndrome or *disease* is restricted to girls who, after a normal birth and development until they are about 6 years old, regress in virtually all phases of their psychomotor development. They gradually lose their language skills, ability to walk, other learned motor activities, and cognitive abilities, i.e., these young girls develop dementia. Although the disorder is diagnosed entirely on clinical grounds and only when girls are at least 5 years old, they have two virtually unique physical characteristics (Fig. 13-16). They display incessant, stereotyped hand movements, typically clapping and wringing. The other characteristic is *acquired microcephaly,* which results from the onset of progressively slower growth of their head while their body continues to have relatively normal growth. In addition, almost all Rett syndrome children have seizures.

The salient feature of Rett syndrome is that its features—loss of language, high incidence of seizures, and stereotyped behavior—mimic autism. However, Rett syndrome children have a pronounced, progressive loss of motor ability; they develop microcephaly; and they retain some interpersonal skills.

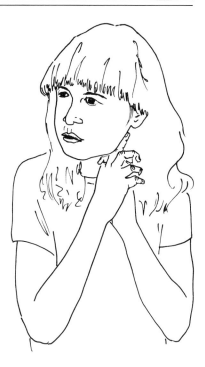

FIGURE 13–16

A 6-year old girl with Rett syndrome has developed repetitive hand-washing and clapping movements, microcephaly, and progressive loss of all forms of communication.

Rett syndrome has been attributed to a faulty gene on the X chromosome. Only females are affected presumably because the chromosome abnormality is fatal to a male fetus. As in the case of fragile X syndrome, the normal X gene in females offers some protection, but ironically it permits the development of this devastating disorder.

REFERENCES

Budden S, Meek M, Henighan: Communication and oral-motor function in Rett syndrome. Dev Med Child Neurol *32*: 51–55, 1990

Coker SB: The diagnosis of childhood neurodegenerative disorders presenting as dementia in adults. Neurology *41*: 794–798, 1991

Czeizel AE, Dudas I: Prevention of the first occurrence of neural-tube defects by periconceptional vitamin supplementation. N Engl J Med *327*: 1832–1835, 1992

Dansky LV, Rosenblatt DS, Andermann E: Mechanisms of teratogenesis: Folic acid and antiepileptic therapy. Neurology *42* (Suppl 5): 32–42, 1992

First LR, Palfrey JS: The infant or young child with developmental delay. N Engl J Med *330*: 478–483, 1994

Hack M, Taylor HG, Klein N, et al: School-age outcomes in children with birth weights under 750 g. N Engl J Med *331*: 753–759, 1994

Kuban KCK, Leviton A: Cerebral palsy. N Engl J Med *330*: 188–195, 1994

Lindhout D, Omtzigt JGC, Cornel MC: Spectrum of neural-tube defects in 34 infants prenatally exposed to antiepileptic drugs. Neurology *42* (Suppl 5): 111–118, 1992

Lubs MLE, Bauer MS, Formas ME, et al: Lisch nodules in neurofibromatosis type 1. N Engl J Med *324*: 1264–1266, 1991

National Institutes of Health Conference: Neurofibromatosis 1 (Recklinghausen disease) and neurofibromatosis 2 (bilateral acoustic neurofibromatosis). Ann Intern Med *113*: 39–52, 1990

Olsson B, Rett A: A review of the Rett syndrome with a theory of autism. Brain Dev *12*: 11–5, 1990

Park TS, Owen JH: Surgical management of spastic diplegia in cerebral palsy. N Engl J Med *326*: 745–749, 1992

Reiss AL, Lee J, Freund L: Neuroanatomy of fragile X syndrome: The temporal lobe. Neurology *44*: 1317–1324, 1994

Rett Syndrome Diagnostic Criteria Work Group: Diagnostic criteria for Rett syndrome. Ann Neurol *23*: 425–428, 1988

Riccardi VM: Neurofibromatosis: Phenotype, Natural History, and Pathogenesis (2nd ed). Baltimore, Johns Hopkins University Press, 1992

Rosa FW: Spina bifida in infants of women treated with carbamazepine during pregnancy. N Engl J Med *324*: 674–677, 1991

Rousseau F, Heitz D, Biacalana V, et al: Direct diagnosis by DNA analysis of the fragile X syndrome of mental retardation. N Engl J Med *325*: 1673–1681, 1991

Rubenstein AE, Korf BR (eds): Neurofibromatosis: A Handbook for Patients, Families, and Health Care Professionals. New York, Thieme Medical Publishers, Inc., 1990

QUESTIONS and ANSWERS: CHAPTER 13

1–11. Match the neurocutaneous disorder (a-d) with its manifestations 1–11.

a.   Tuberous sclerosis
b.   Neurofibromatosis type 1 (NF1)
c.   Sturge-Weber syndrome
d.   Neurofibromatosis type 2 (NF2)

1. Acoustic neuroma

   answer: d

2. Facial lesions vaguely resemble rhinophyma

   answer: a

3. Progressive dementia

   answer: a

4. Neurofibromas

   answer: b

5. Adenoma sebaceum

   answer: a

6. Cauda equina syndrome

   answer: b

7. Intractable epilepsy

   answer: a

8. Café au lait spots

   answer: b

9. Facial angiomatosis

   answer: c

10. Optic glioma

   answer: b

11. Epilepsy

   answer: a, c (rarely b)

12–17. Which of the following disorders cause inattention or episodic changes in mood in children?

12. Migraines

answer: Yes

13. Partial complex seizures

answer: Yes

14. Antihistamines

answer: Yes

15. Cerebral palsy

answer: No

16. Sedative medications

answer: Yes

17. Absences

answer: Yes

18. In which of the following conditions will CT or MRI provide useful diagnostic information?

a. Attention deficit disorder
b. Absences
c. Migraines
d. Hydrocephalus
e. Sturge-Weber syndrome
f. Learning disabilities
g. Tuberous sclerosis
h. Tourette's syndrome
i. Neurofibromatosis type 2

answer: d, e, g, i (MRI may show acoustic neuromas, the CT cannot)

19. Which of the following procedures or developments has helped reduce the incidence of congenital brain injury or abnormality?

a. Prenatal chromosome analysis
b. Neonatal exchange transfusion
c. Fetal cardiac monitoring during labor
d. Amniocentesis
e. Ultrasound examinations
f. Prevention of RH incompatibility
g. Determination of fetal and maternal alpha-fetoprotein

answer: a, b, c, d, e, f, g

20. Children who sustain any brain injury until the age of 5 years are all eligible for assistance by most programs that serve CP children (True/False).

answer: True

21. Is the following sentence true or false? "Children with mental retardation because of a genetic abnormality are usually indistinguishable from those with mental retardation for other reasons."

answer: False. They almost always have overt physical stigmata, such as low-set ears, that are often specific for the particular genetic abnormality.

22. Which of the following are characteristics of Rett syndrome children that are *not* found in autistic children?

a. Only affects girls
b. Stereotyped behavior
c. Loss of language skills
d. Seizures
e. Acquired microcephaly
f. Progressively more pronounced ataxia

answer: a, e, f

23. Which of the following are caused by penetrating head injuries in adults?

a. Aphasia
b. Paresis
c. Cerebral palsy

d. Hyperactivity
e. Seizures
f. Mental retardation

answer: a, b, e

24. A 1-year-old boy has a stroke because of sickle-cell disease. It results in mild right hemiparesis. Which of the following will probably be additional consequences?

a. Chorea
b. Aphasia
c. Seizures

d. Spastic cerebral palsy
e. Stunted growth (growth arrest) of right arm

answer: c, d, e

25–30. Match the disorder (a-d) with its cause (25–30).

a. Cervical cord injury
b. Kernicterus
c. Cerebral anoxia
d. Stroke in utero

25. Choreoathetosis

answer: b

26. Spastic quadriplegia

answer: a or c

27. Spastic hemiparesis

answer: d

28. Deafness

answer: b

29. Seizure disorder

answer: c or d

30. Cortical blindness

answer: c

31–35. Regarding cerebral palsy:

31. List the following types of cerebral palsy (a-e) in order of increasing frequency of the likelihood of mental retardation.

a. Choreoathetosis
b. Spastic diplegia
c. Spastic quadriplegia

d. Spastic hemiplegia
e. Mixed spastic choreoathetosis

answer: a, b, d, c, e

32. Which of the above types of CP has the lowest incidence of seizures?

answer: a

33. Which of the above may not be apparent until as late as 2 years of age?

answer: a

34. Which is the most commonly encountered form?

answer: d

35. In which form are the legs affected more than the arms?

answer: b

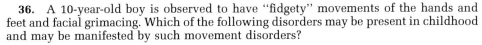

36. A 10-year-old boy is observed to have "fidgety" movements of the hands and feet and facial grimacing. Which of the following disorders may be present in childhood and may be manifested by such movement disorders?

a. Cerebral palsy
b. Rett syndrome
c. Sydenham's chorea

d. Wilson's disease
e. Tourette's syndrome

answer: a, c, d, e

37. With which conditions are meningomyeloceles *not* associated?

a. Spastic paraparesis
b. Mental retardation
c. Incontinence

d. Meningitis
e. Flaccid quadriparesis

answer: a. They are also associated with hydrocephalus and flaccid, not spastic, paraparesis. The defect, which is a congenital neural tube closure defect, occurs in the lower thoracic or lumbar region and does not affect the cervical spinal cord. However, it is usually also reflected in cerebral pathology.

38. Which neurologic conditions are associated with immunodeficiency?

a. Acquired immunodeficiency syndrome (AIDS)
b. Meningomyelocele
c. Sturge-Weber syndrome
d. Ataxia-telangiectasia

answer: a, d. AIDS is associated with a cellular immunodeficiency, and ataxia-telangiectasia is associated with an IgA and IgE immunoglobulin deficiency.

39. Match the condition (a-e) with its clinical features (1-5):

a. Adrenoleukodystrophy
b. Rett syndrome
c. Fragile X syndrome

d. Down's syndrome
e. Meningomyelocele

1. In only girls, autistic behavior, repetitive hand slapping, and acquired microcephaly
2. In only boys, progressive deterioration of mental and motor abilities
3. In boys and girls, short stature, prominent epicanthal folds, single crease, low-set ears, and mental retardation
4. In boys and girls with paraparesis, hydrocephalus, and mental retardation
5. In boys, but less commonly in girls, mental retardation, large ears; and in boys, macro-orchidism

answer: a-2, b-1, c-5, d-3, e-4

40. Match the structures with their origin in the fetal ectoderm or mesoderm.

a. Brain
b. Scalp and face
c. Retina
d. Stomach

e. Vertebrae
f. Spinal cord
g. Dural matter
h. Neural tube

answer: Ectoderm: CNS structures, including the neural tube, and skin: a, b, f, h. Mesoderm: skull, vertebrae, dural matter: e, g

41. Which part of the neural tube does the Dandy-Walker syndrome affect?

a. Cerebrum
b. Cerebellum

c. Lower spinal cord
d. The frontal lobes

answer: a, b. The cerebellum and the posterior cerebrum

42. Which methods reduce the incidence of infants born with a meningomyelocele?

a. Prenatal screening with fetal ultrasound
b. Determining fetal and maternal alpha-fetoprotein

c. Giving the mother folic acid before and during the first trimester
d. Screening for toxins in the environment

   answer: a, b, c

43. Match the genetically based disorder (a-c) with its description (1–11).

a. Rett syndrome
b. Fragile X syndrome
c. Down's syndrome

 1. Repetitive hand movements
 2. Acquired microcephaly
 3. Most frequently occurring disorder
 4. Disorder complicated by Alzheimer's changes
 5. Most common inherited form of mental retardation
 6. The single crease a characteristic
 7. Macro-orchidism a characteristic
 8. Autistic behavior a characteristic
 9. Cognitive deterioration beginning in childhood
10. Occurs exclusively in girls
11. Occurs exclusively in males

   answer: a. 1, 2, 8, 9, 10; b. 5, 7, 8; c. 3, 4, 6

14 Neurologic Aspects of Pain

Neurologists have come to view pain—the most common reason for which people seek medical attention—as a clinical entity, rather than a symptom of physical injury. Multidisciplinary teams, which usually include psychiatrists, are reasonably effective in ameliorating pain, controlling its affective component, suffering, and restoring function. As either individual practitioners or members of a team, psychiatrists should be aware of pain's underlying neuroanatomy and neurochemistry; management with psychotropics and opioids (narcotics);[1] and specific, common causes of pain.

Acute pain results from a particular bodily injury, such as a fracture or surgical procedure. The pain is usually self-limited and, until healing is complete, responsive to opioids or other analgesics. *Chronic malignant pain* is continual pain that results from cancer or other progressively severe illness. *Chronic benign pain* is continual pain from a healed or nonprogressive injury, such as an amputation. Both forms of chronic pain tend to be refractory to simple analgesics, associated with suffering, and accompanied by functional impairments.

Treatment plans are based on a relatively simple model of the neurology of pain transmission. As commonly envisioned, painful stimuli from a bodily injury travel through the peripheral nervous system (PNS) to synapse with central nervous system (CNS) pathways in the spinal cord. Painful stimuli "ascend" predominantly in the lateral spinothalamic tract *to the reticular activating system*, limbic system, *and thalamus*. Stimuli are then relayed to the cerebral cortex and other regions of the brain. Reciprocal CNS pathways, which provide some analgesia, "descend" from the brain through the spinal cord to modulate the stimuli in the ascending pain pathways. Pain that reaches the brain may be further reduced by naturally occurring, powerful, narcotic-like analgesics, the *endogenous opioids* (Table 14–1).

PAIN PATHWAYS

Peripheral

Painful bodily injuries liberate prostaglandins, arachidonic acid, and bradykinin that all stimulate specific peripheral nerve receptors (*nociceptors*). Pain may be alleviated at this very first step while the process is still in the "periphery," with aspirin, acetaminophen, steroids, and nonsteroidal anti-

---

[1]Narcotics are now referred to as "opioids," which includes endogenous as well as synthetic substances. In addition, the term "opioid medications" does not carry a stigma.

TABLE 14-1. GLOSSARY

Beta endorphin: An endogenous opioid, concentrated in the pituitary gland and secreted with ACTH. It consists of amino acid numbers 61–91 of beta lipotropin and gives rise to the enkephalins (see Fig. 14–2).

Beta lipotropin: A 91-amino-acid polypeptide, which may be an ACTH fragment, that gives rise to beta endorphin. However, it has no opioid activity itself, i.e., beta lipotropin is not an endogenous opioid.

Endogenous opioids: Polypeptides (amino acid chains) found within the CNS that create effects similar to those of morphine and other naturally occurring opioids. The effects of endogenous opioids and naturally occurring opioids are characteristically reversed by naloxone.

Endorphins: Endogenous morphine-like substances or opioid peptides; a term virtually synonymous with endogenous opioids.

Enkephalins: Short (5-amino-acid) polypeptide endogenous opioids that include met-enkephalin and leu-enkephalin. They are found primarily in the amygdala, brainstem, and dorsal horn of the spinal cord.

Naloxone (Narcan): A pure opioid antagonist that reverses all effects of endogenous and naturally occurring opioids.

Substance P: An 11-amino-acid polypeptide that is probably the primary pain neurotransmitter at the first synapse of the primary afferent neuron.

inflammatory agents (NSAIDs). These medicines are analgesic in large part because they inhibit the synthesis of prostaglandins or in other ways reduce tissue inflammation.

Nociceptors transmit painful sensations along two types of PNS fibers: A *delta* and C *fibers*. A delta fibers are thinly myelinated and have a small diameter. C fibers are unmyelinated, but are also small.

Pain transmission in these fibers may be dampened by activity in other PNS sensory fibers. According to the well-known *gate control theory*, stimulation of large diameter, heavily myelinated *A beta* fibers, which ordinarily carry vibration and position sensation, inhibit pain transmission by the A delta and C fibers that have little or no myelin. This theory gave rise to *transcutaneous electrical nerve stimulation (TENS)*, in which application of low-voltage electric current presumably reduces pain by stimulating large fibers (see below).

A more direct way of reducing pain is to interrupt (block) the entire peripheral nerve by injecting a local anesthetic or a toxic substance, such as alcohol. *Nerve blocks* are useful in chest and abdominal pain because the thoracic and lumbar nerve roots can be injected with alcohol as they emerge from the spine. However, this technique is usually not feasible for painful limbs because it often causes paresis, as well as analgesia. Nor is it practical in treating facial pain within the first division of the trigeminal nerve (see Fig. 4–11) because analgesia involving the cornea leads to corneal ulcerations.

Sometimes sympathetic plexus or ganglia blockade is helpful. For example, in pancreatic carcinoma, the celiac plexus might be injected with alcohol, and in the shoulder-hand syndrome, the cervical (stellate) ganglia can be injected. These blockades generally are given in conjunction with local anesthetics and physical therapy.

Central

The PNS fibers enter the CNS at the dorsal horn of the spinal cord and synapse in the *substantia gelatinosa* either immediately or after ascending a few segments. At many of these synapses, the fibers release an 11-amino acid polypeptide, *substance P*, which is a major neurotransmitter for pain at the spinal cord level (Fig. 14–1). After the synapse, most pain sensation is trans-

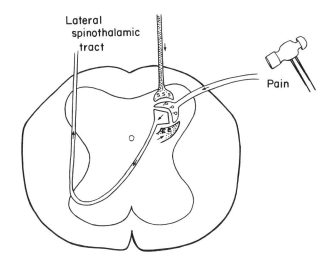

FIGURE 14–1

Painful sensations are conveyed along the *A delta* and *C* fibers of the peripheral nerves. These nerves enter the dorsal horn of the spinal cord where, utilizing *substance P* (P), they synapse. Second-order neurons cross to the contralateral side of the spinal cord and, comprising the *lateral spinothalamic tract*, ascend to the thalamus. Two (*stippled*) pain-dampening analgesic systems play upon the dorsal horn synapse. One tract descends from the brain and releases *serotonin* (S). The other system is composed of spinal interneurons that release *enkephalins* (E).

mitted within the *lateral spinothalamic tract* to the brain (see Figs. 2–6 and 2–14). This crucial tract crosses to the other side of the spinal cord and ascends contralaterally to the injury. The spinal cord contains other, less well-defined pain-transmitting tracts that ascend both ipsilaterally and contralaterally.

Ascending pain-carrying tracts synapse primarily in the thalamus. However, because they also synapse in the reticular activating system, the limbic system, and other regions of the brainstem, pain notoriously affects sleep and mood.

To provide analgesia in carefully selected cases, the lateral spinothalamic tract contralateral to the pain may be severed in a technique called a *cordotomy*. This procedure is particularly useful when patients have intractable cancer-related pain confined to a single limb. However, generalized pain would require a bilateral cordotomy, which is often complicated by respiratory drive impairment (Ondine's curse) and loss of bladder control.

Intraspinal and Descending Modulating Pathways

Providing negative feedback that dampens pain, some PNS fibers synapse onto short neurons, *interneurons*, in the spinal cord that play upon the PNS fibers. The interneurons release powerful, naturally occurring (endogenous) opioid analgesics, *enkephalins* (Table 14–1) that inhibit pain transmission.

Enkephalins' analgesic effects can be reproduced by intraspinal (intrathecal) injections of morphine. Intrathecal narcotic injections can provide long-lasting pain relief in the lower trunk, pelvis, or legs. As with the effects of other narcotics, intrathecal morphine's analgesia can be partially reversed by the powerful opiate antagonist *naloxone.*

Descending analgesic pathways originate in the frontal lobe and hypothalamus. They pass to the gray matter surrounding the third ventricle and aqueduct of Sylvius (*periaqueductal gray matter*). These tracts contain large amounts of endogenous opioids. When the periaqueductal gray matter area is stimulated by implanted electrodes, patients often have profound analgesia.

Analgesic pathways that originate in the brainstem descend in the spinal cord's *dorsolateral funiculus*. They relieve pain by inhibiting spinal cord synapses and ascending pathways. Unlike most other analgesic pathways, they release *serotonin*.

ENDOGENOUS OPIOIDS

Endogenous opioids, often called *endorphins* (endogenous morphine-like substances), are amino acid chains (polypeptides) synthesized in the CNS. They bind to receptors in the limbic system, periaqueductal gray matter, dorsal horn of the spinal cord, and other CNS sites. Synthetic or exogenous opioids, particularly morphine, bind onto the same CNS receptors. Both produce the same effects—analgesia, mood elevation (euphoria), sedation, and respiratory depression.

With long-term administration, increasingly greater quantities of opioids are required to produce effects (*tolerance*)—as if drugs "upregulated" the receptors. Likewise, unpleasant physical signs result from withdrawal or abstinence (*dependence*). Although tolerance and dependence often occur together, each can occur independently. In any case, tolerance and dependence are two physiologic hallmarks of addiction.

Some physicians, in contrast, define addiction in behavioral terms, such as an individual's drug-seeking behavior despite the potential harm both to the individual and to society. These physicians point out that tolerance and dependence are not peculiar to narcotics. Antihypertensive agents, for example, produce tolerance, and their withdrawal typically produces unpleasant symptoms, such as angina and rebound hypertension.

Adhering to the traditional, physiologic perspective, naloxone reverses the effects of endogenous as well as exogenous opioids. Indeed, the opioid antagonist effect of naloxone is so reliable that *naloxone reversibility* is the criterion for determining that an analgesic's effect is mediated by the opioid pathways.

The beta-endorphins and adrenocorticotropin (ACTH) are derived from a large common precursor (Fig. 14–2). The "runners' high" and the initial painlessness described by wounded soldiers are postulated to result from endogenous opioids secreted along with ACTH from the pituitary gland in people who are under stress.

TREATMENTS

Physicians can prescribe a variety of medications that can be administered through different routes. Combined with physical and psychologic treatments, they reduce suffering as well as pain, increase function, and give patients some control over their situation.

Nonopioid Analgesics

Aspirin, other salicylates, NSAIDs, and acetaminophen act predominantly *peripherally* by inhibiting prostaglandin synthesis at the site of injury. They are effective for mild to moderate acute and chronic benign pain (Table 14–

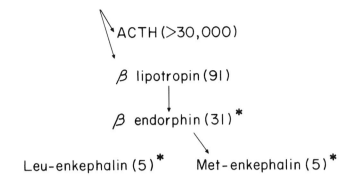

FIGURE 14–2

A large precursor molecule (not pictured) gives rise to ACTH and beta lipotropin, which are often released together. Beta lipotropin gives rise to beta endorphin and met-enkephalin, but another precursor gives rise to leu-enkephalin. (The asterisks denote the important endogenous opioids, and the numbers within parentheses are the amino-acid units in the polypeptide chains.)

2). Two tablets (600 mg) of aspirin, which remains the standard, produce approximately the same analgesia as two common opioids: 65 mg of propoxyphene (Darvon) or 50 mg of oral meperidine (Demerol).

Some NSAIDs are more effective than aspirin and, if given parenterally in large doses, are more effective than those opioids. Not only are NSAIDs effective, but their use is also uncomplicated by tolerance or dependence. In other words, the same dose will provide steady relief for weeks to months, and after a course of treatment, withdrawal does not produce symptoms. Also, these medicines do not induce psychologic side effects. However, once their maximum benefit is achieved, additional quantities will not increase analgesia (the "ceiling effect"). Gastrointestinal bleeding and platelet inhibition are potential complications.

These medications are more effective if a "loading dose" is taken prophylactically. For example, pain can be partly prevented by use of these analgesics before dental procedures, menses, and headaches.

When given in combination with opioids, which act predominantly *centrally*, these medicines enhance each other's analgesia. Simply taking two tablets of aspirin, for example, will increase the potency of either codeine or morphine. Likewise, adding NSAIDs to opioids is helpful in the treatment of metastases to bone, which is a very painful condition.

TABLE 14–2. EXAMPLES OF NONOPIOID ANALGESICS

Acetaminophen (Tylenol and others)
Aspirin
   Choline magnesium trisalicyate (Trilisate)
   Diflunisal (Dolobid)
Nonsteroidal anti-inflammatory agents
   Ibuprofen (Motrin, Advil, Nuprin)
   Indomethacin (Indocin)
   Ketorolac (Toradol)
   Naproxen (Naprosyn)
   Sulindac (Clinoril)

Opioids

Opioids are indicated for acute, moderate, or severe pain, such as pain resulting from a fracture, myocardial infarction, or surgery (Table 14–3). They are also indicated in chronic, malignant pain, especially when it is incessant or distressing enough to cause suffering, depression, or insomnia. Some authors have made a controversial suggestion that opioids are appropriate for chronic, benign pain (see below).

Greater doses or more potent preparations of opioids increase their analgesic potential. In other words, unlike NSAIDs, opioids have no ceiling effect. Their potency can be enhanced, without increasing their side effects, by adding NSAIDs or other nonopioid analgesics; however, combining various opioids provides little additional benefit.

Opioids are not only effective when administered through traditional routes: oral, intramuscular, and intravenous. They can also be given through transdermal (skin patches), intranasal (sprays), rectal (suppositories), and intrathecal and intra-articular (injections) routes. These alternatives offer a more rapid onset of action, steadier medication levels, less reliance on nurses and family members for administration, and more direct access to the painful site.

In a particularly innovative technique, *patient-controlled analgesia (PCA)*, patients themselves regulate a continual or intermittent intravenous opioid infusion. In selected cases, PCA can be administered through an intrathecal device, which produces analgesia in patients' lumbosacral spine and pelvic organs without subjecting them to opioids' CNS side effects. Although expensive, PCA empowers patients, provides a satisfactory, steady state of analgesia, reduces nursing requirements, and permits shorter hospitalizations.

Unless opioids are administered continuously by PCA, patches, or long-acting oral preparations (which is usually preferable), they should be given on a *regular prophylactic* basis, such as every 2 to 4 hours, rather than at the onset of pain. When analgesics must be requested by the patient and then given by nurses only after pain begins, the delayed treatment makes pain more difficult to alleviate, creates a pattern of under- and overtreatment, and prevents a restful sleep-wake schedule. Moreover, the patient, fearful about the recurrence of pain, becomes anxious and preoccupied with obtaining drugs.

TABLE 14–3. EXAMPLES OF OPIOID ANALGESICS

For Mild to Moderately Severe Pain
    Codeine
    Oxycodone (Percocet)
    Propoxyphene (Darvon)
For Moderate to Severe Pain
    Hydromorphone (Dilaudid)
    Levorphanol (Levo-Dromoran)
    Meperidine (Demerol)
    Morphine
Long-Acting Oral Preparations
    Methadone
    Morphine long-acting
      (MS Contin, Oramorph SR, Roxane SR)
Nasal Administration (Spray)
    Butorphanol (Stadol)—mixed agonist-antagonist
Transdermal Administration (Skin Patches)
    Fentanyl (Duragesic)
Transmucosal Administration (lollipops)
    Fentanyl (Fentanyl Oralet)

When injections are used to administer opioids or other medications, the injection should be given into the deltoid or gluteus muscles rather than the surrounding fat because medicines are absorbed faster from muscle than fat, in which they are soluble.

Some physicians, for a variety of reasons, tend to undertreat with opioids. They withhold opioids, prescribe them in insufficient doses, and do not recognize that, as tolerance develops or the underlying disease progresses, more frequent and larger doses are necessary. In fact, although dependence may develop, addiction is an unrealistic consideration for patients who are seriously or terminally ill. Moreover, addiction rarely occurs in patients with a normal premorbid personality who develop a painful illness that requires opioids for several weeks.

Side effects, which rarely occur, can be anticipated. Respiratory depression or hypoventilation—slow, shallow, insufficient breathing—is almost the only potentially life-threatening problem. It usually results from inadvertent overdose, combinations of medications, or pre-existing pulmonary disease. For the psychiatry consultant, opioid-induced mental aberrations can be vexing, especially because they can mimic surgical complications, head trauma, metabolic aberrations including hypoventilation, and, in cancer patients, cerebral metastases. Constipation, which from most patients' perspective is the most bothersome side effect, can be managed with a combination of laxatives, such as senna (Senokot), and stool softeners, such as Docusate sodium (Colace). Nausea, often a devastating problem, may be caused by the underlying illness, radiotherapy, or chemotherapy, as well as the opioids themselves. Patients should be given vigorous and preferably prophylactic treatment with anti-emetic suppositories, injections, or pills; however, antiemetics should be cautiously prescribed because many contain phenothiazines and related dopamine-blocking agents can cause dystonic reactions and parkinsonism (see Chapter 18). Synthetic marijuana, dronabinol (Marinol), and related preparations, such as Nabilone (Cesamet), have been approved as antiemetics, but their benefit is not established and they can cause mental aberrations.

One particular difficulty with opioids is that their blood levels are dependent upon the route of administration. The same dose that is given orally may produce an overdose if given intramuscularly or intravenously. If the situation were reversed, undertreatment may precipitate opioid withdrawal symptoms and recurrence of pain.

The use of certain opioids is fraught with difficulties. Meperidine (Demerol), although one of the most frequently prescribed opioids, is usually unsatisfactory. It is poorly absorbed when taken orally, and changing its route of administration leads to complications. When meperidine is given for several days, especially in patients with renal insufficiency, accumulation of its toxic metabolite, normeperidine, often causes dysphoria, other mental aberrations, tremulousness, myoclonus, and seizures. When taken with monoamine oxidase inhibitors, meperidine can cause a potentially fatal hypertensive encephalopathy. Long-term use, which occurs in recurrent painful conditions, such as sickle-cell crises, as well as addiction, can cause muscle and subcutaneous tissue nodules.

Another problematic opioid is heroin. Not only is its effectiveness in relieving pain and improving mood no greater than an appropriate dose of morphine but also the potential for abuse is much greater. In "Brompton's cocktail" and its variations, heroin is combined with cocaine, chloroform water (for flavor), phenothiazines (for nausea), and gin or another alcoholic beverage.

These concoctions, which have received wide publicity, are no better than morphine and antiemetics in adequate doses.

Finally, opioids with antagonist properties, such as pentazocine (Talwin) and butorphanol (Stadol), have limited use. They were developed, quite rationally, to prevent abuse by incorporating opioid antagonist properties into opioid analgesics; however, they have been abused. Also, they have psychotomimetic properties, and injections of pentazocine lead to skin and muscle necrosis. Because of their opioid antagonism, a change from a morphine-like opioid to one of these mixed agonist-antagonist drugs will, like undertreatment, produce withdrawal symptoms and pain recurrence.

Like any drug, opioids should be discontinued when unnecessary and tapered, rather than stopped abruptly. Sometimes an equivalent dose of methadone can be substituted and then tapered. Patients who agree to a structured program may be given placebos in the final stages of drug withdrawal. As opioids are withdrawn, nonopioid analgesics should be substituted. Physical or mental discomfort from withdrawal might be alleviated by a minor tranquilizer or an ataractic, such as hydroxyzine (Vistaril), or, curiously, clonidine (Catapres).

Adjuvant Medications and Techniques

Antidepressants. Tricyclic antidepressants (TCAs) are the most widely used adjuvant. In contrast, serotonin reuptake inhibitors, particularly fluoxetine, and related antidepressants have not—at least yet—been shown to be effective. TCAs, given at bedtime, help restore a normal sleep-wake schedule. They also produce analgesia, presumably by increasing serotonin concentrations in the descending CNS analgesic pathways. In many cases of chronic pain, TCAs nicely complement opioid or nonopioid analgesics. They are particularly useful in certain painful conditions, such as diabetic neuropathy, migraines, and postherpetic neuralgia.

TCAs are frequently indicated in chronic benign and malignant pain. They are helpful in chronic pain patients without overt depression. In depressed patients, TCAs induce analgesia even before they improve patients' mood. In general, lower dosages of TCAs are required to treat pain than depression.

TCAs also help the affective components of painful illnesses probably because chronic pain is inextricably linked to depression. Chronic pain not only produces signs of depression, including vegetative symptoms and insomnia, but it also often leads to drug and alcohol dependency, counterproductive familial relationships, and exaggeration of physical deficits. Similarly, depression lowers the threshold for pain, increases disability from painful injuries, and makes pain refractory to treatment. In many chronic pain patients, the sequence of pain and depression is unclear. As a practical matter, neurologists typically assume that chronic pain patients have developed depression as a consequence, if not a cause of the pain, and liberally prescribe TCAs.

The most common practice is to begin amitriptyline in a low dose, such as 25 mg, taken at bedtime. Doses are increased gradually, usually to a range of 75 to 150 mg at bedtime. Other TCAs, including imipramine, desipramine, and doxepin, are also useful. However, TCAs by themselves are usually not effective and do not decrease requirements for opioids.

Other Medications. Hypnotics and minor and major tranquilizers often help specific symptoms, such as anxiety, insomnia, and nausea, and thus may indirectly reduce pain and suffering. However, they are usually less effective than TCAs in pain management. Moreover, many of these medicines lead to drug dependency or frank drug abuse that prevents resolution of the pain and disability.

Anticonvulsants—carbamazepine (Tegretol), which is structurally similar to the TCAs, phenytoin (Dilantin), valproate (Depakote), and clonazepam (Klonopin)—are quite effective for specific conditions in which nerves are directly irritated, such as trigeminal neuralgia, diabetic neuropathy, postherpetic neuralgia, and reflex sympathetic dystrophy (see below). For example, carbamazepine relieves trigeminal neuralgia so effectively and specifically that prescribing it is virtually a therapeutic trial. These medications are often used in chronic benign and malignant pain, but with less success.

Stimulation-Induced Analgesia. Scientific studies have found that acupuncture is an effective form of analgesia in some people with mildly to moderately painful injuries. For securing analgesia, the "meridians," the traditional regions where needles are placed, have been shown to be less important than dermatomes (see Figs. 2–15 and 16–2). Since acupuncture induces a rise in CSF endorphins and the analgesia is naloxone-reversible, it is presumed to work in part through the endogenous opioid system (Table 14–4).

A frequently used treatment for chronic musculoskeletal disorders is TENS, a technique in which an electric stimulus is applied to the skin just proximal to the painful region. This technique stemmed from the observation that people instinctually massage a portion of the body proximal to the injury. For example, a person with a sprained ankle will rub the lower leg.

TENS was thought to be analgesic, and the analgesia was believed to result from stimulation of the underlying large, thickly myelinated nerve fibers blocking ascending pain-carrying fibers (the gate control theory) or through the endogenous opioid system. However, subsequent studies have indicated that TENS has no effect, is a placebo, or, at most, provides small amounts of analgesia for only several weeks.

In *dorsal column stimulation*, a technique similar to TENS, electrodes are inserted directly onto the dorsal columns of the spinal cord. Similarly, after initial reports of its analgesic effects, follow-up studies have found that it provides short-lived or no benefit. Moreover, the risks are substantially higher than with TENS.

Stimulation of the CNS has been taken a step further. Neurosurgeons can implant electrodes into the periventricular and periaqueductal gray matter and adjacent brainstem regions. As noted above, stimulation of these sites, which presumably releases endogenous opioids stores, can produce profound analgesia. However, the technique remains investigational

TABLE 14–4.   ANALGESICS MEDIATED BY THE ENDOGENOUS OPIOID SYSTEM[a]

Acupuncture
Opioids
Placebo
Stimulation[b]
   TENS (transcutaneous electrical nerve stimulation)
   Dorsal column stimulation
   Periaqueductal gray matter stimulation

[a]Since these analgesics are partially or entirely reversed by naloxone, their effects are considered to be mediated by the endogenous opioid system. In contrast, analgesia induced by tricyclic antidepressants and hypnosis is not reversed by naloxone.
[b]See text regarding the efficacy.

Placebos, Hypnosis, and Behavioral Therapies. Placebos, which are commonly given by physicians either deliberately or unknowingly when they prescribe ineffectual medications, produce a definite but brief period of analgesia in at least 30 per cent of patients. They are most effective for acute, severe pain, especially when patients have anxiety, and are least effective for continual, mild pain. Contrary to popular notion, a beneficial response to placebo does not mean that a patient's pain is psychogenic. Since the analgesic effect of placebos is partially naloxone-reversible, placebos probably stimulate the endogenous opioid system.

Hypnosis is useful for a limited period in a wide variety of chronic painful conditions including cancer. It differs from placebo therapy because patients' ability to be hypnotized does not correlate with their response to placebos, and hypnosis-induced analgesia is not naloxone-reversible, i.e., hypnosis is not a placebo.

Cognitive therapy, behavior modification, operant conditioning, and other psychologic therapies have been recommended when the response to the usual treatments is insufficient or when the pain is out of proportion to the bodily injury. They have also been used in cases of abnormal behavior, opioid abuse, or when family members have begun to reinforce the pain. Widely used behavioral therapies are relaxation, desensitization, and distraction. Likewise, biofeedback may have a role for certain individuals with chronic pain.

MALIGNANT PAIN

Brain tumors, whether metastatic or primary, cause headaches because of increased intracranial pressure, meningeal irritation, or cranial nerve involvement (see Chapter 19). Other primary tumors, such as lung, breast, kidney, and skin cancer, are agonizingly painful if they metastasize to bone, the epidural space (see Fig. 19–5), or the brachial or lumbosacral plexus. Also, numerous cancer treatments are mildly to moderately painful.

Especially because it is severe, tends to worsen, involves nerves directly, and indicates a poor prognosis, malignant pain is associated with depression, anxiety, and insomnia. If it is associated with dementia or an encephalopathy (delirium), however, cancer patients may have cerebral metastases or a systemic condition, such as toxicity from medications, electrolyte imbalance, sepsis, or organ failure.

In all cases, physicians should monitor their patients' pain regularly—just as regularly as they monitor the platelet count. Patients' reports should generally be accepted without reservation (Fig. 14–3). They should have access to nondrug therapy, such as relaxation techniques, hypnosis and psychotherapy, as well as the full arsenal of medications.

Often local treatment with radiotherapy or opioid injection is satisfactory and avoids systemic and neurologic side effects. Occasionally, surgical procedures, such as a cordotomy and peripheral nerve block, are helpful.

Analgesics in Malignant Pain

The three categories of analgesics—nonopioid, opioid, and adjuvant—should be prescribed early, sometimes pre-emptively, frequently, and generously. If undertreatment in pain management is the greatest physician error, it is egregious in malignant pain.

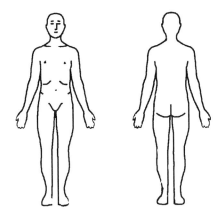

0 – 10 Numeric Pain Intensity Scale

0	1	2	3	4	5	6	7	8	9	10

0
No
Pain

5
Moderate
Pain

10
Worst
Possible
Pain

Visual Analog Scale

No
Pain

Worst
Possible
Pain

FIGURE 14–3

Graphics are replacing verbal descriptions of the site and degree of pain. Patients describe their pain by circling the most intensely painful area on the sketch. Then they are asked either to circle the single number on the Numeric Pain Scale or mark the Visual Analog Scale at the point that describes the intensity of their pain: 0 = No Pain through 10 = The Worst Possible Pain. For children, for whom graphics are particularly useful, scales are based on the smiling face to crying face icons.

Variations of the basic scale measure maximum pain, minimal pain, response to treatment, insomnia, and functional impairment. (Adapted from Jacox et al., 1994.)

A three-step treatment plan based on the World Health Organization Guidelines provides relief in as many as 90 per cent of patients:

- Treat with a nonopioid analgesic until the ceiling is reached.
- Add a long-acting, oral opioid analgesic.
- Combine opioid and nonopioid analgesics with adjuvant medications.

The doses of opioids must be increased as tolerance develops. Although long-acting oral preparations are preferable, transdermal, PCA, or other parenteral administrations may be required for severe pain, continuous administration, or other reasons.

NONMALIGNANT PAIN SYNDROMES

Although agonizing pain is generally associated with malignancies, several nonmalignant pain syndromes create comparable pain, suffering, and disability for many people. Several syndromes are discussed elsewhere in the book: diabetic neuropathy, herniated disks, and low back pain (see Chapter 5); headaches (see Chapter 9); and post-traumatic headaches and whiplash injury (see Chapter 22). Additional syndromes are discussed below.

Treatment can vary widely, but several guidelines can be suggested. Both patients and physicians should accept that most of these conditions are chronic and incurable, but not fatal, illnesses. Their goals should be to achieve living with the pain, reduction of the suffering, and, despite persistent pain, restoration of occupational and social function. All goals should be clearly stated, acceptable to the patient, and attainable within several months.

Medications should usually consist of nonopioid analgesics, especially NSAIDs, combined with TCAs, anticonvulsants, and other adjuvants. If opioid analgesics must be given, they are generally appropriate only for a preplanned, limited period.

Some physicians, however, have advocated prescribing morphine and other opioids for rare individuals who have no alternative treatment for intractable, chronic, nonmalignant pain and do not have abusive, destructive drug-seeking behavior. These physicians believe that opioids are highly effective, relatively safe, and, when used to control pain, not addictive. Rigid drug schedules, "contracts," can be imposed to prevent abuse and to control behavior. The assertion that these medications are not addictive is based on studies showing that patients treated with an opioid for unequivocally severe pain do not experience withdrawal symptoms when the medicine is discontinued and that tolerance does not develop after pain control is reached. In contrast, opioid addiction is characterized by rapidly developing, ever increasing tolerance and, if the opioid is discontinued, withdrawal.

With the possible exception of prescribing inadequate amounts of opioids, many physicians tend to overmedicate patients. They should consider supplementing or replacing medications with nonpharmacologic modalities, such as psychotherapy, hypnosis, cognitive-behavior techniques, and physical therapy.

Physicians should be encouraged to refer patients for psychiatric consultation not only for evaluation for depression but also for other psychologic disturbances and drug abuse. Psychiatrists should evaluate patients (1) who have vegetative symptoms regardless of the apparent connection to the pain; (2) whose pain or disability is refractory to several courses of medical treatment; (3) for whom excessive medications are required; or (4) for whom inpatient treatment or surgical procedures have been unsuccessful. A consultation should be obtained early and as an integral part of the evaluation. It should not be an afterthought, last resort, or a method that merely passes the patient to another physician.

When possible, psychiatrists should examine the physical location of patients' pain. The touching might have a therapeutic benefit, albeit a primitive one. Also, in evaluating any functional disability brought on by the pain, psychiatrists should at least watch the patient sit, walk, and, if possible, use the painful region.

Postmastectomy Axillary Pain

During a mastectomy, surgeons explore the axilla and remove lymph nodes. This portion of the procedure often requires severing the cutaneous branch of the first thoracic nerve root, *the intercostobrachial nerve*. Several weeks later, some women develop searing pain in the axilla extending to the inner aspect of the upper arm, well beyond the incision. This pain can be distinguished from common incision pain, which is only mildly to moderately intense, has an itching quality, and is confined to the incision. Postmastectomy pain, like many other painful disorders, is worse at night. Since shoulder movement provokes the pain, this condition may lead to a "frozen shoulder."

Before embarking on symptomatic treatment, physicians should attempt to diagnose the cause of postmastectomy pain, which can include tumor infiltration of the brachial plexus, infection in the incision, and radiation fibrosis. Patients may benefit from nonopioid analgesics and TCAs. Massaging the painful skin with a damp cloth after applying a vapor-coolant, such as ethyl chloride spray, may also reduce the pain. Patients should exercise to increase shoulder mobility and upper arm strength.

Even though postmastectomy pain does not carry prognostic significance, it intensifies the surgery's psychologic impact. No matter how tempting, pain near the site of a mastectomy should not be attributed to psychogenic factors.

Postherpetic Neuralgia

Acute *Herpes zoster* infection causes a vesicular skin eruption, *shingles*, in the distribution of one or two nerve dermatomes. Although any dermatome may be affected, the thoracic dermatomes and then the first branch of the trigeminal nerve, which includes the cornea, are most commonly affected. The infection is caused by reactivated varicella virus that has lain dormant in dorsal (sensory) nerve root ganglia. It is especially common among people who are older than 65 years even though they are otherwise healthy or in anyone with immunosuppressive illnesses, such as lymphoproliferative disorders and acquired immune deficiency syndrome (AIDS).

The acute infection causes moderate severe burning and unrelenting pain that sometimes precede the vesicles by several days. In most cases, the pain and skin lesions recede within several weeks. During this period, the severe pain justifies the use of opioids. Antiviral agents, such as acyclovir (Zovirax) and famciclovir (Famvir), may speed healing of the vesicles, shorten the duration of the pain, and prevent the spread of the infection into the eye.

As excruciating as the pain of the initial infection may have been, about 20 per cent of patients suffer a more painful secondary phase, *postherpetic neuralgia*. By then, patients are left with a band of numb, scarred skin and, if a major motor nerve has been involved, muscle weakness and atrophy. The pain, which can last for months, tends to be lancinating and so severe that it causes anorexia, insomnia, and mood changes.

Postherpetic neuralgia is unequivocally an indication for a trial of opioids and TCAs. As in other chronic pain syndromes, anticonvulsants have often been suggested, but studies have shown that they are helpful only for certain aspects of the pain. A complementary therapy is an analgesic skin cream containing capsaicin (Zostrix) that depletes substance P.

Reflex Sympathetic Dystrophy (RSD)

RSD is a spectrum of painful disorders that includes *sympathetically maintained pain (SMP)*. These disorders are typically caused by seemingly minor compressive or traction injuries that do not cause overt nerve damage. Causalgia is similar to RSD, but usually follows an obvious injury, such as a gunshot wound, a large peripheral nerve of an arm or leg. Both conditions probably damage autonomic nervous system fibers, as well as peripheral nerves.

RSD is the most important disorder because it is more common in the civilian population and is most apt to be misdiagnosed. It follows within 2 months of an injury. RSD patients develop a relentless burning sensation superimposed on an irritating numbness. Touching or moving an affected region produces greater pain. Patients assiduously protect an afflicted hand by wearing a sling and glove or a foot by using crutches. The entire limb is rendered useless.

In many cases, the extent of the painful area spreads beyond the injury. For example, after several months of left arm pain, a patient may describe similar symptoms in the left leg and then the right leg. Some cases have included tremors and other involuntary movement disorders.

The pain and unusual sensitivity in the affected limb are accompanied by characteristic "trophic" or "sudomotor" changes in which the skin becomes smooth, shiny, pale, and scaly. Fingernails remain uncut and grow to be long and brittle. Although the skin may have excessive sweating, *hyperhidrosis*, it is usually sweatless, cool, and dry. These skin changes, which have been attributed to altered autonomic nervous system innervation, are objective signs of RSD.

The best treatment for causalgia is blockade of the regional sympathetic ganglia with an injection of an anesthetic agent. For example, patients with causalgia of the hand may benefit from blocks of the stellate (sympathetic) ganglion, which is adjacent to the upper cervical vertebrae. Alternatively, an intravenous infusion of bretylium or guanethidine into an affected limb blocks alpha- and beta-adrenergic sympathetic ganglion receptors. Response to sympathetic blocks, although brief, has diagnostic usefulness, as well as potential therapeutic value. TENS and a large variety of drugs provide inadequate relief. Physical therapy is helpful, but patients have trouble complying with programs unless they receive appropriate nerve blocks.

RSD, a unique disorder, probably stems from an interaction between the sympathetic and peripheral nervous systems. The injuries seem to bring about disproportionate pain, suffering, and disability. Symptoms extend far beyond the injury. Patients tend to be totally incapacitated and preoccupied with the limb, which they protect with extravagant methods.

Phantom Limb Pain

Phantom limb pain occurs in an amputated limb. For example, a man may have his leg severed at the thigh in an automobile accident, and weeks later he may still feel pain as though it were centered in his ankle. The pain is often accompanied by nonpainful sensations. For example, patients with amputations still feel that the limb is an integral part of their body, and they sense purposeful movements in their absent hands, fingers, and toes. These sensations can reach the level of a somatic hallucination and are akin to the visual hallucinations perceived by recently blinded people.

Phantom limb pain differs from pain at the site of a surgical incision, called *stump pain*, which is usually attributed to scar tissue and nerve damage (neuromas). Phantom and stump pain, of course, may occur together.

Phantom limb pain varies in quality, severity, and accompanying psychologic symptoms. It usually begins soon after a traumatic amputation of a limb and has a self-limited duration of several weeks. It is more likely to develop in patients older than 35 years, if the limb were chronically painful before the amputation (as occurs with osteomyelitis), or if the amputation were traumatic. Because most cases of phantom pain result from war, the patients are usually young or middle-aged men. Many have lost their ability to walk or work. Some have extensive injuries, including loss of several limbs or their genitalia.

Medical treatment alone is insufficient. Carbamazepine, especially for shooting pains, and conventional analgesics are inconsistently beneficial. TENS and acupuncture have been effective only in isolated cases. TCAs should be tried freely because of the high incidence of depression in patients with this disorder. Some physicians have claimed benefit after stump and forehead muscle relaxation and by inducing the sensation that the phantom limb is shrinking to the point that it disappears.

Chronic pain from phantom limbs, brachial plexus avulsion, and thalamic infarctions (see below) is often attributed to the loss of sensory input and classified *deafferentation pain*. One theory is that the pain results, not from the irritation of nociceptors, but from conversion of the absence of normal sensation to painful sensations. In contrast, pain from direct nerve injury, such as postherpetic neuralgia and diabetic neuropathy, is called *neuropathic pain*. Despite the logic of this classification, it overlaps the roles of the CNS and PNS, effective medications, and nonpharmaceutical therapy.

Thalamic Pain

Thalamic infarctions or other injuries, which themselves are usually painless, initially cause contralateral hemianesthesia. Depending on which nearby structures are damaged, the hemianesthesia may be accompanied by hemiparesis or hemiataxia.

Subsequently, patients sometimes develop a painful condition, also called the *Déjérine-Roussy syndrome*, which is characterized by various painful sensations on the hemianesthetic side of the body. The pain is typically perceived most strongly in the face and hand. In trying to ward off the pain, patients wear hats, long sleeves, and gloves. Similar painful disturbances, called *central pain*, may follow injuries in other portions of the CNS in which sensory systems are destroyed.

In most cases, anticonvulsants and analgesics do not provide sustained relief. Even opioids are rarely satisfactory. Physical therapy and supportive psychotherapy may be temporizing. The pain generally subsides after 6 to 12 months.

REFERENCES

Abramowicz M (ed): Capsaicin—a topical analgesic. Med Lett *34*: 62–63, 1992
Abramowicz M (ed): Butorphanol nasal spray for pain. Med Lett *35*: 105–106, 1993
Abramowicz M (ed): Drugs for pain. Med Lett *35*: 1–6, 1993
Abramowicz M (ed): Oral transmucosal fentanyl citrate. Med Lett *36*: 24–25, 1994
Arbit E (ed): Management of Cancer-Related Pain. Mt. Kisco, NY, Futura, 1993
Aronoff GM (ed): Evaluation and Treatment of Chronic Pain. Baltimore, Williams & Wilkins, 1992
Deyo RA, Walsh NE, Martin DC, et al: A controlled trial of transcutaneous electrical nerve stimulation (TENS) and exercise for chronic low back pain. N Engl J Med *322*: 1627–1634, 1990
Dotson RM: Causalgia--reflex sympathetic dystrophy—sympathetically maintained pain: Myth and reality. Muscle Nerve *16*: 1049–1055, 1993
Jacox A, Carr DB, Payne R, et al: Management of Cancer Pain: Adults Quick Reference Guide. No 9. AHCPR Publication No. 94-0593. Rockville, MD, Agency for Health Care Policy and Research, U.S. Department of Health and Human Services, Public Health Service 1994

Marchand S, Charest J, Li J, et al: Is TENS purely a placebo effect? A controlled study on chronic low back pain. Pain *54*: 99–106, 1993

Max MB: Treatment of post-herpetic neuralgia: Antidepressants. Ann Neurol *35*: S50-S53, 1994

Melzack R: The tragedy of needless pain. Sci Am *262*: 27–33, 1990

Melzack R: Phantom limbs. Sci Am *266*: 120–126, 1992

Meyler WJ, de Jongste MJ, Rolf CA: Clinical evaluation of pain treatment with electrostimulation: A study on TENS in patients with different pain syndromes. Clin J Pain *10*: 22–27, 1994

Patt RB (ed): Cancer Pain. Philadelphia, JB Lippincott, 1993

Portenoy RK: Chronic opioid therapy in nonmalignant pain. J Pain Symptom Manage *5*: S46-S62, 1990

Raj PP (ed): Practical Management of Pain. New York, Mosby-Year Book, 1992

Schwartzman RJ: Reflex sympathetic dystrophy and causalgia. Neurol Clin *10*: 953–973, 1993

Stannard CF: Phantom limb pain. Br J Hosp Med *50*: 583–587, 1993

Turner JA, Deyo RA, Loeser JD, et al: The importance of placebo effects in pain treatment and research. JAMA *20*: 1609–1614, 1994

QUESTIONS and ANSWERS: CHAPTER 14

1–7.   Match the substance with its effect on the pain pathways.

a.   Reduces tissue inflammation
b.   Interferes with prostaglandin synthesis
c.   Provides analgesia by acting within the CNS
d.   Acts as a neurotransmitter of pain in the spinal cord
e.   Is liberated in a spinal cord descending analgesic tract

1.   Morphine

2.   Endogenous opioids

3.   Serotonin

4.   Substance P

5.   Enkephalin

6.   Beta-endorphin

7.   Nonsteroidal anti-inflammatory agents (NSAIDS)

   answer: 1-c, 2-c, 3-e, 4-d, 5-c, 6-c, 7-a, b

8.   Which properties of morphine are *not* shared with endogenous opioids?

a.   Tolerance
b.   Effectiveness in deep brainstem structures and spinal cord
c.   Ability to cause mood changes, as well as analgesia
d.   Reversibility with naloxone
e.   Commercial availability
f.   Respiratory depression

   answer: e

9–17.   What is the composition of these substances?

a.   11-amino-acid polypeptide
b.   5-amino-acid polypeptide
c.   Diacetyl morphine
d.   Greater than 30,000 amino acid polypeptide
e.   An indole
f.   An alkaloid of opium
g.   91-amino-acid polypeptide
h.   31-amino-acid polypeptide

   9.   Leu-enkephalin

   10.   ACTH

11. Morphine

12. Beta endorphin

13. Heroin

14. Beta-lipotropin

15. Met-enkephalin

16. Serotonin

17. Substance P

answer: 9-b, 10-d, 11-f, 12-h, 13-c f, 14-g, 15-b, 16-e, 17-a

18. Which of these fibers do carry pain sensation?

a. A delta   c. A beta
b. C

answer: a, b

19. In which spinal cord tract does most pain sensation ascend?

a. Fasciculus gracilis
b. Fasciculus cuneatus
c. Lateral corticospinal tract
d. Lateral spinothalamic tract

answer: d

20. In which tract do pain-dampening fibers that utilize serotonin descend within the spinal cord?

a. Lateral spinothalamic tract   c. Fasciculus gracilis
b. Dorsolateral funiculus   d. Dentorubral tract

answer: b

21. Which forms of analgesia are mostly naloxone-reversible?

a. Acupuncture   e. Hypnosis
b. Opioid administration   f. Placebo
c. TENS   g. Stimulation of periventricular gray
d. Aspirin   matter
                                h. Intrathecal morphine injections

answer: a, b, c, f, g, h

22. Why would the addition of aspirin or acetaminophen increase the effectiveness of opioids?

a. Aspirin and acetaminophen are also opioids.
b. They actually do not increase analgesia.
c. They stimulate endogenous opioid release.
d. They interfere with prostaglandin synthesis.
e. They increase serotonin reuptake.

answer: d

23. Why are tricyclic and other antidepressants helpful in the treatment of chronic pain?

a. They treat depression.
b. They help restore restful sleep patterns.
c. They probably increase serotonin levels, which decreases pain.
d. They alter autonomic system activity.
e. They themselves are analgesics.

answer: a, b, c, e

24. What are the potential complications of mixed agonist-antagonist opioids, such as pentazocine (Talwin)?

a. Normeperidine accumulation
b. Addiction
c. Delirium
d. Respiratory depression
e. They can precipitate withdrawal in patients using meperidine (Demerol).

answer: b, c, d, e. Also, pentazocine can cause skin and subcutaneous scarring (sclerosis).

25. What are the potential complications of meperidine (Demerol) use?

a. Marked undertreatment when the same dose is given orally as intramuscularly
b. Normeperidine toxicity
c. Overdose when the same dose is given parenterally as orally
d. Stupor
e. Seizures
f. Tremulousness

answer: a, b, c, d, e, f

26. Which one of the following features is *not* a characteristic of reflex sympathetic dystrophy?

a. The sympathetic nervous system is involved.
b. The skin usually becomes shiny and often scaly.
c. The pain is usually relieved with blockade of the sympathetic ganglia.
d. The trunk and abdomen are typically included.
e. Major motor nerves or roots are involved.

answer: d

27. Which features are present in the phantom limb, but not stump (incision) pain?

a. Patients have pain at the site of the amputated limb.
b. Patients have the sensation that the limb is still present.
c. Patients have a sensation that the limb is capable of movement.
d. There is extensive damage to non-neurologic as well as neurologic tissues.

answer: b, c

28. Which of the following is *not* a complication of infarction of the thalamus and its surrounding structures?

a. Hemianesthesia
b. Hemiataxia
c. Patients protecting involved regions, such as their face and arm
d. Abnormal sweating
e. Dysesthesia

answer: d

29. Which of the following statements are true regarding the periaqueductal gray matter?

a. Stimulation of the periaqueductal gray matter produces analgesia.
b. Thiamine deprivation causes hemorrhage into the periaqueductal gray matter.
c. The periaqueductal gray matter surrounds the aqueduct of Sylvius.
d. The aqueduct of Sylvius is the conduit for CSF between the third and fourth ventricles.

answer: a, b, c, d

30. Which of the following statements are true regarding enkephalins?

a. They are tricyclic.
b. They are secondary messengers.
c. Naloxone inhibits enkephalins.
d. They are part of the serotonin system.

answer: c. The enkephalins are peptide neurotransmitters that have a powerful, inhibitory role on spinal cord interneurons. They produce effects similar to morphine because they are part of the opioid system.

31.   Which of the following statements are true regarding serotonin's role in pain and analgesia?

a.   It enhances the serotonin system, which reduces pain, often before affecting mood.
b.   Descending, serotonin-based spinal cord tracts induce analgesia.
c.   In its analgesic role, serotonin is an inhibitory neurotransmitter.
d.   Serotonin is an endogenous opioid

answer: a, b, c

32.   Which statement most closely describes the gate control theory?

a.   Descending pathways inhibit pain.
b.   The periaqueductal gray matter blocks pain transmission to the frontal lobes and limbic system.
c.   Behavioral modification reduces pain-induced suffering.
d.   Stimulation of large diameter, heavily myelinated fibers inhibit pain transmission by small, sparsely myelinated fibers.

answer: d

33.   Which are characteristics of NSAIDs?

a.   They are addictive.
b.   Additional medication produces greater analgesia, i.e., they have no "ceiling."
c.   Patients develop a tolerance to the analgesia.
d.   They can be as effective as opioids.
e.   They can be combined with opioids to produce additional analgesia.
f.   They cause opioid-like psychologic side effects.

answer: d

34.   What are characteristics of tricyclic antidepressants when used in treating chronic pain in depressed patients?

a.   They typically improve pain before altering mood.
b.   Opioid requirements decrease.
c.   One of their main benefits is helping restore a normal sleep-wake schedule.
d.   They are particularly helpful in diabetic neuropathy.
e.   Their analgesic effects relate to their antidepressant effects.

answer: a, c, d

35.   Which of the following are advantages of patient-controlled analgesia (PCA) over analgesia administered on a "by the clock" or an "as needed" basis?

a.   Lower cost
b.   Steady levels of analgesia that avoid under- and overtreatment
c.   Better sleep schedules
d.   Earlier hospital discharge

answer: b, c, d. Despite the expense of training, close monitoring, and equipment, PCA has been a widely accepted and successful innovation in the management of postoperative and chronic malignant pain. It has reduced potential friction between patients, families, physicians, and nurses. However, unless patients have the mental and physical capacity to manipulate the system, PCA will be ineffective. As with conventional administration, PCA opioid doses for patients with pulmonary disease should be assessed carefully.

36.   Where do peripheral nerves carrying pain sensation synapse with ascending spinal cord tracts?

a.   Dorsal columns
b.   Substantia gelatinosa
c.   Lateral spinothalamic tract
d.   Thalamus

answer: b. PNS fibers synapse in the substantia gelatinosa with the lateral spinothalamic tract, which crosses and ascends to synapse in the thalamus.

37.   Which two of the following painful conditions are considered examples of *deafferentation* pain?

a.   Brachial plexus avulsion
b.   Insect stings
c.   Postherpetic neuralgia
d.   Carcinoma metastatic to bones
e.   Thalamic infarction

answer: a, e. When the brain is deprived of normal sensory input, pain is said to result from *deafferentation*. When nerves are directly injured, such as in postherpetic neuralgia, the pain is called *neuropathic*.

38.   A 40-year-old man is dragged by his arm when a passing automobile catches his sleeve. The shoulder is dislocated. After it seems to heal, the arm develops an intense burning sensation that increases on movement or touching. The skin of the hand becomes smooth and dry. He cannot cut his fingernails because the pain is too intense. Which of the following three statements are true concerning his condition?

a.   The disorder is mediated at least in part by the sympathetic nervous system.
b.   The skin changes are an integral part of the condition.
c.   TENS will be effective in most such cases.
d.   Sympathetic blockage will provide temporary relief in most cases.
e.   Shoulder dislocations are painful injuries, but they do not cause nerve injury.

answer: a, b, d. He has developed reflex sympathetic dystrophy (RSD), which probably stems from autonomic nervous system as well as peripheral nerve injury. Shoulder dislocations are often part of traction injuries and often damage the brachial plexus. Aside from temporary relief from sympathetic blockade, treatment is notoriously ineffective.

15 Multiple Sclerosis Episodes

demyeliniz at
r. OPTie N.
4. brain
r. spinal cord

Multiple sclerosis (MS) is the most common disabling neurologic illness of North American and European young adults. With an onset of subtle, evanescent disturbances, MS may initially be misdiagnosed as a psychogenic disorder. When MS reaches its defining characteristic of *multiple episodes of multiple neurologic deficits*, physical disabilities are complicated by various neuropsychologic factors. Despite new tests, the diagnosis of MS and its complications rests on clinical grounds.

ETIOLOGY

An illness of unknown etiology, MS occurs when 1-mm to 3-cm patches of "white matter," the myelin sheaths of central nervous system (CNS) axons, become episodically inflamed, then sclerotic, and eventually stripped of myelin. Demyelinated patches, called *plaques*, are scattered or disseminated throughout the optic nerves, brain, and spinal cord. (MS is consequently called "disseminated sclerosis" in the United Kingdom.) Even though the bodies and axons of the nerves are relatively spared, demyelination impairs impulse transmission and causes neurologic deficits. These deficits seem to resolve as the inflammation subsides; however, with repeated attacks more plaques develop and neurologic deficits accumulate.

The mean age of onset is 33 years. Virtually all cases develop between 15 and 50 years. Some patients suffer their first or subsequent MS attacks after infection, childbirth, head trauma, intervertebral disk surgery, electrical injury, or psychologic stress, but none of these events has been proven to be a cause.

Multiple sclerosis occurs 1.5 times more frequently in women than in men and about 10 times more frequently in close relatives of MS patients than in the general population. Spouses are not especially vulnerable. Although genetic factors are important, they cannot be the entire explanation: Only about 30 per cent of monozygotic twins are concordant for MS, and each twin in the pairs has a different phenotype. In other words, if MS were caused entirely by a genetic abnormality, when one monozygotic twin developed MS, all the other twins would develop the illness (to give 100 per cent concordance) and these twin pairs would have the same clinical manifestations (so that the phenotypes would be similar).

Epidemiologic studies have also suggested an infectious etiology. The incidence of MS is greatest in patients who have lived, at least through age 15, in cool northern latitudes (above the 37th parallel) in the United States and Europe. Likewise, the incidence in Australia is greater in the cool, southernmost region. Specifically, the incidence of MS is higher in Boston than New Orleans; is extremely low in Central Africa and Latin America; and is higher in Northern Europeans who emigrated as adults to Israel than in those who emigrated as children. Several studies have suggested that small indoor dogs may transmit an infectious agent. Also, as in several other chronic debilitating neurologic illnesses, the CSF of MS patients often has a high measles antibody titer and an increased rate of IgG synthesis.

Immunologic abnormalities are clearly present, but their role is unclear. MS patients have an increased frequency of certain HLA and other histocompatibility groups, and decreased suppressor T lymphocytes.

CLINICAL MANIFESTATIONS

The initial manifestations of MS may range from a single trivial impairment lasting several days to a group of debilitating deficits that remains for several weeks and do not fully recede. Moreover, in the initial and subsequent episodes, the areas of CNS involvement, severity of deficits, number of attacks, and the timing are highly variable. On the average, 2 to 3 years elapse before a recurrence (exacerbation) develops. In exacerbations, the initial symptoms, accompanied by additional ones, generally recur. Most MS patients have a course characterized by exacerbations, partial remissions, and accumulated impairments; however, about 10 per cent of patients have a steady deterioration from the outset. Regardless of their initial course, many reach a debilitated state in which they are partially or fully blind, confined to a wheelchair, unable to speak distinctly, and overwhelmed by unwarranted bouts of emotion. On the other hand, about one third of MS patients seem to have no functional disability 10 years after the diagnosis.

Although many different symptoms may occur during the illness, the most frequent ones result from plaques in the white matter tracts of the spinal cord, brainstem, and optic nerves. When the voluminous cerebral white matter has accumulated extensive plaques, late in the course, MS can produce significant mental impairment. Since the cerebral cortical "gray matter," which has no myelin, is relatively spared, MS patients rarely develop signs of cerebral cortical dysfunction, such as seizures or aphasia. Likewise, since the basal ganglia are also devoid of myelin, involuntary movement disorders (see Chapter 18) are virtually never manifestations of MS.

In classic descriptions, the cardinal manifestations of MS—*Charcot's triad*—were dysarthria, nystagmus, and tremor. Currently, the three most troublesome symptoms, "the 3 I's," are incontinence, impotence, and impairment of gait. These symptoms are referable to inflammation of the spinal cord (*myelitis*), which is often the primary or exclusive site of MS. Neurologists apply the term "clinically definite" to patients with two episodes and signs of two lesions, and "clinically probable" to those with one episode or signs of one lesion.

The most frequently encountered symptoms of MS are paresis, sensory disturbances, ataxia, ocular impairments, and bladder and sexual dysfunction (Fig. 15–1). Almost all MS patients develop paresis, if not at the onset of illness, then soon afterward. They usually have paraparesis with hyperactive DTRs and Babinski signs from spinal cord demyelination (see Fig. 2–17), but rarely hemiparesis from cerebral involvement, as found in cerebrovascular accidents (see Figs. 2–3 and 2–4). A characteristic electrical sensation that ex-

INITIAL AND CUMULATIVE MANIFESTATIONS OF MS

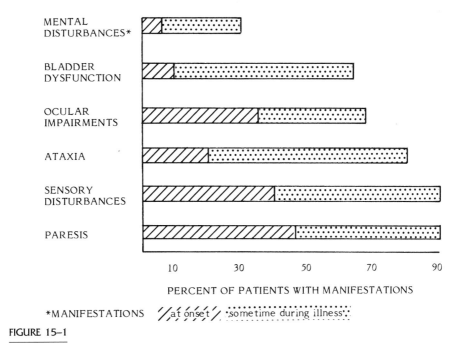

FIGURE 15–1

In this graph of initial and cumulative manifestations of MS, note that mental disturbances are rarely present at the onset.

tends from the neck down the spine when the neck is flexed (*Lhermitte's sign*) frequently indicates spinal cord demyelination. Most importantly, spinal cord demyelination causes spasticity that leads to gait impairment, painful leg spasms, and bladder and sexual disturbances.

The majority of MS patients, including ones with no paresis, describe generalized physical and mental weakness that can reach a state of exhaustion. Their fatigue or "chronic fatigue" has little correlation with their physical impairments and has a problematic relationship to the chronic fatigue syndrome (see Chapter 5).

MS patients regularly develop ataxia and other signs of cerebellar injury. They typically have a prominent broad-based, ataxic gait (see Fig. 2–13); however, when the cerebellar involvement is minimal, patients' only impairment may be in walking heel-to-toe (*tandem gait*). Their ataxia also causes *scanning speech*, which is a variety of dysarthria characterized by irregular cadence and uneven emphasis on words. For example, when asked to repeat a pair of short syllables, such as "ba...ga...ba...ga...," the patient might place unequal stress on different syllables, blur them together, or pause excessively. Other manifestations of MS cerebellar involvement may be intention tremor (see Fig. 2–11), dysdiadochokinesia, and arrhythmic, disconcerting head rocking (*titubation*).

Sensory disturbances are a prominent symptom of MS. Patients often describe hypalgesia or paresthesias, which are sometimes painful, in scattered areas of their limbs or trunk, or below a particular spinal cord level (see Fig. 2–15). Patients may develop sharp facial pains in the distribution of a branch of the trigeminal nerve, which is similar to trigeminal neuralgia. Patients with only sensory disturbances are the ones most liable to be misdiagnosed as harboring a psychogenic condition because sensory complaints often overshadow objective findings and do not conform to commonplace neurologic patterns.

Ocular impairments, which are often early MS manifestations, include impaired visual acuity and disordered ocular motility. Visual acuity impairment results from attacks of *retrobulbar (optic) neuritis*, which is an inflammatory condition of the retrobulbar portion of the optic nerve (see Fig. 12–6). This condition causes a characteristically irregular area of visual loss in one eye, a *scotoma*, that includes the center of vision (*cecocentral scotoma*; Fig. 15–2). Also, the eye is often painful, especially when it is moved, probably because of traction on the inflamed optic nerve. Since the optic disk is unaffected, ophthalmoscopic examination typically reveals no abnormality. This discrepancy between visual loss and normal ophthalmoscopy has given rise to the saying, "The patient sees nothing and the physician sees nothing." As an optic neuritis attack subsides, the pain leaves, and most, if not all, vision returns. However, with repeated attacks, progressive visual loss ensues, and the disk may become atrophic.

Statistics vary on the relationship of optic neuritis and MS. Roughly 25 per cent of MS patients have had overt optic neuritis as their initial symptom, and most had it at some time during their illness. Electrophysiologic studies can show when MS patients have asymptomatic as well as symptomatic optic neuritis. On the other hand, only about 45 per cent of young adults who develop optic neuritis as an isolated condition will later develop MS. Therefore, a single attack of optic neuritis, devoid of other neurologic problems, is not diagnostic of MS.

Multiple sclerosis also causes two ocular movement disturbances: *nystagmus* and the characteristic *internuclear ophthalmoplegia (INO)*, which is also called the *medial longitudinal fasciculus (MLF) syndrome*. Nystagmus results from brainstem or cerebellar MS involvement. Although MS-induced nystagmus is clinically indistinguishable from nystagmus caused by other conditions (see Chapter 12), it frequently occurs in combination with dysarthria and tremor (Charcot's triad).

Internuclear ophthalmoplegia, which causes diplopia on lateral gaze, results when demyelination or other MLF damage interrupts nerve impulse transmis-

FIGURE 15–2

Optic (retrobulbar) neuritis causes impaired vision in a large, irregular area (*scotoma*) in the affected eye (see Fig. 12–6). The optic nerve, which is the only cranial nerve attacked by MS, is susceptible because it has a CNS myelin covering.

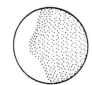

sion to the oculomotor nuclei (Figs. 15–3 and 15–4). Unilateral or bilateral INO, when found in conjunction with other signs of CNS injury, is virtually pathognomonic of MS. Otherwise, an INO may result from systemic lupus erythematosus (SLE or lupus), basilar artery infarctions, botulism, or myasthenia gravis; however, most of these illnesses damage various cranial nerves, as well as the MLF.

Bladder dysfunction, which reflects spinal cord involvement by MS, causes urinary incontinence and is often associated with sexual impairment (see Chapter 16). It results from a combination of paresis, spasticity, and incoordination (*dyssynergia*) of the bladder and sphincter muscles (Fig. 15–5). Patients initially have incontinence during sleep and sexual intercourse. If the disease progresses, they may have intermittent urinary retention and then complete loss of control. Many MS patients need intermittent or continuous catheterization, which burdens them with the risk of infection, as well as esthetic problems.

Sexual impairment, with or without bladder dysfunction, plagues about 85 per cent of MS patients (see Chapter 16). Men often have premature or retrograde ejaculation before erectile dysfunction. With extensive spinal cord damage severe enough to cause paraplegia, men have lowered and abnormal sperm production. Men with erectile dysfunction from MS and other conditions may be helped by injections directly into the penis of papaverine, prostaglandins, and other medications (see Chapter 16).

Women with MS remain fertile. They have no increased incidence of miscarriages, obstetric complications, or fetal malformations. They require cesarean sections for only the usual indications. The incidence of either first MS

MEDIAL LONGITUDINAL
FASCICULUS (MLF)

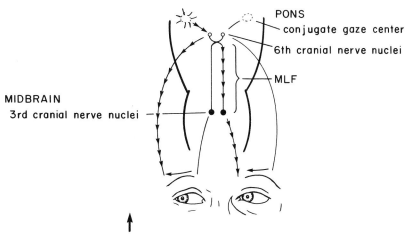

FIGURE 15–3

When looking laterally, the pontine conjugate gaze center stimulates the adjacent abducens (sixth) nerve nucleus and, through the *medial longitudinal fasciculus (MLF)*, the contralateral oculomotor (third) nerve nucleus. Thus, when looking to the right, the right abducens and the left oculomotor nuclei are both stimulated (see Fig. 12–12). The MLF is therefore a crucial link in the complementary innervation of the third and sixth cranial nerve nuclei that is required for lateral, conjugate gaze.

INTERNUCLEAR
OPHTHALMOPLEGIA

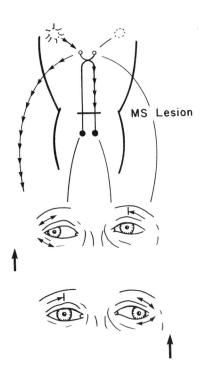

FIGURE 15-4

In *internuclear ophthalmoplegia (INO)*, also called the *MLF syndrome*, interruption of the MLF prevents impulses from reaching the oculomotor (third) nuclei. Since the nuclei themselves are intact, the pupils and eyelids are normal in both eyes. However, when looking to the right, because the oculomotor nuclei are not stimulated, the left eye fails to adduct. The right eye abducts, but nystagmus develops. With bilateral INO, which is characteristic of MS, neither eye adducts and the abducting eye has nystagmus. INO is analogous to the disconnection syndromes that cause aphasia (see Chapter 8) where each center of neurologic activity is normal but the communicating links are severed.

FIGURE 15-5

The urinary outflow of the bladder has two sphincters: An internal sphincter is under the involuntary control of the autonomic nervous system (ANS), and an external sphincter is under voluntary control. Normal urinary bladder emptying (urination) occurs when the detrusor (wall) muscle contracts and *both* sphincter muscles relax. In addition to voluntary action (to relax the external sphincter), urination requires reflex parasympathetic (ANS) activity (to contract the detrusor and relax the internal sphincter). Urinary retention occurs with either anticholinergic medications or excessive sympathetic activity because both inhibit detrusor contraction and internal sphincter muscle relaxation. Retention also occurs with spinal cord injury because the external sphincter is spastic, paretic, and unable to relax (dyssynergia).

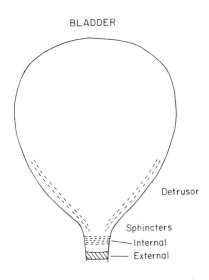

attacks or exacerbations during pregnancy is actually reduced. If they do occur, MS episodes do not affect the pregnancy, and pregnancies do not worsen the long-term course of MS.

On the other hand, during their first 3 postpartum months, mothers who are MS patients are beset with relapses. In addition, the mother passes to her child an increased likelihood of eventually developing the illness.

MENTAL ABERRATIONS

Depression—in the broad sense of the word—is the most common disturbance at the onset of MS. When it does develop, depression can be a psychologic response to the illness, a result of cerebral plaques, or a combination of psychologic and organic factors. In any case, depression is found more frequently in MS patients than in patients with other chronic neurologic and non-neurologic conditions that yield comparable physical impairments. Also, depression is especially frequent during exacerbations, with cerebral involvement, late in the course of the illness, and when cognitive function is impaired. Bipolar affective disorder seems to occur at a higher rate than the general population. The suicide rate of patients in MS clinics is 7.5 times greater than that of a comparably aged group.

In view of the consequences of MS, the apparent elevation of mood in some patients, the so-called euphoria, has been a striking paradox. Certainly, some euphoric patients are protecting themselves psychologically by denial or are masking depression. Others simply are feeling relief as an MS attack subsides. Likewise, after hospitalization, when patients have a remission of symptoms and reduced anxiety, they tend to be overjoyed.

Euphoria, however, is also a result in some patients of advanced cerebral involvement. It is associated with physical deterioration, chronicity of the illness, and subtle, if not overt, intellectual impairment. In particular, the laughing and other superficial aspects of euphoria may be manifestations of pseudobulbar palsy (see Chapter 4). Euphoria may also be induced by treatment with ACTH, prednisone, or other steroid medication (see below, Steroid Psychosis).

Cognitive function may be difficult to assess. Mental status testing is often impeded by slow and inarticulate speech, fatigue, and visual impairments. Large studies of MS patients should be accepted with reservations. They tend to pool MS patients who have had different courses and levels of disease activity. They also tend to pool MS patients with different areas of predominant CNS involvement, even though patients with only spinal cord or optic nerve lesions have a much different profile than those with extensive cerebral lesions. Mild and undiagnosed patients, who would have little or no cognitive impairment, are under-represented.

In the early stages of MS, subtle and nonspecific intellectual changes can be demonstrated using complex neuropsychologic tests, such as the Wechsler Adult Intelligence Scale (WAIS) and the Halstead Category Test. Even the Mini-Mental State Examination (MMSE) may not be sufficiently sensitive.

Overt cognitive impairment often appears late in the course of MS. It is associated with physical impairments, duration of the illness, and certain changes in the brain: enlarged cerebral ventricles, corpus callosum atrophy, periventricular white matter demyelination, total lesion area, and, on positron emission tomography, cerebral hypometabolism. The cognitive as well as physical impairments presumably result from CNS demyelination, rather than from cerebral cortex gray matter degeneration, as in Alzheimer's disease. Although the gray matter is generally spared in MS, it may be undercut, irritated by numerous underlying plaques, or deprived of interconnecting white matter tracts, including the corpus callosum.

The late development of intellectual changes in MS distinguishes it from Alzheimer's disease and CVAs. In Alzheimer's disease, which affects the gray matter exclusively, intellectual impairment occurs first and becomes profound long before the onset of physical impairments. In CVAs, both gray and white matter damage cause simultaneous intellectual and physical impairment. Particularly in multi-infarct (vascular) dementia, intellectual and physical deficits progress together (see Chapter 11).

Although MS mental aberrations occasionally mimic psychosis, the incidence of psychosis in MS patients is remarkably lower than that found in other neurologic illnesses, including Alzheimer's disease, head trauma, and partial complex epilepsy. In MS, psychotic disturbances probably originate partly from intellectual impairment and sensory deprivation. Other contributing factors may be steroid therapy (see below) or systemic infections causing delirium. In general, psychiatrists should initially assume that psychotic behavior and less pronounced mental aberrations in MS patients are organic in origin and are manifestations of cerebral demyelination, medications, or a concomitant physical illness.

LABORATORY TESTS

No particular test is diagnostic of MS. In fact, several tests are required when symptoms are vague, few objective signs are elicited, only a single episode has occurred, or a single CNS area is affected. The currently available tests still produce many false-negative and false-positive results.

Routine cerebrospinal fluid (CSF) analysis during an MS attack will often reveal that the protein concentration is normal (40 mg/100 ml) or only slightly elevated and the gamma globulin portion is elevated (9 per cent or greater), which is a nonspecific reaction. MS is associated more clearly with an increased rate of synthesis of *CSF IgG*; the presence of CSF *oligoclonal bands*, which constitute a discrete IgG protein similar to an antibody; and the presence of CSF *myelin basic protein*, which seems to be a myelin breakdown product. However, these abnormalities may be found in other chronic inflammatory CNS illnesses, such as chronic meningitis, sarcoidosis, postpolio syndrome, neurosyphilis, and Lyme disease. Some of these illnesses thus mimic some laboratory and many clinical features of MS (see below).

Although routine electroencephalograms (EEGs) are not diagnostically helpful, related electrophysiologic testing, *evoked response* or *evoked potential tests,* can reveal characteristic interruptions in the visual, auditory, or sensory pathways. Evoked potential testing is based on repetitive stimulation of these heavily myelinated pathways and detecting the responses with scalp electrodes similar to those used for EEGs. Although individual responses would be so small that they would be lost within the normal electrical cerebral activity and background noise, hundreds of responses are computer-averaged. The averaging cancels out the normal, random electrical activity and displays an otherwise undetectable composite wave pattern. With injury to the pathways, the evoked response is abnormal because of an increased delay (*latency*) between the stimulus and the composite response, as well as distortions in the form of the wave.

Evoked response tests are particularly useful in demonstrating asymptomatic lesions. For example, if a patient has deficits referable only to the spinal cord, but evoked response tests reveal an optic nerve injury, the physician would know that at least two CNS areas were injured and then would be able to consider MS.

Visual evoked responses (VERs), which are designed to reveal visual pathway lesions, are performed by having the patient stare at a rapidly flashing pattern on a television screen and averaging responses detected over the occipital cortex. Abnormalities are found with optic neuritis from MS or any other cause. They are also found with other optic nerve lesions, such as optic nerve gliomas (see Chapter 19) and congenital injuries (see Chapter 13). Since VERs can indicate the site of an interruption in the visual pathway, they are helpful in distinguishing ocular from cortical blindness. When the test is entirely normal, VERs are helpful in identifying psychogenic visual loss (see Chapter 12).

Brainstem auditory evoked responses (BAERs), which measure responses to a series of clicks in each ear, are helpful in indicating MS brainstem involvement. BAERs are also useful in a variety of diagnostic tasks related to hearing: characterizing hearing impairments, diagnosing acoustic neuromas, and evaluating hearing in people unable to cooperate, such as infants and those with autism or psychogenic disturbances.

Somatosensory evoked responses involve the application of various stimuli to the limbs. MS or other spinal cord injury causes abnormal latencies.

Although *computed tomography (CT)* can occasionally demonstrate areas of demyelination, it is not useful in the diagnosis of MS. *Magnetic resonance imaging (MRI)* clearly the superior test, can reveal numerous or widely distributed demyelinated areas indicative of MS plaques (Figs. 15–6 and 20–17). It can detect them in both the cerebral and cerebellar white matter and in structures that are small or encased in bone, such as the optic nerves and spinal cord. It can show plaques that are asymptomatic, as well as symptomatic, thereby indicating that a neurologic disease is disseminated. With gadolinium infusion, the MRI highlights MS plaques. Overall, MRI shows lesions in 90 per cent of patients with unequivocal MS.

MRI findings and the presence of CSF oligoclonal bands and increased CSF IgG are the most reliable laboratory indications of MS. These results permit neurologists, or others who may be inclined, to say that a "clinically definite" or "clinically probable" diagnosis is "laboratory supported."

THERAPY

Systemically administered high-dose ACTH, prednisone, or other steroid medications had been widely used because they were believed, on the basis of scant data, to foreshorten MS attacks and reduce the residual deficits. Treatment of optic neuritis with intravenous methylprednisolone reduces the rate of development of MS over a 2-year period.

Although steroid treatment may lead to mental aberrations, it is rarely complicated by opportunistic infections, such as tuberculosis or cryptococcal meningitis, as happens in lupus or renal transplantation treatment. More potent

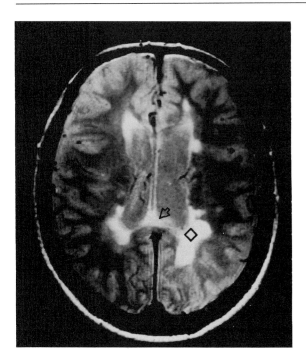

FIGURE 15–6

This MRI scan cuts through the cerebrum of an MS patient. Plaques, identifiable by their increased signal intensity, are multiple, irregular, white, and located in the deeply situated myelin. They are characteristically concentrated in the periventricular region. Of several periventricular plaques, one is marked (*diamond*). Another is located in the posterior limb of the corpus callosum (*arrow*), which is a heavily myelinated, interhemispheric commissure (see Figs. 8–4 and 8–8). However, MRIs often show hyperintense, small, white lesions scattered throughout the brains of entirely healthy people. These "unidentified bright objects" (*UBOs*) are attributable to cerebrovascular vascular disease, infection, and normal variations, but they do not indicate MS.

immunosuppressants, such as cyclosporin, have been advocated; however, their benefit is slight, and they place patients at risk of serious adverse effects.

In a different approach, interferon has been administered in an attempt to modify the immunologic system. Alternate-day injections of interferon beta–1b (Betaseron) have been found to reduce the number, duration, and severity of MS attacks. Moreover, the more benign course is paralleled by fewer plaques on MRI—an objective measure of interferon's benefit. If interferon or similar treatment unequivocally improves the course of MS, then making a definite diagnosis as early as possible will be important.

Physical therapy helps preserve muscle tone, prevent decubitus ulcers, and provide maximum mobility. Depending on the nature of a patient's bladder dysfunction, medication alone, such as imipramine (Tofranil), might be sufficient; however, self-catheterization or sphincter bypass may be necessary. Spasticity, another common problem, usually requires baclofen, diazepam, or muscle relaxants.

Antidepressant medications are useful in many aspects of MS patient care, in addition to their ability to elevate mood. They may improve sleep and reduce some of the pain associated with immobility or spasticity; however, antidepressants with anticholinergic effects must be used cautiously because they may precipitate urinary retention.

STEROID PSYCHOSIS

A wide variety and degree of intellectual, emotional, and behavioral aberrations—loosely termed "steroid psychosis"—can result from treatment of MS with ACTH, prednisone, or other steroid medications. Steroid psychosis also occurs during steroid treatment of various systemic inflammatory conditions, such as lupus, organ transplant rejection, and acute asthma. It is also an occasional manifestation of conditions in which steroids are overproduced, such as Cushing's syndrome. Sometimes athletes who surreptitiously use steroids for energy and body-building develop agitation or personality changes that might fall into the category of steroid psychosis.

When steroid medications are given in high dosage they cause euphoria, ravenous appetite, and insomnia. They also often produce a fine, rapid tremor that mimics anxiety-induced and essential tremors (see Chapter 18). In some cases, which supposedly cannot be predicted by the presence or absence of a premorbid psychiatric disturbance, steroids produce agitation, hallucinations, and delusions. Although rare patients have been described as being depressed, the typical clinical picture is increased physical and mental activity.

Steroid psychosis usually begins 1 to 4 days after starting high-dose steroid treatment. Its incidence increases from 4 per cent of patients receiving less than 40 mg prednisone daily to 20 per cent of patients receiving more than 80 mg daily. When steroid treatment is discontinued, the symptoms recede.

Psychosis in a patient with a systemic inflammatory disease on high-dose steroids poses a clinical dilemma. In illnesses where the brain may be directly involved, such as lupus, abruptly decreasing the steroids might worsen the underlying disease's cerebral involvement. In addition, at a time when the body is under stress and consequently requires increased steroids, stopping them may precipitate adrenal insufficiency. As a general rule, in patients with a systemic inflammatory disease, until the evaluation is completed, steroids should be maintained or increased. On the other hand, in patients with MS, because the benefit of steroids is marginal and they are certainly not life saving, they should be discontinued as soon as possible, being careful not to precipitate adrenal insufficiency. In the interim, in both cases, psychotic disturbances should be treated with tranquilizers or, according to a few reports, lithium. Tricyclic antidepressants may exacerbate steroid-induced mental aberrations.

CONDITIONS THAT MIMIC MS

Other physically incapacitating conditions frequently develop in young people. Several of them can reasonably be confused with MS, at least on a superficial level, because of its protean clinical manifestations.

Guillain-Barré Syndrome

Even though it is a demyelinating illness of the peripheral nervous system (PNS), Guillain-Barré syndrome may resemble MS because it generally strikes young and middle-aged adults and causes paraparesis or quadriparesis (see Chapter 5). However, Guillain-Barré syndrome is monophasic and is characterized by symmetric, flaccid, and areflexia paresis. Moreover, it does not cause brainstem or cerebral dysfunction, such as optic neuritis, INO, or mental aberrations.

The Leukodystrophies

Leukodystrophy (i.e., "white matter degeneration") is the hallmark of a group of genetically transmitted illnesses, the leukodystrophies, that destroy CNS myelin alone or in combination with PNS myelin. Most of these illnesses cause widespread, progressively severe neurologic deficits in infants and children. However, *adrenoleukodystrophy* and *metachromatic leukodystrophy (MLD)* may appear in teenagers or young adults (see Chapter 5). As in MS, the leukodystrophies cause optic, cerebellar, and spinal cord myelin degeneration that leads to blindness, ataxia, and spastic paraparesis or quadriparesis, but the deterioration is slow and unremitting. Also unlike MS, one of the initial symptoms is mental disturbances. These disturbances typically begin with personality changes or other relatively benign aberrations and progress to psychosis and dementia.

A group of rare and nongenetic, but interesting, conditions commonly cause CNS demyelination and the accompanying clinical deficits. *Postinfectious* or *postimmunization encephalomyelitis*, which is rarely and unpredictably caused by vaccination, is a single episode of cerebral and spinal cord injury that is often devastating and permanent. (Postimmunization encephalomyelitis poses a major liability risk for pharmaceutical firms.) *Progressive multifocal leukoencephalopathy (PML)* is a relatively late complication of several illnesses that cause immunologic impairment (including AIDS, see below). Like MS, PML leads to patchy areas of demyelination throughout the CNS. Another example of a non-MS CNS demyelination disease is the infamous *Marchiafava-Bignami syndrome* (see Chapters 7 and 8). This condition, probably induced by excessive, long-term consumption of Italian red wine, consists of degeneration of the heavily myelinated corpus callosum.

Brain Tumors

Brainstem astrocytomas, which occur in children as well as young adults, mimic MS because they invade the corticospinal, cerebellar, and sensory tracts and also the MLF. Cerebral astrocytomas, which occur in young adults and older individuals, cause hemiparesis, but unlike MS they also produce headaches and seizures (see Chapter 19). In general, neoplasms produce steadily worsening symptoms and signs referable to a single CNS area and can be diagnosed with CT or MRI scans.

CNS Infections

Although acquired immune deficiency syndrome (AIDS) usually begins with signs of systemic illness, it may occasionally become apparent through multiple neurologic deficits. Neurologic deficits may be from *human immunodeficiency virus (HIV) encephalitis* or myelitis. As an AIDS complication, they may result from lymphoma, toxoplasmosis, or PML (see Chapter 7). An infection with the related retrovirus HTLV−1, which is endemic in the Caribbean basin, causes a myelitis that can be confused with spinal MS cord involvement. Similarly, Lyme disease may first affect the brain and mimic MS (see Chapter 7).

Inflammatory Diseases

Like MS, lupus and other vascular inflammatory diseases may produce multiple CNS abnormalities in young adults. Although some series consider common symptoms, such as headache or neurosis, as being its first manifestation, lupus rarely causes clear-cut physical neurologic symptoms at its onset. However, approximately 75 per cent of lupus patients eventually develop neurologic complications. The most notorious pattern is a combination of seizures and infarctions, including ones that cause mental aberrations, chorea, and the MLF syndrome—the "three S's: seizures, strokes, and psychosis." These neurologic complications have been attributed to an arteritis produced by immune complexes, but many cases are obviously caused by cardiac valvular disease and a tendency for thrombosis.

Lupus can also cause neuropathy, mononeuropathy multiplex, and other PNS abnormalities. Alternatively, many lupus patients with stupor or coma suffer primarily from infections, rather than lupus cerebritis. In addition, neurologic problems result from the hypertension, uremia, and treatment with immunosuppressant medications. Sjogren's syndrome and, to a lesser extent, sarcoidosis may cause a variety of cognitive changes, other cerebral impairments, facial nerve injury, and peripheral nerve injuries; however, these illnesses can almost always be diagnosed by their extracranial involvement.

Spinal Cord Diseases

In patients with only paraparesis, alternative disorders include combined system disease (B_{12} deficiency), cervical spine degenerative disease, AIDS and HTLV−1 infection, and spinal meningiomas. Thus, neurologists often order an MRI or myelogram, serum B_{12} level determination, and, when indicated, serologic studies.

Psychogenic Disturbances

Despite the many similar neurologic conditions, MS is probably most commonly confused with psychogenic disorders (see Chapter 3). Several symptoms are common to MS and psychogenic disorders: clumsiness, sexual impairments, nonspecific sensory losses, fatigue, and occasionally several weeks of paraparesis or blindness. Indeed, some young paraplegic patients who improved after a course of psychoanalysis may actually have had resolution of an episode of MS. In situations where the diagnosis is unclear on clinical grounds, laboratory tests are indicated. When the diagnosis of MS or other neurologic illness remains uncertain, neurologists tend to use the term "MS suspect."

REFERENCES

Abramowicz M (ed): Interferon beta-1B for multiple sclerosis. Med Lett *35*: 61−62, 1993

Beck RB, Cleary PA, Anderson MM, et al: A randomized, controlled trial of corticosteroids in the treatment of acute optic neuritis. N Engl J Med *326*: 581−588, 1992

Birk K, Ford C, Smeltzer S, et al: The clinical course of multiple sclerosis during pregnancy and the puerperium. Arch Neurol *47*: 738−742, 1990

Franklin GM, Nelson LM, Filley CM, at al: Cognitive loss in multiple sclerosis. Arch Neurol *46*: 166−167, 1989

Futrell N, Schultz LR, Millikan C: Central nervous system disease in patients with systemic lupus erythematosus. Neurology *42*: 1649−1657, 1992

Goldstein PJ, Stern HJ (eds): Neurological Disorders of Pregnancy, 2nd rev. ed. Mt. Kisco, NY, Futura Publishing, 1992

Hall RCW, Popkin MK, Stickney SK, et al: Presentation of the steroid psychoses. J Nerv Ment Dis *167*: 229–23, 1979

Hietaharju A, Yli-Kerttula U, Hakkinen V: Nervous system manifestations in Sjogren's syndrome. Acta Neurol Scand *81*: 144–152, 1990

Honer WG, Hurwitz T, Li DKB, et al: Temporal lobe involvement in multiple sclerosis patients with psychiatric disorders. Arch Neurol *44*: 187–190, 1987

Joffe RT, Lippert GP, Gray TA, et al: Mood disorder and multiple sclerosis. Arch Neurol *44*: 376–378, 1987

Kurtzke JF, Hyllested K: Multiple sclerosis in the Faröe Islands. Neurology *36*: 307–328, 1986

Kurtzke JF, Beebe GW, Norman JE: Epidemiology of multiple sclerosis in US veterans: III. Migration and the risk of MS. Neurology *35*: 672–678, 1985

Lee KH, Hashimoto SA, Hooge JP, et al: Magnetic resonance imaging of the head in the diagnosis of multiple sclerosis. Neurology *41*: 657–660, 1991

McFarland HF: Editorial: Twins studies and multiple sclerosis. Ann Neurol *32*: 722–723, 1992

Menkes JH: The leukodystrophies. N Engl J Med *322*: 54–55, 1990

Minden SL, Schiffler RB: Affective disorders in multiple sclerosis. Arch Neurol *47*: 98–104, 1990

Mumford CJ, Wood NW, Kellar-Wood H, et al: The British Isles survey of multiple sclerosis in twins. Neurology *44*: 11–15, 1994

Omdal R, Mellgren SI, Husby G: Clinical neuropsychiatric and neuromuscular manifestations in systemic lupus erythematosus. Scand J Rheumatol *17*: 113–117, 1988

Poser CM, Roman GC, Vernant JC: Multiple sclerosis or HTLV–1 myelitis? Neurology *40*: 1020–1022, 1990

Rao SM, Leo GJ, Bernardin L, et al: Cognitive dysfunction in multiple sclerosis. Neurology *41*: 685–691, 1991

Sadovnick AD, Eisen K, Ebers GC, et al: Cause of death in patients attending multiple sclerosis clinics. Neurology *41*: 1193–1196, 1991.

Scheinberg LC, Holland NJ (eds): Multiple Sclerosis: A Guide for Patients and Their Families, 2nd ed. New York, Raven Press, 1987

Schwankhaus JD, Katz DA, Eldridge R, et al: Clinical and pathologic features of an autosomal dominant, adult-onset leukodystrophy simulating chronic progressive multiple sclerosis. Arch Neurol *51*: 757–766, 1994

Scott TF: Neurosarcoidosis: Progress and clinical aspects. Neurology *43*: 8–12, 1993

Shapiro EG, Lockman LA, Knopman D, et al: Characteristics of the dementia in late-onset metachromatic leukodystrophy. Neurology *44*: 662–665, 1994

Silberg DH: Multiple sclerosis: Approaches to management. Ann Neurol 36 (suppl), 1994

Steinman L: Autoimmune disease. Sci Am 107–114, (Sept) 1993

Stenager EN, Stenager E: Suicide and patients with neurologic diseases. Arch Neurol *49*: 1296–1303, 1992

Swirsky-Sacchetti T, Mitchell DR, Seward J, et al: Neuropsychological and structural brain lesions in multiple sclerosis. Neurology *42*: 1291–1295, 1992

The IFNB Multiple Sclerosis Study Group: Interferon beta–1b is effective in relapsing-remitting multiple sclerosis. Neurology *43*: 655–661, 1993

van den Burg W, van Zomeren AH, Minderhoud JM, et al: Cognitive impairment in patients with multiple sclerosis and mild physical disability. Arch Neurol *44*: 494–501, 1987

QUESTIONS and ANSWERS: CHAPTER 15

1–5. Over four days, a 25-year-old policeman developed paraparesis. Then his left eye became painful and blind. On examination, his left pupil reacts slowly to light, his legs have hyperactive deep tendon reflexes (DTRs), and bilateral Babinski signs accompany the paraparesis.

1. Which of the following disorders are likely causes of his neurologic deficits?

a. Spinal cord tumor
b. Psychogenic distrubances
c. MS
d. Postvaccination or postinfectious encephalomyelitis
e. Wilson's disease

> **answer:** c and d. The policeman might have either MS affecting the optic nerve and spinal cord or a demyelinating inflammatory reaction to an infection or vaccination, especially one for smallpox or rabies. In contrast, spinal cord tumors would create spastic paraparesis, but of course not visual impairment. Psychogenic disturbances might lead to visual and motor complaints; however, people

with them cannot mimic abnormal pupil reactions, DTR abnormalities, or Babinski signs. Wilson's disease produces movement disorders and changes in mental status.

2. Which regions of the CNS are most likely to be involved?

a. Right occipital lobe and thoracic spinal cord
b. Thoracic spinal cord and left optic nerve
c. Sacral spinal cord and left optic nerve

> ***answer:*** b. The patient has retrobulbar neuritis and thoracic myelitis (spinal cord inflammation).

3. After three weeks, he becomes ambulatory and finds that his vision is almost normal. One year later, however, he develops dysarthria, ataxia, nystagmus, and tremor of the arms. Where is the new lesion?

a. Cerebrum
b. Cerebellum
c. Brainstem
d. Spinal cord

> ***answer:*** b, c

4. Although a diagnosis cannot be made with complete assurance, this patient's illness is typical of a certain disorder. What is it?

> ***answer:*** MS

5. After 6 months, that episode subsides completely. Three years later, however, he develops paraparesis, urinary and fecal incontinence, and complete loss of sensation below the umbilicus. He also develops intention tremor, scanning speech, and nystagmus. What diagnostic procedure is indicated?

a. CT of the head
b. Visual evoked responses
c. Myelography
d. MRI of the head
e. CSF analysis

> ***answer:*** b, d, e. Neurologic deficits have recurred in the cerebellum, spinal cord, and possibly the brainstem. In one of the previous attacks, the optic nerve was involved. Since CNS neurologic deficits have appeared at least twice and in at least two locations, the illness is "disseminated in time and place." MS can now be diagnosed as "clinically definite."
>
> The clinical diagnosis can be "supported" by various laboratory tests. Visual evoked and brainstem evoked responses are highly credible. MRI scans of the brain and spinal cord should reveal plaques and exclude other structural lesions, such as tumors. CSF analysis for oligoclonal bands and IgG concentration can also be used to support a clinical diagnosis. However, CT of the head and spinal cord, even with infusion of contrast material, is often too insensitive to detect plaques, but it can exclude most tumors. Myelography is suitable only for structural lesions of the spinal canal, such as herniated disks and spinal meningiomas.

6. Which of the following substances is associated with optic neuritis?

a. Tobacco
b. Oral contraceptives
c. Ethyl alcohol
d. Methyl alcohol
e. Penicillin
f. Heroin

> ***answer:*** a, c, d

7. Which of these conditions is associated with optic neuritis?

a. Rubella
b. Gonorrhea
c. MS
d. Combined system disease
e. Sarcoidosis
f. Vasculitis
g. Syphilis

> ***answer:*** c, d, e, f, g. In other words, MS is not the only cause of optic neuritis.

8. Which of the following conditions may lead to internuclear ophthalmoplegia?

a. MS
b. Subdural hematoma
c. Hysteria
d. Lupus erythematosus
e. Pontine gliomas
f. Brainstem infarctions

   answer: a, d, e, f. Several possible causes are presented to warn clinicians that these neurologic signs are not peculiar to MS.

9–12. A 60-year-old man has difficulty walking and lower back pains that radiate to the trunk and legs. He walks with a broad-based gait, but he has no dysmetria or intention tremor. Although strength in his legs is normal, his deep tendon reflexes are absent. He has lost position sense (but not pain or touch sense) in the feet. He has small pupils that are unreactive to light.

9. What is the origin of the gait disturbance?

a. Cerebellar damage
b. Spinal cord compression
c. MS
d. Dysfunction of tracts of the spinal cord

   answer: d. The gait disturbance is entirely explainable by loss of proprioception in his legs. Neurologists might say that he has a "sensory ataxia." Loss of reflexes and pupillary abnormalities indicate that the disease is not psychogenic.

10. Although his pupils were small and unreactive to light, they constricted when he looked at a closely held object. What is the pupillary disturbance called?

   answer: He has pupils with lack of light reaction and preserved accommodation—Argyll-Robertson pupils.

11. He had dysfunction of two parts of the nervous system, but why can he not be diagnosed as having MS?

   answer: He could not be diagnosed as having MS mostly because he has had only one episode of the illness. In addition, the pupil abnormality is not generally accepted as a sign of MS, and he is much older than average for the onset of the illness. The most likely diagnosis is tabes dorsalis from syphilis.

12. What laboratory test would be best in confirming a diagnosis of CNS syphilis?

   answer: Keeping in mind that many serum and CSF test results are false negative, the most reliable test for confirming CNS syphilis is a positive CSF VDRL.

13–17. A 32-year-old man reported that 2 years before his current admission he had a 10-day episode of blindness and right hemiparesis. He underwent a CT scan of the head, but no diagnosis was made. He is currently admitted to the neurology service for paraparesis. Although he cannot perceive pain below the waist, he can distinguish warm from cold and has vibration and position sensation. He does not have incontinence. Deep tendon, plantar, anal, and cremasteric reflexes are normal.

13. If the patient's paraparesis is from MS, which of the following signs would usually be present?

a. Urinary incontinence
b. Erectile dysfunction
c. Brisk DTRs
d. Brisk anal and cremasteric reflexes
e. Babinski signs

   answer: a, b, c, e. MS usually does not cause a hemiparesis. When MS causes myelitis, it leads to signs upper motor neuron injury: brisk or hyperactive DTRs, Babinski signs, and a loss of superficial reflexes, such as the anal and cremasteric reflexes. When MS patients have paraparesis, they usually have urinary incontinence and erectile dysfunction.

14. In the second episode, what is indicated by his preservation of temperature sensation, despite the loss of pain perception?

a. Lateral spinothalamic tract impairment
b. Posterior column impairment
c. A peripheral neuropathy
d. None of the above

answer: d. Pain and temperature sensation both travel in the spinothalamic tract. Although the sensory loss in MS may be inconsistent, this man's discrepancy defies the laws of neurology.

15. In MS, blindness is usually the result of retrobulbar or optic neuritis that often leads to optic atrophy. In this situation, what are the pupillary reactions?

a. The pupils are normally reactive to light.
b. The light reflex is impaired.

answer: b. With any optic nerve injury that cause blindness, the pupils are less reactive to light: Often they are completely unreactive. Moreover, in acute optic neuritis, patients have pain when they move their eyes.

16. With spinal cord injuries, how are the cremasteric and anal reflexes altered?

answer: Cremasteric and anal reflexes, both superficial reflexes, are suppressed by both central and peripheral nervous system injuries. Their loss cannot determine the site of neurologic damage, but it indicates an organic cause of erectile dysfunction.

17. What is the origin of the patient's multiple symptoms that have occurred multiple times?

answer: Few illnesses cause recurring symptoms and signs. This patient does not have signs of MS. A normal CT scan in a patient suspected of having MS is inconsequential. (Only CT scans performed after a several hour delay following infusion of a double dose of contrast agent in patients suspected of having cerebral involvement are credible.) An MRI is superior. Since the diagnosis is not established and it could be a psychogenic disorder, further testing is indicated.

18–24. Match the ocular movement disorder (18–24) with the most likely cause (a-g).

a. Wernicke's encephalopathy
b. Labyrinthitis
c. Psychogenic disorders
d. Myasthenia gravis
e. MS
f. Midbrain infarction
g. None of the above

18. Pupillary dilation, ptosis, and paresis of adduction

answer: f

19. Bilateral ptosis

answer: d

20. Bilateral horizontal nystagmus

answer: a, b, e

21. Bilateral horizontal nystagmus, unilateral paresis of abduction, and areflexic DTRs

answer: a

22. Nystagmus in abducting eye and paresis of adduction of the other eye

answer: e (MLF syndrome)

23. Ptosis bilaterally, paresis of adduction of one eye, and normal pupils

answer: d

24. Nystagmus in adducting eye and paresis of abduction of the other eye

answer: g

25–28. Match the laboratory results (25–28) with the conditions (a-f).

a. MS in its chronic phase
b. MS in its acute phase
c. Psychogenic disorders

d. Generalized myasthenia gravis
e. Fungal meningitis
f. Myasthenia with underlying thymoma

25. Anti-ACh receptor antibodies

answer: d, f

26. CSF oligoclonal bands

answer: a, b, and e

27. CSF myelin basic protein

answer: b and e

28. Anti-striated muscle antibodies

answer: f

29. Of the natives of the following cities, who would have the highest and the lowest MS incidence?

a. New Orleans
b. Boston
c. Philadelphia

answer: Highest-Boston; lowest-New Orleans

30. Which of the following people have the highest and lowest incidence of MS?

a. Native Israelis (Sabras)
b. European immigrants to Israel
c. Black Africans

answer: Highest-European immigrants; lowest-Black Africans

31. In which situations do visual evoked responses (VERs) show prolonged latencies or otherwise abnormal patterns?

a. Asymptomatic optic neuritis
b. Retrobulbar neuritis
c. Most patients with long standing MS

d. Patients with psychogenic blindness
e. Optic nerve gliomas

answer: a, b, c, e

32. In MS patients, with which finding(s) is urinary incontinence associated?

a. Leg spasticity
b. Ataxia
c. Spasticity of the external sphincter of the bladder
d. Sexual impairment
e. Internuclear ophthalmoplegia (MLF syndrome)

answer: a, c, d. Urinary incontinence, sexual impairment, and spastic paraparesis all result from MS-induced myelitis.

33. Which symptoms typically develop only late or not at all in the course of MS?

a. Pseudobulbar palsy
b. Internuclear ophthalmoplegia
c. Optic neuritis
d. Bladder dysfunction

e. Neurologic-induced psychotic behavior
f. Depression
g. Sexual dysfunction
h. Dementia

answer: a, e, h

34. Which of the following conditions often leads to multiple CNS lesions in young adults?

a. Lupus
b. AIDS
c. Myasthenia gravis
d. Bacterial endocarditis
e. Postvaccination demyelination (encephalomyelitis)

   answer: a, b, d, e

35. Which of the following conditions may lead to the appearance of euphoria in MS patients?

a. Pseudobulbar palsy
b. Medications
c. Cerebellar cortex demyelination
d. Cerebral demyelination
e. Depression
f. Remission of an acute attack
g. Partial complex seizures
h. Optic nerve demyelination

   answer: a, b, d, e, f

36. Although the geographic studies suggest that an environmental factor causes MS, they may actually reflect susceptibility in certain genetic pools (races). Which one of the following types of studies suggests a genetic predilection?

a. VER
b. HLA
c. Israeli immigrant
d. Spousal

   answer: b. The Israeli studies indicated that geography was a greater risk factor than gene pool. The failure of spouses to contract MS indicated that adults were not infective.

37. Which of the following cells produce CNS myelin?

a. Glia cells
b. Neurons
c. Schwann cells
d. Oligodendroglia
e. Lymphocytes

   answer: d. Oligodendroglia produce CNS myelin. Schwann cells produce peripheral nervous system myelin. Both varieties of myelin act primarily as insulators of electrochemical nerve transmission. Certain illnesses usually attack one or the other variety of myelin.

38. In a patient who suddenly developed paraparesis, urinary incontinence, and a T10 sensory level, which test is the best for detecting a CNS lesion in addition to the obvious one in the spinal cord?

a. CSF oligoclonal bands
b. CSF myelin basic protein
c. EEG
d. CT of the head
e. VERs

   answer: e. CSF oligoclonal bands and myelin basic protein might be present because of spinal cord involvement. EEGs and CTs are too insensitive.

39. Of the following, which two tests are the most reliable confirmation of the clinical diagnosis of MS?

a. MRI of the head
b. VERs
c. CSF studies for oligoclonal bands
d. CSF studies for myelin basic protein
e. CT of the head

   answer: a and c. The combination of an MRI showing plaques and the detection of oligoclonal bands in the CSF is generally accepted as the most reliable test. VERs, although often used, may be abnormal because many non-neurologic illnesses can cause abnormalities. VER studies add support to a diagnosis of MS only in individual cases.

40. Which one of the following descriptions best characterize the MRI changes of MS?

a. Multiple, white areas scattered in the cerebrum
b. Conversion of the cerebral hemisphere white matter to gray
c. Loss of the myelin signal throughout the corpus callosum
d. Periventricular, high-intensity abnormalities

> ***answer:*** d. MS is characterized by relatively large patches (plaques) in the cerebellar and cerebral periventricular white matter, including the corpus callosum. Plaques can even be visualized in the optic nerves and spinal cord. Scattered, small white matter hyperintense lesions—unidentified bright objects (UBOs)—are a nonspecific finding.

41. A 30-year-old man is brought to the Emergency Room because he is acutely confused and agitated. No additional history is available. He has nystagmus and a broad-based, unsteady gait. He has no Babinski signs. The general medical evaluation, routine blood tests, and a CT scan of his head are all normal. Of the following, which should be the next step?

a. Transfer the man to a tertiary care facility for an MRI.
b. Administer steroids.
c. Since no disease is diagnosable, do not do anything.
d. Draw blood for toxicology studies and administer thiamine.

> ***answer:*** d. Even though he has nystagmus and gait ataxia, this man probably does not have MS. MS does not cause acute confusion and agitation. Also, when MS does occur, it almost always causes Babinski signs. Instead, he has signs of Wernicke's encephalopathy. That diagnosis would be supported by a history of alcohol intoxication and a sixth nerve palsy; however, more cases are incomplete than are classic. Since irreparable damage may occur if Wernicke's encephalopathy remains untreated and the treatment is benign, neurologists administer thiamine to individuals who have any inkling of the condition. They are fond of the adage, "We give thiamine to all patients with nystagmus. We even give it to visitors."

42. During which obstetric period is MS most likely to become exacerbated?

a. First trimester
b. Second trimester
c. Third trimester
d. First 3 postpartum months

> ***answer:*** d. The first 3 postpartum months are associated with MS exacerbations. The pregnancy is associated with some protection.

43. What is the effect of one or more pregnancies on the course of a woman's MS?

a. Her functional status deteriorates with each succeeding pregnancy.
b. Her functional status is better with each succeeding pregnancy.
c. There is little or no effect.

> ***answer:*** c. Contrary to previous thinking, pregnancy and delivery have little effect on the mother's MS.

44. Which other statement regarding pregnancy and MS is true?

a. MS causes a high rate of spontaneous abortions.
b. Obstetric complications are frequent.
c. Fetal malformations are common.
d. Cesarean sections are indicated in most deliveries.
e. Offspring have a greater risk than the general population of developing MS.

> ***answer:*** e. Children of MS patients have an increased incidence of the illness.

45. Which MS features are associated with cognitive impairment?

a. Physical impairments
b. Duration of the illness
c. Enlarged cerebral ventricles
d. Corpus callosum atrophy
e. Periventricular demyelination
f. Total lesion area
g. Cerebral hypometabolism

> ***answer:*** All

46. If MS resulted from an abnormal gene and 50 MS patients each had a monozygotic twin, how many people in total would have MS?

a. 25
b. 50
c. 75

d. 100
e. 200

answer: d. If the illness were genetically determined, both sibs of each of the twin pairs would be affected. In other words, with 100 per cent concordance, the 50 patients and their sibs would all have MS.

47. What is the approximate actual concordance rate of MS among monozygotic twins?

a. 25 per cent
b. 50 per cent
c. 75 per cent

d. 100 per cent
e. 200 per cent

answer: a. Most studies describe an MS concordance rate for monozygotic twins of 25 to 30 per cent and for dizygotic twins of 5 per cent.

16 Neurologic Aspects of Sexual Function

Whatever its psychology, sexual function depends on two major neurologic pathways that are complex and delicate: one is a virtual highway between the brain and the genitals and the other mostly a short reflex loop between the genitals and spinal cord. Both involve the central nervous system (CNS), the peripheral nervous system (PNS), and the autonomic nervous system (ANS).

The brain converts various cerebral stimuli, including sleep-related events, into sexually arousing neurologic impulses. Some impulses travel down the spinal cord, which is also part of the CNS, and exit at its sacral region to be carried by the *pudendal nerve*, which is part of the PNS (Fig. 16–1). As if diverted to a parallel route, some impulses leave the low thoracic and upper lumbar segments of the spinal cord to join the *sympathetic* ANS. Others leave the lower sacral segments to join the *parasympathetic* ANS. Increased ANS activity reduces the tone of the genital arteries' wall muscles. Relaxed arteries dilate, increasing genital blood flow. Increased blood flow in men inflates the penis and produces an erection. In women, it produces clitoral engorgement.

A complex series of ANS-mediated events produces an orgasm. Afterward, restoration of normal arterial wall muscle tone constricts blood flow and leads to detumescence. Although the sympathetic and parasympathetic components of the ANS have different roles in sexual function and depend on different neurotransmitters—acetylcholine in the parasympathetic and monoamines in the sympathetic—they are complementary and vulnerable to similar injuries.

In the other, simpler pathway, impulses from genital stimulation pass through the dorsal and then pudendal nerves to the spinal cord. Some impulses, in a *genital-spinal cord reflex*, synapse in the sacral region of the spinal cord and return, via the ANS, to the genitals. Others ascend through the spinal cord to join other cerebral stimuli.

NEUROLOGIC IMPAIRMENT

Without accepting a strict distinction between neurologic and psychogenic sexual impairment, a neurologic origin is reliably indicated by elements of the patient's history (Table 16–1) and routine neurologic examination (Table 16–2). Either spinal cord or peripheral nerve injury might lead to a pattern of weakness and sensory loss below the waist or one confined to the genitals, anus, and buttocks—the "saddle area" (Fig. 16–2). Plantar and deep tendon reflex (DTR) testing will indicate which system is responsible: spinal cord injury causes hyperactive DTRs and Babinski signs, whereas peripheral nerve injury causes hypoactive DTRs and no Babinski signs. Both CNS and PNS

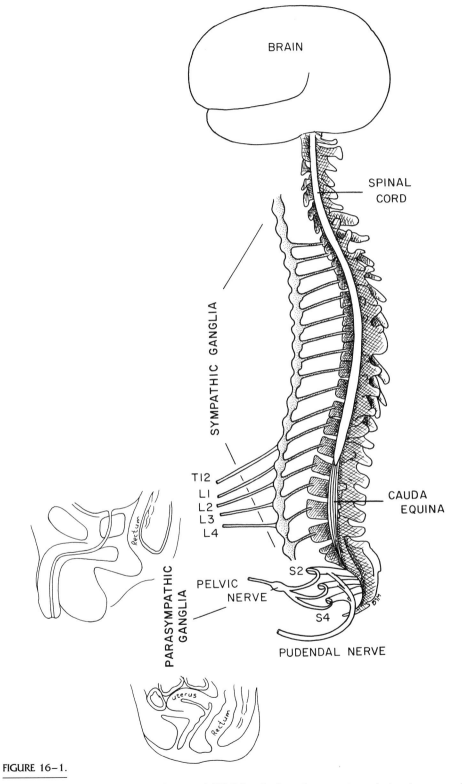

FIGURE 16–1.

The genitals are innervated by the sacral (S2-S4) spinal cord segments and also, in a complementary manner, by the sympathetic and parasympathetic components of the autonomic nervous system (ANS). Branches of the pudendal nerve supply the genital muscles and skin. The ANS innervates the genitals, reproductive organs, bladder, sweat glands, and artery wall muscles.

TABLE 16–1. INDICATIONS OF NEUROLOGIC SEXUAL IMPAIRMENT

Continual erectile dysfunction
　Absence of morning erections
　No erection or orgasm during masturbation or sex with different partners
Related somatic complaints
　Sensory loss in genitals, pelvis, or legs
　Urinary incontinence
Certain neurologic conditions
　Spinal cord injury
　Diabetic neuropathy
　Multiple sclerosis
　Herniated intervertebral disk
　Use of medications

TABLE 16–2. SIGNS OF NEUROLOGIC SEXUAL IMPAIRMENT

Signs of spinal cord injury
　Paraparesis or quadriparesis
　Leg spasticity
　Sensory level
　Urinary incontinence
Signs of autonomic nervous system injury
　Orthostatic hypotension or lightheadedness
　Anhidrosis in groin and legs
　Urinary incontinence
　Retrograde ejaculation
Signs of peripheral nervous system injury
　Loss of sensation in the genitals, "saddle area," and legs
　Paresis and areflexia in legs
　Scrotal, cremasteric, and anal reflex loss[a]

[a]Also found with spinal cord injury.

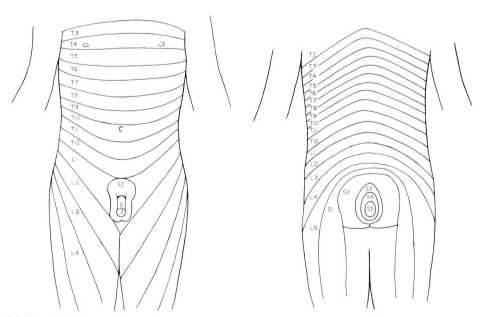

FIGURE 16–2.

The sacral dermatomes (S2–S5) innervate the skin overlying the genitals and anus, but the lumbar dermatomes innervate the legs.

impairment lead to loss of the relevant "superficial reflexes": scrotal, cremasteric, and anal (Fig. 16–3).

Signs of ANS impairment, which may be subtle, are important. For example, *orthostatic hypotension*, usually defined as a fall of 10 mm Hg in blood pressure on standing, is strong evidence of diabetic, medication-induced, or spontaneous ANS impairment. Other signs are *anhidrosis*, lack of sweating, in the groin and legs that is usually found with hairless and sallow skin, and *urinary incontinence*. Finally, *retrograde ejaculation* can be detected if microscopic examination of urine obtained after orgasm reveals sperm.

Neurologic-induced sexual impairment is frequently accompanied by urinary and fecal (double) incontinence because the bladder, bowel, and genitals share an almost common spinal cord, peripheral nervous system, and ANS innervation. The anus, like the bladder (see Fig. 15–5), has two sphincters: (1) an internal sphincter, the more powerful one that is under the involuntary control of the ANS and (2) an external sphincter, which is under voluntary control through the pudendal nerves and other branches of the S3 and S4 peripheral nerve roots.

Laboratory Tests

During REM sleep, from infancy to old age, normal men have erections and other manifestations of ANS activity, such as tachycardia. This activity occurs regardless of the dream's overt content. Normal men have three to five erections lasting about 30 minutes each night. In a standard test, the *nocturnal penile tumescence (NPT) study*, erections are monitored during 1 to 3 nights and correlated with rapid eye movement (REM) sleep. (The "poor man's" simple "stamp test" consists of affixing a ring of several postage stamps around

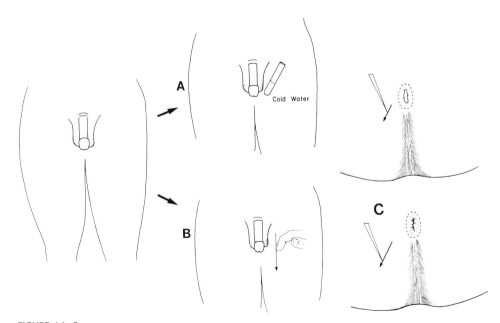

FIGURE 16–3.

A, The *scrotal reflex.* Normally when a cold surface is applied to the scrotum, the testicle retracts and the skin surface contracts. *B,* The *cremasteric reflex.* Likewise, when the inner thigh is stroked, the testicle retracts and the skin surface contracts. *C,* The *anal reflex.* When the perianal skin is scratched, the anus tightens.

the base of the penis at bedtime: if the ring is found to be broken open in the morning, the man is assumed to have had erections.)

During NPT studies, many men with sexual impairment, when freed from social and psychologic influences, are found to have erections. However, a failure to have erections during this test does not necessarily mean that erectile dysfunction is neurologic. Profoundly depressed men and others who may have sleep disorders, but who are otherwise neurologically intact, may not have erections when sleeping. Contrary to the traditional assumption that erectile dysfunction generally results from psychogenic impairment, NPT and other physiologic studies have shown that at least 50 per cent of men with erectile dysfunction have underlying neurologic or other physical abnormalities.

Physicians can assess the blood pressure and blood flow in the dorsal artery of the penis with a small blood pressure cuff, Doppler-based sonography, and other instruments. These tests are particularly important in men with peripheral vascular disease, atherosclerosis, diabetes, or pelvic injuries. Electrophysiologic studies, similar to nerve conduction velocities (see Chapter 6), can detect nerve damage. Also, radioimmunoassay of serum prolactin and gonadotropic hormone concentrations can reveal abnormalities in the hypothalamic-pituitary-gonadal axis.

Mechanical and Physiologic Treatment of Erectile Dysfunction

Several techniques can produce credible erections in a man with erectile dysfunction resulting from neurologic injury, vascular insufficiency, or certain other physiologic abnormalities. An effective, noninvasive device is a suction pump that simply draws blood into a flaccid penis. Once an erection is created, a rubberband-like ring is put around the base of the penis to prevent blood from escaping and deflating the erection.

A more dramatic, physiologically based technique of drawing blood into the penis is injecting vasoactive medicines into the base of the corpus cavernosum (the erectile tissue). These "intracavernous injections" produce erections that permit enjoyable intercourse and orgasms. The vasoactive medicines are combinations of a smooth muscle relaxant, papaverine; the alpha-adrenergic blocker, phentolamine (Regitine); and prostaglandin E1, also called *alprostadil* (Prostin). After intercourse, the erections usually subside spontaneously. If prolonged erections (priapism) do not subside, they can be aborted with the vasoconstrictor epinephrine, which is an alpha-adrenergic receptor agonist. Intracavernous injections are so regularly successful that they have even produced erections in men thought to have psychogenic erectile dysfunction. (In the future, vasodilator medications, such as nitroglycerin, may be applicable as creams.)

Delicate and tedious arterial reconstructive procedures are often performed. However, except in men with localized vascular injuries, the results are disappointing. Surgically implanted devices, such as rigid or semi-rigid rods or a balloon-like apparatus, can mimic an erection. Unfortunately, they are costly and prone to mechanical failures, infections, or aesthetic difficulties.

NEUROLOGIC ILLNESSES ASSOCIATED WITH SEXUAL IMPAIRMENT

Although most patients with certain neurologic illness have predictable sexual impairments, those with other illnesses, even when incapacitated in many ways, have no sexual impairment. Some textbooks, although technically correct, list dozens of illnesses that can impair sexual function; however, only a few are responsible for the majority of cases.

Spinal Cord Injury

Every year, hundreds of teenagers and young adults sustain spinal cord injuries from automobile, diving, horseback riding, and trampoline accidents; knife or bullet wounds; and multiple sclerosis (MS; see Chapter 15). The spinal cord is also subject to congenital injury, such as the myelomeningocele (see Chapter 13). Depending on the level of the spinal cord injury and whether or not the cord is completely transected, patients have an easily recognizable triad of symptoms:

- paraparesis or quadriparesis with spasticity, hyperactive reflexes, and Babinski signs
- sensory loss up to a certain level (Fig. 16–2)
- bladder, bowel, and sexual difficulties

In addition, when the upper cervical cord is damaged, the breathing centers are impaired and the sympathetic nervous system is released from CNS control. Although cerebral sexual functions should remain intact, spinal cord injury is typically associated with a diminished libido and other psychologic difficulties.

Upper Spinal Cord Injury. When the cervical spinal cord is severed, quadriparesis develops. When the thoracic portion is severed, paraparesis develops. In both of these upper spinal cord injuries, ascending sensory impulses are interrupted, and patients cannot sense genital stimulation.

With upper spinal cord lesions, the genital-spinal cord reflex remains intact. Patients retain the capacity for having genital arousal and orgasm. However, they are unable to appreciate the arousal, and men's erections are usually too weak for intercourse. Moreover, their orgasms may produce an excessive, almost violent ANS response, *autonomic hyperreflexia*, which causes hypertension, bradycardia, nausea, and lightheadedness. Autonomic hyperreflexia can even lead to an intracerebral hemorrhage.

Most spinal cord injury patients lose bladder and bowel control. Their urinary incontinence and constipation require catheters and enemas. Urinary tract, genital, and decubitus infections are constant threats. Although men become infertile because of inadequate and abnormal sperm production, women continue to ovulate, menstruate, and retain their capacity to conceive and bear children.

With incomplete spinal cord injuries, as typically occur in MS and many nonpenetrating injuries, neurologic deficits are less pronounced. Still, because of the delicate nature of the neurologic pathways, problems with genital arousal and anorgasmy plague most patients.

Lower Spinal Cord Injury. When the lumbar or sacral spinal cord is transected or congenitally deformed, both the descending tracts and genital-spinal cord reflex are interrupted. Neither cerebral nor genital stimulation produces arousal or orgasm. As in upper spinal cord transection, patients have paraparesis and double incontinence. Nevertheless, the ANS sometimes continues to innervate the genitals, fertility in both men and women are preserved, and breast sensation and its erotic capacity are preserved (and possibly enhanced) because upper chest innervation is unaffected.

Poliomyelitis and Other Exceptions

Several neurologic illnesses that spare sexual function can be so devastating that the untrained physician might assume that these people are "impotent." Before vaccinations virtually eradicated the illness, poliomyelitis (polio), a motor neuron disease of the spinal cord, caused numerous children and young adults to have lifelong trunk and limb paresis that was frequently severe enough to confine them to braces or wheelchairs (see Chapter 5). Polio does not damage the intellect, sensation, involuntary muscle strength, or the ANS. Most importantly from a sexual viewpoint, its victims, who may still suffer marked handicaps in other spheres, have normal sexual function, genital sensation, bladder and bowel control, fertility, and libido.

As if the weak arms and legs were not enough of a burden, middle-aged adults who contracted polio in childhood develop increased limb weakness with fasciculations, the *postpolio syndrome* (see Chapter 5). They retain normal bladder, bowel, and sexual function. The other, more devastating motor neuron disease, amyotrophic lateral sclerosis (ALS), likewise does not damage these functions.

In a different situation, extrapyramidal illnesses (see Chapter 18), despite causing difficulties with mobility, also do not impair sexual desire, sexual function, or fertility. For example, Parkinson's disease patients have an intact sexual drive that may be acted upon once dopa-repleting medications are introduced. Moreover, illness-induced loss of inhibition, as in frontal lobe trauma and Alzheimer's disease, can lead to sexual aggressiveness.

Diabetes Mellitus

Sexual impairment, especially retrograde ejaculation and erectile dysfunction, eventually affects almost 50 per cent of diabetic men. It is the first sign of diabetes in about 5 per cent of patients. Diabetic sexual impairment results from ANS and PNS injury and also from atherosclerosis of the arteries of the genitals (see below). Similar sexual problems are found in alcoholics. Since the bladder and genitals have common ANS innervation, erectile dysfunction and urinary incontinence typically coincide in diabetics. The bladder of affected patients is typically large, flaccid, and poorly controlled (Fig. 16–4). Patients with diabetes-induced sexual dysfunction generally also have other signs of ANS impairment, such as anhidrosis and orthostatic hypotension. However, they do not necessarily have other complications of diabetes, such as retinopathy, nephropathy, or peripheral vascular disease. Diabetic sexual impairment should not directly lessen the libido, but psychologic repercussions, as in spinal cord injury, can be debilitating. Although many diabetic men with erectile dysfunction have low testosterone concentrations, testosterone therapy generally has only a placebo effect.

The few available descriptions of sexual impairment in diabetic women are conflicting. For example, Kolodny et al. (1979) found that 35 per cent of diabetic women had anorgasmy and that sexual impairment was related to neuropathy; however, other authors found that diabetic women were no more prone than nondiabetic ones to sexual impairment and that diabetic women, even with profound neuropathy, had full sexual function. Vaginal infections are undoubtedly more common in diabetic women, and although these women remain fertile, pregnancies are more often complicated by miscarriages and fetal malformations.

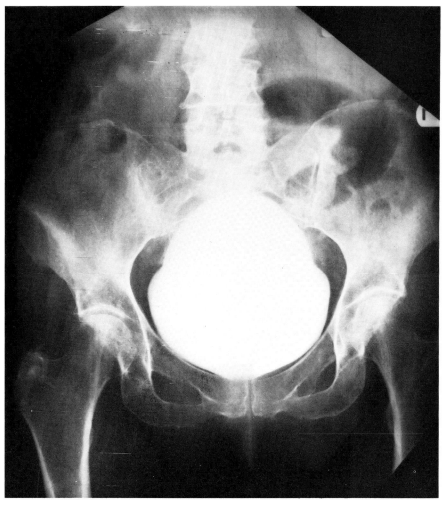

FIGURE 16–4.

A patient had diabetes mellitus complicated by impotence and urinary incontinence, which are typically associated with a large, flaccid bladder. His intravenous pyelogram (IVP) reveals a distended bladder, which is the large white circular area.

Multiple Sclerosis

Sexual impairment can be the sole symptom of MS (see Chapter 15). When it causes only vague sensory disturbances, MS can lead to the misdiagnosis of a psychogenic disturbance. At the other extreme, when MS is devastating, sexual impairment becomes a relatively unimportant aspect. In typical cases, multiple sclerosis causes premature ejaculation, erectile dysfunction, retrograde ejaculation, and anorgasmy. In the early stages of MS, patients might have few extrasexual deficits, but when episodes develop repeatedly, the incidence of sexual impairment, urinary incontinence, and extrasexual deficits all rise dramatically.

In women, fertility is preserved. Pregnancies do not affect the course of MS, and similarly, MS does not complicate the pregnancy or lead to fetal malformations. However, deliveries may be more complicated, and the first 3 months of the postpartum period have been associated with MS exacerbations. Men's fertility is impaired because of decreased sperm production.

Medication-Induced Impairment

Although over a hundred medications are implicated, only a few categories consistently impair sexual function. Antihypertensive medications are the most common offenders: clonidine (Catapres), thiazide diuretics, and beta-blockers (e.g., propranolol, Inderal). Fortunately, the newer antihypertensive medications—angiotensin-converting enzyme (ACE) inhibitors and the calcium-channel blockers—do not cause impairment.

Virtually all antidepressant and antipsychotic medications—even the newer ones—cause sexual impairment (Table 16–3). Often given to counteract the parkinsonian side effects of phenothiazines, anticholinergic medications cause sexual impairment and other bothersome symptoms: dry mouth, orthostatic hypotension, accommodation paresis (see Fig. 12–4), and urinary hesitancy (see Fig. 15–5). Trazodone (Desyrel) and clozapine (Clozaril) can cause priapism. Finally, contradicting the triad of "sex, drugs, and rock-and-roll," alcohol, minor tranquilizers, and all narcotics impair sexual function.

Miscellaneous

Vascular disease of the arteries of the penis, more than any other organic condition, leads to erectile dysfunction. This etiology can be suspected in men who have peripheral vascular disease and the predisposing conditions for atherosclerosis: age greater than 65 years, hypertension, diabetes, coronary artery disease, and, naturally, cerebrovascular disease. When evaluations indicate vascular disease in the penis, arterial reconstructive procedures, including grafting, can be attempted. However, when vascular disease or surgery has caused nerve damage or spinal cord infarction, the prognosis is poor.

Men with low testosterone levels, usually as part of panhypopituitarism, have erectile dysfunction accompanied by reduced libido. Indiscriminate use

---

TABLE 16–3.   PSYCHIATRIC MEDICATIONS ASSOCIATED WITH SEXUAL DYSFUNCTION[a]

Tricyclic and heterocyclic antidepressants
    Amitriptyline (Elavil[b])
    Clomipramine (Anafranil)
    Imipramine (Tofranil[b])
    Nortriptyline (Aventyl[b])
    Trazodone (Desyrel[c])
Monamine oxidase inhibitors
    Isocarboxazid (Marplan)
    Phenelzine (Nardil)
    Tranylcypromine (Parnate)
Other antidepressants
    Amoxapine (Asendin)
    Fluoxetine (Prozac)
    Lithium
Antipsychotics
    Chlorpromazine (Thorazine[b])
    Clozapine (Clozaril[c])
    Haloperidol (Haldol[b])

[a]Decreased libido, erectile dysfunction, or anorgasmy. For a fuller listing of medications, see Abramowicz M (1992).
[b]And other brands.
[c]Can cause priapism.

of testosterone can be counterproductive because it can increase libido in men who still cannot achieve erections. Elevated prolactin levels can also lead to erectile dysfunction and reduced libido. In cases of elevated prolactin levels with or without low testosterone levels, prolactin-secreting pituitary adenomas should be sought with an MRI of the brain.

Prostate surgery that damages the pudendal nerves is another common cause of erectile dysfunction. Transurethral prostatectomy (TURP), for example, leads to impotence in 4 to 12 per cent of cases. Other common pelvic and lower abdominal surgical procedures, especially sympathectomies, also cause impotence.

Herniated lumbar intervertebral disks occasionally compress the sacral nerve roots (see Chapter 5). Patients with herniated disks have distressing, radiating low back pain. Examination usually reveals signs of nerve root compression, such as loss of DTRs, urinary retention, and Lasègue's sign (see Fig. 5–7). Compared to the acute pain and other impairments, sexual impairment is a minor part of the patient's problem.

Survivors of myelography, laminectomy, and related operations on the lower spine sometimes develop nerve root injury from surgical trauma or postoperative *arachnoiditis* (inflammation of the covering of the nerve roots). These patients often suffer from chronic low back pain, sexual unarousability, and extensive nerve root damage.

LIBIDO

From a neurologic viewpoint, the *limbic system* is the source of the libido (Fig. 16–5). When it is damaged, usually through injury of the frontal or temporal lobe, hypothalamus, or the entire brain, the libido is usually reduced.

Pure limbic system injury is rarely encountered. The closest example is the *Klüver-Bucy syndrome* that consists of bilateral anterior temporal lobectomies, which necessarily include removal of both amygdalae, in rhesus monkeys. The monkeys display increased heterosexual and homosexual activity, aggression, and other behavioral changes. Their increased sexuality is accompanied by unnatural tranquillity, continual tactile activity, and placing inedible objects in their mouth, which is called "psychic blindness" or *oral exploration* (similar to visual agnosia, Chapter 12).

A modified form of this syndrome, the *human Klüver-Bucy syndrome*, has been described in children and adults who have sustained bilateral temporal lobe damage from *Herpes simplex* encephalitis, Pick's disease, infarctions of both posterior cerebral arteries, head trauma, and Alzheimer's disease. People with the Klüver-Bucy syndrome, like the experimental monkeys, are placid, tend to eat excessively, and show oral exploration. However, only about one half of them have any increase in heterosexual activity or masturbation, and most of them only make suggestive gestures. Also, despite their oral tendencies, they rarely become obese. Although Klüver-Bucy syndrome patients' sexual proclivities have been noteworthy, they are more handicapped by other manifestations of temporal lobe injury, such as memory impairment (amnesia), aphasia, and dementia. Children who develop the Klüver-Bucy syndrome, which usually results from hypoxia, are most impaired by the amnesia.

Increased sexual activity can result from certain medications that act as stimulants, including hallucinogens, amyl nitrate, and L-dopa compounds, such as Sinemet. A different mechanism that produces increased sexual activ-

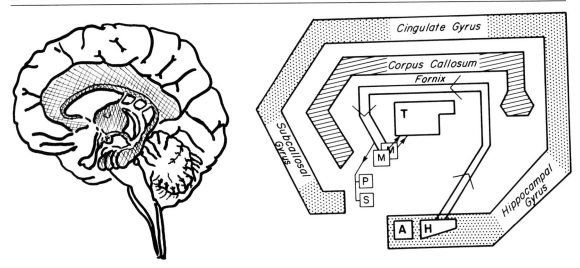

FIGURE 16–5.

(*Left*), The *limbic system* (shaded) is a circuit deep in the brain that connects with the overlying cerebral cortex. (*Right*) This schematic portrayal of the *limbic system* shows its main features:

Hippocampus (H) with the adjacent amygdala (A)

↓

Fornix

↓

Mamillary bodies (M) that send off a mamillothalamic tract

↓

Anterior nucleus of the thalamus (T)

↓

Cingulate gyrus that connects to the overlying cerebral cortex and back to the hippocampus ↑

ity is damage to centers that normally inhibit sexual activity. People with Alzheimer's disease and Parkinson's disease, for example, may seem to develop increased sexual activity as the result of an increased libido, but a loss of inhibition is actually responsible.

Otherwise, most neurologic damage decreases the libido. Lesions of the pituitary, hypothalamus, and diencephalon have occasionally been associated with hypersexuality, but usually these injuries generally cause hyposexuality and appetite changes. For example, the Wernicke-Korsakoff syndrome and transient global amnesia, conditions in which limbic system structures are injured, are characterized by amnesia, not libido changes.

Partial complex epilepsy, which characteristically originates in temporal lobe dysfunction, is sometimes associated with simple, nonerotic, sexual actions. During seizures, patients may seem to engage in rudimentary masturbation or even partially undress; however, they do not engage in heterosexual activity. During interictal periods, these epilepsy patients are prone to hyposexuality (see Chapter 10).

The libido is vulnerable, indirectly if not directly, to neurologic impairments because lack of sexual satisfaction seems to decrease demand. For example, men with MS or diabetes who have chronic erectile dysfunction, as through a "negative feedback loop," often ignore their sexual desires. The classic question posed to people with sexual dysfunction—"Is the problem decreased libido or impotence?"—becomes the question of the chicken and the egg.

Although the libido resists mild fatigue, hunger, and fear, it is almost always dampened by pain. In addition, patients with chronic pain may have an associated depression or use of potent analgesics that produces sexual dysfunction.

REFERENCES

Abramowicz M (ed): Intracavernous injections for impotence. Med Lett *32*: 116–117, 1990

Abramowicz M (ed): Drugs that cause sexual dysfunction: An update. Med Lett *34*: 73–78, 1992

Boller F, Frank E: Sexual Dysfunction in Neurologic Disorders: Diagnosis, Management, and Rehabilitation. New York, Raven Press, 1982

Comfort A (ed): Sexual Consequences of Disability. Philadelphia, George F. Strickley Co, 1978

Dechesne BH, Schellen AM: Sexuality and Handicap: Problems of Motor Handicapped People. Springfield, IL, Charles C. Thomas, 1986

Ford JR, Duckworth B: Physical Management of the Quadriplegic Patient. Philadelphia, F. A. Davis, 1987

Hale G (ed): Sex Instruction for the Physically Handicapped. Philadelphia, W.B. Saunders Press, 1979

Kolodny RC, Masters WH, Johnson VE: Textbook of Sexual Medicine. Boston, Little, Brown, 1979

Krane RJ, Goldstein I, DeTejada IS: Impotence. N Engl J Med *321*: 1648–1659, 1989

Lilly R, Cummings JL, Benson DF, et al: The human Klüver-Bucy syndrome. Neurology *33*: 1141–1145, 1983

Madoff RD, Williams JG, Caushaj PF: Fecal incontinence. N Engl J Med *326*: 1002–1007, 1992

Monat RK: Sexuality and the Mentally Retarded: A Clinical and Therapeutic Guidebook. San Diego, College-Hill Press, 1982

Mooney TO, Cole TM, Chilgren RA: Sexual Options for Paraplegics and Quadriplegics. Boston, Little Brown, 1975

Morales A, Condra M, Reid K: The role of nocturnal penile tumescence monitoring in the diagnosis of impotence: A review. J Urol *143*: 441–446, 1990

Singer C, Weiner WJ (eds): Sexual Dysfunction: A Neuro-Medical Approach. Armonk, NY, Futura Publishing Company, 1994

Tonsgard JH Harwicke N Levine SC: Klüver-Bucy syndrome in children. Pediatr Neurol *3*: 162–165, 1987

QUESTIONS and ANSWERS: CHAPTER 16

1. A 40-year-old man complains of long-standing erectile dysfunction. He has severe low back pain, mild hypertension, and borderline diabetes. Which conditions should be considered as possible causes of his sexual dysfunction?

a. Herniated lumbar intervertebral disk
b. Antihypertensive medications
c. Diabetic neuropathy
d. Psychogenic factors
e. All of the above

> **answer:** e. This man might have sexual impairment because of the various medical or psychogenic disorders.

2. A 24-year-old man who complains of premature ejaculation also had episodes of unsteady gait, diplopia, and paraparesis. Which of the following might a neurologic examination reveal?

a. Internuclear ophthalmoplegia
b. Absent abdominal reflexes
c. Ataxia of gait
d. Babinski signs
e. Hyperactive deep tendon reflexes

> **answer:** a, b, c, d, e. The patient is likely to have MS with cerebellar, brainstem, and spinal cord involvement. Between episodes, when the patient is likely to have residual neurologic signs (a-e), he may also have sexual dysfunction. Premature ejaculation and impotence are often manifestations—and possibly the only manifestations—of quiescent MS that has affected the spinal cord. Virtually any insult of the spinal cord disrupts the intricate and delicate sexual pathways.

3. Which of the following conditions might cause retrograde ejaculation?

a. Ovarian dysfunction
b. Diabetic autonomic neuropathy
c. Psychogenic influence
d. Use of guanethidine (Ismelin)
e. Sexual inexperience

answer: b, d. In retrograde ejaculation, semen is propelled by involuntary mechanisms into the bladder instead of the urethra. It is always the result of neurologic, muscular, or other organic impairment.

4. In which illnesses might a physician assume that sexual dysfunction has a neurologic basis?

a. Dominant hemisphere infarctions
b. Nondominant hemisphere infarctions
c. Parkinsonism
d. Poliomyelitis
e. Amyotrophic lateral sclerosis
f. None of the above

answer: f. Although each of these illnesses may cause weakness, the patient's sexual drive, genital sensation, and orgasmic reactions are all preserved.

5. In which illness is medication-induced sexual dysfunction likely to be encountered?

a. Psychosis
b. Migraine headache
c. Hypertension
d. Low back pain
e. Duodenal ulcer

answer: a, c, e. Medications that cause sexual impairments are usually antihypertensive medications and those with anticholinergic properties, including neuroleptics and ulcer therapies.

6. During sleep, when do erections and emissions occur?

answer: Erections and orgasm occur during REM sleep. Erections are also characteristically present on awakening.

7. In which situations is fertility lost?

a. Women with cervical spinal cord transection
b. Men with cervical spinal cord transection
c. Men with diabetes mellitus and neuropathy
d. Women with diabetes mellitus and neuropathy

answer: b. Men with upper spinal cord injury have reduced concentration and abnormalities of their sperm. Women are able to conceive and bear children despite spinal cord injury. Both men and women with diabetes remain fertile.

8. In which conditions are erections still possible?

a. Severe diabetic autonomic neuropathy
b. Use of clonidine (Catapres) or enalapril (Vasotec)
c. Sacral spinal cord transection
d. Cervical spinal cord transection
e. Upper thoracic spinal cord transection
f. Multiple sclerosis

answer: b, d, e, f. Erections are possible if the lumbosacral spinal cord and the sacral autonomic nervous system are intact. Thus, men with either severe diabetic autonomic neuropathy or sacral spinal cord damage are unable to have erections. When the spinal cord damage is incomplete, as in patients with MS, or is located in the cervical region, erectile function may be preserved. Although sexual dysfunction often results from medications, the new antihypertensives (b) usually do not cause sexual dysfunction.

9. In which conditions are cremasteric reflexes lost?

a. Severe diabetic autonomic neuropathy
b. Psychogenic difficulties
c. Sacral spinal cord injury
d. Frontal meningiomas

answer: a, c. Cremasteric reflexes require that the pudendal nerves, autonomic nervous system, and lower spinal cord be intact. Loss of these reflexes indicates a neurologic impairment.

10. One month after falling down a flight of stairs, a 35-year-old man complains of low back pain and impotence. Examination reveals loss of pinprick sensation from the waist down to the toes, but intact position, vibratory, and warm-cold sensation. Deep tendon and cremasteric reflexes are intact, and plantar reflexes are flexion. To what condition could the impotence be attributed?

a. Spinal cord injury
b. Autonomic nervous system dysfunction
c. Peripheral neuropathy
d. Multiple sclerosis
e. None of the above

answer: e. The lack of objective neurologic deficit indicates that no neurologic injury has occurred. In fact, the dissociation of pinprick and warm-cold sensation cannot be caused by a structural lesion because both sensations travel in the same nerve pathways.

11. In monkeys, which are components of the Klüver-Bucy syndrome?

a. Psychic blindness
b. Apathy
c. Frontal lobectomy
d. Loss of amygdalae
e. Increased homosexual, heterosexual, and autosexual activity

answer: a, b, d, e. After temporal lobectomy including removal of the amygdalae, monkeys have oral exploratory behavior. They are said to have visual agnosia because they do not identify objects by their appearance even though their vision is intact. The monkeys characteristically lose extreme emotion. Sometimes appearing fearless, they are actually apathetic. Most striking, they have increased and indiscriminate sexual activity.

12. In humans who have had bilateral temporal lobe damage, which of the following conditions are almost always found?

a. Memory impairment
b. Placing food and inedible objects in their mouths
c. Hypersexuality
d. Rage attacks
e. Aphasia

answer: a, b, e. The human variety of the Klüver-Bucy syndrome is characterized by impaired language function and memory, the tendency to eat excessively, and, like monkeys, placing inedible objects in their mouths. Contrary to expectations, these people have little increased sexual appetite or violent outbursts. Even though they put inanimate objects into their mouth, they are usually not obese.

13. Which conditions damage the limbic system?

a. *Herpes simplex*
b. Alcoholism
c. TIAs of the posterior cerebral arteries
d. *Herpes zoster*

answer: a, b, c. Since the amygdala and hippocampus are in the temporal lobe, these limbic system structures are vulnerable to conditions that damage the temporal lobe. *Herpes simplex* virus, which has a predilection for the frontal and temporal lobes, is a frequent cause of encephalitis characterized by memory impairment and partial complex seizures. Although *Herpes zoster* often causes painful neuralgia in the trigeminal nerve distribution, it usually does not infect the CNS. Posterior cerebral TIAs cause ischemia of the temporal lobes. These TIAs induce episodes of confusion and memory impairment that are called "transient global amnesia." Chronic alcohol abuse can cause the Wernicke-Korsakoff syndrome, which is associated with hemorrhage into the mamillary bodies and other parts of the limbic system.

14. Which of the following are consequences of pituitary tumors?

a. Headaches

b.   Hyperprolactinemia
c.   Optic atrophy
d.   Homonymous superior quadrantanopia

answer: a, b, c, d

15.   In normal males, which of the following are associated with REM-induced erections?

a.   Dreams with no overt sexual content
b.   Most dreams with even frightful or anxiety-producing content
c.   Increased pulse and blood pressure
d.   Increased cerebral blood flow
e.   An EEG that appears, aside from eye movement artifact, as though the patient were awake

answer: a, b, c, d, e

16.   In the treatment of men with erectile dysfunction, injections into the corpus cavernosum of which substances will produce an erection?

a.   Epinephrine
b.   Phentolamine
c.   Papaverine
d.   Morphine

answer: b, c. Men who have erectile dysfunction because of multiple sclerosis, diabetes, and many other illnesses can obtain an erection by injections of phentolamine (Regitine), papaverine, or prostaglandins into the dorsum of the penis. Persistent erections are terminated by an epinephrine injection, but the injections can be complicated by priapism. They must be used with caution in men with vascular disease. The injections are so effective that they may be applicable in certain men who are thought to have psychogenic erectile dysfunction.

17.   What is the origin of the sympathetic autonomic nervous system supply of the sexual organs?

a.   Lower cranial nerves
b.   Cervical and upper thoracic spinal cord
c.   Lower thoracic and upper lumbar spinal cord
d.   Sacral spinal cord

answer: c

18.   What is the origin of the parasympathetic autonomic nervous system supply of the sexual organs?

a.   Lower cranial nerves
b.   Cervical and upper thoracic spinal cord
c.   Lower thoracic and upper lumbar spinal cord
d.   Sacral spinal cord

answer: d

19.   What is the effect of hyperprolactinemia?

a.   Increased libido
b.   Decreased libido
c.   Priapism
d.   Erectile dysfunction

answer: b

20.   Which of the following cause priapism?

a.   Trazodone (Desyrel)
b.   Clozapine (Clozaril)
c.   Papaverine intracavernous injections
d.   Epinephrine intracavernous injections
e.   Phentolamine intracavernous injections

answer: a, b, c, e. Epinephrine intracavernous injections terminate iatrogenic erections.

21. Which President had survived poliomyelitis (polio) as a young man?

a. Carter
b. T. Roosevelt
c. F.D. Roosevelt
d. J.F. Kennedy

answer: c. FDR required heavy braces for his legs and eventually was confined to a wheelchair. Polio is an example of a neurologic illness that causes massive physical impairments, but spares intellectual abilities.

22. Which of the following sequences is the generally described path of the limbic system?

a. Fornix, mamillothalamic tract, amygdala, anterior nucleus of the thalamus, cingulate gyrus.
b. Cingulate gyrus, mamillary bodies, mamillothalamic tract, anterior nucleus of the thalamus, hippocampus and adjacent amygdala
c. Hippocampus and adjacent amygdala, fornix, mamillary bodies, mamillothalamic tract, anterior nucleus of the thalamus, cingulate gyrus
d. Hippocampus and adjacent amygdala, mamillothalamic tract, fornix, hippocampus and adjacent amygdala, mamillary bodies, anterior nucleus of the thalamus, cingulate gyrus

answer: c

23. During sexual function, which of the following act as the neurotransmitter for sympathetic nervous system activity? parasympathetic nervous system activity?

a. Acetylcholine
b. Monoamines
c. Serotonin
d. Dopamine

answer: a, b. Monoamines are the neurotransmitters in the sympathetic system and acetylcholine in the parasympathetic. The actual genital engorgement may be modulated by nitric oxide.

17 Sleep Disorders

The scientific study of sleep, from its inception, has stemmed from a hybrid of psychiatry and neurology. Sleep and its stages are now defined by a combination of clinical observations and physiologic information. The chief source of physiologic information is a device, the *polysomnogram* (*PSG*), that in sleeping people simultaneously records (a) cerebral activity through several electroencephalogram (EEG) channels; (b) ocular movement through an electrooculogram (EOG); (c) muscle movement and tone, through an electromyogram (EMG); (d) vital signs; and (e) other physiologic parameters.

Almost the entire discipline rests on the distinction between two phases of sleep detected by the PSG. In one phase, *rapid eye movement* (*REM*) *sleep*, dreaming and flaccid limb paralysis accompany eye movements that are rapid, conjugate, and predominantly horizontal. The other phase, *nonrapid eye movement* (*NREM*) *sleep*, consists of relatively long stretches of essentially dreamless sleep accompanied by eye rolling and, approximately every 15 minutes, repositioning movements (Table 17–1).

NORMAL SLEEP

REM Sleep

Since most people who are awakened during a REM period report that they were having a dream, REM sleep has become synonymous with dreaming. Dreams during REM sleep are intellectually complex, at least on a superficial level, and rich in visual imagery. The vigorous eye movements are attributed to people watching or feeling themselves participating in a dream.

Except for the eye movements and normal breathing, people are immobile and their muscle tone is virtually absent. Muscles are paretic, flaccid, and areflexic. EMGs show no electric activity in the chin and limb muscles (Fig. 17–1). This paralysis is fortuitous because it normally prevents people from acting on their dreams.

Nevertheless, so much autonomic nervous system activity takes place in REM sleep that it has been called "activated" or "paradoxical." REM sleep produces increased pulse, blood pressure, intracranial pressure, cerebral blood flow, and muscle metabolism, and, in men, erections regardless of the content of their dreams. REM-induced autonomic activity has been implicated in the increased incidence of myocardial infarctions and ischemic cerebrovascular accidents from 6:00 AM to 11:00 AM.

The EEG is also surprisingly active. Aside from eye-movement artifact, the REM-induced EEG is similar to EEGs in wakefulness. Overall, in REM sleep, the bodily activities and EEG, except for the EMG, are more similar to wakefulness than in NREM sleep.

TABLE 17–1. NORMAL SLEEP

Stage	Bodily Movements	Ocular Movements	EMG	EEG
NREM				
1 Light	Persistent face and limb tone with repositioning every 15–20 minutes	Slow, rolling	Continual activity	Loss of alpha (8–12 Hz) activity
2 Intermediate	Same	Same	Further reduction	Sleep spindles and K complexes
3 Slow-wave, deep, delta	Same	Same	Same	Increased proportion of slow-wave (1–3 Hz) activity
4 Slow-wave, deep, delta	Same	Same	Greatest proportion of slow-wave activity	
REM Activated, paradoxical	Flaccid, areflexic paresis, except for brief face and limb movements	Rapid, conjugate	Silent	Low voltage fast with ocular movement artifacts

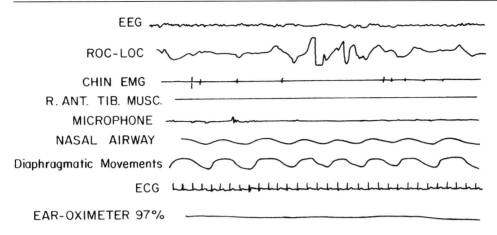

FIGURE 17-1

Polysomnography (PSG) of REM sleep displays nine channels, and even more could have been added. The EEG has low-voltage, fast activity, which is similar to activity of people when they are awake. The electro-oculogram (EOG) channel—OC-LOC—reflected several rapid eye movements (REM) by large-scale, quick fluctuations. Electromyograms (EMGs) of the chin and right anterior tibialis muscles show virtually no activity, which indicates an absence of muscle movement and tone. The microphone detected a little noise, which might be a snore. The regular, undulating airway and diaphragm recordings indicate normal breathing and air movement.

Although the particular brainstem nuclei that trigger it cannot be specified, REM sleep is associated with increased acetylcholine (cholinergic) activity. Similarly, REM sleep is enhanced by cholinergic agonists, such as nicotine, and suppressed by anticholinergic medications. It is associated with decreased dopamine, norepinephrine, and epinephrine (adrenergic) activity.

NREM Sleep

NREM sleep, in contrast to REM sleep, is divided into four stages that are distinguished by progressively greater depths of unconsciousness and slower, higher-voltage EEG patterns. In NREM sleep, the eyes have slow, rolling motions, and thinking is brief, rudimentary, and readily forgotten. Bodily repositioning movements are conspicuous. Muscle tone is present, and DTRs can be elicited. EMG activity is detectable in the chin and limb muscles (Fig. 17–2).

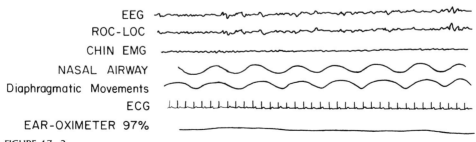

FIGURE 17-2

PSG of stage I NREM sleep reveals slow EEG activity, not the higher-voltage, very slow EEG activity of slow-wave NREM sleep. The ROC-LOC channel shows no substantial ocular movement, i.e., no REM activity. Continual, low-voltage EMG activity in the chin muscles reflects muscle tone. Breathing and cardiac activity are normal.

Although people in NREM sleep have a generalized decrease in autonomic nervous system function accompanied by hypotension and bradycardia, important hypothalamic-pituitary (neuroendocrine) activity ensues. The daily secretion of growth hormone occurs almost entirely during NREM sleep, about 30 to 60 minutes after sleep begins. Likewise, the serum prolactin concentration is highest soon after sleep begins. In contrast, cortisol is secreted in five to seven discrete late nighttime episodes, which accumulate to yield the day's highest cortisol concentration at about 8:00 AM.

Overall, the third and fourth stages of NREM sleep, which are called *slow-wave*, *delta*, or *deep NREM* sleep, provide most of the physical recuperation derived from a night's sleep. As if the immediate role of sleep were to revitalize the body, slow-wave sleep occurs predominantly in the early night. After "squeezing in" slow-wave sleep at the beginning of the night, remaining sleep becomes lighter and dream filled.

NREM sleep is associated with increased serotonin activity, but a decrease in other metabolic activities. The main scheme, however, seems to be that wakefulness is induced or maintained by increased adrenergic activity, NREM sleep by a decreased generalized metabolic activity, and REM sleep by increased cholinergic activity.

Sleep Patterns

After retiring, people usually fall asleep within 10 to 20 minutes. The interval is called *sleep latency* and is an indication of sleepiness. During daytime, it is actually shortest at 4:00 PM and is influenced by numerous psychologic and physical factors. In general, sleep latencies are longest in adolescents and successively shorter in adults, elderly people, college students and patients with specific sleep disorders (Table 17–2).

Once asleep, normal individuals enter NREM sleep and pass in succession through its four stages. After 90 minutes to 120 minutes of NREM sleep, they enter the initial REM period. The interval from falling asleep to the first REM period is called *REM latency*. Determining the REM latency can be helpful in diagnosing many sleep disorders, especially narcolepsy (Table 17–3).

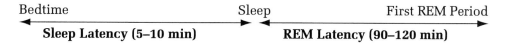

Bedtime   Sleep   First REM Period

Sleep Latency (5–10 min) **REM Latency (90–120 min)**

TABLE 17–2.   SLEEP LATENCY CHANGES IN SLEEP DISORDERS[a]

Shortened Sleep Latency[a]
  Alcohol- and drug-induced sleep
  Narcolepsy
  Sleep apnea
  Sleep deprivation
Prolonged Sleep Latency[a]
  Delayed sleep phase syndrome
  Inadequate sleep hygiene
  Psychiatric disorders
    Acute schizophrenia
    Major depression
    Mania
  Restless leg syndrome

[a]Normal sleep latency is 10 to 20 minutes.

TABLE 17–3.   CAUSES OF SHORTENED OR SLEEP-ONSET REM LATENCY[a]

Alcohol, hypnotics, and sedative withdrawal
Depression
Narcolepsy
Sleep apnea
Sleep deprivation[b]

[a]Normal REM latency is about 90 to 120 minutes.
[b]As part of REM rebound.

The NREM-REM cycle repeats itself throughout the night with a periodicity of about 90 minutes. REM periods occur four or five times nightly and are progressively longer and more frequent (Fig. 17–3). In later sleep, body temperature falls to the day's lowest point (the nadir). The final REM period can merge with awakening. Thus, a person's final dream may be influenced by surrounding morning household activities, and on awakening, men usually have erections.

Important changes can be observed after sleep deprivation, as occurs in adults who have worked all night or when children skip their customary afternoon nap. Those people have a short sleep latency, increased sleep time, and more slow-wave sleep. Also, they have a characteristic *REM rebound* in which the first REM period occurs soon or immediately after falling asleep (*sleep-onset REM*), subsequent REM periods are longer than normal, and REM sleep occupies a greater proportion of sleep time. In other words, after missing sleep, people usually fall asleep almost immediately, soon start to dream a great deal, and sleep late the next morning. As could be anticipated, REM rebound also occurs after withdrawal from REM-suppressing substances, such as antidepressants and alcohol, and in several sleep disorders (Table 17–3).

Effects of Age

The first REM-NREM cycles appear at about 20 weeks in the fetus. Neonates sleep 16 to 20 hours a day, with about 50 per cent of that time spent in REM

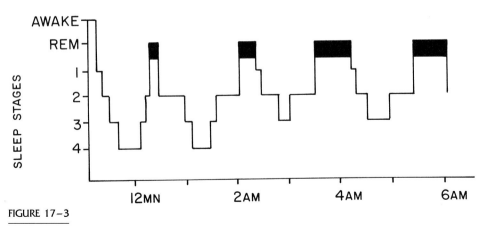

FIGURE 17–3

In the conventional representation of a normal night's sleep pattern—sleep architecture—the first REM period starts about 90 minutes after sleep begins and is only about 10 minutes long. (In this example, the REM latency is about 90 minutes, but sleep latency cannot be determined.) Later in the night, REM periods recur more frequently and have longer duration. NREM sleep progresses through regular, progressively lighter stages.

sleep. As individuals mature, they spend less total time sleeping and proportionately less in dreaming. Young children spend 10 to 12 hours sleeping during the night and in afternoon naps, with about 30 per cent in REM sleep. Adolescents, teenagers, and college students have erratic sleep patterns that are strongly influenced by social "cues." Adults average 6 to 8 hours of total sleep time with 20 to 28 per cent in REM sleep. Adults who are accustomed to relatively little sleep increase the proportion of slow-wave NREM sleep. In other words, the *quantity* of their slow-wave NREM sleep tends to be preserved at the expense of their REM and lighter stages of NREM sleep.

The elderly sleep somewhat less than young adults. Their nighttime sleep is shorter and fragmented by multiple brief awakenings, especially in the early morning. They recoup their sleep during daytime naps not only after meals, in the late afternoon, and other periods of normal sleepiness, but irresistibly at any time, including during social activities. In addition, their sleep onset and awakening times tend to be earlier than normal. In what is termed *phase-advanced* sleep, they go to sleep in the early evening and awaken in the early morning.

Just as remarkable, the elderly have decreased total REM time, and their REM periods, instead of being longer and more frequent in the later night, do not change in duration or frequency. Moreover, during REM sleep, often because of their use of hypnotics and certain medications, such as L-dopa, the elderly have relatively frequent nightmares. Also, NREM sleep, especially its slow-wave phase, diminishes. In fact, the slow-wave phase almost disappears in people older than 75 years. Unlike in younger adults, reductions in their sleep are taken at the expense of slow-wave NREM.

In addition, people older than 55 years are prone to certain sleep disorders, including various leg movement disorders, REM behavior disorder, and sleep apnea syndrome (see below). Also, they are subject to medication-induced sleep disturbances; medical disorders, especially cardiovascular disturbances and pain; dementia and other neurologic illnesses; and depression.

SLEEP DISORDERS

Neurologists, as well as the "sleep community," follow the newly revised, comprehensive *International Classification of Sleep Disorders*, which is consistent with the *Diagnostic and Statistical Manual-IV (DSM-IV)*. It recognizes three major categories of sleep disorders (Table 17–4): (1) dyssomnias, (2) parasomnias, and (3) neurologic/psychiatric disorders.

Dyssomnias

The dyssomnias incorporate two traditional groups. One is roughly equivalent to insomnia or too little sleep and includes *disorders of initiating or maintaining sleep (DIMS)*. The other is *disorders of excessive sleepines (DOES)*. Although these disorders are prominent symptoms of many sleep problems, the dyssomnias are now divided into *Intrinsic*, *Extrinsic*, and *Circadian Disorders*.

Intrinsic Sleep Disorders. Intrinsic Sleep Disorders are important neurophysiologic disturbances that usually come to medical attention because of *excessive daytime sleepiness (EDS)* or, less important, insomnia.

TABLE 17–4. SLEEP DISORDERS[a]

1. Dyssomnias
   A. Intrinsic
      Narcolepsy
      Sleep Apnea Syndrome
      Periodic Limb Movements
      Restless Legs Syndrome
      Hypersomnias
   B. Extrinsic
      Inadequate Sleep Hygiene
      Environmental Sleep Disorder
      Hypnotic-, Stimulant-, Alcohol-, and Toxin-Dependency
   C. Circadian
      Time Zone Change (Jet Lag)
      Shift Work
      Delayed Sleep Phase
2. Parasomnias
   A. Arousal
      Sleep Terrors
      Sleepwalking
   B. Sleep-Wake Transition
      Rhythmic Movement Disorder
      Sleep Talking
   C. Parasomnias with REM Sleep
      Nightmares
      Sleep Paralysis
      REM Sleep Behavior Disorder
   D. Other Parasomnias
      Bruxism
      Enuresis
3. Neurologic/Psychiatric Disorders
   A. Psychiatric
      Psychoses
      Depression
      Alcoholism
   B. Neurologic
      Dementia
      Parkinson's disease
      Epilepsy
      Headaches
   C. Other

[a]Major categories and examples in the classification by the American Sleep Disorders Association, 1991.

NARCOLEPSY. Narcolepsy, the most dramatic of the Intrinsic Disorders, starts in 90 per cent of patients between their adolescence and 25th year, with men and women being affected equally. Its salient feature is EDS that takes the form of brief, irresistible sleep episodes (attacks). Mimicking normal naps, sleep attacks usually occur when patients are bored, comfortable, and engaged in monotonous activities. However, as the disease progresses in some patients, multiple attacks occur daily and take place when patients are standing, having a lively interchange, and engaged in activities that require constant attention, including driving. Attacks can occur 12 to 24 times weekly. Each usually lasts less than 15 minutes, but can be easily interrupted by noise or movement. Despite its brevity, the sleep is refreshing. However, short episodes cause momentary amnesia, confusion, and autonomic behavior.

Secondary symptoms, which develop late in the course of the illness, are manifestations of disordered REM sleep: *cataplexy*, *sleep paralysis*, and *sleep hallucinations*. These symptoms, together with the sleep attacks, form the *narcoleptic tetrad*. However, the more common condition is restricted to a *narcolepsy-cataplexy syndrome*.

Cataplexy consists of episodes, lasting 30 seconds or less, of sudden weakness that can be precipitated by laughter, anger, surprise, fright, or other heightened emotional states. The episodes begin about 4 years after the onset of narcolepsy, can occur one to four times daily, and affect up to 70 per cent of narcolepsy patients. Most often, in symptoms that could easily be dismissed, cataplexy induces only brief periods of weakness that is limited to certain muscles. For example, patients' knees buckle, their jaw drops open, or their head nods. In its most sensational but rare form, patients slump to the floor as their entire body musculature becomes limp. Whether a group of muscles or the entire musculature is involved, affected muscles become flaccid and areflexic; however, patients breathe normally, have full ocular movements, and, unless they have a simultaneous sleep attack, remain alert.

Sleep paralysis and sleep hallucinations, the other symptoms accompanying narcolepsy, affect only about 10 per cent of patients, develop several years after the onset of narcolepsy, and can occur independently. In other words, only 10 per cent of narcolepsy patients have the full narcoleptic tetrad. These symptoms may be present on awakening (hypnopompic) or while falling asleep (hypnagogic). In sleep paralysis, patients are unable to move for several seconds on awakening or when falling asleep, but they can breathe and move their eyes. Similarly, with sleep hallucinations, patients have vivid, dreamlike sensations on awakening or falling asleep. (They qualify as an organic cause of visual hallucinations [see Chapters 9 and 12].) Most important, since clinical features of the narcolepsy tetrad appear as REM sleep and the PSG shows REM-like EEG and EMG activity—low-voltage fast EEG activity and absent EMG activity—it can be envisioned as REM sleep intruding into people's wakefulness (Fig. 17–4).

The standard test for narcolepsy is the *multiple sleep latency test* (*MSLT*). Using PSG recording techniques, the MSLT determines sleep latency and REM latency during four or five "nap opportunities" presented at 2-hour intervals during daytime. Compared to the normal adult sleep latency of 10 to 20 minutes, narcoleptic patients have a sleep latency of 5 minutes or less. Notably, rather than following the normal, preliminary 90 minutes of NREM stages of sleep, REM sleep in narcolepsy characteristically starts immediately or within 10 minutes of falling asleep. These short REM latencies fall into the category of *sleep-onset REM periods* (*SOREMPs*). More than 70 per cent of narcoleptic patients have two or more SOREMPs on their MSLT.

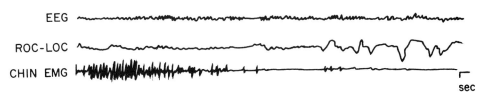

FIGURE 17–4

During the start of a narcoleptic attack, the PSG shows the almost immediate onset of REM sleep accompanied by the loss of (chin) muscle EMG activity. The multiple sleep latency test (MSLT) would show similar, characteristic sleep-onset REM periods (SOREMPs). However, one SOREMP does not make a diagnosis of narcolepsy.

In addition, nighttime sleep in narcolepsy is restless and interrupted by multiple, brief, spontaneous awakenings. Thus, narcolepsy patients' EDS partly reflects their inadequate nighttime sleep.

Narcolepsy undoubtedly rests on a genetic predisposition. Virtually 100 per cent of white and Japanese narcolepsy patients, compared to about 25 per cent of controls, have a certain major histocompatibility complex designated human leukocyte antigen (HLA) DR2, which is located on chromosome 6 (see Appendix 3). This is the closest known link between any illness and an HLA antigen. The DQwl antigen is found almost as often in blacks with narcolepsy. Whereas most cases of narcolepsy are associated with these HLA antigens, some have followed head trauma, multiple sclerosis, or tumors in the diencephalon. Narcolepsy also occurs in ponies and dogs who have been bred in research colonies.

Treatment for narcolepsy and its associated disturbances relies on a combination of stimulants for EDS and REM-suppressing tricyclic antidepressants for cataplexy. Medicines suggested for daytime sleep attacks are pemoline (Cylert), methylphenidate (Ritalin), and amphetamines; for cataplexy, chlorimipramine, imipramine, protriptyline (Vivactil), and possibly fluoxetine; and for nighttime sleep, benzodiazepines, such as triazolam (Halcion). Patients should maintain regular bedtimes, take strategic daytime naps, and avoid potentially dangerous situations.

SLEEP APNEA.   Sleep apnea, one of the most common causes of EDS, is characterized by multiple, 10-second to 2-minute interruptions in breathing (apnea) during sleep that induce partial awakenings. Patients are usually unaware of the awakenings because they are usually brief and incomplete. Nevertheless, they lead to EDS with superimposed, multiple, and, unlike narcolepsy, relatively long, unrefreshing naps.

Sleep apnea includes an *obstructive* and *central* variety. Obstructive sleep apnea is caused by upper airway obstruction usually from thickened soft tissues of the pharynx, congenital cranial deformities, hypertrophied tonsils or adenoids, trauma, and other pharyngeal abnormalities. The central variety, which is rare, results from reduced or absent ventilatory effort, presumably because of an inconsistent central nervous system (CNS) respiratory effort. It has been described in patients with lateral medullary infarctions (see Fig. 2–10), bulbar poliomyelitis, and other injuries to the medulla, which is the site of the respiratory drive. (In the DSM-IV, sleep apnea—at least the central variety—is a prime example of a "Breathing-related sleep disorder.")

Both varieties can result in arterial blood oxygen desaturation (hypoxia), with oxygen saturation as low as 40 per cent, cardiac arrhythmias, and pulmonary and systemic hypertension. Directly or indirectly, sleep apnea causes morning headache and confusion. It also may cause persistent intellectual impairments and depression.

The patients' breathing ceases intermittently during the episodes of sleep apnea. As breathing resumes at the end of an apneic episode, patients have loud, irregular snoring as part of a resuscitative mechanism. Loud snoring, when combined with EDS and irresistible napping, is virtually diagnostic.

Patients are typically but not exclusively middle-aged, hypertensive, and overweight men. Older children, adolescents, and young adults can be affected as well. Even young children who have enlarged tonsils may have sleep apnea. In all age ranges, males are affected much more than females.

The diagnosis of sleep apnea can be confirmed by a PSG that shows periods of apnea, arousals, and hypoxia. In the obstructive variety, air flow is absent despite chest and diaphragm respiratory movements (Fig. 17–5). Because of sleep deprivation, sleep latency is short, REM latency is short, and SOREMPs appear. During the night, episodes of sleep apnea occur in either phase of sleep, but they are more pronounced in REM sleep.

The initial management of this condition, in almost all cases, is to lose weight, stop smoking, and stop using hypnotics and alcohol. Also, if patients refrain from sleeping on their back, their airway tends to remain patent. Ventilation by nasal continuous positive airway pressure (CPAP) will alleviate respiratory impairments, but the device is cumbersome. Insertion of a tongue-retaining device or a small nasopharyngeal tube each night can sometimes secure an airway. In the past, tracheostomies were performed to bypass the pharynx, but now surgeons can perform simpler procedures, such as a uvulopalatopharyngoplasty (UPPP), jaw abnormality correction, or, in children, tonsillectomy. For central sleep apnea, protriptyline or medroxyprogesterone may be useful.

PERIODIC LIMB MOVEMENT DISORDER AND RESTLESS LEG SYNDROME. *Periodic limb movement disorder*, also called *nocturnal myoclonus* or, when confined to the legs, *periodic leg movements*, consists of regular (periodic), episodic movements of the legs or, less often, of the arms during sleep. The movements are most often stereotyped, brief (0.5 to 5.0 seconds), bilateral dorsiflexion movements of the foot, toes, and sometimes the hips. They take place at 20- to 40-second intervals, for periods of 10 minutes to several hours primarily during NREM sleep (Fig. 17–6). Since periodic limb movements continually arouse patients, the disorder, as do narcolepsy and sleep apnea, leads to daytime EDS.

During periodic limb movements, EMG leads show regular muscle contractions that lead to arousals. The disorder usually develops in individuals older than 55 years. It can occur in association with sleep apnea and other sleep disorders, use of antidepressants, withdrawal from various medications, or medical illnesses, such as uremia. Treatment with benzodiazepines or L-dopa may be helpful.

Restless leg syndrome—which also induces leg movements, occurs in the same age group, and leads to EDS and insomnia—consists of unpleasant sen-

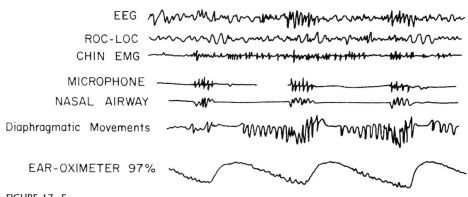

FIGURE 17–5

During sleep apnea the PSG shows that, during a period of NREM sleep, the oxygen saturation falls. Then, as diaphragmatic movements reach a crescendo, loud snoring begins. After strenuous diaphragm movements, air moves through the nasal airway and oxygen saturation improves. During the hypoxic phase, the EEG becomes faster and has higher voltage, which indicates a partial arousal.

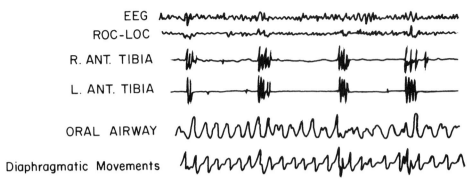

EEG
ROC-LOC
R. ANT. TIBIA
L. ANT. TIBIA
ORAL AIRWAY
Diaphragmatic Movements

FIGURE 17-6

Periodic limb movements, which usually occur during NREM sleep, can be seen in approximately 30-second intervals of synchronous anterior tibialis EMG activity. The muscle contractions dorsiflex the patient's ankles. Until its name was changed, this patient's disorder is easily recognized as the term "periodic leg movements."

sations (dysesthesias or painful paresthesias) in the legs that compel patients to move their legs and feet. The dysesthesias may be present all day, but are worse with prolonged sitting, resting in bed, and especially before sleep. They ordinarily produce a burning feeling, aches, or nonspecific discomforts. Restless leg syndrome may be the result of an autosomal dominant trait in one third of cases, but similar sensations and movements are often a manifestation of peripheral neuropathy induced by diabetes, uremia, or various medications (see Chapter 5). Sometimes the disorder is assocated with pregnancy. The dysesthesias and movements delay the onset of sleep (prolong sleep latency) and interrupt it. No medication is consistently effective, but L-dopa, hypnotics, analgesics, and antidepressants may be helpful.

Both of these disorders are different from the sensation of falling and generalized bodily jerk that affects virtually all people at some time as they "fall" asleep. These movements, *sleep starts*, which are also called *hypnic* or *hypnagogic jerks*, occur in the twilight of sleep, as if REM-like flaccid paralysis jumped into stage 1 or 2 NREM sleep. They are not associated with periodic movements or any illness, but in view of the time of onset, they are considered a "sleep-wake transition disorder parasomnia."

HYPERSOMNIAS.   Several other disorders are also characterized by EDS. The Kleine-Levin syndrome, *periodic hypersomnia*, is a rare sleep disorder in which patients, who are predominantly adolescent males, have lengthy but otherwise normal sleep. Sleep lasts for periods of several days to 2 weeks, three or four times yearly. Patients awaken during these periods to eat great quantities of food and display unusual behavior, typically hypersexuality and irritability. At the same time they are slow, withdrawn, and apathetic. No laboratory abnormality proves that the disorder is clearly "organic."

Encephalitis, brain tumors, hypothalamic injuries, and head trauma (see postconcussive syndrome, Chapter 22) cause EDS. Although these conditions can induce sleepiness, patients often sleep poorly at night, and they have other signs of cerebral dysfunction, such as personality changes and intellectual impairment.

Extrinsic Sleep Disorders.   In this category can be found sleep disorders that result from personal, social, or drug and alcohol-related factors. Removing these factors should restore a normal sleep-wake schedule. Whereas the intrinsic disorders are manifestations of disordered neurophysiology, the extrinsic disorders result from these factors interfering with an otherwise normal brain.

Inadequate Sleep Hygiene comprises insomnia or EDS associated with irregular sleep schedules; use of caffeine, alcohol, and certain medications at night; performing exercise, mental challenging, or anxiety-provoking activities before bed; and engaging in other counterproductive activities. Related conditions, such as an Environmental Sleep Disorder, also result from outside interference with proper, restful sleep. In most of these conditions, the PSG shows prolonged sleep latency, which is the physiologic counterpart of "tossing-and-turning" in bed, frequent arousals, and advanced (early morning) awakening.

Hypnotic-, Stimulant-, Alcohol-, or other Toxin-Dependency is a major cause of both insomnia and EDS. These disorders are defined by the use of various substances for their hypnotic effect, but they exclude frank addiction, such as alcoholism. The PSG, in general, shows a short sleep latency, disrupted sleep, fragmented or suppressed REM phases, and an increased proportion of slow-wave sleep.

Sleep impairment may also be caused by medicines that have unappreciated stimulant effects, such as steroids, aminophylline, or pseudoephedrine (Actifed). The most common stimulant is caffeine. Coffee has 60 to 175 mg of caffeine per cup; tea, 25 to 100 mg; cola drinks, 25 to 60 mg; weight-loss drugs, 100 to 200 mg; and headache medicines, 130 mg in two aspirin-compound tablets. Many Americans easily and often inadvertently ingest so much caffeine (250 to 500 mg per day) that they develop *caffeinism*: insomnia, agitation, tremulousness, palpitations, gastric distress, and diuresis.

When certain medications are withdrawn, patients may initially have insomnia, increased sleep disruption, greater EDS, and psychologic agitation. When finally able to fall asleep, they may have REM rebound—as though their previously suppressed REM sleep were trying to catch up. Abrupt withdrawal from alcohol or barbiturates, especially short-acting ones, may lead to generalized, tonic-clonic seizures and delirium tremens (DTs).

Circadian Rhythm Disorders. Both neurophysiologic and external factors can alter sleep's daily sleep-wake schedule. These factors can create *circadian rhythm disorders*, which were called "sleep-wake schedule disorders" in the DSM-III. The best known example is the *Time Zone Change (Jet Lag) Syndrome*. In this condition, people who rapidly traverse at least two time zones develop insomnia and EDS that are often accompanied by changes in digestion and other autonomic behavior, malaise, and inattentiveness. They may feel as though their mind and body were adhering to the schedule of their city of origin.

Going from east to west is easier because travelers can more easily postpone (delay) their night's sleep than fall asleep earlier (advance it). To reduce the toll, travelers should shift their sleep-wake schedule to their destination city's day-night schedule by adopting it before the trip or immediately accepting it on arrival. On long west-to-east flights, taking a hypnotic will advance the sleep schedule to conform to the new time zone. In either direction, the traveler can facilitate the adjustment by exposure to daylight. (Light is more powerful than noise in entraining people to a time schedule.)

A related cause of insomnia and EDS is *Shift Work Sleep Disorder*. A well-known example is the worker who begins work on a night shift suffering daytime fatigue and inattention, with an inability to fall asleep. Although most workers can make the transition after several days, some may be unsuccessful because their internal schedule is too ingrained or they continue to follow their old schedule on weekends or holidays.

In contrast to the previous disorders that result from outside scheduling, the *Delayed Sleep Phase Syndrome* results from a neurophysiologic delay in falling asleep, i.e., prolonged sleep latency. Because sleep is normal in quality and length, the late hour of sleep postpones the time that they would naturally awaken. Nevertheless, their school, work, or social requirements result in their awakening after insufficiently long sleep.

In a unique "chronotherapy" treatment of the delayed sleep phase syndrome, patients delay their sleep-time by 30 to 180 minutes successively each night. They postpone (further delay) their sleep-onset time—with activities, coffee and other stimulants, and light—by *almost* 24 hours. They eventually fall asleep at an appropriate time, such as 11 PM, and, with effort, maintain that bedtime.

Parasomnias

Behavioral aberrations, the *parasomnias*, orginiate in neurophysiologic dysfunction and intrude into otherwise normal sleep. Parasomnias are usually associated with full or partial arousal, the sleep-wake interface, and NREM sleep. They are not considered sleep disorders, per se—and they are noticeably absent as causes of alterations in sleep and REM latency (Tables 17–2 and 17–3).

Arousal Disorders. One group of parasomnias, which are provoked by arousals during slow-wave sleep, occur overwhelmingly during the first 2 hours of sleep when this phase predominates. They are not manifestations of dreams or REM sleep abnormalities.

An important example is *Confusional Arousals*. This parasomnia consists of disorientation and amnesia when the individual is roused from slow-wave sleep. It is relevant for physicians who are awakened for medical decision making and find that they are confused and, in the morning, unable to recall conversations they held.

SLEEP TERRORS. Completely different from nightmares (see below), sleep terrors in children are episodes in which they suddenly, after a partial or full awakening, behave as though they were in great danger. The children stare, moan, and sometimes speak a few words with their eyes fully open and their pupils dilated. They characteristically sweat, hyperventilate, and have tachycardia. They resist their parents' attempts to wake them up, put them back to sleep, or comfort them. They often leave their parents' arms to walk aimlessly. The terror lasts for several minutes and ends abruptly with a return to deep sleep. Despite the episode's vivid and awesome features, children do not recall it in the morning.

As a reflection of PSG studies showing their occurrence in slow-wave sleep, sleep terrors tend to develop several hours after bedtime and after sleep deprivation. Noises or other disruptions during slow-wave sleep can arouse children and precipitate the episodes. Unlike dreams, sleep terrors are unrelated to frightening events of the day, and no REM activitiy is detectable during the episode. Also, sleep terrors usually take place only a few times a month.

Sleep terrors can be prevented in some children by enforcing an afternoon nap and avoiding sleep disruptions, such as loud noises. Similarly, predisposed children should be limited to a few sips of water at bedtime to avoid awakening to urinate.

SLEEPWALKING.   Sleepwalking (somnambulism) usually consists just of sitting or standing, but can include more complex activities. During a typical episode, children walk slowly, with their eyes open, along familiar pathways. Although they seem to be partially awake, they cannot be aroused fully. When questioned, they are confused, inappropriate, and amnestic.

Both sleep terrors and sleepwalking usually develop in early childhood, affect boys more often than girls, and cease before puberty. Treatment of an episode is not feasible because of its brevity, but when they occur several times a week, prophylactic benzodiazepine or imipramine may be worthwhile. Their impact can be reduced by reassuring the parents that the episodes will cease by themselves and that they do not result from pain, abuse, or emotional disturbance.

Children are liable to have more than one variety of parasomnia and display complex behavior during any of them. Although parasomnias might be confused with a partial complex seizure (see Chapter 10), these seizures tend to be stereotyped, undergo secondary generalization, and be followed by (postictal) confusion. A PSG during a parasomnia or seizure is diagnostic. Parasomnias are not associated with psychiatric disturbances in children. However, when they develop in adults, they can be associated with both psychiatric disturbances and CNS pathology.

Sleep-Wake Transition Disorders.   As people fall asleep, enter stage 1, and then progress through the various sleep stages, they are subject to certain parasomnias. Occasionally the disorders are peculiar to certain stages or transitions.

In one disorder, *Rhythmic Movement Disorder*, infants, children, and occasionally adults have rhythmic, repetitive, stereotyped movements of their head, trunk, or entire body while lying in bed during the initial stages of falling asleep and during daytime naps. The movements usually begin in infancy and disappear by age 5. They usually consist of slow *head banging* on the pillow. However, they can persist into the teenage years and be a relatively violent rocking from side to side or back and forth.

Another example is *Sleep Talking*. The common phenomenon of people "talking" in their sleep is an overstatement because they merely say a few words that are difficult to distinguish. It occurs in adults and children and in all sleep stages. This parasomnia is benign and usually independent of dreams, but can be associated with sleepwalking and REM sleep behavior disturbance (see below).

Parasomnias with REM Sleep

NIGHTMARES.   In contrast to sleep terrors, *nightmares* are essentially dreams that have a frightening content, i.e., "bad dreams." They contain complex imagery that the dreamer is able to recall when awakened during the nightmare or on arising in the morning. Nightmares are usually unaccompanied by any bodily movement other than mild tachycardia or other autonomic response, or vocalizations except for crying. Often a nightmare ends by itself, or it can be interrupted by awakening the dreamer. After becoming fully awake, the dreamer has a slow, difficult return to sleep.

Unlike sleep terrors, nightmares occur during REM periods. They may be precipitated by certain medications, such as L-dopa, as well as by emotional factors. Nightmares often develop when REM activity is increased, such as after sleep deprivation, alcohol withdrawal, and discontinuing medications. Therefore, evaluation of frequent nightmares would include exploring not only the circumstances and content of the dreams but also the potential abuse of medications, alcohol, and drugs.

REM SLEEP BEHAVIOR DISORDER. During normal REM sleep, even during nightmares, the bodily musculature is motionless, flaccid, and areflexic. The immobility seems to protect people from participating in their dreams. In comparison, in the *REM Sleep Behavior Disorder*, the normal immobility and flaccidity are lost. People with this disorder, who are usually men older than 65 years, thrash, hit, and make running movements during REM sleep. They are potentially injurious to themselves and their bed partner.

The violent motor activity seems to result from people "acting out" dreams. In contrast to normal REM sleep, their muscles have tone and strength. The disorder is associated with lacunar infarcts of the brain and with REM rebound, especially from medication withdrawal. Clonazepam is an effective treatment.

Other Parasomnias

BRUXISM. Sleep-related, stereotyped, forceful teeth grinding or clenching, *bruxism*, is a parasomnia; however, it is also associated with dementia, mental retardation, and Parkinson's disease. Although bruxism occurs in all sleep stages, it occurs mainly in the transition from wakefulness to sleep and during light sleep. Bruxism makes a loud, disconcerting sound and leads to wearing away of teeth, headaches, and temporomandibular joint dysfunction. Nighttime dental devices are helpful.

ENURESIS. Bed-wetting (enuresis) is considered a parasomnia in children older than 5 years and in all adults. Like bruxism, it is not restricted to a particular sleep stage or transition. Enuresis occurs mostly in slow-wave sleep during the first third of the night. Boys are affected more than girls. In children and some adults, enuresis can be treated with imipramine or by behavior modification therapy devices, such as ones that complete a low-voltage electric circuit to "alert" a child who wets the bed.

In adults, enuresis can result not only from a parasomnia but also from a variety of neurologic and urologic conditions. For example, it can result from degenerative cerebral disease and thus can be associated with dementia. In addition, it can be the residue of a seizure. Also, nighttime incontinence can result from spinal cord damage, as with multiple sclerosis; cauda equina injuries, as with meningomyeloceles; and autonomic nervous system damage, as with diabetes.

Neurologic/Psychiatric Disorders

Psychiatric Disorders. *Schizophrenia*, schizophreniform disorder, and other functional psychoses are associated with both insomnia and EDS. However, probably because of the diverse nature of psychiatric illnesses, fluctuations in their activity and severity, and patients' exposure to antipsychotic medications, PSGs are inconsistent. PSG results often overlap with normal values and are too variable to serve as a biologic marker. Nevertheless, in acute schizophrenia, the PSG generally shows a decreased total sleep time, increased sleep latency, and frequent, long awakenings that reflect restlessness ("decreased sleep efficiency"). It also shows normal or slightly reduced REM sleep. Patients with chronic schizophrenia, in contrast, have essentially normal sleep patterns and, interestingly, can distinguish their dreams from hallucinations.

Depression, also associated with insomnia and EDS, has characteristic, but not diagnostic REM abnormalities. A typically short REM latency (less than 60 minutes) is followed by an abnormally long, intense REM period. Subsequent REM periods occur in relatively quick succession, leaving the latter half of the night virtually devoid of REM sleep. Although the total amount of REM sleep is about the same as in normal individuals, the reduction in total sleep time is extracted from slow-wave sleep. In *mania*, sleep latency can be excessive (seemingly infinite), REM sleep can be abolished, and total sleep time can be reduced markedly.

In addition, depressed individuals have neuroendocrine abnormalities related to their sleep stage abnormalities. Their body temperature nadir occurs several hours earlier than normal. Likewise, they have an earlier excretion of cortisol and the norepinephrine metabolite MHPG. Overall, the earlier onset of so many features of sleep—the first REM period, the bulk of REM sleep, the temperature nadir, and nocturnal hormone excretion—is the result of the forward movement of the normal circadian rhythm called a *phase-shift advance.* When depressed people fall asleep, they seem to skip into the middle of the normal sleep and neuroendocrine cycle. This perspective is consistent with a briefly effective treatment of depression being one night of sleep deprivation and phase advancing by 3 to 5 hours.

Alcoholism is also associated with insomnia and EDS. The clinical and PSG data are variable. In the first half of the night, alcoholic individuals generally have a short sleep latency, less REM sleep, and increased slow-wave sleep, as though they were collapsing into stupor. In the second half, they have increased REM and periods of wakefulness, as though they emerged into delirium. The net effect is decreased total and slow-wave sleep. Alcohol withdrawal, which is similar to withdrawal from other hypnotic substances, leads to insomnia and REM rebound.

Neurologic Disorders

DEMENTIA.   Dementia (see Chapter 7), at least in its moderate stages, disrupts patient's sleep-wake cycle and produces nighttime thought and behavioral disturbances. During the night, patients tend to become confused, agitated, and disoriented, especially in new surroundings. They wander about the house and may actually leave it. PSGs show increased stage 1 NREM sleep, fragmentations, and decreased efficiency. Despite the prediction that decreased cholinergic activity in Alzheimer's disease would lead to decreased and delayed REM activity, the PSGs do not correlate with that pattern. Moreover, PSGs do not correlate with Alzheimer's disease or other etiologies of dementia.

PARKINSON'S DISEASE AND OTHER MOVEMENT DISORDERS.   During the night, the physical problems of *Parkinson's disease* (see Chapter 18—tremor, rigidity, and bradykinesia—are characteristically absent during sleep; however, its mental features are prominent. A combination of dementia and side effects from L-dopa and other medications induces nighttime hallucinations and physical agitation. These symptoms are the most troublesome aspect of the illness for the patient's family and the commonest reason for transferring the patient to a nursing home. These mental aberrations may be related to dopamine receptor and locus ceruleus abnormalities.

Reducing the number and dosage of medications and administering them earlier in the evening may be helpful; however, that strategy may worsen the physical problems in the morning and possibly for the entire day. Similarly, common neuroleptics reduce nighttime hallucinations and agitation, but they also worsen the physical symptoms and lead to sedation. Clozapine may be a superior medication, but not a panacea, compared to other neuroleptics for this dilemma. Hypnotics have a limited role.

Although other basal ganglia-related involuntary movement disorders, such as athetosis and chorea, also disappear during sleep, several involuntary movements persist or are even induced by sleep. Most of them appear in no particular stage and have no demonstrable cause. Those that are primarily or exclusively sleep related include periodic limb movements, restless leg syndrome, and hypnic jerks (see above). Those that are commonly seen during the day, but continue in sleep especially during partial arousals, are tics, palatal myoclonus, generalized dystonia, and focal dystonias, including blepharospasm and hemifacial spasm.

EPILEPSY.   Some seizures occur primarily or exclusively in sleep (see Chapter 10). For example, about 45 per cent of patients with primary generalized epilepsy have seizures predominantly during sleep. Primary generalized seizures develop within stages 1 and 2 of NREM sleep, which occurs during the first 2 hours of sleep and on awakening. Although partial seizures also appear during sleep, they occur more frequently during the daytime and, when they occur at night, are less restricted to NREM sleep.

Moreover, sleep deprivation precipitates seizures in susceptible patients. Obtaining an EEG after enforced sleep deprivation elicits sharp waves and a variety of spike-and-sharp wave activity in more than one third of epileptic patients who have no such abnormalities on routine EEGs.

Among their many actions, anticonvulsants promote normal sleep. They raise the efficiency of sleep by reducing arousals and increasing slow-wave sleep. On the other hand, even at therapeutic blood concentrations, anticonvulsants can lead to EDS.

HEADACHES.   Another neurologic disorder clearly associated with sleep is vascular headaches (see Chapter 9). Migraines and, even more so, cluster headaches seem to be precipitated by REM phases. In some people, these headaches appear only during REM periods, but in most, they begin during early morning intense REM sleep and continue after awakening. Thus, excessive sleep or other conditions that increase REM sleep are associated with headaches. As would be predicted, medications that suppress REM sleep reduce headaches.

OTHER DISORDERS.   Of the various medical conditions that are precipitated by sleep, cardiovascular disorders are the most important. Angina pectoris and myocardial infarctions take place much more often during REM sleep, when pulse and blood pressure are often elevated and erratic, than during NREM sleep. Thrombotic cerebrovascular accidents (CVAs) are more frequent during NREM sleep and are thus found disproportionately on awakening. Those CVAs, but not cerebral hemorrhages, occur during NREM, when pulse and blood pressure are relatively low.

Attacks of asthma, exacerbation of chronic obstructive lung disease, gastroesophageal reflux, and peptic ulcer disease tend to develop during sleep. Some of the problems may be related to the patient's position, but the attacks occur with equal frequency in either sleep phase. All of these nighttime disturbances interrupt sleep and lead to EDS.

INSOMNIA

The traditional problem of insomnia—an inability to fall asleep or to remain asleep—is a nonspecific symptom common to many sleep disorders in the new classification. Insomnia is also prevalent in certain groups: people with medical and neurologic illnesses, drug and alcohol abuse, psychiatric disorders, and those older than 65 years. Nevertheless, with many people complaining of insomnia, PSGs show a normal pattern and duration of sleep. This discrepancy may indicate a psychologic disturbance that can approach a delusion.

When true insomnia is induced by a transient disturbance, such as grief, it may respond to a limited course of sleeping pills (hypnotics). However, hypnotics are rarely effective if taken for longer than one month. Patients with sleep apnea and certain respiratory problems may retain CO_2 if they are sedated. Also, the elderly, who are prone to insomnia, unadvisedly take inordinate quantities of both prescription and over-the-counter hypnotics and become psychologically if not physically dependent on them. In particular, when people with Alzheimer's disease and many other neurologic illnesses take hypnotics, instead of being sedated, they may, in a "paradoxical reaction," develop agitation and other mental aberrations.

Nonprescription hypnotics are less effective and potentially more hazardous than prescription hypnotics. For example, antihistamines can produce delirium, mental aberrations, and dystonic reactions. Alcohol may cause an initial sleep that is stuporous and then REM rebound with early awakening. Tryptophan, which may be the "active ingredient" in warm milk, is not proven to be an effective hypnotic, and contaminated tryptophan pills may have caused the eosinophilia-myalgia syndrome (see Chapter 6).

Despite potential complications, benzodiazepines are effective and the mainstay of treatment. They increase total sleep time and reduce fragmentation. Surprisingly, the total sleep increase is only about 10 per cent, and they decrease valuable slow-wave NREM sleep. Depending on their duration of action and if the patient is elderly, benzodiazepines can cause anterograde amnesia, insomnia in the early morning, daytime anxiety, EDS, and psychomotor impairments. They have been linked to a tendency to hip fractures from falls and, in extreme cases, withdrawal seizures.

REFERRAL FOR A POLYSOMNOGRAM

In evaluating most patients who have sleep disorders, a thorough medical-psychiatric evaluation should be sufficient (Table 17–5). Physicians must accept restrictions in referring patients for a polysomnogram (PSG). It is useful in few disorders, and it is expensive. As a general rule, a PSG is not cost effective in evaluating patients with insomnia unless it is treatment resistant, induces mental aberrations, associated with sleep apnea, or endangers health.

On the other hand, a PSG will provide a diagnosis, confirm a clinical impression, justify surgery, or indicate a prescription of potent medications in the following disorders: sleep apnea syndrome, narcolepsy-cataplexy, REM behavior disorder, periodic limb movements, and parasomnias that are potentially injurious. Also, it is useful for detecting neurologic disorders that develop exclusively during sleep, such as seizures.

Alternatively, a preliminary, inexpensive screening procedure that might be diagnostic of some of these disorders is to make a home videotape of several nights' sleep with a luminescent clock in the background. Many elements can then be detected: sleep times and awakenings, random or periodic jaw or limb movements, seizures, snoring, apnea, many parasomnias, and nightmares. (Similarly, home videotaping is especially helpful in children suspected of having episodic movement disorders, seizures, tics, or behavioral disturbances. Home cameras are sufficient because they are quiet, inconspicuous, and can record for 8 hours under low light conditions.)

TABLE 17–5.   SALIENT HISTORICAL FEATURES OF PATIENTS WITH INSOMNIA AND OTHER SLEEP DISORDERS[a]

A.   Nighttime sleep
   1.   What are the usual times that you try to fall asleep, actually fall asleep, and awaken?
   2.   Do you awaken during the night? How often? How long? What do you do when awake?
   3.   When asleep, do you have any of the following interruptions?
     Nightmares or night terrors, sleepwalking, bed-wetting
     Loud or irregular snoring
     Cessation of breathing
     Restless or painful legs
     Leg or other limb movements
     Headaches, chest pain, or other medical symptoms
   4.   Was the nighttime sleep restful?
B.   Daytime sleep
   1.   Do you take afternoon or evening naps?
     Are they restful?
     Are they irresistible?
     Do they occur at inappropriate times?
   2.   Do you lose bodily tone or have episodic muscle weakness?
     Do you suddenly weaken, especially after laughter or excitement?
     Does a single muscle group, such as those in the jaw or knees, suddenly weaken?
C. If left to your own schedule:
   1.   Would you be more alert in the morning or night?
   2.   How much sleep would you get?
D.   General health
   1.   Do you suffer from medical, neurologic, or psychiatric illness?
   2.   Do you take any prescription or over-the-counter medications or drugs?
   3.   Do you use alcohol?
   4.   Do you use coffee or other caffeine-containing beverage?

[a]A reliable history may be obtained only from a bed partner who, as in other conditions, may be suffering more than the patient.

The usefulness of the MSLT is confined to confirming disorders of EDS, particularly narcolepsy where it shows SOREMPs. The expense is justifiable because of the amphetamines and other powerful medications used to treat the disorder. An MSLT may also confirm EDS induced by sleep apnea and periodic limb movements, but those diagnoses rest on PSG findings.

REFERENCES

Abramowicz M (ed): Oral hypnotic drugs. Med Lett *31*: 23–24, 1989
Albarede JL, Morley JE, Roth T, et al (eds): Sleep Disorders and Insomnia in the Elderly. New York, Springer Publishing, 1993
Aldrich MS: Narcolepsy. Neurology *42* (suppl 6): 34–43, 1992
Alvarez B, Dahitz, Vignau J, et al: The delayed sleep phase syndrome. J Neurol Neurosurg Psychiatry *55*: 665–670, 1992
American Sleep Disorders Association: The International Classification of Sleep Disorders Diagnostic and Coding Manual. Rochester, MN, American Sleep Disorders Association, 1990
Askenasy JJ: Sleep in Parkinson's disease. Acta Neurol Scand *87*: 167–170, 1993
Culebras A: The neurology of sleep. Neurology *42* (suppl): 6–8, 1992
DiMario FJ, Emery ES: The natural history of night terrors. Ann Neurol *20*: 440, 1986
Fish DR, Sawyers D, Allen PJ, et al: The effect of sleep on the dyskinetic movements of Parkinson's disease, Gilles de la Tourette syndrome, Huntington's disease, and torsion dystonia. Arch Neurol *48*: 210–214, 1991
Gillen JC, Byerley WF: The diagnosis and management of insomnia. N Engl J Med *322*: 239–248, 1990
Kavey NB, Whyte J, Resor SR, et al: Somnambulism in adults. Neurology *40*: 749–752, 1990
Moore-Ede MC, Czeisler CA, Richardson GS: Circadian time keeping in health and disease. N Engl J Med *309*: 469, 530, 1983
Prinz PN, Vitiello MV, Raskind MA, et al: Geriatrics: Sleep disorders and aging. N Engl J Med *323*: 52–526, 1990

Silvestri R, Domenico PD, DiRosa AE, et al: The effect of nocturnal physiological sleep on various movement disorders. Movement Dis 5: 8–14, 1990

Walters AS, Hening WA, Chokroverty S: Review and videotape recognition of idiopathic restless legs syndrome. Movement Dis 6: 105–110, 1991

QUESTIONS and ANSWERS: CHAPTER 17

1–15. Is the statement true or false?

1. Normal sleep begins with the first stage of NREM sleep and progresses through the four NREM stages before the first period of REM sleep occurs.

answer: True

2. Since REM sleep usually begins about 90 to 120 minutes after the onset of sleep, normal REM latency is 90 to 120 minutes.

answer: True

3. The bulk of REM sleep occurs in the early evening, whereas the bulk of NREM sleep occurs in the early morning.

answer: False

4. The normal sequence of NREM-REM sleep recurs with a periodicity of about 90 minutes.

answer: True

5. REM sleep is a period of decreased physical and mental activity.

answer: False

6. Stages 3 and 4 of NREM sleep, which are called slow-wave, delta, or deep sleep, provide great physical restfulness.

answer: True

7. Sleep always begins with stage 1 of NREM sleep.

answer: False

8. Aside from the artifact caused by eye movement, the REM sleep EEG is similar to the one found in wakefulness.

answer: True

9. The EEG during NREM sleep is characterized by slow activity.

answer: True

10. In general, the proportion of REM sleep remains constant from birth to old age.

answer: False

11. Most people's sleep-wake schedules are determined by social and occupational factors, rather than by internal, physiologic mechanisms.

answer: True

12. NREM sleep increases with increasing age.

answer: False

13. Some productive, vigorous, and well-rested people sleep as little as 5 hours nightly.

answer: True

14. When a daily activity, such as falling asleep, tends to occur earlier in the cycle, the change in time is said to be a phase advance.

   answer: True

15. Infant boys have penile erections during REM sleep.

   answer: True

16. In the night after sleep deprivation, which of the following can be expected to occur?
   a. Sleep may begin with a period of REM activity.
   b. Epileptiform discharges may emanate from the temporal lobe of patients with partial complex (psychomotor) seizures.
   c. Total sleep time will increase.
   d. There will be an increase in time spent in REM sleep.
   e. Stages 1 and 2 of NREM sleep will increase more than slow-wave sleep.

   answer: a, b, c, d

17–24. Which of the following characteristics are associated with (a) sleep terrors, (b) nightmares, (c) both, or (d) neither?

17. Onset during stages 1 and 2 of NREM sleep

   answer: d

18. Onset during slow-wave sleep

   answer: a

19. Onset during REM sleep

   answer: b

20. A variety of common dreams, albeit "bad" ones

   answer: b

21. Amnesia for content

   answer: a

22. May be precipitated by loud noises during first NREM period

   answer: a

23. Cannot be interrupted

   answer: a

24. Associated with somnambulism

   answer: a

25–42. Which of the following phenomena typically occur during (a) REM sleep, (b) NREM sleep, (c) either phase, or (d) neither phase?

25. Sleepwalking (somnambulism)

   answer: b

26. Areflexic DTRs

   answer: a

27. EEG delta waves

   answer: b

28.   Bed-wetting (enuresis)

   answer: b

29.   Sleep terrors

   answer: b

30.   Cluster headache

   answer: a

31.   REM sleep behavior

   answer: a

32.   Migraine headache

   answer: a

33.   Nightmares

   answer: a

34.   Bruxism

   answer: c

35.   Restless leg movements

   answer: c

36.   Parkinson tremor

   answer: d

37.   Muscular contraction (tension) headaches

   answer: d

38.   Hemiballismus

   answer: d

39.   Body repositioning

   answer: b

40.   Tics

   answer: c

41.   Low-voltage, fast EEG activity

   answer: b

42.   Head banging

   answer: c

43–47.   Is each statement true or false?

43.   Narcolepsy typically begins in middle age when normal afternoon fatigue becomes prominent.

   answer: False. About 90 per cent of cases develop between adolescence and age 25 years.

44.   Sleep apnea is a disorder only of adults.

   answer: False. Children and teenagers, especially ones with nasopharyngeal abnormalities, have the illness.

45. Sleep apnea is associated with morning headaches and cardiovascular disorders.

answer: True

46. Sleep apnea sometimes leads to cognitive impairments and poor school performance.

answer: True

47. Hypnopompic refers to phenomena that occur on awakening, and hypnagogic refers to phenomena that occur on falling asleep.

answer: True

48. With which of the following is narcolepsy associated?

a. Cataplexy
b. Hallucinations

c. Sleep paralysis
d. Sleep-onset REM

answer: a, b, c, d

49. A 27-year-old woman had the onset over 48 hours earlier of lethargy, fever, temporal lobe seizures, and lymphocytic pleocytosis of the CSF. Which of the following illnesses is most likely?

a. Hypothyroidism
b. Schizophrenia

c. *Herpes simplex encephalitis*
d. Metastatic carcinoma

answer: c. *H. simplex* is the most common cause of nonepidemic encephalitis, which often causes sleepiness or lethargy as its first symptom.

50. At what time of the day is sleep latency the shortest?

a. 11:00 AM
b. 1:00 PM

c. 4:00 PM
d. 11:00 PM

answer: c

51. Which characteristic(s) is (are) common to the sleep patterns seen in depression and after sleep deprivation?

a. Increased sleep latency
b. Shortened REM latency

c. Sleep terrors
d. Interruptions in sleep

answer: b

52. Which conditions are characterized by short sleep latency?

a. Alcohol- and drug-induced sleep
b. Narcolepsy
c. Sleep apnea

d. Sleep deprivation
e. Depression
f. Delayed phase syndrome

answer: a, b, c, d

53. Which conditions are associated with sleep-onset REM periods (SOREMPs)?

a. Restless leg syndrome
b. Alcohol and hypnotic withdrawal
c. Depression
d. Narcolepsy

e. Sleep apnea
f. Sleep deprivation
g. Periodic leg movements
h. Alcohol-induced sleep

answer: b, c, d, e, f

54. With which physiologic changes are REM sleep associated?

a. Absent respirations
b. Lower pulse and blood pressure
c. Increased intracranial pressure

d. High-voltage, slow EEG activity
e. Absent limb and chin EMG activity
f. Penile erections

answer: c, e, f

55. In depressed patients, which of the following are typical?

a. Delay in the nighttime body temperature nadir
b. Advance of REM activity
c. Advance of cortisol excretions
d. Delay in MHPG excretion

answer: b, c

56. What are the consequences of alcohol withdrawal?

a. Hallucinations
b. Excessive dreaming
c. Increased REM sleep
d. Tendency to have seizures
e. Insomnia

answer: a, b, c, d, e

57. Which of the following conditions often begin before 25 years of age?

a. Delayed sleep phase syndrome
b. Head banging
c. Kleine-Levin syndrome
d. Sleep apnea syndrome
e. Narcolepsy
f. REM behavior disorder

answer: a, b, c, e

58. Which of the following are effective treatments for the delayed sleep phase syndrome?

a. Continually advancing the bedtime
b. Continually delaying the bedtime
c. Light therapy (phototherapy)
d. Stimulants

answer: b, c

59. In which conditions will the MSLT show SOREMPs?

a. Nightmares
b. Sleep terrors
c. Narcolepsy
d. Sleep apnea
e. REM sleep disorder

answer: c, d

60. Which factor(s) determine most people's sleep schedule?

a. Early learning
b. Social and occupational demands
c. Endocrine excretions
d. Personality type
e. Physiologic "clocks"

answer: b

61. What are the possible effects of withdrawal from medications that have hypnotic effects?

a. Insomnia
b. Excessive daytime sleepiness
c. REM rebound
d. Heightened awareness
e. Vivid dreams
f. Seizures

answer: a, b, c, d, e, f

62. Almost all narcolepsy patients have the major histocompatibility complex antigen HLA DR$_2$. Which one of the following statements regarding this finding is *false*?

a. It indicates that narcolepsy has a genetic etiology.
b. The short arm of the chromosome 6 is implicated.
c. Almost all people with this antigen have narcolepsy.
d. Multiple sclerosis patients also have significantly increased proportion of certain HLA antigens.
e. The association is one of the closest in medicine.

answer: c

63. Which of the following conditions are associated with increased sleep latency?

a. Delayed phase syndrome
b. Inadequate sleep hygiene
c. Certain psychiatric disorders
d. Narcolepsy
e. Restless leg syndrome

answer: a, b, c, e

64. In which conditions do people involuntarily grind their teeth in a loud, noisy, and continuous fashion?

a. Meige's syndrome
b. Mental retardation
c. A parasomnia, bruxism
d. Parkinson's disease

answer: b, c, d

65. Which are the beneficial effects of benzodiazepines?

a. Increase in total sleep time of 10 per cent
b. Increase in total sleep time of 30 per cent
c. Increase in total sleep time of 50 per cent or more
d. Reduced fragmentation
e. Increase in slow-wave NREM sleep

answer: a, d

66. Which are the side effects of benzodiazepines?

a. Hip fractures from an increased tendency to fall
b. Anterograde amnesia
c. With long-acting preparations, daytime sleepiness
d. With short-acting preparations, insomnia in the morning and daytime anxiety
e. Lowered seizure threshold
f. Further impairment of sleep apnea syndrome and chronic obstructive lung disease

answer: a, b, c, d, f

67. For which conditions is routinely obtaining a PSG appropriate?

a. Sleep apnea syndrome
b. Narcolepsy
c. Insomnia
d. Restless leg syndrome
e. Alcohol-induced insomnia
f. REM behavior disorder
g. Periodic limb movements
h. Exclusively nocturnal epilepsy
i. Nocturnal migraines

answer: a, b, f, g, h

68. A 36-year-old man moved into town 2 weeks ago. He complains that several months ago he began to develop irresistible sleep episodes even though he was in dangerous positions, sudden collapse, and experienced paralysis and hallucinations when awakening. He requests a refill of his amphetamine prescription until he can find a new sleep disorder specialist. The medicine was exhausted since he moved, and all of his symptoms have reached crisis proportions. What should be the next step?

a. Refill the amphetamine prescription.
b. Refer him to a sleep specialist.
c. Order urine testing for amphetamine metabolites.
d. Order HLA testing.

answer: All or any one of the choices is appropriate. However, the diagnosis of narcolepsy-cataplexy is unlikely because he is relatively old to have just developed the entire constellation of the tetrad. Narcolepsy usually begins in the late teens or early twenties, and then, beginning with cataplexy, the other symptoms develop over the next 5 to 10 years. Amphetamine addicts tend to list all the symptoms and indicate that the situation is dire.

69. By what age do children usually give up daytime naps?

a. 3 years
b. 5 years
c. 7 years
d. 9 years

answer: b

70. By what age do children usually control their bladder during the night?

a. 3 years
b. 5 years
c. 7 years
d. 9 years

answer: b. Children usually stop wetting their bed between ages 2 and 4 years. The best treatment for those who continue, assuming they have no neurologic or psychiatric abnormalities, is behavioral therapy.

71. Which of the following disorders interfere with falling asleep, but do not interrupt sleep once it begins?

a. Delayed sleep phase syndrome
b. Sleep apnea
c. Alcohol abuse
d. Seizures
e. Night terrors

answer: a. This disorder is relatively common in young adults.

18 Involuntary Movement Disorders

The involuntary movement disorders consist of a group of conditions, rather than specific illnesses. For example, tremor can be caused by several different illnesses. These disorders are important because many occur frequently, provide instructive clinical-anatomic correlations, and can be induced by psychiatric medications. Moreover, dementia and depression are closely associated with several disorders and may precede or overshadow the movements. On the other hand, certain disorders cause extraordinary physical disabilities, but little or no mental disturbances.

This chapter briefly reviews the anatomy and physiology of the basal ganglia, which are the basis of most movement disorders. It then describes the common classic disorders that are attributable to basal ganglia abnormalities: Parkinson's disease, athetosis, chorea, hemiballismus, Wilson's disease, and dystonia. Next, it describes disorders that do not conform to classic patterns and for which the origins are not definitely known: focal dystonias, tremors, tics, Tourette's syndrome, and myoclonus. It concludes with a review of neuroleptic-induced and psychogenic conditions.

Several themes run through the discussions of the various movement disorders.

- The diagnosis of many conditions remains entirely clinical because laboratory confirmation is possible only in certain illnesses. As with neurocutaneous disorders, the diagnosis of these disorders rests on a "diagnosis by inspection."
- Certain involuntary movement disorders are accompanied by dementia.
- Certain involuntary movement disorders are inherited.

THE BASAL GANGLIA

The basal ganglia are essentially composed of five subcortical, macroscopic nuclei (Figs. 18–1 and 18–2):

- the *caudate nucleus* and the *putamen*, which constitute the *corpus striatum (striatum)*
- the *globus pallidus*
- the *subthalamic nucleus* (*corpus of Luysii*)
- the *substantia nigra*

Intricate tracts link the basal ganglia to each other and to thalamic nuclei, conjugate oculomotor circuits, and the frontal lobe. Projections from the basal ganglia constitute the *extrapyramidal tract*, which is complementary to the

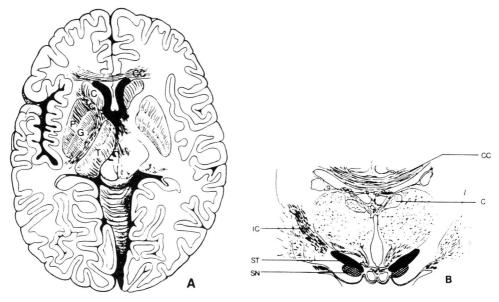

FIGURE 18–1

A, In this axial view, which is the plane shown in CT and MRI studies, the basal ganglia can be seen in relation to the brain. The heads of the caudate nuclei (C) indent the anterior horns of the lateral ventricles. The caudate and putamen (P) are considered the *corpus striatum* or *striatum.* The globus pallidus (G) and putamen (P) form the *lenticular nucleus,* named for its resemblance to an old-fashioned lens. The lenticular nucleus is separated from the thalamus (T) by the posterior limb of the internal capsule (IC). *B,* In this coronal view of the diencephalon, the substantia nigra (SN) and the subthalamic nuclei (ST) are below the thalamus. In fresh specimens, all the nuclei are large enough to be readily identified, and the substantia nigra is black.

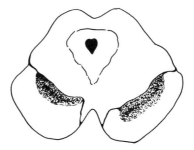

FIGURE 18–2

The midbrain, which lies just caudal to the diencephalon (see Fig. 18–1B), contains the prominent pair of elongated, pigmented substantia nigra (*stippled*). In Parkinson's disease, these and other pigmented nuclei lose their pigment. The midbrain also contains the prominent aqueduct of Sylvius, which is surrounded by the periaqueductal gray matter and the dorsal raphe nucleus (site of serotonin activity, see Chapter 21).

The aqueduct appears as an inverted, midline triangle in the superior portion. Cerebrospinal fluid (CSF) passes from the third ventricle, through the aqueduct, and to the fourth ventricle. The periaqueductal gray matter is subject to microscopic hemorrhages in the Wernicke-Korsakoff syndrome.

pyramidal or corticospinal *tract* (see Chapter 2). Although both tracts are intimately involved with motor activity, the extrapyramidal tract influences the corticospinal tract only indirectly—through the thalamus. Also, the extrapyramidal tract is confined to the brain and does not descend into the spinal cord.

Of the various basal ganglia tracts, the most important one, from a clinical viewpoint, is the *nigrostriatal tract* (Fig. 18–3). This tract extends from the substantia nigra to the corpus striatum (striatum) and provides dopamine innervation. Its function is impaired by Parkinson's disease, psychiatric illness, and exposure to various medications and illicit drugs.

While the pyramidal tract generates voluntary movements, the extrapyramidal tract helps select, inhibit, and sequence complex movements. It maintains appropriate muscle tone and adjusts posture. As in other injuries of the brain (except for ones in the cerebellum), unilateral injuries of the basal ganglia induce clinical abnormalities in the contralateral limbs. In most cases, basal ganglia injuries produce involuntary movements, rigidity or other abnormality in muscle tone, impaired postural reflexes, and slowed or absent movement (*bradykinesia* or *akinesia*).

GENERAL CONSIDERATIONS

The involuntary movement disorders have several common clinical features. The movements are increased by anxiety, exertion, fatigue, and stimulants, including caffeine. They can be momentarily suppressed by intense concentration. Also, they are decreased by relaxation and, in some cases, by

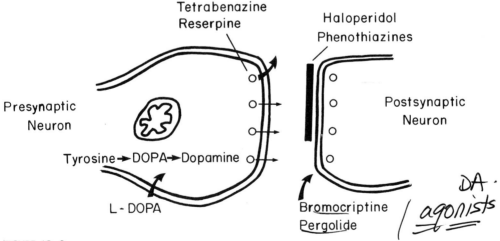

FIGURE 18–3

In the presynaptic neuron, tyrosine is metabolized to dopa and then to the neurotransmitter dopamine. In Parkinson's disease, the absence of tyrosine hydroxylase results in insufficient dopa and then a marked reduction in dopamine. Although D-dopa does not cross the blood-brain barrier, L-dopa (levodopa), which is given as an oral medication, will penetrate the barrier and substitute for endogenous dopa in dopamine production. Dopamine can be depleted from its presynaptic sites by reserpine and by tetrabenazine, an experimental drug in the United States.

A similar, but weaker, dopamine-like effect on the postsynaptic neuron can be mimicked by agonists, such as bromocriptine and pergolide, that act directly on postsynaptic dopamine receptors. The dopamine receptors, which have several subsets, are blocked specifically or generally by many neuroleptics.

biofeedback. With a few exceptions—myoclonus, tics, focal dystonias, and specific sleep-related disorders (see Chapter 17)—they are absent during sleep.

[handwritten margin note: except: • myocleonus • tics • focal dyston]

In many disorders, when only extrapyramidal damage occurs, patients have neither signs of pyramidal (corticospinal) tract damage—paresis, spasticity, hyperactive reflexes, and Babinski signs—nor signs of cerebral cortex damage (dementia and seizures). Patients may be debilitated by uncontrollable movements and inarticulate speech, but they remain fully alert, intelligent, and, possibly by using unconventional means, able to communicate.

Another important consideration is that patients with movement disorders are liable to be misdiagnosed as having psychogenic disorders (see below and Chapter 3). The error is usually made when the movements are bizarre; apparent only during anxiety; absent during sleep; or suppressed by concentration, hypnosis, or amobarbital. An erroneous diagnosis is especially apt to occur when dementia is a component of the illness, in which case both the movements and dementia may appear psychogenic.

PARKINSON'S DISEASE

There are three cardinal features of Parkinson's disease:

- tremor
- rigidity
- bradykinesia

The initial and ultimately most debilitating physical feature of Parkinson's disease is akinesia or bradykinesia. The poverty of movement results in the classic *masked face* (Fig. 18–4), paucity of trunk and limb movement (Figs. 18–5 and 18–6), and impairment of activities of daily living, including eating, dressing, and bathing.

It is usually accompanied by *cogwheel rigidity* (Fig. 18–7). Although rigidity may also be found in other extrapyramidal disorders, it should not be confused with spasticity, which is a sign of corticospinal tract disease (see Chapter 2).

The Parkinson's disease tremor is usually the most conspicuous feature of the illness; however, it is the least incapacitating and least associated with dementia. The tremor has a regular rate and primarily involves the hands and

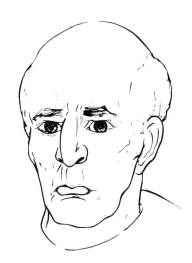

FIGURE 18–4

The facial akinesia of Parkinson's disease patients is characterized by decreased blinking and facial expression. In addition, their widened palpebral fissures and lack of head motion give them a "stare." This facial appearance has been called a "masked facies," a Latin term for "face" or "countenance," but the term *masked face* is becoming more widely used.

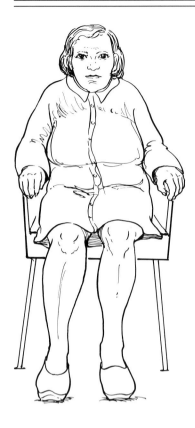

FIGURE 18–5

Parkinson's disease patients typically sit motionless with their legs uncrossed and their feet flat. Their arms, which are rarely used for gesturing, remain on the chair or in their lap. In contrast to normal individuals and those with chorea, Parkinson's disease patients do not shift their weight from one hip to another or make any unnecessary movements.

feet. Because the tremor is most evident when patients sit quietly with their arms supported, it is called a *resting tremor* (Fig. 18–8). This tremor differs from cerebellar tremor (see Fig. 2–11) and essential tremor.

In Parkinson's disease, as opposed to medication-induced movement disorders, tremor, rigidity, and bradykinesia typically develop in an asymmetric or unilateral pattern—*hemiparkinsonism*—for years before they appear bilaterally. Even when Parkinson's disease patients develop bilateral signs, the side initially involved continues to display more pronounced impairment.

In addition to developing bilateral signs as Parkinson's disease progresses, patients often lose their postural reflexes, which are the compensatory mech-

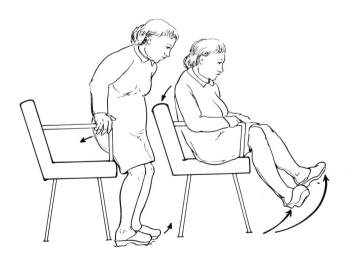

FIGURE 18–6

Patients with akinesia and rigidity cannot rapidly flex their spine, hips, or knees. When sitting, they tend to rock slowly and solidly backward into a chair. Unable to bend rapidly, their feet rise several inches off the floor. "Sitting *en bloc*" is an early, reliable manifestation of parkinsonism.

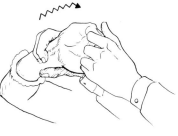

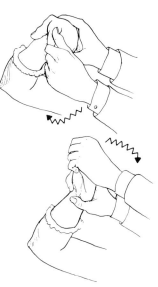

FIGURE 18-7

Cogwheel rigidity, which can be elicited by rotating the patient's wrist, is characterized by increased tone in all directions of movement and superimposed ratchet-like resistance.

anisms that alter muscle tone in response to change in position. Postural reflex loss, in combination with akinesia and rigidity, results in a gait impairment, called *marche à petit pas* or *festinating gait,* that is characterized by shuffling, short steps, and a tendency to accelerate (Fig. 18-9). Of the several characteristic gait abnormalities (see Table 2-4), the festinating gait is most similar to gait apraxia (see Fig. 7-7) because both gait disorders are characterized by small steps and slowed movements. However, gait apraxia is associated with impaired voluntary leg motion, spasticity, and incontinence.

FIGURE 18-8

The *resting tremor* is a relatively slow (4 to 6 Hz) to-and-fro flexion movement of the wrist, hand, thumb, and fingers that is most apparent when patients sit comfortably. The cupped hand's appearance of shaking pills gave rise to the name "pill-rolling" tremor. The tremor is exaggerated or sometimes apparent only when patients are anxious. However, it may be momentarily reduced during voluntary movement or by intense concentration. It is absent during sleep.

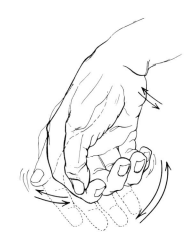

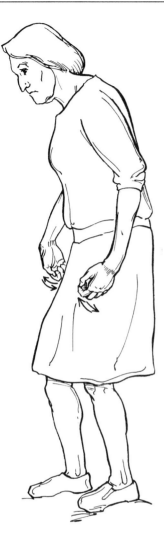

FIGURE 18–9

When Parkinson's disease patients walk, they are said to have a *festinating gait*, in which they take short steps and accelerate their pace. Also, if they take several steps backward, they may have retropulsion, in which they are unable to stop. When walking, they move en bloc, in that they do not swing their arms, look about, or have other normal accessory movements. Likewise, when turning en bloc, they simultaneously move their head, trunk, and legs.

In addition, Parkinson's disease patients' voices often become *hypophonic* (low in volume), *monotonous* (devoid of the normal fluctuations in pitch and cadence), and tremulous. Their handwriting similarly becomes *micrographic* (Fig. 18–10), i.e., small and tremulous.

Another aspect of the illness is that L-dopa (levodopa) treatment reverses the symptoms and signs. A firm clinical diagnosis of Parkinson's disease requires a positive response to L-dopa because there is no readily available confirmatory laboratory test.

Mental Aberrations

15-20%

Dementia Dementia is not an initial symptom of Parkinson's disease. Even in advanced, incapacitating Parkinson's disease, many patients, who must be carefully identified, have their full cognitive capacities. *Diffuse Lewy body disease* (see Chapter 7), a different illness, presents with dementia accompanied by rigidity and other signs of Parkinson's disease.

As Parkinson's disease progresses and patients age, dementia is an increasingly common complication. Dementia occurs in 15 to 20 per cent of all Par-

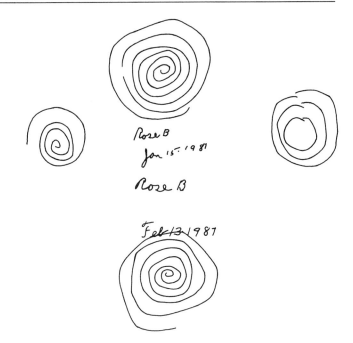

FIGURE 18–10

Micrographia from Parkinson's disease is evident in the patient's upper three spirals, date, and signature. In the lower examples, after treatment, the excursions were larger, bolder, and relatively free of tremor.

kinson's disease patients, and in 40 per cent of patients older than 70 years. Dementia most commonly occurs when Parkinson's disease develops in older patients, has a rapid progression, and is not alleviated by medications. It increases in proportion to physical impairments, especially the bradykinesia.

The dementia is sometimes labeled a "subcortical dementia" because of inattention, poor motivation, and difficulty shifting mental sets offset by gait impairments and the absence of aphasia (see Chapter 7); however, the cognitive impairments, except for a few features, are nonspecific. One such feature, which is possibly merely a side effect of the medications, is that the cognitive impairments and behavior disturbances fluctuate throughout the day. Another is the slow speed of thinking, *bradyphrenia*, which is the cognitive counterpart of bradykinesia.

The cause of the dementia is not established, but unlike the motor disabilities, it is not entirely attributable to dopamine deficiency. Not only do L-dopa and other antiparkinsonian medications fail to alleviate the dementia, but they also frequently precipitate psychosis. Other factors that might induce dementia in Parkinson's disease patients may be cholinergic depletion in the nucleus basalis or Lewy bodies in the cerebral cortex. Of course, these patients may have other common illness that develop in people over 65 years and cause dementia, such as Alzheimer's disease.

Psychosis. At least 10 per cent of Parkinson's disease patients exhibit psychotic thought and behavior. The psychosis is closely associated with dementia, older age, long-standing illness, physical disability, and excessive levels of antiparkinsonian medications.

Visual hallucinations, delusions, and chronic confusion are the most common manifestations. Patients' sleep-wake cycles are disturbed, often markedly. Patients can be abusive and express paranoid ideation that may extend to their physicians. Compared to the other major physical and mental impairments of Parkinson's disease—motor disability and dementia—hallucinations and delusions are the greatest reason why families place patients in nursing homes.

Psychotic symptoms in Parkinson's disease, however, may differ from those in schizophrenia and toxic-metabolic encephalopathy (see Delirium, Chapter 7). Parkinson's disease's visual hallucinations may arise independently from psychotic thought—probably because they really result from L-dopa or other medications (see Table 12–3, Organic Causes of Visual Hallucinations). Auditory hallucinations are rare. Mental aberrations may be accompanied by physical manifestations of excessive medications, such as dyskinesias.

The psychosis in Parkinson's disease is most often attributable to a combination of dementia, antiparkinsonian medications, and toxic-metabolic encephalopathy from other illnesses, such as pneumonia. Also, certain aspects of Parkinson's disease, such as the sleep disturbance and visual hallucinations, exacerbate mental aberrations.

Because antiparkinsonian medications routinely cause mental aberrations, the first step in treatment is to reduce their total dose, often by eliminating night-time administration. Of course, the physical impairments may worsen, but night-time rigidity is a relatively small problem. Another strategy is to add minor tranquilizers to re-establish a normal sleep-wake schedule. Although the concurrent use of L-dopa and classic dopamine antagonist neuroleptics should generally be avoided because they interfere with each other and worsen the patient's physical condition, the addition of neuroleptics may be necessary to avoid exhaustion, injury, and disturbing mental aberrations. The *atypical* neuroleptic clozapine, which can be administered along with L-dopa, can control the psychosis without exacerbating the physical impairments.

Depression. Depression affects almost 50 per cent of Parkinson's disease patients. Some symptoms, such as despair, may occur early in the course of the illness when the overall picture is not classic depression. Unequivocal depression is associated with a history of depression and, as with psychosis, dementia and physical disability. The patient's age, duration of illness, and antiparkinsonian medications are less important factors.

The symptoms of depression in Parkinson's disease patients are difficult to separate from illness-related disability, sleep disturbance, and side effects of medicines. In addition, anxiety, panic attacks, and, most importantly, dementia may confound the clinical picture. Psychiatrists must cautiously apply the Beck Depression Inventory and the Hamilton Rating Scales because of the overlapping symptoms.

Attempting to tease out distinctive traits, some authors suggest that certain symptoms are indicative of depression in Parkinson's disease: anorexia, sleep disturbance, and sadness without guilt or self-reproach. In any case, the suicide rate is low.

The neurotransmitter abnormality in depression has not been established. Low cerebrospinal fluid levels of 5-hydroxyindoleacetic acid (5-HIAA) suggest that diminished serotonin may be responsible, but it is not a sufficiently reliable finding to be diagnostic.

The best initial treatment is to optimize standard antiparkinsonian medications, L-dopa, dopamine agonists, and a monoamine oxidase (MAO) inhibitor, *selegiline* (*deprenyl* [Eldepryl]). In high doses, selegiline produces amphetamine-like activity and the other drugs each have some antidepressant activity. Tricyclic antidepressants and trazodone produce some benefit, but their effects are inconsistent and their anticholinergic side effects might impair patients' memory. Not only has fluoxetine (Prozac) received mixed, mostly negative reviews in this situation, it might exacerbate the motor disabilities. MAO inhibitor antidepressants should not be given to Parkinson's disease patients taking L-dopa or selegiline. In fact selegiline should not be given along with fluoxetine, other serotonin reuptake inhibitors, tricyclic antidepressants, or MAO inhibitors.

Electroconvulsive therapy (ECT) has been successful and safe for depressed Parkinson's disease patients. It reduces the illness' cardinal features, although only for a few weeks, and alleviates depression.

In contrast to the high incidence of dementia and depression in Parkinson's disease, manic-depressive illness and schizophrenia are rare. The coexistence of Parkinson's disease and schizophrenia, also rare, is important not only as a clinical point, but also because it belies the classic "dopamine hypothesis of schizophrenia." This theory predicts that these two conditions, one from decreased and the other from increased dopamine activity, would be mutually exclusive.

Medications should be supplemented by realistic counseling of the family, as well as of the patient. Sometimes support groups are helpful, but most patient-members are in advanced stages. Patients in the initial stage of the illness who visit a support group are often devastated.

Pathology of Parkinson's Disease

In Parkinson's disease, nigrostriatal tract neurons slowly degenerate. The brain loses its ability to convert tyrosine into L-dopa, which would normally be converted into dopamine (Fig. 18–3). Once 80 per cent of these neurons degenerate, insufficient dopamine is produced and symptoms appear. The striatal neurons, which are coated with dopamine receptors, remain intact and responsive to dopamine and its agonists. In other words, the primary pathology in Parkinson's disease is death of the nigrostriatal tract's *presynaptic*, dopamine-producing neurons.

The characteristic neuropathologic finding of Parkinson's disease, which is immediately evident on gross examination of the brain, is loss of the normal pigment in certain nuclei: the substantia nigra, locus ceruleus, and the vagus motor nuclei. These depigmented nuclei's neurons contain microscopic eosinophilic, intracytoplasmic inclusions, called *Lewy bodies*.

The defect is not, however, exclusively in dopamine transmission. Serotonin (5-hydroxytryptophan [5-HT]) concentrations are reduced in the brain and CSF.

Parkinson's disease patients who have dementia have histologic and biochemical changes similar to those found in Alzheimer's disease (see Chapter 7). Microscopic inspection in both conditions reveals senile plaques, abundant neurofibrillary tangles, and loss of neurons. Likewise, cholinergic neurons are depleted in the nucleus basalis, and choline acetyltransferase (ChAT) is decreased markedly.

Positron emission tomography (PET) using fluorodopa demonstrates decreased dopamine activity in the basal ganglia. Although these changes are detectable in presymptomatic individuals as well as in those with established disease, PET is not suitable for clinical practice (see Chapter 20). Other tests, such as magnetic resonance imaging (MRI), computed tomography (CT), and routine serum and CSF tests, fail to reveal significant abnormalities. The diagnosis therefore remains based on the patient's clinical features and response to treatment.

Causes of Parkinson's Disease

Innumerable cases of Parkinson's disease, "postencephalitic Parkinson's disease," were attributed to the worldwide epidemic of encephalitis of 1917–1918. Toxic substances have been thought to cause Parkinson's disease based on the landmark discovery (in the 1970s) of *methyl-phenyl-tetrahydro-pyridine* (*MPTP*), a meperidine analogue byproduct of illicit narcotic manufacture. MPTP causes a fulminant and often fatal Parkinson disease-like condition in drug abusers. It is highly toxic to dopamine neurons and is used to produce the standard animal model of Parkinson's disease. Other substances produce clinical and pathologic signs of basal ganglia damage, particularly herbicides, cyanide, manganese, and carbon monoxide. Head trauma, but only if it causes coma or is repetitive, may have a role. Parkinson's disease clearly does not result from cerebrovascular infarctions (strokes).

One unequivocal risk factor is older age: The mean onset of the illness is approximately 60 years. Another risk factor is a family history of Parkinson's disease. On the other hand, the concordance rate in twins is too low for Parkinson's disease to be solely a Mendelian (chromosomal) genetic condition.

Current hypotheses center on mitochondrial abnormalities, which have already been found to underlie numerous neurologic illnesses (see Mitochondrial Myopathies, Chapter 6 and Appendix 3). Mitochondrial abnormalities would explain why many familial cases do not follow a Mendelian pattern. Suggested mitochondrial problems include defects in the mitochondrial respiratory chain and the presence of cytotoxic *free radicals.* Free radicals are atoms or molecules that are highly unstable because they contain a single, unpaired electron. To complete their electron pairs, free radicals snatch away electrons from neighboring atoms or molecules. The removal of electrons causes oxidization. The pathologic process has been called "oxidant stress." An example of a toxic free radical is methylphenylpyridinium (MPP$^+$), which is the metabolic product of MPTP formed by MAO. Pretreatment of animals with MAO inhibitors prevents their developing MPTP-induced Parkinson's disease, presumably by inhibiting MPP$^+$ formation.

Parkinsonism

Parkinson's disease's cardinal features, often accompanied by postural instability, constitute the clinical condition *parkinsonism*. Several illnesses may be responsible for parkinsonism. In particular, parkinsonism—accompanied by dementia at the onset—is a manifestation of diffuse Lewy body disease (see Chapter 7), dementia pugilistica (see Chapter 22), and many MPTP cases. Parkinsonism is also found in a group of disorders known as "parkinson plus" or *multisystem atrophy*, that are characterized by degeneration of the striatal *postsynaptic* neurons and other systems.

Medication-Induced Parkinsonism. Probably the most common cause of parkinsonism is the administration of classic, *typical* dopamine-blocking neuroleptics, such as phenothiazines and haloperidol. These medications' tendency to induce parkinsonism is related to their affinity for (tendency to block) D$_2$ dopamine receptors in the caudate nucleus.

At therapeutic doses, risperidone (Risperdal) has only a minimal tendency to cause parkinsonism. Clozapine (Clozaril), which has the lowest affinity for D$_2$ receptors of all the antipsychotic medications, does not produce parkinsonism. In contrast, amoxapine (Asendin), a unique antidepressant in this regard, interferes with dopamine and induces parkinsonism.

For the typical neuroleptics, the clinical similarity is so great between Parkinson's disease and neuroleptic-induced parkinsonism that the physical examination provides few distinguishing guidelines. One is that neuroleptic-induced parkinsonism causes symmetric, bilateral signs from the onset. Another is that neuroleptics induce face and limb dyskinesia and akathisia along with parkinsonism. A related issue is that the low coincidence of Parkinson's disease and schizophrenia indicates that schizophrenic patients with parkinsonism probably have either neuroleptic-induced parkinsonism or a neurologic disorder other than Parkinson's disease.

For neuroleptic-induced parkinsonism, the symptoms are related to the medication's dose and antipsychotic strength. Trying to counteract the symptoms with anticholinergics remains controversial because of their side effects. If anticholinergics are given, they should be withdrawn after 3 months to determine if they are still necessary. L-Dopa should be avoided because it can precipitate a toxic psychosis. Neuroleptic-induced parkinsonism typically persists for months. At least 10 per cent of the patients with more persistent symptoms are actually harboring Parkinson's disease: the neuroleptics merely unveil the disorder.

Medication-induced parkinsonism is also produced by non-psychiatric dopamine-blocking medications, such as metoclopramide (Reglan), trimethobenzamide (Tigan), prochlorperazine (Compazine), and promethazine (Phenergan). They can cause neuroleptic malignant syndrome, oculogyric crisis, and other signs of dopamine blockade, as well as parkinsonism.

Parkinsonism in Young Adults. Although Parkinson's disease can begin in individuals as young as 21 years, when it seems to develop in teenagers and young adults, physicians should consider the alternatives: Wilson's disease, the juvenile form of Huntington's disease, medications, and illicit drugs. In these conditions, parkinsonism is often accompanied or even overshadowed by dementia, psychosis, depression, personality disorders, and other psychiatric symptoms.

Therapy of Parkinson's Disease

Medication. The current medical treatment for Parkinson's disease primarily attempts to maintain normal dopamine activity. Orally administered L-dopa, "precursor replacement," is the most effective treatment in the first 3 to 5 years of the illness. In this period, sufficient (greater than 20 per cent) nigrostriatal neurons must be intact to convert L-dopa to dopamine. A decarboxylase inhibitor, carbidopa, is usually given in combination with L-dopa to maximize nigrostriatal L-dopa concentration (Fig. 18–11).

When dopamine production becomes insufficient, L-dopa can be supplemented with dopamine agonists (Fig. 18–3). These medicines are ergot derivatives that stimulate D_2 dopamine receptors, but have different properties regarding the D_1 receptor.

Despite their remarkable effectiveness, L-dopa and dopamine agonists almost inevitably lead to treatment-limiting "dopamine toxicity." After 5 years of Parkinson's disease, presynaptic neurons generally cannot properly store and release dopamine. Then L-dopa and the agonists often cause sleep disturbances, dyskinesias, and mental aberrations. The dyskinesias consist of buccal-lingual movements, chorea, akathisia, dystonia, and rocking trunk movements

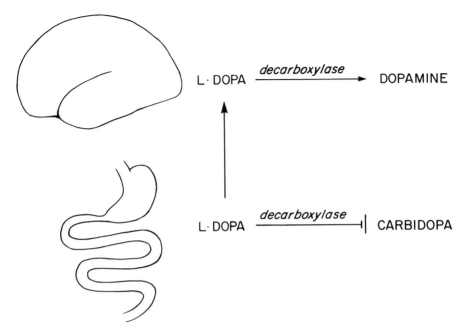

FIGURE 18–11

Carbidopa is a *dopa decarboxylase inhibitor* that prevents the metabolism of L-dopa to dopamine. Because it cannot cross the blood-brain barrier, carbidopa does not interfere with the nigrostriatal dopamine production. Medications that combine L-dopa and carbidopa, such as Sinemet, allow L-dopa to be converted to dopamine almost exclusively in the brain. In addition to raising basal ganglia dopamine levels, carbidopa keeps dopamine's systemic side effects to a minimum. For example, carbidopa reduces the conversion of L-dopa to norepinephrine in the heart.

that are similar to tardive dyskinesia. Despite the apparent problems with dyskinesias, which include embarrassment, exhaustion, and discomfort, most patients usually choose to bear with them, rather than to reduce the drug dosage and return to rigidity and bradykinesia. Both the physical and mental side effects of these therapies can be suppressed with clozapine.

Anticholinergics may reduce tremor in Parkinson's disease and other forms of parkinsonism presumably by balancing the dopamine depletion or blockade (Fig. 18–12). Otherwise they offer little benefit and routinely produce serious side effects: dry mouth, constipation, urinary retention, and mental aberrations, including memory impairment, confusion, and agitation. In addition, anticholinergics potentially cause three problems: exacerbating a cholinergic deficit in an undiagnosed case of Alzheimer's disease, worsening or hastening the development of tardive dyskinesia, and precipitating psychotic behavior in patients with marginal or frank dementia.

Amantadine (*Symmetrel*) produces a modest improvement in rigidity and bradykinesia through an unknown mechanism of action. It is a benign medicine that rarely produces confusion or hallucinations unless the patient has underlying dementia or is also being treated with anticholinergics.

A complementary strategy is administering selegiline. Because of its antioxidant effect, this medicine is thought to prevent cell death and preserves both naturally occurring and medically derived dopamine. It is partly metabolized to amphetamine, which provides a mild antidepressant benefit and stim-

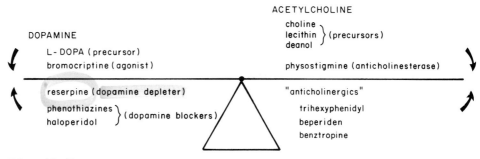

FIGURE 18-12

The countervailing effects of dopamine and acetylcholine can be pictured as a balanced scale. In this model, the left side of the scale would be pulled upward when there is dopamine depletion, as in Parkinson's disease; however, it would be realigned by dopamine precursors, dopamine agonists, or anticholinergics—Parkinson's disease treatments. In conditions where excessive dopamine activity is postulated, such as chorea, the left side would be pushed further downward. In this situation, it could be realigned by substances that either antagonize dopamine or enhance acetylcholine.

ulates dopamine release (see Chapter 21). Also, it may reduce free radical formation. More important, as well as reversing symptoms, selegiline may actually retard the progression of the disease, i.e., selegiline may have a "neuroprotective" effect. Unlike MAO inhibitors used for depression, which are type A or mixed A and B, selegiline is a MAO type-B inhibitor and does not leave patients vulnerable to hypertensive crises. However, it causes potentially fatal interactions with most antidepressants. (SE SDR .)

- Alpha tocopherol (vitamin E), an antioxidant and free radical scavenger, should theoretically protect dopamine from destruction by intrinsic and extrinsic toxins, including MPP^+ and other free radicals. However, a major study showed that tocopherol alone or combined with selegiline did not slow the progression of Parkinson's disease.

Surgery.   Surgical procedures—transplantation and ablative lesions—have been introduced because Parkinson's disease is a progressive illness that is so far unresponsive to neuroprotective therapies. In a dramatic innovation, neurosurgeons transplanted patients' own adrenal medulla cells, which are capable of synthesizing dopamine, into the basal ganglia or ventricular system of the brain. However, the procedure has a high mortality rate and is frequently complicated by permanent major mental aberrations.

Transplantation of fetal mesencephalon (midbrain) cells into the basal ganglia has a higher success rate and lower morbidity and mortality rate. Even though foreign cells are utilized, they are partly hidden from the patient's immunologic system by the blood-brain barrier, i.e., the brain is an "immunologically privileged site." Fetal cell transplantation is more successful in MPTP-induced parkinsonism than in Parkinson's disease patients. Now that federal restrictions have been removed, fetal research can proceed in the United States.

In ablative procedures, neurosurgeons place lesions by stereotactic control in the patient's thalamus or globus pallidus. Stereotactic ablation of a portion of the globus pallidus, a *pallidotomy,* shows considerable promise. Although similar procedures have also been introduced for other movement disorders, including athetosis and dystonia, they have not been particularly successful.

ATHETOSIS

Athetosis is a slow, regular, continual twisting of the muscles. The movements are typically bilateral and symmetric, and affect predominantly the distal parts of the limbs (Fig 18–13). Athetosis is often combined with chorea, *choreoathetosis*. Athetosis is at one end of a spectrum with hemiballismus at the other, where movements are progressively greater in amplitude and irregularity. The distinctions are entirely clinical.

Athetosis almost always is a congenital problem that becomes apparent in early childhood. Although not observable in infants, athetosis usually results from perinatal hyperbilirubinemia (kernicterus), hypoxia, or prematurity, i.e., *choreoathetotic cerebral palsy* (see Chapter 13). There is no genetic factor.

Athetosis is closely associated with mental retardation, but when perinatal damage is confined to the basal ganglia, some patients have normal intelligence. Most important, patients with disabling movement disorders and a garbled voice may still have normal intelligence.

Dopamine antagonists suppress the movements, but their long-term use may lead to complications. Neurosurgeons have placed lesions in the thalamus and the basal ganglia, but few patients are helped.

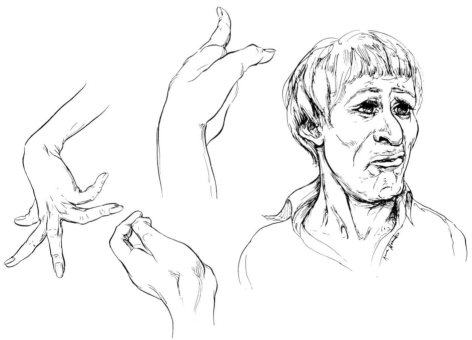

FIGURE 18–13

In athetosis, the face has incessant grimacing and fractions of smiles that alternate with frowns. Neck muscles contract and rotate the head. Laryngeal contraction and irregular chest and diaphragm muscle movements cause dysarthria that has an irregular cadence and nasal pitch. Fingers writhe constantly and tend to assume hyperextension postures while the wrists rotate, flex, and extend. These movements prevent writing, buttoning, and other fine hand movements, but they usually permit gross shoulder, trunk, and hip movements.

CHOREA

Huntington's Disease   AD   CR.4.

The most infamous cause of chorea is Huntington's disease, which was previously called "Huntington's chorea." Huntington's disease is an autosomal dominant genetic illness characterized by chorea and dementia that becomes apparent when patients are 35 to 40 years old. However, approximately 10 per cent of patients develop symptoms in childhood and 25 per cent over the age of 50 years. Adults with the illness succumb to aspiration and inanition one to two decades after the diagnosis, but children succumb twice as rapidly.

Between 2 and 6 per 100,000 persons suffer from Huntington's disease, making it a relatively frequent cause of dementia in middle-aged adults (see Chapter 7). Although families of all races and ethnic backgrounds have been diagnosed as having Huntington's disease, most cases in the United States have been traced to several 17th–century English immigrants.

The world's largest Huntington's disease pedigree lives in a Venezuelan village, where more than 100 affected individuals have shared the same genetic pool, environment, and lack of neuroleptic exposure. Extensive studies have described affected children, heterozygous individuals (carriers) in the presymptomatic state, and several homozygous patients. (Homozygous and heterozygous patients are phenotypically similar.)

Clinical Features.   In contrast to athetosis, which consists of slow writhing movements, chorea consists of random, discrete, brisk movements that cause jerks of the pelvis, trunk, and limbs (Fig. 18–14). Likewise, the face has intermittent frowns, grimaces, and smirks (Fig. 18–15). Pelvic thrusts and other abnormal movements give the gait an irregular, herky-jerky pattern (Fig. 18–16) that contradicts the etymology of *chorea* (Greek, "dance").

In its earliest stage, chorea is often so subtle that it mimics the nonspecific movements that result from anxiety, restlessness, discomfort, or clumsiness.

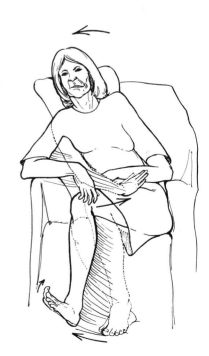

FIGURE 18–14

Patients with chorea, such as this woman who has Huntington's disease, have intermittent and brisk pelvic, trunk, and limb movements that are often a wrist flick, a forward jutting of the leg, or a shrugging of the shoulder. Patients with chorea are sometimes said to have movements that are *choreiform*, which is the adjectival form of the word.

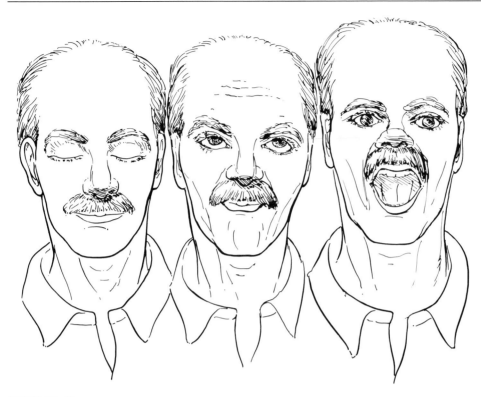

FIGURE 18-15

Huntington's disease patients have unexpected, inappropriate, and incomplete facial expressions, including frowns, eyebrow raising, and smirks.

Chorea may then consist of only excessive face or hand gestures, frequent weight shifting, continual leg crossing, or twitching fingers (Fig. 18–17). Although not clearly identifiable, the movements cause *motor impersistence*, which leads to clumsiness, the inability to hold objects firmly, and the inability to extend the hand or tongue for more than several seconds.

Another early, reliable sign is abnormal *saccades*—purposeful, rapid, conjugate eye movement. Patients typically cannot look smoothly toward an object. They must even first blink or jerk their head. Once moving, the eyes track the object slowly and irregularly. (Patients with schizophrenia also have abnormal saccades.)

The dementia in adults typically begins one year either before or after the chorea. The dementia first causes inattentiveness, erratic behavior, and impaired judgment followed by clear-cut cognitive impairments. As with Parkinson's disease, Huntington's disease dementia is often cited as an example of a subcortical dementia; however, neuropsychologic testing and pathologic examination reveal cortical as well as subcortical abnormalities.

Dementia is accompanied by a change in affect in the majority of patients. Most of them have depression with occasional, transient manic features. Patients are prone to commit suicide.

A preliminary diagnosis can be based on the patient having chorea, dementia, and a relative with a similar disorder. Definitive DNA testing is available for patients and asymptomatic, potential carriers, including a fetus. This testing is necessary to exclude illnesses that mimic Huntington's disease and to

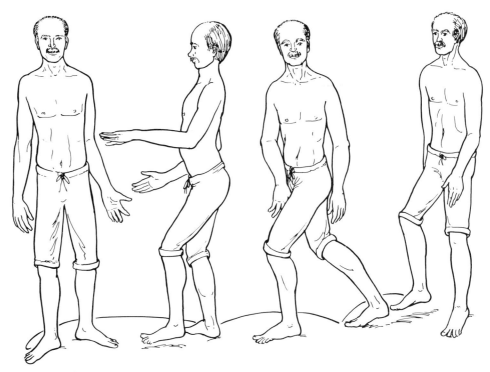

FIGURE 18–16

The gait in Huntington's disease is not rhythmic or graceful, but lurching and contorted. The abnormality results from intermittent, unexpected trunk and pelvic motions, spontaneous knee flexion, lateral swaying, and a variable cadence.

confirm a clinical diagnosis. Although highly accurate, the DNA testing cannot predict the age when symptoms will develop in carriers. DNA testing is more reliable and easier to perform than linkage analyses. Neuropsychologic tests cannot distinguish presymptomatic gene carriers from normal individuals.

When chorea is mild, it may be suppressed by dopamine antagonists, such as the neuroleptics, or dopamine depletors, such as tetrabenazine. The dementia is unaffected by any treatment.

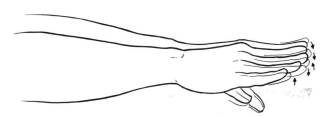

FIGURE 18–17

When extended, the arms and hands of Huntington's disease patients make fidgety "piano playing" movements that consist of momentary finger and wrist flexion and extension. Motor impersistence can be demonstrated by a patient intermittently squeezing if asked to grasp two of the examiner's fingers ("milk maid's sign") and by intermittent, involuntary withdrawal of the tongue when attempting to protrude it for 30 seconds ("Jack-in-the-box tongue"). These classic, graphic terms reflect 200 years of physicians' diagnoses based solely on clinical manifestations.

Juvenile Huntington's Disease. In 10 per cent of Huntington's disease cases, dementia and personality changes appear before patients are 15 years old. This "juvenile" variety of Huntington's disease is characterized not by chorea, but by rigidity, dystonia, and akinesia. These symptoms create childhood parkinsonism. The juvenile variety also differs from the adult form because it is usually transmitted from the patient's father, causes seizures, and leads to a rapid demise.

Pathology. A spectacular medical advance has been made with the discovery that the genetic abnormality consists of an excessive number of repeats of the nucleotide base triplet CAG (*trinucleotide repeats*) in the short arm of chromosome 4. In contrast to the normal complement of about 20 repeats (with the range of 11 to 34 repeats), Huntington's disease is associated with 37 or more repeats and its juvenile variety with 60 or more repeats. In general, the more numerous the repeats, the younger the age of onset of symptoms.

The trinucleotide repeats are not only numerous but are also unstable. An affected father's gametes tend to generate increased repeats, although the mother's gametes maintain similar numbers. Since children of an affected father have a larger number of repeats, the disease is more likely to develop in his children.

Other illnesses with underlying trinucleotide repeats, which may exceed 100 times greater than normal, are myotonic dystrophy (see Chapter 6) and fragile X syndrome (see Chapter 13). As in Huntington's disease, myotonic dystrophy tends to appear in younger family members in successive generations, i.e, *anticipation*.

The genetic defect is believed to influence N-methyl-D-aspartate (*NMDA*) receptors. When excessively stimulated by glutamate and other excitatory amino acids, NMDA receptors are deleterious to neurons, i.e., NMDA receptors cause "excitotoxicity" (see Chapter 21). They may also be responsible for neuron death in stroke and epilepsy.

On a biochemical level, Huntington's disease is characterized by degeneration of gamma-aminobutyric acid (GABA)-producing neurons of the corpus striatum. In the caudate nuclei, where the changes are most pronounced, the GABA concentrations are reduced to less than 50 per cent of normal.

The characteristic gross pathologic finding is atrophy of the caudate nuclei. Their loss permits the lateral ventricles to balloon outward and become so voluminous that they are called "bat wing ventricles" (see Fig. 20−12). As the illness progresses, the cerebral cortex also undergoes atrophy. PET studies demonstrate caudate hypometabolism early in the illness. CT and MRI scans show the caudate atrophy, which correlates with the severity of dementia.

Other Varieties of Chorea

Sydenham's chorea (*St. Vitus' dance*) is a "major diagnostic criterion" of rheumatic fever that begins 2 to 6 months after the carditis and has an average duration of 2 months. It almost exclusively affects children between the ages of 5 and 15 years. In children older than 10 years, girls are affected twice as frequently as boys. With the decreasing incidence of rheumatic fever, Sydenham's chorea has become rare except for small outbreaks.

Nevertheless, Sydenham's chorea remains an important condition. It is sometimes the only sign of a serious illness. Since chorea develops months after the carditis, the movements often surprisingly strike otherwise healthy children. Undiagnosed cases may be referred to psychiatrists because children may seem to suddenly develop irritability, strange behavior, or overwhelming anxiety. Child psychiatrists have to distinguish Sydenham's chorea from tics, dystonia, and withdrawal-emergent dyskinesia, as well as from psychiatric conditions.

Children who develop Sydenham's chorea have an insidious onset of grimaces, limb movements, and other stigmata of chorea (Fig. 18–18). As during most illnesses, children may have listlessness, irritability, and emotional lability. They do not develop frank cognitive impairments or major psychiatric disorders, but detailed testing reveals that about 50 per cent of them have permanent minor psychologic disturbances. The few postmortem examinations have disclosed extensive microscopic hemorrhages.

Chorea recurs in about 20 per cent of patients with subsequent attacks of rheumatic fever. Also, women who had Sydenham's chorea in childhood, who start to take oral contraceptives or conceive, may have a recurrence of chorea. In addition, close relatives of Sydenham's chorea patients are liable to develop chorea under any of those same circumstances.

The etiology of Sydenham's chorea is probably a cerebrovascular inflammation that can be triggered by streptococcal infections. The movements are thought to recur because of a permanently increased sensitivity to dopamine when estrogen levels are elevated during female puberty, use of oral contraceptives, and pregnancy. Sedating dopamine antagonists suppress the movements and give the child some rest.

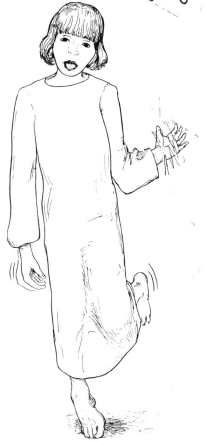

FIGURE 18–18

Children with Sydenham's chorea may appear to have coy smiles and brief grimaces. They walk with a playful sashay. However, the chorea can be made obvious if the children attempt to hold a fixed position, such as standing at attention or standing on the ball of one foot.

Oral contraceptive-induced chorea is a rare reaction to oral estrogen-containing contraceptives. In this condition, chorea develops in teenaged women several months after starting a contraceptive and resolves after the contraceptive is stopped. This variety of chorea is not associated with mental abnormalities.

Chorea gravidarum, another rarely occurring variety of chorea, almost always develops in young primigravidas in the first two trimesters of pregnancy. Many patients or their close relatives have had Sydenham's chorea, oral contraceptive-induced chorea, or a prior episode of chorea gravidarum. Women with this condition frequently become so exhausted that it precipitates a spontaneous abortion or necessitates a therapeutic one. In any case, all symptoms resolve within several days after delivery or termination of the pregnancy.

Many other causes of chorea have been described (Table 18–1). In most of them, structural lesions, metabolic derangements, or inflammatory conditions, such as systemic lupus erythematosus (SLE), have injured the basal ganglia. In some, dopamine activity is increased.

HEMIBALLISMUS

Hemiballismus is intermittent, gross movements of one side of the body that are similar to those found in chorea, except that they are unilateral and more of a flinging (ballistic) motion (Fig. 18–19). Since the cause of hemiballismus is usually a small lesion in the (contralateral) subthalamic nucleus, which is nowhere near the cerebral cortex, hemiballismus is not accompanied by mental abnormalities, visual impairments, paresis, or other corticospinal tract signs. The most common etiology in individuals older than 65 years is an occlusion of a small perforating branch of the basilar artery. In these cases, hemiballismus can be suppressed with dopamine-blocking neuroleptics. In young adults, the most common cause is AIDS-associated toxoplasmosis in the subthalamic nucleus.

TABLE 18–1. CAUSES OF CHOREA

Basal ganglia lesions
  Perinatal injury, e.g., anoxia, kernicterus
  Cerebrovascular accidents
  Tumors, abscesses, toxoplasmosis[a]
Genetic disorders
  Huntington's disease
  Wilson's disease
Metabolic derangements
  Hypocalcemia
  Hepatic encephalopathy
Drugs
  Oral contraceptives[b]
  L-dopa compounds, precursors, and agonists
  Cocaine, amphetamine, methylphenidate
  Neuroleptics
Inflammatory conditions
  Sydenham's chorea
  Systemic lupus erythematosus (SLE)

[a]AIDS causes chorea when toxoplasmosis involves the basal ganglia.
[b]Estrogens from contraceptives or pregnancy (chorea gravidarum) cause chorea.

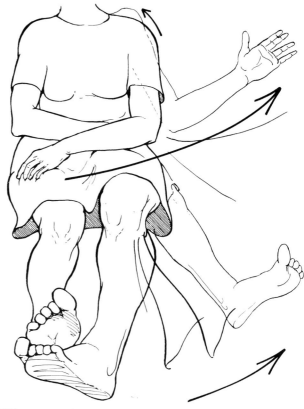

FIGURE 18-19

Hemiballismus is sudden and large-scale movements of the limbs on one side of the body. Patients often attempt to suppress the movements by pressing their body or unaffected limbs against the involuntarily moving ones. They also attempt to camouflage the involuntary movements by converting them into apparently purposeful movements. For example, if a patient's arm were to fly upward, he or she might incorporate the movement into a gesture, such as waving to someone.

WILSON'S DISEASE   AR.   CR13

16y.old

Wilson's disease (*hepatolenticular degeneration*) is an autosomal recessive genetic illness attributable to a defect on chromosome 13. It is characterized by dementia and other neuropsychologic changes, a variety of involuntary movements, and hepatic insufficiency. The cause is insufficient copper excretion that results in destructive copper deposits in the brain, liver, cornea, and other organs. As its formal name implies, the illness damages the brain's lenticular nuclei (Fig. 18-1).

Symptoms become evident at the average age of 16 years. Dementia, which may begin before the movements, can be overshadowed by personality changes, conduct disorders, mood disturbances, or thought disorders. The movements, which are likewise highly variable, usually consist of rigidity, akinesia, dystonia, or the characteristic *wing-beating* tremor (Fig. 18-20), but other manifestations can be tremors and ataxia. The various movements tend to occur in combination and be accompanied sometimes by corticospinal or corticobulbar tract signs. With its various neurologic manifestations, Wilson's disease can mimic Parkinson's and Huntington's diseases and neuroleptic-induced dystonia. Each may induce parkinsonism and dystonia in young adults.

Non-neurologic signs are often as obvious as neurologic ones. For example, liver involvement leads to cirrhosis, and copper deposition in the cornea produces a Kayser-Fleischer ring (Fig. 18-21).

The protean manifestations of Wilson's disease require that physicians test for this illness, despite its infrequent occurrence (1 per 100,000 persons), in young adults who develop a wide variety of conditions, including tremor, par-

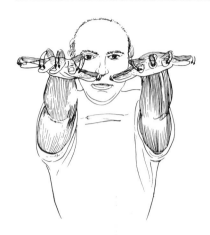

FIGURE 18–20

Although Wilson's disease may induce parkinsonism, dystonia, and dysarthria, it characteristically produces a *wing-beating tremor*, which is coarse and centered on the shoulders. Patients with this tremor, as its name implies, move their arms as though they were attempting to fly.

kinsonism, dystonia, atypical psychosis, dementia, dysarthria, or chronic hepatitis. Since the Kayser-Fleischer ring can be observed in virtually all patients with neurologic symptoms, suspected patients should undergo a slit–lamp examination. A diagnostic finding, even when the illness does not affect the brain, is a very low concentration of serum ceruloplasmin (the serum protein to which copper adheres). A chelating agent, such as penicillamine, when administered early enough, can reverse the mental deterioration, movement disorders, and non-neurologic manifestations in about 50 per cent of cases.

DYSTONIA

Dystonia Musculorum Deformans

Dystonia musculorum deformans, or *torsion dystonia*, is a group of conditions characterized by *dystonia*, which is involuntary twisting or turning (torsion) movements, sustained at the height of muscle contraction. The limb (appendicular) and neck, trunk, and pelvis (axial) muscles are contorted most commonly. The movements create *dystonic postures* that are often precipitated or exacerbated by voluntary actions, such as walking. Although dystonia becomes progressively more severe over the years and patients become physically incapacitated, their mental abilities remain intact. As in choreoathetosis, children with dystonia have terribly disabling movements that can mask a normal intellect.

Dystonia musculorum deformans stems from a gene located on chromosome 9. Although the illness is inherited in an autosomal dominant pattern, the

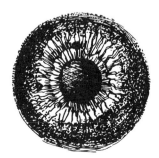

FIGURE 18–21

The Kayser-Fleischer ring, which is pathognomonic of Wilson's disease affecting the brain, is a green-brown pigment in the periphery of the cornea. It is most obvious at the superior and inferior margins of the cornea where it obscures the fine structure of the iris. In the early stages of Wilson's disease, when the ring is forming, it can be seen only with an ophthalmologist's slit lamp.

penetrance is so low that initial studies erroneously indicated that the inheritance was recessive. The illness is found predominantly among Ashkenazi (Eastern European) Jews. In them, torsion of a hand or foot typically develops in 8– to 14–year–old children (Fig. 18–22). Over the next several years, the dystonia also affects the other limbs, pelvis (tortipelvis), trunk, and neck (torticollis) (Fig. 18–23).

Dystonia, whether caused by dystonia musculorum deformans or another etiology, can be suppressed briefly by *tricks*, such as skipping, walking backward, dancing (with or without music), or pressing the affected body part. Dystonic movements tend to trigger compensatory movements, which sometimes makes the patients' appearance bizarre. Probably more frequently than any other involuntary movement disorder, dystonia is mistakenly diagnosed as a psychogenic disturbance (see Psychogenic Movements).

Despite no identifiable abnormality of the blood chemistry, EEG, MRI or CT, or brain tissue, the diagnosis of dystonia musculorum deformans can be achieved through DNA testing. Inconsistently effective medications have included anticholinergics, baclofen, and carbamazepine. Thalamotomy is a last resort. Unlike other movement disorders, studies of CSF and autopsy material have implicated norepinephrine metabolism abnormalities.

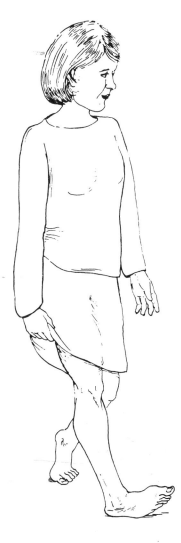

FIGURE 18–22

Patients with dystonia musculorum deformans (torsion dystonia) typically first have involuntary inturning (torsion) of one foot. In this case, because of torsion of the right ankle and hip, the girl's foot slowly twists inward and onto its side when she walks.

As in other cases of dystonia, the dystonic posture can be overlooked or misinterpreted. The movement is sometimes momentary and incomplete. Moreover, in a "sensory trick," the gait abnormality can be suppressed by her walking backward, skipping, or dancing.

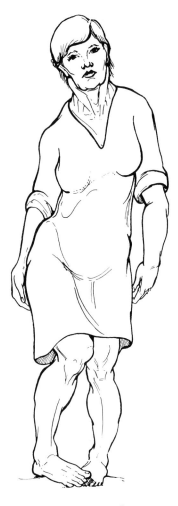

FIGURE 18-23

As dystonia musculorum deformans encompasses the remaining limb and axial musculature, patients develop grotesque, dystonic postures. Because of their continuous exertion, their muscles hypertrophy, and their subcutaneous fat is lost. The postures in this condition are similar to those in Wilson's disease and tardive dystonia.

Other Causes of Generalized Dystonia. *Dopa-responsive dystonia*, a condition described by Segawa and colleagues and often named after them, also causes dystonia in children and is inherited in an autosomal pattern. Nevertheless, this disorder is distinct from dystonia musculorum deformans and childhood Parkinson's disease. Its inheritance, which is not more frequent among Jews, is attributable to an abnormality on chromosome 14; the dystonia has a marked diurnal variation, being pronounced in the late afternoon and evening, but virtually absent by the morning. Most important, small doses of L-dopa ameliorate the dystonia. Thus, giving L-dopa to children who have developed dystonia has become a standard therapeutic-diagnostic strategy.

Dystonia, as mentioned previously, can also be a prominent symptom of neurologic illnesses that primarily cause other involuntary movements. Such *symptomatic* or *secondary dystonia* can, for example, be found in Wilson's disease, juvenile Huntington's disease, tardive dystonia, and several rare degenerative neurologic illnesses.

Within the last group *Lesch-Nyhan syndrome* is most notable. It is a sex-linked recessive genetic illness in which 2- to 6-year-old children develop dystonia, self-mutilation and other bizarre behavior, mental retardation, corticospinal tract signs, seizures, and hyperuricemia. The basic abnormality is a deficiency of an enzyme required for urea metabolism, hypoxanthine-guanine phosphoribosyl transferase (HGPRT).

The following conditions are often included in discussions of involuntary movement disorders. However, their clinical characteristics are considerably different from those of the conditions already discussed. Moreover, investigations have failed to find structural abnormalities of the basal ganglia, definite neurotransmitter imbalances, or, with the exception of Tourette's syndrome, a beneficial response to dopamine or ACh manipulation.

Focal Dystonias

[handwritten: Tx w/ Botulinum toxin !]

In contrast to generalized dystonia, *focal dystonias* typically occur sporadically, develop in middle–aged and older adults, and involve muscles either in the head (*cranial dystonia*), neck (*cervical dystonia*), or arm (*limb dystonia*). Certain focal dystonias are *task-specific* as they are precipitated exclusively by performing a particular action, such as writing. As with generalized dystonia, mental abilities are preserved, and the diagnosis is entirely clinical.

Many focal dystonias have been attributed to psychogenic factors or tardive dyskinesia because the dystonic movements are particularly bizarre, easily conform to psychoanalytic interpretations, and appear similar to neuroleptic-induced movements. In fact, most patients with focal dystonias have had no exposure to neuroleptics. Except for one condition, hemifacial spasm, the cause is unknown.

[handwritten: → prohibits the release of ACH at the neuro-musc. junct- ↓↓ weakens the muscle (which is dystonic)]

Botulinum A toxin (Botox) injections into affected muscles have been dramatically successful in each of these conditions (Fig. 18–24). Botulinum can also be used in generalized dystonia, but only to treat one particularly troublesome muscle group. Systemic medications provide little benefit, especially compared to their side effects.

Cranial Dystonias. *Blepharospasm*, which is easily recognizable and frequently occurring, consists of bilateral, simultaneous contractions of the orbicularis oculi and sometimes the frontalis muscles (Fig. 18–25). Patients unconsciously learn "sensory tricks" that temporarily suppress the contractions (Fig. 18–26). Like most other focal dystonias, blepharospasm is particularly amenable to botulinum treatment.

Meige's syndrome is a similar but more extensive condition that consists of contractions of the lower as well as the upper facial muscles, but it usually

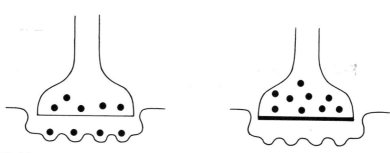

FIGURE 18–24

Left, At the normal neuromuscular junction, acetylcholine (ACh) vesicles (*black dots*) are released from the presynaptic membrane, bind to postsynaptic membrane receptors, and trigger muscle contractions. In focal dystonias, which are characterized by intense muscle contractions, the neuromuscular system seems to be hyperactive. *Right,* Botulinum A toxin (Botox) injected into muscles binds irreversibly onto the presynaptic membrane of the neuromuscular junction. It interferes with the release of the ACh packets and thereby weakens the injected muscle. The injections reduce dystonic contractions for about 3 months while permitting normal muscle function. Botulinum A toxin injections must be repeated after that time.

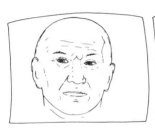
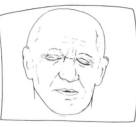
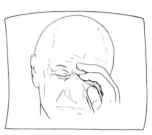

FIGURE 18–25

This elderly gentleman has blepharospasm in which his orbicularis oculi (eyelid) muscles have prolonged (average duration, 5 seconds) bilateral contractions. During spasms, his vision is blocked, and he resorts to prying open his eyelids.

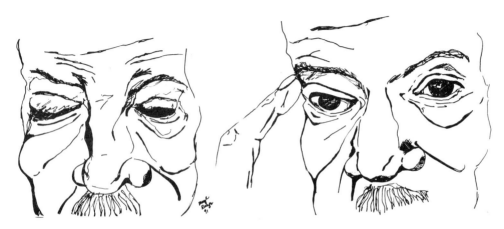

FIGURE 18–26

Left, A 70-year-old man with blepharospasm cannot open his eyelids. The contracted, elevated forehead muscles show that he is making an subconscious attempt to open them. *Right*, He has instinctively learned the sensory trick of pressing one eyebrow (a *geste antagoniste*), which alleviates the spasms for several minutes.

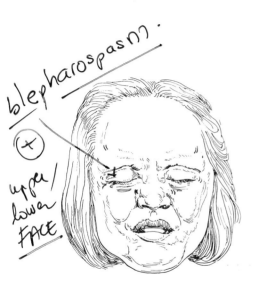

[handwritten annotations: "blepharospasm?", "⊕", "upper/lower FACE"]

[handwritten annotations: "Dx μ ≠ w/TD", "Meige: ⌐symmetric / ⌐upper face / ⌐absence tongue protrusion"]

FIGURE 18–27

This patient with Meige's syndrome has blepharospasm accompanied by comparable lower face and orbicularis oris muscle contractions. Meige's syndrome movements differ from the oral-buccal-lingual movements of tardive dyskinesia with respect to their symmetry, predominant involvement of the upper face, and absence of tongue protrusions.

includes blepharospasm (Fig. 18–27). Since Meige's syndrome involves oral-buccal dyskinesias, it is usually considered in the differential diagnosis of tardive dyskinesia.

Hemifacial spasm, a completely different cranial dystonia, consists of spasms of the muscles on one side of the face that are supplied by the ipsi-lateral facial nerve (the seventh cranial nerve) (Fig. 18–28). The spasms occur intermittently one to ten times per minute and disfigure the face. Unlike other generalized and focal dystonias, as well as the classic movement disorders, hemifacial spasms readily persist into stages 1 and 2 of NREM sleep and occasionally into deeper stages.

Some cases are caused by misdirected regrowth of the facial nerve after injuries or inflammations, such as Bell's palsy. In most cases, hemifacial spasm is caused by an aberrant vessel or other structural lesion compressing the facial nerve at its origin from the pons (see Fig. 4–13). Neurosurgeons can alleviate hemifacial spasm in these cases by performing a microvascular decompression, in which they insert a cushion between the vessel and nerve. (In a similar procedure, microvascular decompression of the trigeminal nerve [the fifth cranial nerve] provides dramatic relief of trigeminal neuralgia [see Fig. 9–5]. Trigeminal neuralgia patients, who are in severe pain, will much sooner undergo neurosurgery than hemifacial spasm patients, who are disfigured.)

Cervical Dystonias. Spasmodic torticollis is a focal dystonia in which the sternocleidomastoid and adjacent neck muscles undergo involuntary, painful contractions that rotate the patient's head and neck (Figs. 18–29 and 18–30). The contractions have an initial duration of several seconds to several minutes, but, as the disease progresses, the head and neck continuously turn. Spasmodic torticollis is occasionally a component of dystonia musculorum deformans, but it usually occurs alone. Similar neck muscle contractions can be a transient side effect of neuroleptics or L-dopa. The condition can also result from a cervical nerve root irritation ("wry neck"). Cases of spasmodic torticollis and other forms of dystonia have allegedly resulted from head and neck injuries, especially "whiplash" from motor vehicle accidents.

Spasmodic dysphonia, previously called "spastic dysphonia," is a distinctive speech abnormality caused by a sudden, involuntary contraction of the larynx muscles when patients speak. Their voice is intermittently and abruptly

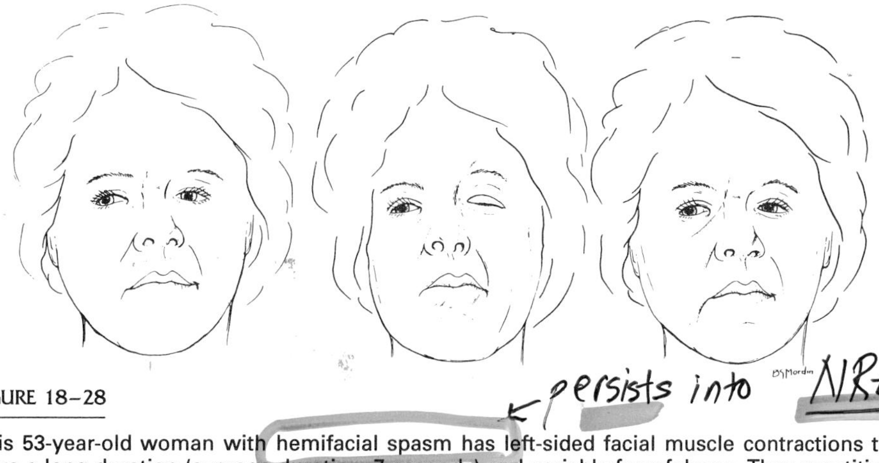

FIGURE 18–28

This 53-year-old woman with hemifacial spasm has left-sided facial muscle contractions that have a long duration (average duration, 7 seconds) and variable forcefulness. They repetitively squeeze shut her left eyelids and pull her mouth to her left side.

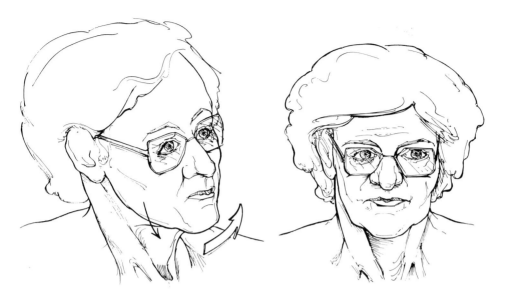

FIGURE 18-29

In spasmodic torticollis, most patients have a rotation of their head in a downward and lateral sweep because of continuous contraction of the sternocleidomastoid muscle. (Most patients' head and neck movement is predominantly lateral, but sometimes it is backward [in extension, *retrocollis*] or forward [in flexion, *anterocollis*]; however, movement in any direction falls into the rubric of "torticollis.") Lateral neck movements are accompanied by shoulder elevation, as though the head and shoulder were being pulled toward each other. Continuous contractions also result in muscle hypertrophy and pain.

strained—as if they were trying to speak while being strangled. Nevertheless, they can shout, sing, and whisper: These varieties of speech bypass the larynx and rely on the lips, mouth, and tongue. Likewise, patients can normally use neighboring muscles to swallow and breathe.

Spasmodic dysphonia often occurs within the context of other cranial and cervical dystonias and head tremors. Clinical evaluation can distinguish it from vocal cord tumors, psychogenic voice disorders, and pseudobulbar

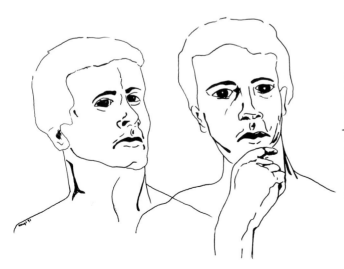

FIGURE 18-30

The involuntary rotation of spasmodic torticollis can be overcome by a great deal of voluntary effort. As with blepharospasm and other focal dystonias, spasmodic torticollis patients instinctively learn sensory tricks, such as applying slight counter-rotational pressure against the chin, which temporarily stops the movement. Moreover, the maneuver camouflages the involuntary movements by striking a studious pose.

palsy (see Chapter 4). Spasmodic dysphonia is treated quite effectively by electromyography-guided botulinum injections through the front of the throat directly into the larynx.

Limb Dystonias. Limb dystonias usually affect the upper rather than the lower extremities. *Occupational* spasms or *cramps* are hand muscle contractions that begin shortly after engaging in a repetitive activity that is often the basis of the patient's livelihood; however, patients can use the same hand to perform similar functions. The cramps may or may not be painful. The best known example is *writer's cramp* (Fig. 18–31). Other artistic or creative professions are often afflicted: Musicians develop *pianist's* or *violinist's cramps*. However, more mundane professions, brick laying for example, can also be complicated by the disorder.

ESSENTIAL TREMOR *in action.*

Patients with *essential tremor*, which is sometimes called an "action" or "postural tremor," have fine oscillations of 6 to 9 Hz at their wrist, hand, or fingers. The tremor is characteristically elicited by certain actions or positions (Fig. 18–32). As in other varieties of tremor, the oscillations are in a single plane. Patients may have head shaking (titubation), usually in a "yes" or "no" pattern, and a tremor in their voice.

Essential tremor most often develops in young and middle-aged adults and affects about 400 per 100,000 people older than 40 years. In one variety, *benign familial tremor*, the tremor is inherited in an autosomal dominant pattern. The tremor appears the same when it develops in people older than 65 years, but it is then called *senile tremor*.

In some patients, the amplitude of the tremor is suppressed by alcohol-containing beverages. Although no cure or completely effective treatment is available, β-adrenergic blockers, such as propranolol (Inderal), and often primidone (Mysoline) can suppress it. Propranolol blocks both β-1 and β-2 adrenergic sympathetic nervous system receptor sites. Metoprolol (Lopressor), which also suppresses the tremor, blocks β-1 adrenergic sites. Essential tremor's response to β-blockers suggests that it results from excessive β-adrenergic activity.

Several similarly appearing tremors, which also may originate in excessive adrenergic system activity, respond to β-blockers. These tremors result from anxiety, stage fright (performance anxiety), hyperthyroidism, use of steroids, use of β-adrenergic-stimulating agents, such as isoproterenol (Isuprel), and use of amitriptyline or lithium (see below).

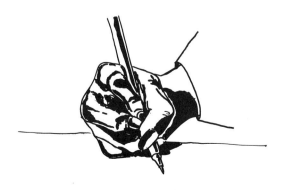

FIGURE 18–31

An author with a writer's cramp develops finger and hand muscle spasms within minutes after starting to write, but not when she uses the same hand to type, eat, or button clothing. In her case, the cramps are painless. Writer's cramp is a classic task-specific or occupational dystonia. It differs from fatigue-induced cramps, which occur after hours of performing the task and prohibit the limb from being used for other purposes. She can dictate the material that she cannot write, indicating that she has writer's cramp and not the psychologic phenomenon of "writer's block."

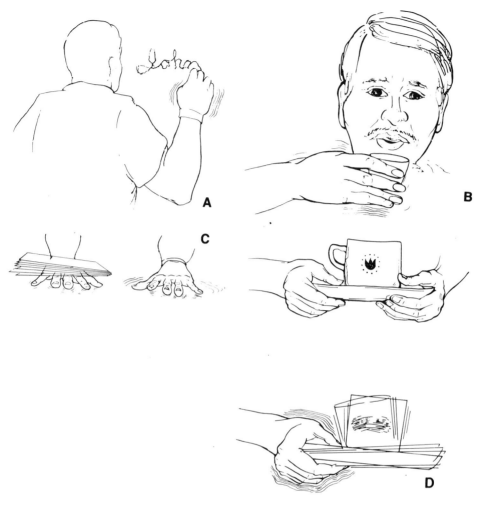

FIGURE 18-32

An essential tremor, which is typically absent when hands are resting, may be elicited by having a patient *A,* write his name, *B,* drink from a filled glass, *C,* support an envelope on his outstretched hand, or *D,* transfer a cup and saucer from one hand to the other.

Dµ #

The pill rolling tremor of Parkinson's disease, in contrast, occurs at rest, is diminished by the initiation of movements, and is relatively slow (see Fig. 18–8). It is also usually accompanied by rigidity and akinesia. Cerebellar dysfunction causes an intention tremor that is coarse, irregular, and elicited by gross actions (see Fig. 2–11). The tremors of Wilson's disease remain difficult to categorize, but they can appear similar to those in Parkinson's disease, cerebellar disease, or essential tremor. Overall, in young adults who develop a tremor, Wilson's disease is the most important disorder to consider.

TICS

Tics are rapid, repetitive, nonrhythmic *stereotyped* movements of functionally related muscle groups. They may be *simple* or *complex* and *motor* or *vocal.* *Simple motor tics* include a head toss, prolonged eye blink, shoulder jerk, and asymmetric smile. *Complex motor tics* are complete movements, such as touching or hitting oneself, jumping, stomping, or skipping. *Simple vocal tics* are short, inarticulate sounds, such as throat clearing, grunting, and sniffing. *Complex vocal tics* are words or at least fractions of words. Other tics can involve the patient moving in response to an urge or uncomfortable sensation (sensory tics), repeating words (echolalia), mimicking movements (echopraxia or echokinesis), or touching themselves or others. (Neurologic terminology, although not codified, is consistent with the *Diagnostic and Statistical Manual of Mental Disorders [DSM–IV]*.)

As in the classic movement disorders, the frequency and intensity of tics are increased by excitement, anxiety, and fatigue. Likewise, tics may be decreased or abolished for minutes to hours by voluntary suppression with intense concentration. In fact, of all the involuntary movement disorders, tics are the most suppressible by intense concentration, but afterward they rebound in a flurry. In contrast to classic movement disorders, tics are stereotyped, vary in pattern and intensity over weeks or months (often seeming to remit entirely or respond to treatment), and persist during sleep (see Chapter 17).

Simple motor tics develop in about 5 per cent of school-aged children, but by the end of adolescence, most affected children will have a spontaneous remission. Boys are affected three times more often than girls. A disproportionate number of children with tics have a close relative with one or more tics.

Tics in Adults

In addition to the tics that have persisted since childhood, otherwise healthy 40– to 60–year–old adults sometimes develop tics as a transient or chronic problem. Although tics in children usually tend to involve only the head or neck, those in adults involve the chest, diaphragm, entire trunk, and limbs, i.e., the more caudal structures. In addition, tics in adults tend to have a longer duration, be more complex, and occur in combination with other tics.

Tics in adults may be a symptom of various neurologic illnesses: encephalitis, Parkinson's disease, neuroleptic treatment (tardive tics), and the use of cocaine or other psychoactive substances. Dramatic bursts of obscenities—ordinarily found in severe cases of Tourette's syndrome—may result from non-dominant hemisphere injury (see Chapter 8) and the disordered and frustrated speech of someone with aphasia (see Chapter 7).

Tourette's Syndrome

In Gilles de la Tourette's (Tourette's) syndrome—by DSM-IV definition—a combination of vocal and multiple motor tics develops before the age of 18 years and lasts longer than 1 year (Fig. 18–33). This syndrome affects boys two to three times more frequently than girls, becomes apparent on average at age 7 years, and is present in 90 per cent of patients by age 13 years. In affected children, the tics are often greatest at the beginning of the school year and least during the summer months. By the time they are adults, about 30 per cent of patients undergo a complete remission, and another 30 per cent undergo a substantial improvement. When the illness persists, tics change in distribution, vary in intensity, and undergo transient remissions.

The cardinal feature of Tourette's syndrome is vocal tics, which are repetitive, stereotyped sounds that the patients blurt rapidly, irresistibly, and com-

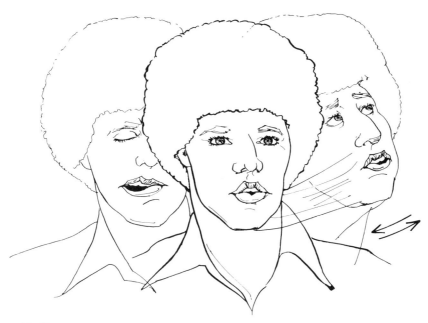

FIGURE 18–33

In a typical Tourette's syndrome case, a young man has multiple motor tics, including head jerking (head toss), grimacing of the right side of his mouth (half-smile), and depression of his forehead (frowning). The motor tics are accompanied by vocal tics of throat clearing and a short blowing sound. Tics continue throughout the day, being only slightly affected by conversation, eating, and social situations.

    Intense concentration—more than in any other involuntary movement disorder—can suppress the tics. On the other hand, tics are like breathing: They are unnoticed by the individual and can be suppressed at will, but afterward, they return forcefully.

    Tics often occur in rapid succession or in combination and have lightning-like rapidity. Various tic repetitions and combinations can persist for several seconds and generate complex movements. After several months, each tic may recede or be replaced by another tic.

pulsively. Throughout the course of the illness, vocal tics of most patients are simple. The tics usually consist of inarticulate sounds, such as sniffing, throat clearing, or clicks; however, many patients eventually make loud and disconcerting noises, such as grunting, snorting, or honking. When vocal tics become complex, they can culminate in unprovoked outbursts of obscene words, *coprolalia*. Although most such explosions contain only fractions of obscene words, such as "shi," "fu," or "cun," some consist of strings of unequivocal obscenities. Moreover, coprolalia is often accompanied by intrusions of obscene thoughts, *mental coprolalia*, or the involuntary performance of obscene movements or gestures, *copropraxia* (Fig. 18–34).

    Ever since the original description of the illness, physicians and the public have overemphasized the feature of coprolalia. It is not a diagnostic criterion for the illness. Less than 10 per cent of patients have coprolalia, and in these cases its onset is about 6 years after the development of the tics.

    Also in contrast to the original literature on the disorder, children with Tourette's have normal intelligence and no propensity toward psychosis. However, between 10 to 50 per cent have an obsessive-compulsive disorder (OCD). In addition, almost 50 per cent have elements of an attention-deficit hyperactivity disorder (ADHD). According to some authors, tics in as many as one third of ADHD–Tourette's syndrome children have been provoked or exacer-

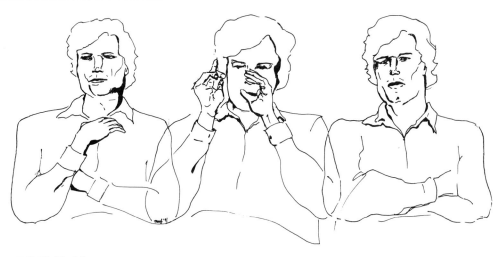

FIGURE 18–34

Copropraxia, in a typically furtive and compulsive, but not sexual or aggressive manner, complicates this young man's Tourette syndrome.

bated by methylphenidate (Ritalin), amphetamines, or pemoline (Cylert)— *All of which* stimulants that block the reuptake of norepinephrine and dopamine; however, *↑ NE, DA.* if the ADHD and tics are both expressions of the same genetic abnormality, *N.B.* exposure to stimulants before the appearance of tics would be merely a coincidence. The data concerning associated behaviors must be examined critically because some studies have included Tourette's syndrome symptoms, such as complex motor tics, as evidence of OCD or ADHD, and do not account for possible overlap between those two diagnoses.

About 50 per cent of patients have soft neurologic signs, and 13 to 50 per *50% = soft* cent have minor, nonspecific EEG abnormalities. CT and MRI scans are normal. *Neurol signs* PET scans show decreased glucose utilization in the inferior frontal and cin- *13–50% =* gulate cortex, but this pattern is also not distinctive. As with many other move- *nonspec EEG abn.* ment disorders, the diagnosis rests in the hands of clinicians. They should be able to diagnose Tourette's syndrome when tics are subtle and do not include *– CT/MRI = ne* coprolalia. *DA ↑* *PET ⊕*

Etiology. Studies have indicated that a single autosomal dominant gene makes carriers vulnerable to Tourette's syndrome. Penetrance is almost complete (100 per cent) in boys, but only about 50 to 70 per cent in girls. With the concordance for Tourette's syndrome far less than 100 per cent for monozygotic twins, nongenetic factors must be important.

The immediate cause of Tourette's syndrome seems to be dopamine hypersensitivity. Dopamine-blocking neuroleptics, particularly haloperidol, suppress the tics. On the other hand, dopamine–enhancing substances, such as cocaine and medical stimulants, exacerbate or provoke tics, at least in some individuals. As if a feedback loop sensed excessive dopamine stimulation, the spinal fluid contains reduced dopamine metabolic products, such as HVA.

Treatment. Medications are usually not indicated for children with single tics, and guidelines are not established for adults with either single or multiple motor tics without verbal tics. In fact, many Tourette patients have mild manifestations that do not require medications.

When indicated, treatment of Tourette's syndrome with haloperidol suppresses the vocalizations and most motor tics in about 80 per cent of patients.

Although haloperidol often causes transient dystonia and gynecomastia in young men, it rarely if ever induces tardive dyskinesia in Tourette's syndrome patients. Other dopamine antagonists, such as fluphenazine (Prolixin) and pimozide (Orap), are also effective. Likewise, although it has drawbacks, tetrabenazine has been effective. An alpha-adrenergic agonist, clonidine (Catapres), had been a popular treatment carrying few side effects, but its purported usefulness has been challenged. Botulinum injections might be used for individual, particularly bothersome motor tics.

Treatment of other symptoms, particularly OCD and ADHD, requires different medications supplemented by nonmedical therapy. The treatment should be aimed at the most pressing symptom. Thus, the use of fluoxetine for OCD and stimulants for ADHD may be justified.

Related Conditions

Several other disorders are also characterized by stereotyped, repetitive, apparently purposeless, involuntary movements. Compared to tics, these movements, *stereotypies*, tend to be more complex, rhythmic, and performed in place of routine activities. They may result from a wide variety of neurologic conditions that involve serious mental disturbances, as well as from psychiatric illnesses.

The classic neurologic example of a stereotypy is the incessant hand washing motions of Rett syndrome (see Fig. 13–14). Similarly, hand shaking, body rocking, and face slapping stereotypies are common features of autism. Some stereotypies may even mimic tardive dyskinesia. ≈ like

Stereotypies are closely associated with mental retardation and blindness. In these conditions, the stereotypies may serve a purpose in that they stimulate individuals who have sensory deprivation. They are also a manifestation of amphetamine intoxication (see Chapter 21).

MYOCLONUS

Myoclonus differs from the classic movement disorders in several respects. The movements consist of irregular, shock-like, and usually generalized muscle contractions. They originate from motor neuron abnormalities in the cerebral cortex, brainstem, or spinal cord—rather than in the basal ganglia. Myoclonus persists when patients are asleep or comatose. *Action myoclonus* can be elicited by the patient's voluntary movement. *Stimulus-sensitive myoclonus* can be elicited by the examiner stimulating the patient with noise, touch, or light.

CORTEX → When myoclonus results from extensive cerebral cortex damage it is associated with dementia, delirium, and seizures. For example, myoclonus is found in the AIDS-dementia complex and Alzheimer's disease. Also, myoclonus is the most prominent physical manifestation of both subacute sclerosing panencephalitis (SSPE) and Creutzfeldt-Jakob disease, which are characterized by myoclonus, dementia, and periodic EEG complexes (see Chapters 7 and 10). Myoclonus also commonly results from metabolic derangements, such as anoxia, uremia, penicillin toxicity, and meperidine (Demerol) toxicity. In most of these conditions, clonazepam (Klonopin) or sometimes valproate (Depakene) can suppress it.

Palatal myoclonus, an entirely different disorder, consists of uninterrupted symmetric contractions of the soft palate. Unlike other movement disorders, the muscle contractions occur regularly and rapidly (120 to 140 times per minute) and are present during sleep as well as wakefulness. Palatal myoclonus, unlike generalized myoclonus, results from small brainstem infarctions that involve the inferior olivary nucleus. Like other disorders confined to the brainstem, especially the medulla, it is not associated with dementia.

MOVEMENT DISORDERS FROM DOPAMINE-BLOCKING NEUROLEPTICS

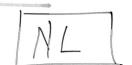

Classic or *typical* dopamine-blocking neuroleptics cause the neuroleptic-malignant syndrome (see Chapter 6), lower the seizure threshold, alter the EEG (see Chapter 10), and produce retinal abnormalities (see Chapter 12). In addition, they can cause a variety of striking involuntary movement disorders that are often called "extrapyramidal reactions." Non-psychiatric, dopamine-blocking medications can produce the same disorders.

The atypical neuroleptics are almost problem free with respect to movement disorders. Clozapine has not been reported to cause extrapyramidal reactions, such as parkinsonism or tardive dyskinesia. Moreover, it may suppress tardive dyskinesia. Risperidone, at therapeutic doses, causes negligible parkinsonism and has not been complicated by tardive dyskinesia.

Neurologists divide most dopamine-blocking disorders into two major groups—*acute* and *tardive dyskinesias* (Table 18–2). The acute dyskinesias develop within days of initiating or increasing the dose of the neuroleptic. They subside spontaneously or in response to decreasing the neuroleptic dose or adding anticholinergic medications. The tardive dyskinesias develop late—as their name indicates—at least 6 months after initiating the neuroleptic. In contrast, they rarely subside spontaneously and are resistant to treatment.

Acute Dyskinesias

Acute Dystonias. Acute dystonic reactions consist of abruptly developing limb or trunk dystonic postures, repetitive jaw and face muscle contractions, tongue protrusion, torticollis, or oculogyric crisis (Fig. 18–35). Any combi-

FIGURE 18–35

During an oculogyric crisis, the patient's eyes roll upward or sideward. When these movements follow the administration of dopamine-blocking neuroleptics, especially if they are aborted by anticholinergics, they can be attributed to the neuroleptic.

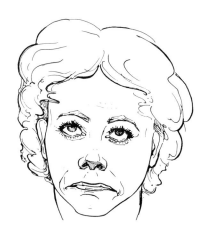

nation of these muscle groups may be involved. Unlike other movement disorders, acute dystonic reactions are painful.

Compared to middle-aged and older individuals, adolescents and young adults seem to be more susceptible and have more severe reactions. They often have forceful, dramatic trunk, neck, and limb extension with prominent retrocollis. Other, serious neurologic disorders—seizures, meningitis, and localized and generalized tetanus—can cause similar postures.

Acute dystonic reactions may be prevented by giving oral anticholinergics. They can be aborted by intravenous anticholinergic or antihistamine medications, such as diphenhydramine (Benadryl) 50 to 100 mg or trihexyphenidyl 2 mg IV, followed by oral anticholinergics for several days.

Their beneficial response to anticholinergic medications indicates that acute dystonic reactions most likely result from excessive cholinergic activity. Alternatively, they result from a paradoxical excessive dopamine sensitivity because the dopamine blockade transiently stimulates dopamine receptors, or as initial neuroleptic doses fall off, the dopamine receptors are left completely exposed.

Parkinsonism.   Neuroleptic-induced parkinsonism was discussed in the previous section which differentiated parkinsonism from Parkinson's disease.

Akathisia.   Akathisia is continual, almost regular leg movements while lying, sitting, or standing (Fig. 18–36). Unlike other movement disorders (ex-

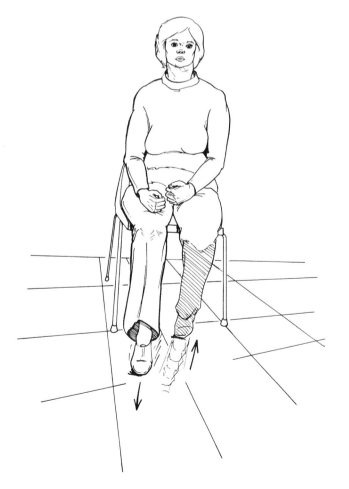

FIGURE 18–36

Akathisia usually consists of continual, fairly regular, to-and-fro sliding leg movements, repeated leg crossings, or lateral knee movements. Leg movements are especially prominent when a neuroleptic causes akinesia of the upper trunk, arms, and face, as in this case. Repetitive arm movements, such as scratching, hair smoothing, and rubbing, may be manifestations of akathisia.

cept for tics), akathisia is partly a response to distressing feelings. Patients complain of having an urge to move, restlessness, and an intense desire to walk.

Their leg movements resemble dopamine-induced movements, as occur in excessive L-dopa treatment (Sinemet toxicity) and those produced by fluoxetine. Akathisia may be easily distinguished from the restless leg syndrome and polyneuropathy-induced leg movements by its lack of paresthesias. Perhaps most commonly, akathisia is mistaken for anxiety, agitated depression, or an insufficiently treated psychiatric disturbance because the sensations can exceed the movements.

As neuroleptic treatment continues, akathisia recedes. It can be alleviated by reducing the neuroleptic dosage. A variety of medications reportedly reduce akathisia: propranolol, benzodiazepines, opioids (propoxyphene, codeine), and anticholinergics.

Tardive Dyskinesias

Oral-Buccal-Lingual Variety. The *oral-buccal-lingual, choreic*, or *orofacial syndrome* variety is so frequently occurring that it has become the generic description for all tardive dyskinesias; however, several varieties of tardive as well as acute dyskinesias should be recognized (Table 18–2). The common oral-buccal-lingual variety consists of tongue, jaw, and lower face movements that are either stereotyped or irregular, i.e., stereotypies or chorea (Fig. 18–37). They are generally painless, are not provoked by urges to move, and do not interrupt speaking, eating, or breathing.

Its frequency and severity are proportional to patients' age, at least until age 60 years. The incidence remains constant throughout neuroleptic exposure, which results in an increasing prevalence with increasing age. The prevalence is greater in women than men, especially for individuals older than 65 years. Individuals with pre-existing brain disease are also especially at risk.

Causes. Despite its limitations, the *dopamine receptor hypersensitivity theory* remains popular and is consistent with several of tardive dyskinesia's major clinical features (Fig. 18–38). For example, tardive dyskinesias begin only a relatively long time (months) after typical dopamine-blocking neuroleptics are instituted, when denervation hypersensitivity would be expected to develop. The dyskinesias are similar, although not identical, to those produced

TABLE 18–2.   NEUROLEPTIC-INDUCED MOVEMENT DISORDERS

Acute dyskinesias
    Oculogyric crisis and other dystonias
    Parkinsonism
    Akathisia
Tardive dyskinesias
    Oral-buccal-lingual[a]
    Dystonia
    Akathisia
    Tics
    Tremor
    Stereotypies
Neuroleptic malignant syndrome
Withdrawal emergent dyskinesias

    [a]Commonly referred to as "tardive dyskinesia."

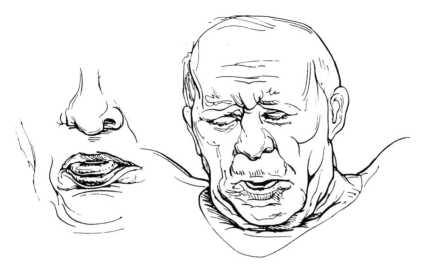

FIGURE 18–37

The oral-buccal-lingual variety of tardive dyskinesia consists of repetitive tongue movements accompanied by continual jaw and facial muscle contractions, i.e., chorea of the tongue, jaw, and lower face. The movements, which may be stereotyped, typically include tongue darting, lip smacking, kissing, lip puckering, chewing, and sometimes blepharospasm.

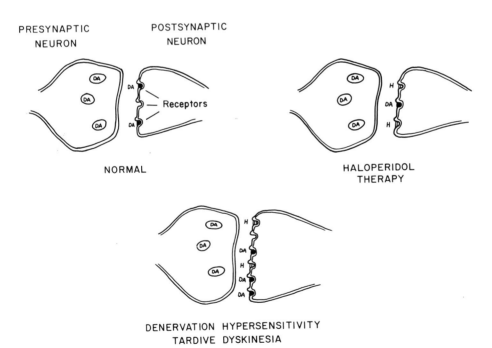

FIGURE 18–38

The denervation hypersensitivity theory proposes that when postsynaptic dopamine receptors are occupied by typical neuroleptics, such as haloperidol, dopamine receptor blockade leads to physiologic denervation. In response, postsynaptic receptor sites eventually become more numerous and more sensitive (hypersensitive). Once hypersensitivity is established, minute quantities of dopamine—either released from the presynaptic neuron, able to evade the blockade, or present in the ambient fluid—trigger receptor-mediated responses.

by excessive L-dopa. They are worsened by maneuvers that expose the post-synaptic neuron to increased dopamine concentrations: reducing the dosage of these neuroleptics, stopping them (withdrawal-emergent syndrome, see below), or adding L-dopa. Likewise, tardive dyskinesias are suppressed by increasing the neuroleptic dosage, which would reduce dopamine receptor exposure. Also, many months after the neuroleptics are discontinued, some cases remit spontaneously, suggesting that dopamine sensitivity can revert to normal.

The theory is consistent with the reports that the atypical antipsychotic medication, clozapine, does not induce parkinsonism or tardive dyskinesias: Clozapine does not block D_2 dopamine receptors.

Alternatively, abnormal GABA activity in the striatum might be responsible. Another theory is that the glutamate system spurs excitotoxicity through the NMDA receptors.

Treatment.   The treatment of tardive dyskinesia is aimed at reducing dopamine activity. Preliminary reports suggest that clozapine might actually suppress tardive dyskinesia induced by other antipsychotic medications. Dopamine depletors, such as reserpine, alpha-methylparatyrosine, and tetrabenazine, have been helpful in some cases, presumably because they reduce dopamine receptor stimulation. One method is to give reserpine 0.25 mg per day with a gradual increase to 5.0 mg per day until a clear benefit or a complication ensues. Use of these medications, however, might be complicated by hypotension, depression, sleep disturbances, or parkinsonism.

As a last resort, physicians can increase the dosage of a dopamine-blocking neuroleptic, substitute a more potent neuroleptic, or reinstate a neuroleptic if it had been discontinued. These plans, of course, may create a vicious cycle in which recurrence of the dyskinesia again requires additional medication.

Although anticholinergics may prevent neuroleptic-induced parkinsonism and acute dystonia, older (but not recent) reports have reported that they worsen this variety of tardive dyskinesia. In either case, anticholinergics do not help, and their use may be complicated by confusion and memory impairment.

A different strategy has been to counterbalance dopamine hypersensitivity with enhanced ACh activity. Physostigmine, which prolongs ACh activity, and ACh precursors, such as deanol (Deaner), lecithin, or choline, have all been administered. However, except for brief periods, they have not been helpful. Various other medications, including GABA agonists, such as valproate (Depakote) and baclofen (Lioresal); a calcium channel blocker, diltiazem (Cardizem); lithium; and clonazepam are not consistently helpful.

Botulinum toxin injections cannot yet be administered for dyskinesias that involve the tongue. Injecting its main muscles (genioglossus and geniohyoid) would require a passage through the upper part of the neck, which contains vital structures. Moreover, it would entail a risk of inducing throat weakness and the tongue slipping back to occlude the airway.

Tardive Dystonia.   A related condition, *tardive dystonia* consists of sustained, powerful, twisting, and predominantly extensor postures (Fig. 18–39). Its incidence is constant over time, and dystonia can develop after a relatively short neuroleptic exposure, sometimes as little as 3 months, as well as after chronic use.

As with many of the tardive dyskinesias, tardive dystonia is often accompanied by other neuroleptic-induced movements, including oral-buccal-lingual dyskinesia, blepharospasm, and akathisia. Tardive dystonia is other-

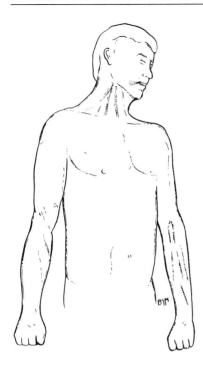

FIGURE 18–39

Tardive dystonia, in a 35-year-old man who has been receiving neuroleptic treatment for several years, consists of prolonged twisting and extension of his arms, extension of his head and neck (retrocollis), and arching of his back. This tardive dyskinesia is accompanied in the majority of cases by choreiform oral-buccal-lingual movements, blepharospasm, or other tardive dyskinesia. Tardive dystonia differs from idiopathic or torsion dystonia in its tendency for retrocollis rather than torticollis and the simultaneous appearance of other tardive dyskinesia.

wise similar to the dystonia in Wilson's disease, torsion dystonia, and juvenile Huntington's disease.

Tardive dystonia, in contrast to choreic oral-buccal-lingual dyskinesia, partially responds to anticholinergics. It is otherwise refractory to treatment. Although dopamine depletion and dopamine receptor blockade have little effect, this disorder has been attributed to dopamine hypersensitivity.

Because tardive dystonia is usually more disabling than other tardive dyskinesias, aggressive measures are justified. Clozapine may also be helpful in suppressing tardive dystonia. Typical neuroleptics can be reinstituted or increased.

Botulinum toxin injections are useful for certain muscle groups, such as those in the neck, which might be particularly troublesome. Injecting the entire spinal musculature is impractical.

Other Tardive Dyskinesias.   *Tardive akathisia*, which appears similar to the acutely developing disorder, persists long after initiation of neuroleptic therapy and, in fact, may appear only after the neuroleptic is withdrawn. Tardive akathisia is often accompanied by oral choreiform movements and other tardive dyskinesias. Emphasizing that tardive akathisia, like acute akathisia, stems from uncomfortable sensations, one neurologist, oversimplifying the situation, quipped that patients with tardive dyskinesia are distressed because they move, but those with tardive akathisia move because they are distressed.

Tardive as well as acute akathisia sometimes can be alleviated by opioids and propranolol. Reported benefits from reserpine, tetrabenazine, amantadine, anticholinergics, and other medications are unconfirmed.

Patients may have *tardive tics* that involve vocalization and breathing, such as grunts and loud, irregular gasping. They can have *tardive oculogyric crises*, *tardive tremors*, and other tardive movements. As with tardive dystonia and akathisia, all these dyskinesias are typically accompanied by oral choreiform movements.

Withdrawal-Emergent Syndrome

As its name suggests, withdrawal-emergent syndrome (WES) consists of excessive, involuntary, rapid dyskinesias following the abrupt cessation of prolonged neuroleptic administration. Mimicking Sydenham's chorea, WES produces generalized choreiform movements with motor impersistence and restlessness, affects only children, and usually lasts less than 6 weeks. Cases lasting longer than 6 months probably represent tardive dyskinesia. For intolerable dyskinesias, physicians might have to reinstitute the neuroleptic and then slowly withdraw it.

Non-Neuroleptic Facial Dyskinesias

Other Medications. Whereas L-dopa medications can cause dyskinesias, dopamine-depleting medications, such as reserpine and tetrabenazine, cause parkinsonism.

Tricyclic antidepressants, because of their anticholinergic properties, cause ocular accommodation impairment (see Fig. 12–4), narrow–angle glaucoma (see Fig. 12–7), and urinary hesitancy or retention (see Fig. 15–4). In addition, about 10 per cent of patients taking them develop a fine tremor that appears similar to essential tremor and also responds to propranolol. The antidepressant amoxapine has dopamine antagonist properties and can induce parkinsonism; however, almost no other antidepressant causes parkinsonism or other sign of extrapyramidal dysfunction.

In contrast, even at therapeutic concentrations, lithium routinely causes a tremor and subtle extrapyramidal dysfunction. At higher concentrations, lithium causes a coarse tremor, but it can be suppressed by propranolol. At excessive concentrations, lithium also causes akinesia, cogwheel rigidity, and dysarthria.

Stimulants—cocaine, methylphenidate, amphetamines, and pemoline—exaggerate, precipitate, or cause tics. Anticonvulsants also cause movement disorders, but generally only at toxic blood concentrations.

Non-Iatrogenic Movements. Abnormal tongue, jaw, and facial movements are, of course, not peculiar to tardive dyskinesia. *Buccolingual dyskinesia of the elderly* is observable in individuals much older than 65 years, especially those with dementia. Also, in edentulous older individuals who have *edentulous orofacial dyskinesia*, the absence of teeth presumably deprives the tongue of its expectable proprioceptive feedback. This dyskinesia is correctable by properly fitting dentures.

Stereotyped movements of the face, mouth, or tongue have been observed in schizophrenic patients who have never received neuroleptics. Such movements may also be found in patients who take L-dopa, antidepressants, and other medications. Patients with chorea, Meige's syndrome, blepharospasm, and tics also have similar movements.

Thus, before initiating neuroleptic treatment, the psychiatrist might record the presence or absence of abnormal movements and distinguish between tardive dyskinesias and other involuntary movement disorders. Although it has some limitations, the *Abnormal Involuntary Movement Scale (AIMS)* is a suitable device (Fig. 18–40). It has several drawbacks. It attempts to assess dyskinesias that fluctuate in intensity during the day; the measurements are gross; akinesia (lack of movement), which is an important sign, is not recognized;

				PATIENT NUMBER	DATA GROUP	EVALUATION DATE	

DEPARTMENT OF HEALTH AND HUMAN SERVICES
PUBLIC HEALTH SERVICE
Alcohol, Drug Abuse, and Mental Health Administration
NIMH Treatment Strategies in Schizophrenia Study

**ABNORMAL INVOLUNTARY
MOVEMENT SCALE
(AIMS)**

PATIENT NUMBER DATA GROUP EVALUATION DATE

— — — — aims   M M   D D   Y Y

PATIENT NAME

RATER NAME

RATER NUMBER

— — —

EVALUATION TYPE *(Circle)*

1 Baseline   4 Start double-blind   7 Start open meds   10 Early termination
2 2-week minor   5 Major evaluation   8 During open meds   11 Study completion
3   6 Other   9 Stop open meds

INSTRUCTIONS: Complete Examination Procedure (reverse side) before
making ratings.
MOVEMENT RATINGS: Rate highest severity observed.

Code: 1 = None
2 = Minimal, may be extreme normal
3 = Mild
4 = Moderate
5 = Severe

				(Circle One)			
FACIAL AND ORAL MOVEMENTS:	1.	**Muscles of Facial Expression** e.g., movements of forehead, eyebrows, periorbital area, cheeks; include frowning, blinking, smiling, grimacing	1	2	3	4	5
	2.	**Lips and Perioral Area** e.g., puckering, pouting, smacking	1	2	3	4	5
	3.	**Jaw** e.g., biting, clenching, chewing, mouth opening, lateral movement	1	2	3	4	5
	4.	**Tongue** Rate only increase in movement both in and out of mouth, NOT inability to sustain movement	1	2	3	4	5
EXTREMITY MOVEMENTS:	5.	**Upper** *(arms, wrists, hands, fingers)* Include choreic movements, (i.e., rapid, objectively purposeless, irregular, spontaneous), athetoid movements (i.e., slow, irregular, complex, serpentine). Do NOT include tremor (i.e., repetitive, regular, rhythmic)	1	2	3	4	5
	6.	**Lower** *(legs, knees, ankles, toes)* e.g., lateral knee movement, foot tapping, heel dropping, foot squirming, inversion and eversion of foot	1	2	3	4	5
TRUNK MOVEMENTS:	7.	**Neck, shoulders, hips** e.g., rocking, twisting, squirming, pelvic gyrations	1	2	3	4	5
GLOBAL JUDGMENTS:	8.	Severity of abnormal movements	None, normal 1 Minimal 2 Mild 3 Moderate 4 Severe 5				
	9.	Incapacitation due to abnormal movements	None, normal 1 Minimal 2 Mild 3 Moderate 4 Severe 5				
	10.	Patient's awareness of abnormal movements Rate only patient's report	No awareness 1 Aware, no distress 2 Aware, mild distress 3 Aware, moderate distress 4 Aware, severe distress 5				
DENTAL STATUS:	11.	Current problems with teeth and/or dentures	No 1 Yes 2				
	12.	Does patient usually wear dentures?	No 1 Yes 2				

ADM 117
Rev. 11-85

FIGURE 18–40

The *Abnormal Involuntary Movement Scale (AIMS)* guides the examiner through inspection for dyskinesias of the face, jaw, tongue, trunk, and limbs. The physician is asked to record observations when the patient is at rest, extending the tongue or limbs, or performing certain activities, such as finger tapping, standing, or walking. In addition, the examiner is asked to check for rigidity. This revision of the original (Guy, 1976), requests that patients remove their shoes and socks, and it does not rate as less severe those movements that are activated. However, tests for akinesia, tremor, and dysarthria are omitted. *Illustration continued on opposite page*.

EXAMINATION PROCEDURE

Either before or after completing the Examination Procedure observe the patient unobtrusively, at rest (e.g., in waiting room).

The chair to be used in this examination should be a hard, firm one without arms.

---

1. Ask patient to remove shoes and socks.

2. Ask patient whether there is anything in his/her mouth (i.e., gum, candy, etc.) and if there is, to remove it.

3. Ask patient about the <u>current</u> condition of his/her teeth. Ask patient if he/she wears dentures. Do teeth or dentures bother patient <u>now</u>?

4. Ask patient whether he/she notices any movements in mouth, face, hands, or feet. If yes, ask to describe and to what extent they <u>currently</u> bother patient or interfere with his/her activities.

5. Have patient sit in chair with hands on knees, legs slightly apart, and feet flat on floor. (Look at entire body for movements while in this position.)

6. Ask patient to sit with hands hanging unsupported. If male, between legs, if female and wearing a dress, hanging over knees. (Observe hands and other body areas.)

7. Ask patient to open mouth. (Observe tongue at rest within mouth.) Do this twice.

8. Ask patient to protrude tongue. (Observe abnormalities of tongue movement.) Do this twice.

9. Ask patient to tap thumb, with each finger, as rapidly as possible for 10-15 seconds; separately with right hand, then with left hand. (Observe facial and leg movements.)

10. Flex and extend patient's left and right arms (one at a time). (Note any rigidity.)

11. Ask patient to stand up. (Observe in profile. Observe all body areas again, hips included.)

12. Ask patient to extend both arms outstretched in front with palms down. (Observe trunk, legs, and mouth.)

13. Have patient walk a few paces, turn, and walk back to chair. (Observe hands and gait.) Do this twice.

FIGURE 18–40

(*Continued*)

and the test does not distinguish among chorea, dystonia, tics, and stereotypies.

PSYCHOGENIC MOVEMENTS

Commonly accepted indications of a psychogenic movement are (1) the absence of movements when patients believe themselves to be unobserved *or* (2) relief with nonpharmacologic treatment, such as placebos, physical therapy, psychotherapy, or physical therapy. Other indications include a variable location, intensity (*incongruency*), or occurrence (paroxysms) of the movements; the coexistence of psychogenic weakness or sensory loss (see Chapter 3), a somatization disorder, or other relevant psychiatric condition; and outstanding litigation.

Virtually every variety of movement disorder has been considered psychogenic, but dystonia and tremors are the ones most commonly diagnosed as such. In psychogenic dystonia, the movements tend to be bizarre, inconsistent in location and incongruent, paroxysmal, and associated with psychogenic weakness and sensory loss. Psychogenic tremor characteristically develops in two planes, has a variable frequency, and, because of fatigue, a diminishing amplitude during long examinations. When a psychogenic tremor affects one arm, it often switches sides when the affected arm is restrained. It may not interfere with activities requiring the same muscles.

Instead of being psychogenic in the usual sense, some movements seem to be culturally determined. For example, the "Jumping Frenchmen of Maine," a group of otherwise healthy French-Canadian descendants, respond to unexpected loud noises by leaping upward, screaming, or throwing any object that they might be holding.

On the other hand, making the diagnosis of a psychogenic movement disorder is perilous. As discussed previously (see above and Chapters 3 and 18), true involuntary movements may be misdiagnosed when they are bizarre, complicated by compensatory movements, or modified by tricks. The following disorders may be self-limited, suppressed, or reduced by various interventions, including concentration, hypnosis, amobarbital, or solitude: tics, torticollis, Parkinson's tremor, and dystonia.

Alternatively, in psychiatric patients with unusual movements, medications may be responsible for bizarre but partly controllable movements, such as acute dystonic reactions and tardive dystonia. Also, in these patients, involuntary movements may intensify the psychiatric disturbances to such an extent that the entire situation is deemed psychiatric.

Another reason for caution in diagnosing psychogenic movement disorders is that outside of referral centers, they are actually rare. Psychogenic movement disorders are rarer than psychogenic seizures or psychogenic hemiparesis. Few patients have seen movement disorders that might be a model for psychogenic behavior. Even fewer have the strength and determination to sustain movements. (Try it yourself.)

SUMMARY

Many involuntary movement disorders are still diagnosed exclusively by their clinical features, the family history, the patient's age at the onset of the illness (Table 18–3), the presence or absence of dementia (Table 18–4), or exposure to neuroleptics (Table 18–2). Laboratory tests are available for Huntington's and Wilson's diseases, SSPE, Lesch-Nyhan syndrome, and dystonia musculorum deformans. The study of involuntary movement disorders has benefited from many major recent medical advances: the treatment of Parkinson's disease with transplantation and ablative surgery, identification of the DNA trinucleotide repeat in Huntington's disease and other illnesses, linking of abnormal chromosomes to various diseases (see Appendix 3), recognition of obsessive-compulsive disorder in Tourette's syndrome, and introduction of botulinum toxin treatment for focal dystonias. Although tardive dyskinesia treatment remains largely ineffective, the atypical neuroleptics may prevent its development.

TABLE 18–3.   COMMONLY CITED MOVEMENT DISORDERS THAT BEGIN IN CHILDHOOD OR ADOLESCENCE

Early childhood
  Athetosis or choreoathetosis
  Lesch-Nyhan syndrome[a]
Childhood
  Childhood-onset Parkinson's disease
  Dopa-responsive dystonia
  Dystonia musculorum deformans (childhood-onset variety)[a]
  Myoclonus from subacute sclerosing panencephalitis (SSPE)
  Sydenham's chorea
  Tourette's syndrome[a]
  Withdrawal-emergent dyskinesia
Adolescence
  Wilson's disease[a]
  Huntington's disease (juvenile form)[a]
  Essential tremor[a]
  Medication- and drug-induced movements
  Tardive dyskinesias

[a]Genetic transmission is established.

TABLE 18–4.   COMMONLY CITED MOVEMENT DISORDERS THAT ARE ASSOCIATED WITH MENTAL ABNORMALITIES[a]

Young children
  Athetosis or choreoathetosis[b]
  Lesch-Nyhan syndrome
  Rett syndrome
Older children and adolescents
  Myoclonus from SSPE
  Wilson's disease
  Huntington's disease[c]
Adults
  AIDS[d]
  Huntington's disease[c]
  Myoclonus from Creutzfeldt-Jakob disease, rarely Alzheimer's disease
  Parkinson's disease

[a]Dementia, depression, or psychotic behavior.
[b]Despite severe movement disorders, many choreoathetosis patients will not have mental abnormalities (Chapter 13).
[c]Sydenham's chorea may cause persistent but only minor abnormalities.
[d]Depending on the presence of encephalitis or toxoplasmosis, AIDS can cause parkinsonism, chorea, tremor, or myoclonus.

REFERENCES

Parkinsonism

Abramowicz M (Ed): Drugs for parkinsonism. Med Lett *35*: 31–34, 1993
Abramowicz M (Ed): Surgical treatment of Parkinson's disease. Med Lett *35*: 103–104, 1993
Caley CF, Friedman JH: Does fluoxetine exacerbate Parkinson's disease? J Clin Psychiatry *53*: 278–282, 1992
Calne DB: Treatment of Parkinson's disease. N Engl J Med *329*: 1021–1027, 1993
Cummings JL: Depression and Parkinson's disease: A review. Am J Psychiatry *149*: 443–454, 1992
Duvoisin RC: Parkinson's Disease: A Guide for Patient and Family (3rd ed). New York, Raven Press, 1991
Ebmeier KP, Calder SA, Crawford JR, et al: Clinical features predicting dementia in idiopathic Parkinson's disease. Neurology *40*: 1222–1224, 1990
Faber R, Trimble MR: Electroconvulsive therapy in Parkinson's disease and other movement disorders. Movement Disord 6: 293–303, 1991
Friedman A, Sienkiewicz J: Psychotic complications of long-term levodopa treatment of Parkinson's disease. Acta Neurol Scand *84*: 111–113, 1991

Goetz CG, Stebbins GT: Risk factors for nursing home placement in advanced Parkinson's disease. Neurology *43*: 2227–2229, 1993

Goetz CG, DeLong MR, Penn RD, et al: Neurosurgical horizons in Parkinson's disease. Neurology *43*: 1–7, 1993

Guze BH, Barrio JC: The etiology of depression in Parkinson's disease patients. Psychosomatics *32*: 390–395, 1991

Mayeux R, Chen J, Mirabello E, et al: An estimate of the incidence of dementia in idiopathic Parkinson's disease. Neurology *40*: 1513–1517, 1990

Olanow CW: Oxidation reactions in Parkinson's disease. Neurology *40* (suppl 3): 32–37, 1990

Pate DS, Margolin DI: Cognitive slowing in Parkinson's and Alzheimer's disease patients: Distinguishing bradyphrenia from dementia. Neurology *44*: 669–674, 1994

Pfeiffer RF, Kang J, Graber B, et al: Clozapine for psychosis in Parkinson's disease. Movement Disord *5*: 239–242, 1990

Schapira AHV: Evidence for mitochondrial dysfunction in Parkinson's disease—A critical appraisal. Movement Disord *9*: 125–138, 1994

Segawa M, Nomura Y, Tanka S, et al: Hereditary progressive dystonia with marked diurnal fluctuation. Adv Neurol *50*: 367–376, 1988

Steur EN: Increase of Parkinson disability after fluoxetine medication. Neurology *43*: 211–213, 1993

Chorea

Folstein SE: The psychopathology of Huntington's disease. Assoc Res Nerv Ment Dis *69*: 181–191, 1991

Gusella JF, MacDonald ME, Ambrose CM, et al: Molecular genetics of Huntington's disease. Arch Neurol *50*: 1157–1163, 1993

Kremer B, Goldberg P, Andrew SE, et al: A worldwide study of the Huntington's disease mutation: The sensitivity and specificity of measuring CAG repeats. N Engl J Med *330*: 1401–1406, 1994

LaSpada AR, Paulson HL, Fischbeck KH: Trinucleotide repeat expansion in neurologic disease. Ann Neurol *36*: 814–822, 1994

Lipe H, Schultz A, Bird TD: Risk factors for suicide in Huntington's disease: A retrospective case-controlled study. Am J Med Genet *48*: 231–233, 1993

Penny JB, Young AB, Shoulson I, et al: Huntington's disease in Venezuela: 7 years of follow-up on symptomatic and asymptomatic individuals. Movement Disord *5*: 93–99, 1990

Strauss ME, Brandt J: Are there neuropsychologic manifestations of the gene for Huntington's disease in asymptomatic, at-risk individuals? Arch Neurol *47*: 905–908, 1990

Tian JR, Zee DS, Lasker AG, et al: Saccades in Huntington's disease. Neurology *41*: 875–881, 1991

Wiggins S, Whyte P, Huggins M, et al: The psychological consequences of predictive testing for Huntington's disease. N Engl J Med *327*: 1401–1405, 1992

Wilson's Disease

Brewer GJ, Yuzbasiyan-Gurkan V: Wilson disease. Medicine *71*: 139–164, 1992

Jackson GH, Meyer A, Lippmann S: Wilson's disease. Psychiatric manifestations may be the clinical presentation. Postgrad Med *95*: 135–138, 1994

Stremmel W, Myerrose KW, Niederau C: Wilson disease: Clinical presentation, treatment, and survival. Ann Intern Med *115*: 720–726, 1991

Dystonia (Non-Neuroleptic)

Bressman SB, Leon DD, Kramer PL, et al: Dystonia in Ashkenazi Jews: Clinical characterization of a founder mutation. Ann Neurol *36*: 771–777, 1994

Calane DB: Dopa-responsive dystonia. Ann Neurol *35*: 381–382, 1994

Jankovic J, Brin MF: Therapeutic uses of botulinum toxin. N Engl J Med *324*: 1186–1194, 1991

Jankovic J, Leder S, Warner D, et al: Cervical dystonia: Clinical findings and associated movement disorders. Neurology *41*: 1088–1091, 1991

Kaufman DM: Facial dyskinesias. Psychosomatics: *30*: 263–268, 1990

Krauss JK, Mohadjier M, Braus DF, et al: Dystonia following head trauma. Movement Disord *7*: 263–272, 1992

Lee MS, Rinne JO, Ceballos-Bauman A, Thompson PD, et al: Dystonia after head trauma. Neurology *44*: 1374–1378, 1994

Therapeutics and Technology Assessment Subcommittee of the American Academy of Neurology: Assessment: The clinical usefulness of botulinum toxin-A in treating neurologic disorders. Neurology *40*: 1332–1336, 1990

Tsui JKC, Bhatt M, Calne S, et al: Botulinum toxin in the treatment of writer's cramp. Neurology *43*: 183–185, 1993

Essential Tremor

Koller WC, Vetere-Overfield B: Acute and chronic effects of propranolol and primidone in essential tremor. Neurology *39*: 1587–1588, 1989

Koller WC, Busenbark K, Miner K, et al: The relationship of essential tremor to other movement disorders: Report on 678 patients. Ann Neurol *35*: 717–723, 1994

Lou JS, Jankovic J: Essential tremor: Clinical correlates in 350 patients. Neurology *41*: 234–238, 1991

Martinelli P, Gabellini AS, Gulli MR, et al: Different clinical features of essential tremor: A 200-patient study. Acta Neurol Scand *75*: 106–111, 1987

Tics, Tourette's Syndrome, and Related Disorders

Chase TN, Friedhoff AJ, Cohen DJ (Eds): Advances in Neurology, Vol. 58: Tourette Syndrome: Genetics, Neurobiology, and Treatment. New York, Raven Press, 1992

Como PG, Kurlan R: An open-label trial of fluoxetine for obsessive-compulsive disorder in Gilles de la Tourette's syndrome. Neurology *41*: 872–874, 1991

Gatto E, Pikielny R, Micheli F: Fluoxetine in Tourette's syndrome. Am J Psychiatry *151*: 946–947, 1994

Goldenberg JN, Brown SB: Coprolalia in younger patients with Gilles de la Tourette syndrome. Movement Disord *9*: 622–625, 1994

Jankovic J, Fahn S: The phenomenology of tics. Movement Disord *1*: 17–26, 1986

Meiselas KD, Spencer EK, Oberfield R, et al: Differentiation of stereotypies from neuroleptic-related dyskinesias in autistic children. J Clin Psychopharmacol *9*: 207–209, 1989

Shapiro AK, Shapiro ES: Evaluation of the reported association of obsessive-compulsive symptoms or disorder with Tourette's syndrome. Compr Psychiatry *33*: 152–165, 1992

Singer HS, Walkup JT: Tourette syndrome and other tic disorders. Medicine *70*: 15–32, 1991

Medication-Induced and Related Movement Disorders

Abramowicz M (Ed): Drugs for psychiatric disorders. Med Lett *36*: 89–96, 1994

Burke RE, Fahn S, Jankovic J, et al: Tardive dystonia: Late-onset and persistent dystonia caused by antipsychotic drugs. Neurology *32*: 1335–1146, 1982

Burke RE, Kang UJ, Jankovic J, et al: Tardive akathisia: An analysis of clinical features and response to open therapeutic trials. Movement Disord *4*: 157–175, 1989

Cardoso FEC, Jankovic J: Cocaine-related movement disorders. Movement Disord *8*: 175–178, 1993

FitzGerald PM, Jankovic J: Tardive oculogyric crises. Neurology *39*: 1434–1437, 1989

Guy W: Abnormal Involuntary Movement Scale (AIMS). In ECDEU Assessment Manual for Psychopharmacology. U.S. Department of Health, Education, and Welfare, pp. 534–37, 1976

Hardie RJ, Lees AJ: Neuroleptic-induced Parkinson's syndrome. J Neurol Neurosurg Psychiatry *51*: 850–854, 1988

Kang UJ, Burke RE, Fahn S: Natural history and treatment of tardive dystonia. Movement Disord *1*: 193–208, 1986

Kaufman DM: Use of botulinum toxin injections for spasmodic torticollis of tardive dyskinesia. J Neuropsychiatry Clin Neurosci *6*: 50–53, 1994

Lang AE, Weiner WJ: Drug-Induced Movement Disorders. Mt. Kisco, NY, Futura Publishing Co, 1992

Lieberman JA, Saltz BL, Johns CA, et al: The effects of clozapine on tardive dyskinesia. Br J Psychiatry *158*: 503–510, 1991

Sachdev P: Clinical characteristics of 15 patients with tardive dystonia. Am J Psychiatry *150*: 498–500, 1993

Stacy M, Jankovic J: Tardive tremor. Movement Disord *7*: 53–57, 1992

Wojcik JD, Falk WE, Fink JS, et al: A review of 32 cases of tardive dystonia. Am J Psychiatry *148*: 1055–1059, 1991

Psychogenic Movement Disorders

Fahn S, Williams DT: Psychogenic dystonia. Adv Neurol *50*: 431–455, 1988

Koller WC, Biary NM: Volitional control of involuntary movements. Movement Disord *4*: 153–156, 1989

Koller W, Lang A, Vetere-Overfield B, et al: Psychogenic tremors. Neurology *39*: 1094–1099, 1989

Owens DG: Dystonia—a potential psychiatric pitfall. Br J Psychiatry *156*: 620–634, 1990

Saint-Hilaire MH, Saint-Hilaire JM, Granger Luc: Jumping Frenchmen of Maine. Neurology *36*: 1269–1271, 1986

QUESTIONS and ANSWERS: CHAPTER 18

1–4. Complete the sentence.

1. In general, movement disorders:

a. Are present intermittently 24 hours a day.
b. Are absent during sleep.
c. May be suppressed by intense voluntary effort.
d. Are made worse by anxiety.
e. Originate in basal ganglia abnormalities.

   answer: b, c, d

2. Gilles de la Tourette's (Tourette's) syndrome is characterized by:

a. Multiple motor tics.
b. Single motor tics.
c. Vocal tics.
d. Variation of the pattern and intensity of tics over many months or years.
e. Constant pattern of verbal and motor tics.
f. Frequent obsessive-compulsive traits.
g. Frequent attention deficit disorders.
h. Progressive cognitive impairment.
i. Family members with a similar or less pronounced condition.

   answer: a, c, d, f, g, i

3. Obscenities in Tourette's syndrome are:

a. Present in all cases.
b. Clearly present in less than one quarter of the cases.
c. Usually develop as an initial symptom.
d. A late manifestation when they occur.
e. May be accompanied by echolalia.

   answer: b, d, e

4. Tourette's syndrome develops:

a. Usually before 5 years of age.
b. Usually before 13 years of age.
c. Predominantly in white Anglo-Saxon Protestants.
d. In girls more than boys.

   answer: b

5. By which two methods is dopamine deactivated?

a. Decarboxylation
b. Oxidation
c. Reuptake
d. Hydroxylation
e. Reduction

   answer: b, c. Most dopamine undergoes reuptake, but some of it is metabolized by monoamine oxidase (MAO) and other enzymes.

6–9. Match the tremor with the examination that will elicit it.

a. Finger-nose test
b. Psychologic stress
c. Extending arms and hands
d. Observing the patient's hands when they are at rest

6. Essential tremor

   answer: c

7. Cerebellar tremor

answer: a

8. Parkinson's disease tremor

answer: d

9. Lithium-induced tremor

answer: c

(Psychologic stress exacerbates most neurologic disorders, including tremors.)

10–15. Match the tremor with an effective therapy (therapies).

a. L-dopa
b. Propranolol (Inderal)
c. Amantadine (Symmetrel)

d. Trihexyphenidyl (Artane)
e. Primidone (Mysoline)
f. None of the above

10. Essential

answer: b, e

11. Cerebellar

answer: f

12. Parkinson's disease

answer: a, c, d (L-dopa may be less effective than anticholinergics)

13. Stagefright

answer: b

14. Hyperthyroidism

answer: b

15. Delirium tremens

answer: f

16–20. Pick the correct answer(s).

16. Spasmodic torticollis:

a. May actually consist of retrocollis and anterocollis as well as torticollis.
b. Develops in childhood.
c. May be relieved by sectioning the sternocleidomastoid and adjacent muscles.
d. May be resisted by applying slight pressure to the chin.
e. Whether a manifestation of tardive dystonia or an idiopathic condition, may respond to botulinum toxin injections.

answer: a, d, e

17. A 37-year-old woman is entirely well, but one of her parents had died of Huntington's disease. What chance does she have of developing the illness?

a. 0 %
b. 25%
c. 50%

d. 75%
e. 100%

answer: b. Since one of her parents had Huntington's disease, at birth this patient had a 50 per cent chance of developing the illness. If she were asymptomatic at age 100 (or even 75) years, the chance of her developing the illness would be virtually 0 per cent.

In all abnormal gene carriers, the average age when Huntington's disease becomes symptomatic is 37 years. Therefore, at age 37 years, 50 per cent of the individuals have become symptomatic. This patient therefore has only a 25 per cent chance. (With DNA studies, genetic abnormalities can be identified at any age and in utero.)

18. Which statements are true regarding the development of dystonia musculorum deformans (DMD) in adolescents:

a. Patients eventually have involvement of the trunk and neck muscles, but limb muscles are usually first affected.
b. At its onset, the disorder may be confused with Wilson's disease.
c. Patients may present with tortipelvis.
d. MRI studies reveal brainstem abnormalities.
e. The inheritance is mostly autosomal dominant with varying degrees of penetrance.
f. Among Eastern European (Ashkenazi) Jews, the disease is so prevalent that further testing is unnecessary.

answer: a, b, c, and e. At the least, children should be tested for Wilson's disease and dopa-responsive dystonia.

19. Which statement regarding surgery for Parkinson's disease is false?

a. In transplantation, mesencephalic fetal cells are inserted into the basal ganglia.
b. Transplanted cells enjoy an "immunologically privileged site."
c. Stereotactic lesions in the globus pallidus, a "pallidotomy," usually offers considerable benefit with minimal risk.
d. The United States prohibits government funding of research utilizing fetal cells, except from miscarriages.
e. Adrenal medulla cells synthesize dopamine, but autologous transplants were unsuccessful.

answer: d

20. Chronic dystonia of the head and neck muscles in young adults may result from:

a. Dystonia musculorum deformans
b. Wilson's disease
c. Huntington's disease
d. Neuroleptic medications, i.e., tardive dystonia

answer: a, b, c, d

21–31. Match the symptoms (21–31) with the movement disorder (a-c).

a. Athetosis
b. Chorea
c. Hemiballismus

21. Unilateral involvement

answer: c

22. Bilateral involvement

answer: a, b

23. Most often associated with dementia

answer: b

24. Associated with mental retardation and seizures

answer: a

25. Continual movements

answer: a

26. Intermittent movements

answer: b, c

27. Greatest movement in distal portions of the extremities

answer: a

28. Prominent involvement of facial muscles

answer: a, b

29. Exacerbated by anxiety

answer: a, b, c

30. Dance-like quality to gait

answer: b

31. Patients suppress movements by mechanical pressure

answer: c

32–40. Match the description (32–40) with the illness (a-d):

a. Huntington's disease	c. Wilson's disease
b. Sydenham's chorea	d. None of the above

32. Recessive sex-linked inheritance

answer: d

33. Autosomal recessive inheritance

answer: c

34. Autosomal dominant inheritance

answer: a

35. May develop in children

answer: a, b, c

36. Not associated with progressive mental deterioration

answer: b

37. Mental changes may precede involuntary movements

answer: a, c

38. Movements may be ameliorated by neuroleptics

answer: a, b, c

39. Presence of Kayser-Fleischer ring

answer: c

40. Associated with rheumatic fever

answer: b

41–49. Match the underlying abnormality (41–49) with the condition (a-h).

a. Huntington's disease	e. Choreoathetotic cerebral palsy
b. Wilson's disease	f. Parkinsonism
c. Hemiballismus	g. Myoclonus
d. Creutzfeldt-Jakob disease	h. SSPE

41. Cerebral cortical anoxia or uremia

    answer: g

42. Toxoplasmosis

    answer: c

43. Perinatal kernicterus

    answer: e

44. Low serum ceruloplasmin

    answer: b

45. Infarction of the subthalamic nucleus

    answer: c

46. Nigrostriatal depigmentation

    answer: f

47. Probably caused by an infectious agent

    answer: d, h

48. Atrophy of the caudate heads

    answer: a

49. Cavitary lesions of the globus pallidus and putamen

    answer: b

50–53. Are these statements true or false?

50. Only one neuroleptic-induced movement disorder may occur at a time.

    answer: False

51. Tetrabenazine and reserpine deplete dopamine from the presynaptic neurons.

    answer: True

52. Phenothiazines induce oculogyric crises and other acute dystonias only when used as an antipsychotic medication.

    answer: False

53. Tardive dyskinesia rarely develops when haloperidol is used for Tourette's syndrome.

    answer: True

54–55. A 29-year-old man has been hospitalized intermittently for the previous 3 years for progressively severe schizophrenia. He has been readmitted because of paranoid hallucinations. His treatment has been resumed with dopamine-blocking neuroleptics. Several weeks later, a visiting physician notices that the patient has intermittent, forceful contractions of all the head and neck muscles that last several seconds. His neck tends to retrovert. Likewise, his limbs involuntarily extend forward. His tongue protrudes intermittently for several seconds. The patient remains alert during these movements, which appear bizarre and "psychotic" to the neurologists.

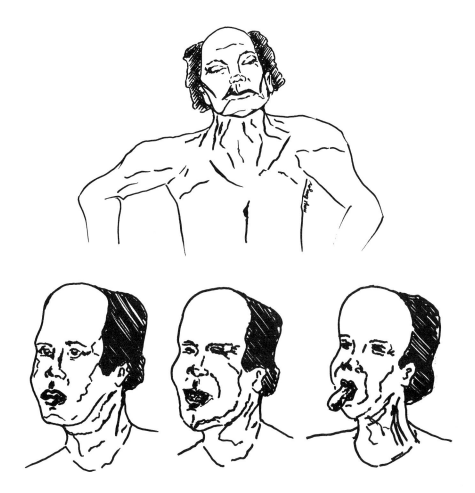

54.   Which single condition is unlikely to cause dystonia in this individual?

a.   Wilson's disease
b.   Chronic neuroleptic use (tardive dystonia)
c.   Torsion dystonia
d.   Multiple sclerosis

answer: d.

Multiple sclerosis only rarely produces a movement disorder. The other choices can each produce dystonia with bizarre features. Wilson's disease and tardive dystonia are associated with mental abnormalities.

55.   Which of the conditions listed in Question 54 is associated with forceful, prolonged tongue movements?

answer: b.

Tardive dystonia is often accompanied by classic, choreiform buccolingual dyskinesia. Classic oral-buccal-lingual tardive dyskinesia tongue movements are brief and irregular, i.e., choreiform.

56   Which single statement is true regarding the trinucleotide (CAG) repeats in Huntington's disease?

a.   The pathologic sequence is located on chromosome 4.
b.   Normal individuals do not have any repeats at the site of the genetic abnormality.

c. The repeats in affected individuals are stable.
d. An affected mother's gene would be more unstable than an affected father's.

answer: a.

Normal individuals have about 20 repeats of the CAG trinucleotide. Huntington's disease patients have 37 or more repeats. The father's gametes are highly unstable and that instability leads to the father being more apt to have a child with juvenile Huntington's disease.

57. Which three illnesses are *not* associated with trinucleotide repeats?

a. Myotonic dystrophy
b. Depression
c. Fragile X syndrome
d. Alzheimer's disease
e. Huntington's disease
f. Duchenne's muscular dystrophy

answer: b, d, f

58. What is the term applied when a genetic illness produces symptoms in younger victims in successive generations?

a. Anticipation
b. Suppression
c. Dys-inhibition
d. None of the above because it does not happen

answer: a.

Anticipation occurs in Huntington's disease, myotonic dystrophy, and several other illnesses. It results from unstable trinucleotide repeats.

59. Which disorders often develop in adolescence and are associated with dementia, which might present with personality change?

a. Creutzfeldt-Jakob disease
b. Wilson's disease
c. Choreoathetotic cerebral palsy
d. Huntington's disease
e. SSPE
f. Essential tremor

answer: b, d, e

60. In which ways does the juvenile variety of Huntington's disease differ from its adult variety?

a. Children may have marked rigidity.
b. In children, the striatum is preserved.
c. The outcome is not fatal.
d. Children may appear to have parkinsonism.
e. Seizures are relatively frequent.
f. Chorea is absent or minimal.
g. Children may appear to have dystonia.
h. The affected chromosome is different.
i. Affected children are more likely to be boys, and their father is more likely to have been the affected parent.
j. Most individuals with 60 or more CAG trinucleotide repeats have juvenile rather than adult Huntington's disease.

answer: a, e, f, g, i, j

61–65. Match the patients' description (61–65) with the neurologic disturbances (a–g) that are often initially diagnosed as psychogenic.

a. Blepharospasm
b. Writer's cramp
c. Spasmodic dysphonia
d. Meige's syndrome
e. Oromandibular dystonia
f. Anxiety-induced tremor (e.g., stage fright)
g. Aphasia
h. Spasmodic torticollis

61. A 70-year-old man develops a high-pitched squeaky voice that forces him to speak in a whisper. Nevertheless, he can sing in a normal volume and pitch.

answer: c

62. An actor begins to have a high-pitched voice and hand tremor while on stage.

answer: f

63. Continual forced bilateral eyelid closure prevents a 70-year-old man from seeing.

answer: a

64. A middle-aged woman develops continual face, eyelid, and jaw contractions.

answer: d

65. An author develops hand cramps when writing with a pen, but he can type, play tennis, and button his shirts.

answer: b

Meige's syndrome, oromandibular dystonia, and spasmodic dysphonia are varieties of cranial dystonia. Spasmodic dysphonia and spasmodic torticollis are varieties of cervical dystonia. Neuroleptic exposure often precedes the development of cranial and cervical dystonias; however, many patients have no history of medicine exposure, psychiatric illness, or any other indication that their movements are a variety of tardive dyskinesia.

66. Which two structures constitute the corpus striatum?

a. Caudate
b. Putamen
c. Globus pallidus

d. Subthalamic
e. Substantia nigra

answer: a, b

67. Which one of the following characteristics does not pertain to the nigrostriatal tract?

a. It links the substantia nigra to the corpus striatum.
b. The substantia nigra are normally black, but in Parkinson's disease they are hypopigmented.
c. It produces about 80 per cent of the dopamine of the brain.
d. Tyrosine is converted to dopa in this tract.
e. Its origin cannot be seen with the naked eye.
f. Its major metabolic end product is HVA.
g. Degeneration of most of the presynaptic neurons leads to Parkinson's disease.

answer: e

68. Sinemet is a combination of L-dopa and which other substance?

a. Carbidopa, a dopa decarboxylase inhibitor
b. Bromocriptine (Parlodel)
c. Anticholinergics

answer: a

69. A 25-year-old man has had lifelong involuntary slow, twisting movements of his face, mouth, trunk, and limbs. The neck muscles have become hypertrophied. He performs poorly on standard intelligence tests. Which two of the following statements regarding his condition are true?

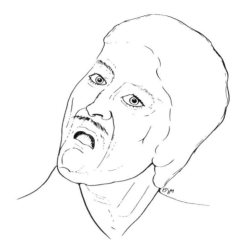

a. His condition might be inherited by his children.
b. He probably performs poorly, in part, because he is dysarthric and unable to use his hands.
c. He probably has lesions in the basal ganglia.
d. His condition is not associated with cognitive impairments.

> ***answer:*** b, c. He probably has congenital athetosis—a variety of cerebral palsy (CP) that becomes apparent between ages 2 and 4 years and is associated with mental retardation. Children with all forms of cerebral palsy tend to be underestimated and undereducated. Dystonia musculorum, which appears late in childhood, is usually inherited as an autosomal dominant condition that is not associated with cognitive impairment.

70. Which of the following statements describe the Lesch-Nyhan syndrome?

a. It is characterized by the onset of dystonia and other movements in children aged 2 to 6 years.
b. It is an autosomal dominant genetic illness.
c. Brain HVA and CAT concentrations are low.
d. The basic deficit is a deficiency of HGPRT.
e. Hyperuricemia is present.

> ***answer:*** a, c, d, e

71. In which conditions is myoclonus found?

a. Cerebral anoxia
b. SSPE
c. Creutzfeldt-Jakob disease
d. Alzheimer's disease
e. Meperidine (Demerol) use
f. Psychogenic disturbances
g. Uremia

> ***answer:*** a, b, c, d (rarely), e, g

72. What is the mechanism of action that permits propranolol to suppress essential tremor?

a. It slows the cardiac output.
b. It is a mild sedative.
c. It blocks both β-1 and β-2 adrenergic sympathetic nervous system receptor sites.
d. It blocks both β-1 adrenergic sympathetic nervous system receptor sites.
e. It suppresses the synthesis of norepinephrine.

> ***answer:*** c. Propranolol is a relatively nonspecific adrenergic blocker, but it is useful in suppressing essential tremor and migraine headaches. However, it may precipitate asthma and congestive heart failure in susceptible individuals. Moreover, its use is frequently complicated by depression and cognitive impairments.

73. Which one of the following is *not* a characteristic of MPTP-induced parkinsonism?

a. MPTP provides a laboratory model of Parkinson's disease.
b. Pretreatment with monoamine oxidase inhibitors protects animals.
c. Patients respond, at least temporarily, to L-dopa replacement.
d. MPTP is toxic only if oxidized by a monoamine oxidase.
e. MPTP is a byproduct of hydrocarbon manufacturing.

   answer: e. Methyl-phenyl-tetrahydro-pyridine (MPTP), a meperidine analogue, is a byproduct of illicit narcotic manufacturing. MPTP is actually not the toxin. It must be converted to MPP⁺ by MAO. The reaction can be prevented with MAO inhibitors.

74. When botulinum A toxin is used to treat blepharospasm, Meige's syndrome, and other orofacial dyskinesias, which mechanism is involved?

a. Botulinum, like tetrabenazine, depletes dopamine.
b. Botulinum binds to the postsynaptic neuron.
c. Botulinum prevents the release of ACh from the presynaptic neuromuscular junction neuron.
d. Botulinum penetrates the blood-brain barrier.

   answer: c

75. Which is the most accurate test for Huntington's disease?

a. Genetic linkage analysis
b. Restriction length fragments
c. Measuring CAG nucleotides
d. PET scans

   answer: c. DNA testing for repeats of the trinucleotide CAG is highly accurate. In general, the number of repeats cannot determine the age when symptoms will develop; however, more than 60 repeats indicate that the illness will develop in childhood.

76. Which statement is false regarding saccades?

a. The term refers to rapid, purposeful, conjugate eye movements.
b. Saccades are abnormal in Huntington's disease and schizophrenia.
c. Abnormal saccades are an early, reliable sign of Huntington's disease.
d. When abnormal, saccades might be initiated by patients jerking their heads.
e. Wernicke-Korsakoff syndrome is characterized by abnormal saccades.

   answer: e

77. Which statement is false regarding the NMDA receptor?

a. It is a type of glutamate receptor.
b. Its inactivity is causally related to Huntington's disease.
c. It may be involved in neurologic damage in epilepsy and stroke.
d. It is a receptor for excitatory neurotransmitters

   answer: b

78. Which structure undergoes the greatest atrophy in Huntington's disease?

a. GABA-producing neurons of the striatum
b. GABA-producing neurons of the cerebral cortex
c. ACh-producing neurons of the striatum
d. ACh-producing neurons of the cerebral cortex
e. NMDA receptors

   answer: a. The striatum consists of the caudate and the putamen. In Huntington's disease, the heads of the caudate nuclei atrophy. Also, GABA concentration in the striatum decreases by 50 per cent.

79. An intravenous drug addict, who has been given neuroleptics, develops dystonic movements that affect his entire body. He is febrile and is found to have a deep infection in his left thigh muscles. His breathing becomes strained because of laryngeal and pharyngeal contractions. His face assumes prolonged contractions. His jaw is pulled backward. Anticholinergics and antihistamines do not correct the problem. Which conditions may have developed?

a. Acute dystonic reaction to neuroleptics
b. Seizures

c. Meige's syndrome
d. An infectious complication of drug abuse

> *answer:* d. Although neuroleptic-induced dystonia is possible, the history of his drug abuse, trismus (lockjaw), and the infection indicate that he may have classic, generalized tetanus. Drug addicts who share dirty needles are prone to tetanus. Immunization lasts for about 10 years. When it wears off, patients can develop tetanus that is either generalized or restricted to the limb with the infection, "regional tetanus." Affected limbs have spontaneous or stimulus-sensitive muscle spasms that mimic dystonia.

80. Which of the following conditions or medications elevate the serum prolactin concentration?

a. Use of clozapine
b. Use of pergolide
c. Use of haloperidol
d. Primary generalized seizures
e. Partial complex seizures

f. Petit mal seizures
g. Pituitary adenoma
h. L-dopa
i. Risperidone

> *answer:* c, d, e, g, i. Prolactin is a pituitary hormone, but not a neurotransmitter. Its secretion into the systemic circulation is normally inhibited by dopamine. Dopamine agonists as well as dopamine inhibit its secretion. In contrast, dopamine blockade, as occurs with many neuroleptics, enhances prolactin secretion, which produces elevated serum prolactin levels. Seizures that involve the limbic system also trigger a transient prolactin release. Many pituitary adenomas, prolactinomas, secrete prolactin. These adenomas can be shrunk and their prolactin secretion suppressed with bromocriptine.

81. A 50-year-old woman, who has been taking antidepressants for 10 years, complains that her face pulls to her left. The movements are uncomfortable but not painful, are more intense during anxiety, and are able to last for several seconds. The eyelid closure prevents her from driving her car. Which one of the following conditions is probably causing her movements?

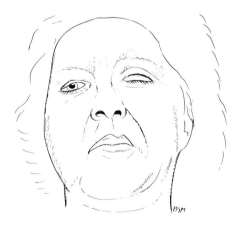

a. An aberrant blood vessel at the cerebellopontine angle
b. Partial complex seizures
c. Dopamine blocking neuroleptics

d. Psychogenic mechanisms
e. Antidepressants

> *answer:* a. She has hemifacial spasm that is caused in most cases by an aberrant blood vessel compressing the facial nerve as it exits from the brainstem.

82. Which two structures constitute the lenticular nuclei?

a. Caudate
b. Putamen
c. Globus pallidus
d. Subthalamic
e. Substantia nigra

answer: b, c

83. Which one of the following nuclei is not part of the set of the others?

a. Substantia nigra
b. Locus ceruleus
c. Dorsal motor nuclei
d. Anterior thalamic nuclei

answer: d. The anterior and other thalamic nuclei are not normally pigmented. The other nuclei, which are basal ganglia, are normally pigmented, but lose their color in Parkinson's disease.

84. A 72-year-old man is brought by his family for evaluation of dementia that developed along with mild rigidity and bradykinesia during the previous several months. Which of the following statements are valid and applicable to this case?

a. Parkinson's disease often causes dementia early in its course.
b. His cerebral cortex, as well as substantia nigra, probably contains Lewy bodies.
c. He probably has depression.
d. He probably has Alzheimer's disease.

answer: b. He probably has diffuse Lewy body disease. Parkinson's disease, at its onset, usually does not cause depression or dementia. Alzheimer's disease usually does not present with either pyramidal or extrapyramidal signs.

85. In the treatment of depression in Parkinson's disease patients, which of the following statements are false?

a. Fluoxetine may cause a potentially fatal interaction with selegiline.
b. Fluoxetine may worsen Parkinson's disease's physical manifestations.
c. Selegiline has an antidepressant effect.
d. Tocopherol is often helpful.

answer: d. Tocopherol is vitamin E, which has no benefit on either the mental or physical manifestations of Parkinson's disease. Selegiline is metabolized, in part, to amphetamine.

86. Which of the following complications is the most common reason why families place Parkinson's disease relatives in nursing homes?

a. Hallucinations and delusions
b. Depression
c. Rigidity
d. Akinesia

answer: a. Sleep disturbances, which usually accompany or result from hallucinations or delusion, are another major reason for nursing home placement.

87. Of the following dopamine receptors, with which do all dopamine agonists interact positively?

a. D_1
b. D_2
c. Both
d. Neither

answer: b. Effective antiparkinsonian dopamine agonists stimulate D_2, but they may either stimulate or inhibit D_1.

88. With which feature of Parkinson's disease is dementia least associated?

a. Older age
b. Rapid progression of the illness
c. Poor response to dopamine medications
d. Tremor
e. Akinesia

answer: d. Of the cardinal features, dementia is *least* closely associated with tremor. If dementia occurs at the onset of an illness with parkinsonism, consider diffuse Lewy body disease in individuals older than 50 years (see Chapter 7). In young adults, consider Wilson's disease, juvenile Huntington's disease, and drug abuse.

89. A 70-year-old man, under treatment for depression for 10 years, has begun to develop intermittent contractions of the orbicularis oculi. His medications were tricyclics until 2 years ago when serotonin reuptake inhibitors were substituted. He had a good response to the change. He had two courses of ECT. The involuntary movements impair his ability to read and intensify the depression. What would be the best treatment?

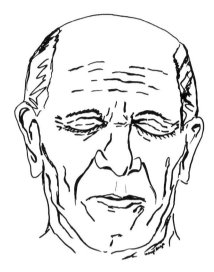

a.   Return to the tricyclic antidepressants.
b.   Prohibit any further ECT.
c.   Reduce the dose of the serotonin reuptake inhibitors.
d.   Add anticholinergic medications.
e.   None of the above.

   answer: e. The patient has developed blepharospasm, but it is probably not a side effect of either the antidepressants or ECT. (Although blepharospasm may follow treatment with dopamine-blocking neuroleptics, in most cases it is an idiopathic condition.) Regardless of its origin, botulinum toxin injections into the affected muscles will alleviate the blepharospasm and permit the antidepressant treatment to continue.

90–92. Match the neurotransmitter (90–92) with its metabolic product(s) (a-c).

a.   HVA
b.   5-HIAA
c.   VMA

90.   Norepinephrine

   answer: c

91.   Dopamine

   answer: a

92.   Serotonin

   answer: b

93.   Which two features are not regularly associated with palatal myoclonus?

a.   Persistence at night   d.   A 4- to 8-Hz regular tremor
b.   Persistence during stupor and coma   e.   Dementia
c.   Injury to the medulla

answer: d, e. Palatal myoclonus results from infarctions, inflammations, or other injuries of the inferior olivary nucleus, which is located in the inferior portion of the medulla. Its frequency is 120 to 140 contractions/minute or 2 to 2.5 Hz. Although it is associated with stupor and coma, palatal myoclonus is not associated with dementia.

94. Which three movements are typically preceded by sensations that compel patients to move?

a. Chorea
b. Tics
c. Restless leg syndrome
d. Akathisia
e. Dystonia

answer: b, c, d

95. Unlike typical neuroleptics, clozapine does not induce parkinsonism. The sparing of which receptor explains this freedom?

a. D_1 dopamine
b. D_2 dopamine
c. D_3 dopamine
d. NMDA
e. GABA

answer: b

96. Which of the following is not a characteristic of free radicals?

a. They contain single, unpaired electrons.
b. They are stable.
c. They snatch away electrons from neighboring atoms or molecules.
d. Removal of electrons oxidizes atoms or molecules.
e. Methylphenylpyridinium (MMP^+) is a free radical.

answer: b

97. Which three characteristics distinguish visual hallucinations in Parkinson's disease from those in schizophrenia?

a. In Parkinson's disease, visual hallucinations often arise independent of psychotic thought.
b. In Parkinson's disease, visual hallucinations are almost never accompanied by auditory hallucinations.
c. In Parkinson's disease, visual hallucinations are often accompanied by dyskinesias.
d. In Parkinson's disease, visual hallucinations are symptoms at the onset of the illness.

answer: a, b, c. Visual symptoms in Parkinson's disease are precipitated or caused by L-dopa medications, but are typically found in older patients with longstanding disease that is complicated by dementia.

98. Which two characteristics of dementia are associated with Parkinson's disease?

a. It responds to L-dopa.
b. Its incidence is constant in various age groups.
c. Thought processes are typically slow.
d. Patients have difficult shifting mental sets.
e. Aphasia and apraxia are commonly associated with the dementia.

answer: c, d. Bradyphrenia and lack of initiative are common manifestations, but these cognitive impairments do not respond to L-dopa. The incidence of dementia in Parkinson's disease increases with age. The dementia conforms more to a subcortical than cortical pattern.

99. What are the two most important implications of dystonia developing in the hand of a 9-year-old boy, rather than a 49-year-old-man?

a. The dystonia will respond to botulinum toxin injections.
b. A therapeutic trial of L-dopa should be administered.

c.   The prognosis is much worse in the boy.
d.   The boy is likely to have had kernicterus.

answer: b, c. Botulinum will be helpful in the hand muscles of either the boy or man. A therapeutic trial of L-dopa should be administered because the child, but not the man, might have dopa-responsive dystonia. Children who develop virtually any dystonia are likely to go on to develop generalized dystonia from either dystonia musculorum deformans (DMD) or an underlying neurologic illness, such as Huntington's or Wilson's disease. Adults who develop dystonia usually do not progress beyond a focal dystonia. Congenital movement disorders, such as athetosis from kernicterus, become apparent before 4 years of age.

19 Brain Tumors and Metastatic Cancer

Brain tumors command unique attention because of their unpredictable onset and potentially tragic consequences. They frequently develop insidiously in young and middle-aged adults in whom they may produce depression, thought disorders, or cognitive impairment without overt physical symptoms. A brain tumor epitomizes an organic cause of psychiatric symptoms.

VARIETIES

Primary Brain Tumors

Primary brain tumors develop within the brain tissue (*parenchyma*) or its coverings (*meninges*) and are named after their original cell line (Table 19–1). Most of these tumors arise from the brain's numerous, mostly small, *glial cells*, which include *astrocytes* and *oligodendrocytes*. Glial cells form the central nervous system (CNS) connective tissue and provide its mechanical, biochemical, and immunologic support. Oligodendrocytes, in addition, produce the myelin insulation for CNS neurons. (Schwann cells produce the myelin insulation for the peripheral nervous system [PNS].) However, unlike neurons, glial cells do not generate electrophysiologic signals.

If glial cells undergo malignant transformation, they form *gliomas*. This group of tumors consists mostly of the *astrocytoma*, which arises from the astrocyte, and its more malignant variety, *glioblastoma multiforme*. Astrocytomas affect children as well as adults, are relatively noninvasive, and develop in the cerebrum, optic nerves, and the structures of the posterior fossa (cerebellum, pons, and medulla).

Astrocytomas are common brain tumors in children, in whom they tend to be cystic and located in the cerebellum. Because they may be removed totally, their cure rate is about 90 per cent. In contrast, astrocytomas in adults usually occur in the cerebrum, infiltrate extensively, and evolve into more malignant forms, such as the glioblastoma. Total surgical removal is practical only if the surrounding brain can be sacrificed. Although cure rates are low, combined surgery and radiotherapy routinely prolong life for 10 years.

Glioblastomas are highly malignant and infiltrating glial tumors, occur almost only in adults, develop in the cerebrum, and grow rapidly. They spread across the corpus callosum (Figs. 19–1A and 20–6). Surgical excision is often attempted, but cure is rarely achieved. Radiotherapy, steroids, and chemotherapy reduce the size and subsequent regrowth of the tumor. They may enable a brief (6 month to 1 year), physically comfortable survival; however,

TABLE 19–1.   PRIMARY BRAIN
                        TUMORS

Gliomas
  Astrocyte tumors
    Astrocytomas
    Glioblastomas
  Oligodendroglioma
Meningiomas[a]
Lymphomas
Medulloblastomas
Pituitary adenomas[a]
Acoustic neuroma[a]

[a]Relatively benign histology.

persistence of the tumor, radiotherapy, and other treatments produce progressive mental deterioration.

Oligodendrocytes, the other major group of glial cells, also give rise to primary brain tumors. These cells lead to *oligodendrogliomas*, which are rarely occurring and slowly growing.

Meningiomas are tumors that arise from the meninges of the CNS. Unlike gliomas, they do not arise within the parenchyma of the CNS. Meningiomas produce symptoms by compressing the underlying brain or spinal cord without infiltrating the parenchyma (Figs. 19–1B and 20–5). They grow slowly and develop almost exclusively in adults. Meningiomas are associated with neurofibromatosis type 1.

Often meningiomas are small and innocuous and must not necessarily be removed. On the other hand, since slowly growing lesions can be asymptomatic, meningiomas over the frontal lobes can grow to an extraordinary size before they cause problems. Many can be totally removed by surgery.

Another variety of primary brain tumor is the *primary cerebral lymphoma*. These tumors develop within the brain parenchyma, but not from astrocytes. Although systemic lymphoma commonly spreads to the CNS, the primary cerebral lymphoma is a neoplasm that develops exclusively in the brain. It is often a consequence of an impaired immunologic system and is thus seen in patients with the acquired immune deficiency syndrome (AIDS) and those receiving immunosuppressive therapy for renal and cardiac transplants. In AIDS patients, cerebral lymphomas are particularly aggressive. In addition, they are difficult to distinguish from cerebral toxoplasmosis (see Figs. 20–7 and 20–18) and cytomegalic inclusion disease because the clinical, CT (computed tomography), and MRI (magnetic resonance imaging) signs of these conditions are similar (see Chapter 7). Treatment of the lymphoma, whatever its cause, includes radiotherapy and chemotherapy. Although diagnostic biopsies are performed, surgical excision is not feasible.

Metastatic Tumors

Metastatic tumors, which are more common than primary brain tumors, spread hematogenously to the brain or spinal cord. (Metastases do not spread to the brain by lymphatic channels because the brain does not have a lymphatic system.) Metastatic tumors tend to be multiple, surrounded by edema, and rapidly growing. Their multiplicity, combined volume, and edema combine to form a burdensome mass (Figs. 19–1C and 20–6). The most common metastatic brain tumors originate from cancer of the lung, breast, kidney, and skin (malignant

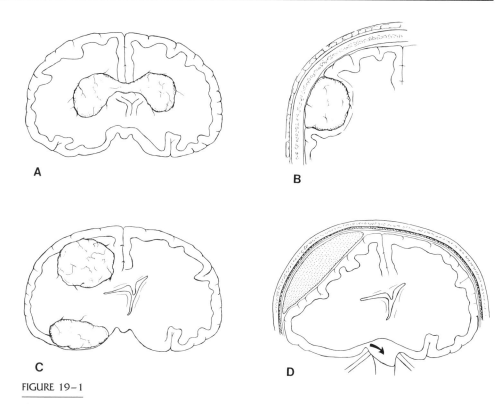

A

B

C

D

FIGURE 19–1

A, A *glioblastoma* is a highly malignant tumor that typically infiltrates. Sometimes it spreads in a "butterfly pattern" from one cerebral hemisphere through the corpus callosum to the other (see Fig. 20–6A). *B, Meningiomas* grow slowly from the meninges overlying the brain or spinal cord (see Fig. 20–5). They compress and irritate, but do not infiltrate the CNS. *C, Metastatic tumors,* usually multiple and surrounded by edema, destroy large areas of brain and raise intracranial pressure (see Fig. 20–6B). *D, Subdural hematomas*, typically located over the cerebral hemisphere (see Figs. 20–10 and 20–11), compress the underlying brain. Acute, rapidly expanding subdural hematomas push the brainstem and ipsilateral oculomotor (third cranial) nerve through the tentorial notch. That process, which also occurs with epidural hematomas (see Chapter 22), *transtentorial herniation*, constitutes an immediately life-threatening condition. In contrast, small or slowly growing meningiomas and subdural hematomas cause relatively few physical symptoms because they are "extra-axial," i.e., situated outside of the brain.

melanomas). In contrast, gastrointestinal, pelvic, and prostatic cancers spread to the brain rarely or only late in their course because these organs' portal vein drainage diverts metastases to the liver. Whatever the origin of the metastatic cancer, steroids, which dramatically reduce the edema, and radiotherapy are palliative. Surgical removal of a single metastasis is sometimes appropriate.

Overall, about 15 per cent of cancer patients develop cerebral metastases, but the incidence is increasing because there is more sensitive detection, many forms of chemotherapy do not penetrate the blood-brain barrier, and cancer patients live longer. Occasionally, the discovery of a metastatic brain tumor is the first indication that a person has cancer. Patients with metastatic brain tumors have complex neurologic problems from CNS and PNS metastases, non-neurologic metastases, and many forms of treatment.

INITIAL PHYSICAL SYMPTOMS

Although mental symptoms occur more frequently, the physical symptoms—seizures, headaches, and lateralized signs—are a more reliable indication of a brain tumor. Seizures do not result from tumors of the brainstem, cerebellum, or spinal cord, but they are the initial symptom of cerebral tumors in approximately one half of patients. Looking at the issue from the opposite perspective, in people older than 50 years, seizures are caused almost equally by brain tumors and strokes. When seizures are a manifestation of a brain tumor, they are partial elementary or partial complex seizures, which often undergo secondary generalization, rather than either absences (petit mal) or other primary generalized seizures (see Chapter 10).

Another aspect of tumor-induced seizures relates to electroshock therapy (ECT). If a patient harboring a brain tumor were to undergo ECT, it might produce multiple, uninterrupted, life-threatening seizures (*status epilepticus*). Large, presumably undetected brain tumors might produce transtentorial herniation during ECT.

Headaches occur frequently as an initial manifestation of brain tumors, but fewer than 1 out of 1000 people with headaches have a tumor. Moreover, brain tumor headaches are not distinctive. They usually mimic tension-type headaches because they are diffuse, dull, relatively mild, and responsive to mild analgesics, including aspirin. Sometimes brain-tumor-induced headaches mimic migraines because they may be predominantly unilateral and worse in the early morning hours when they awaken patients from sleep.

When intracranial pressure increases, tumor headaches intensify and are associated with nausea and vomiting. The increased intracranial pressure also causes generalized physical and mental dysfunction. Pressure transmitted along the optic nerve to the optic disks causes *papilledema* (Fig. 19–2). The physician should bear in mind that the notorious triad of headache, nausea or vomiting, and papilledema occurs relatively late, if at all, in the course of brain tumors. Only a minority of brain tumor victims have papilledema during an initial examination: Its absence should not be taken as evidence against the presence of a brain tumor.

Tumors of the CNS cause common physical neurologic deficits, such as hemiparesis and other lateralized signs, that follow the usual clinical correlations (see Chapters 2 and 4). In most cases, at the initial medical evaluation, however, tumors do not cause pronounced physical deficits because they are small, slowly growing, or located in "silent areas" of the brain; namely the right frontal and both anterior temporal lobes.

Tumors that arise from cranial nerves, although rare, result in readily recognizable distinct deficits. For example, optic nerve gliomas cause optic at-

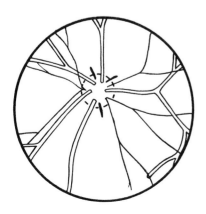

FIGURE 19–2

Papilledema is characterized by reddening of the optic disk, which loses its distinct margin, and by distention of the retinal veins. The disk is elevated, and hemorrhages appear at its edge. (Compare this disk to the normal optic disk in Figure 4–3.)

rophy with blindness. Acoustic neuromas cause unilateral progressive hearing loss and tinnitus.

Meningiomas are a special case. As discussed previously, small meningiomas are frequent, and large meningiomas can be asymptomatic. Nevertheless, meningiomas tend to develop in certain locations and produce characteristic signs. A meningioma arising from the falx, a *parasagittal meningioma*, can compress the medial motor cortex and cause spastic paresis of one or both legs. Meningiomas arising from the sphenoid wing, *sphenoid wing meningiomas* (see Fig. 20–5), can cause paresis of eye movement, proptosis, and damage of the adjacent temporal lobe. Likewise, *olfactory groove meningiomas* can compress the immediately adjacent olfactory and optic nerves and the overlying frontal lobe (see Foster-Kennedy Syndrome, Chapter 4). These tumors characteristically cause anosmia, unilateral blindness, and, when large, frontal lobe dysfunction (see below and Chapter 7).

INITIAL MENTAL SYMPTOMS

Mental symptoms, which vary tremendously, depend on the tumor's location, size, and rate of growth. Unless intracranial pressure is raised, most symptoms are attributable to unilateral or bilateral frontal lobe involvement with rapidly growing tumors, such as a glioblastoma. With increased intracranial pressure, patients successively develop impaired concentration, slowness of thought, lethargy, and then unconsciousness.

Frontal tumors without increased intracranial pressure produce psychomotor retardation with emotional dulling, loss of initiative, and a reduced capacity to execute complex mental tasks. Despite the apathy, cognitive capacity may be spared. Rarely, however, these tumors impair normal inhibitory systems. In these cases, patients may quickly react to any irritation, tend to use profane language, cry with little provocation, and jump from topic to topic.

Mental changes from tumors differ in subtle ways from mental changes in the early stages of Alzheimer's disease (see Chapter 7). In tumor patients, personality changes tend to be prominent while cognitive capacity is preserved. In Alzheimer's disease patients, memory and judgment deteriorate before the personality changes occur. Moreover, Alzheimer-induced cognitive changes develop insidiously over years and are unaccompanied by lateralized deficits.

The distinction between tumor-induced mental changes and depression may be even more subtle. Guidelines, which are admittedly simplistic, suggest that tumors should be considered in an apparently depressed individual who is older than 50 years, if the history is inconsistent with an affective disorder, there is a history of a cancer, or the symptoms include impairment of cognitive, language, or physical function.

In a patient with a known brain tumor, a psychiatrist should attempt to determine how much of the patient's abnormal mental state is psychogenic, neurologic, or iatrogenic (Table 19–2). Being able to achieve an overview, a psychiatrist might help cancer patients, their families, and other physicians by weighing the benefits against the side effects of various treatments; arranging for health care proxies if patients lose their cognitive capacity; assessing analgesics, hypnotics, and antidepressants; and providing supportive psychotherapy.

TABLE 19–2.   EVALUATION OF CANCER PATIENTS WITH MENTAL ABERRATIONS

What is the primary tumor?
  Lung, breast, kidney, malignant melanoma[a]
Where are metastases known to be present?
  Brain, liver, lung, spine
Does the patient have symptoms or signs of a cerebral lesion?
  Headache, seizures, hemiparesis, papilledema
What treatments have been given?
  Radiation: total dose
  Chemotherapy: medications and antiemetics
  Analgesics: daily dose, route, indication, recent changes
  Psychotropics: antidepressants, hypnotics, tranquilizers
  Others: steroids, cimetidine
What is the patient's general status?
  Pain control
  Sleep schedule and restfulness
  Nutrition, weight change, and appetite
  Temperature
What are the results of important laboratory tests?
  Complete blood count
  Serum calcium concentration
  CT or MRI scan

[a]Cancers that tend to metastasize.

Causes of Mental Symptoms

Direct Effects of Brain Tumors. Tumors produce symptoms referable not only to the areas of the brain where they develop but also to adjacent regions where they infiltrate or spread their edema. Furthermore, when intracranial pressure is increased (normally it is below 200 mm H_2O), it impairs the function of the entire brain. Thus, purported associations between tumors in specific areas and certain neuropsychologic syndromes are tenuous or only general guidelines.

Several factors raise intracranial pressure. The mass effect of the tumor and its surrounding edema raises intracranial pressure because the brain is encased within the rigid skull and, unlike the liver with metastases, has virtually no room to expand. Increased intracranial pressure can also result from metastases blocking the flow or reabsorption of cerebrospinal fluid (CSF). Most commonly, metastases in the cerebellum obstruct CSF flow through the fourth ventricle and precipitate *obstructive hydrocephalus*. A similar situation, *carcinomatous meningitis*, occurs when cancer cells coat the meninges at the base of the brain. In addition to these cells impeding reabsorption of CSF and thus causing *communicating hydrocephalus*, they strangulate cranial and spinal nerves.

Medications and Other Treatments. Medications, notoriously narcotics, cause confusion, lethargy, or stupor. For example, the metabolic products of meperidine (Demerol) can result in a toxic psychosis. On the other hand, too little or poorly prescribed narcotics can result in unrelieved suffering, restless sleep, and drug-seeking behavior. Similarly, hypnotics—obviously often essential in patients with pain, discomfort from tests and various tubes, insomnia, and anxiety—can cause dulling, confusion, and disorienting changes in the sleep-wake cycle.

Other medications likely to induce mental changes in cancer patients are antiemetics that contain antihistamines or phenothiazines, cimetidine (Tagamet), anticonvulsants, steroids, and psychotropics. Although the side effects of common medications are usually predictable, sometimes their mental side effects in cancer patients are unexpected. For example, patients might have undiagnosed liver metastases that slow the metabolism of drugs. A patient whose body mass is reduced might be given a relatively large dose of medicine. When several organs are involved, several specialists are each likely to order different medications. Furthermore, multiple medications not only cause mental changes but also interfere with each other's intended benefits.

On the other hand, with few exceptions, chemotherapy agents do not cause mental status changes because they cannot penetrate the blood-brain barrier. An unfortunate exception is methotrexate when administered with craniospinal radiotherapy for childhood leukemia. Although given to protect children from leukemia invasion of the CNS, methotrexate often injures the brain and induces confusional states, learning disabilities, and other permanent intellectual impairment.

Another debilitating aspect of chemotherapy, which is partly neurologic in origin, is the vomiting that it induces (*chemotherapy-induced emesis*). Chemotherapy agents, among their many actions, trigger the brain's *chemoreceptor zone*, which initiates vomiting through the adjacent *vomiting center*. The chemoreceptor zone is located in the *area postrema* of the medulla and is one of the few regions of the brain that is unprotected by the blood-brain barrier. Since it is freely accessible to any blood-borne chemical, the chemoreceptor zone is readily activated by morphine, heroin, and high doses of L-dopa as well as the chemotherapeutic agents.

Another iatrogenic cause of mental changes, particularly dementia, is cranial or "whole brain" radiotherapy. Especially when administered in high doses over a short time, radiation can cause necrosis of small cerebral arteries that results in a series of small, stroke-like cerebral infarctions, termed *radiation necrosis* or *radiation arteritis*. An analogous complication can occur when the spine or mediastinum is radiated: radiation necrosis of the spinal cord, *radiation myelitis*.

Characteristically, the physical and mental deficits suddenly begin about 6 to 18 months after completion of a course of cranial radiotherapy. They often accumulate in a stepwise pattern over several more months to result in irreversible dementia, hemiparesis, and dysarthria. Cranial radiation given to children for acute leukemia leads to mental retardation, dementia, and growth retardation and other hypothalamic-pituitary deficiencies.

Failure of Vital Organs. Medications or metastases can also cause renal, pulmonary, or hepatic failure. The organ failure, usually in the late stages of cancer, can lead to a toxic-metabolic encephalopathy (see Chapter 7). Ectopic hormone production from certain cancers can cause metabolic aberrations. Excess parathyroid hormone production causes hypercalcemia. Inappropriate antidiuretic hormone (ADH) secretion can cause hyponatremia and other electrolyte abnormalities.

Inflammatory and Infectious Conditions. Systemic cancer can also induce antibody-mediated CNS inflammatory disorders, termed *paraneoplastic syndromes* or *remote effects of carcinoma*. In these conditions, patients may have a subacute cerebellar degeneration or other impairments of the CNS. On occasions that are rare but interesting, patients have limbic system involvement, *limbic encephalitis,* that causes memory impairment, personality changes, and alterations in the sensorium.

Cancer patients are susceptible to various bacterial infections when they have indwelling intravenous lines and urinary catheters. These infections are likely to develop in patients with radiotherapy- and chemotherapy-induced immunosuppression. Mental aberrations induced by various infections are difficult to diagnose when, as often occurs, they are unaccompanied by fever and leukocytosis. In addition, immunosuppressed patients are susceptible to fungi, particularly *Cryptococcus*, and other opportunistic organisms.

Similarly, viruses can affect patients who have received intensive chemotherapy. Several can cause a patchy loss of myelin in the brain. For example, *progressive multifocal leukoencephalopathy (PML)*, which is probably caused by a papovavirus, results in diffuse mental and physical impairments late in the course of an illness (see Chapter 7).

DIAGNOSTIC TESTS FOR BRAIN TUMORS

Testing for brain tumors and most neurologic conditions begins with a thorough history and physical, but this clinical evaluation may overlook tumors that are slowly growing, located in silent areas, or cause only nonspecific mental changes, including depression. Despite their expense, CTs are the most reliable, ultimately cost-effective, routine diagnostic procedure (see Chapter 20). Most important, they can detect virtually all of the tumors that might present with depression, psychosis, or similar mental disorder. Also, they are usually sufficient to identify other intracranial lesions, including CVAs, subdural hematomas, and arteriovenous malformations (AVMs).

Although CTs are a satisfactory screening device, MRIs, which are costly, are more sensitive and are necessary to detect optic or acoustic nerve tumors, pituitary adenomas, multiple metastases, PML, and small posterior fossa lesions. If a tumor is detected, an MRI is often necessary to determine its exact location, internal structure, and involvement of the surrounding brain.

In comparison, EEGs are simply not useful for detecting tumors or other structural lesions (see Chapter 10). Even with some large meningiomas, EEGs may show few or only nonspecific abnormalities. However, the EEG remains a good test for detecting toxic-metabolic encephalopathy, particularly hepatic encephalopathy. Arteriography is rarely required because CTs and MRIs are so accurate.

A lumbar puncture (LP) to analyze CSF is usually not performed when a brain tumor or other intracranial mass lesion is suspected. In these cases, the CSF is usually not diagnostic because it is usually either normal or only nonspecific abnormal (see Chapter 20). Moreover, an LP can precipitate transtentorial herniation (Fig. 19–3). However, an LP is indicated when patients are suspected of having carcinomatous meningitis or a chronic, infectious meningitis. In those cases, large volumes of CSF must be examined for carcinoma cells, cultured for fungi, and tested for *Cryptococcus* antigens.

RELATED CONDITIONS

Pituitary Adenomas

Although pituitary adenomas are also considered tumors of the brain, their clinical manifestations, histology, and treatment are entirely different from the brain tumors that have been discussed so far. Classic studies described major mental, physical, and visual abnormalities as common manifestations of pi-

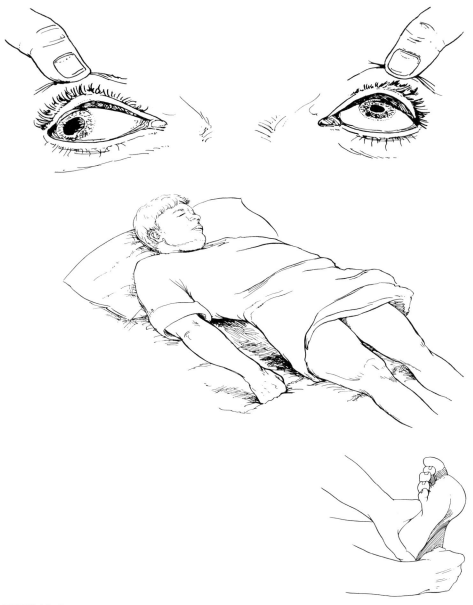

FIGURE 19–3

A patient in *transtentorial herniation* from a right-sided subdural hematoma, as in **19–1D**, has coma, decerebrate (extensor) posture, Babinski signs, and a dilated right pupil. This catastrophe has resulted from the right temporal lobe compressing the right-sided oculomotor nerve and brainstem through the tentorial notch.

tuitary adenomas; however, those symptoms resulted from massive pituitary tumors that produced extraordinary secretions of hormones, expanded out of the sella to encroach on the adjacent temporal lobes and optic chiasm, or obstructed the flow of CSF through the third ventricle. Now these adenomas are detected early in their course, when they are "microscopic," by using readily available diagnostic tests that include MRIs and hormone radioimmunoassay, which are practical applications of two Nobel Prize-winning concepts.

The majority of pituitary adenomas are either *prolactinomas*, which secrete prolactin, or *chromophobe adenomas*, which are nonsecretory. Pituitary adenomas occur almost only in adults and rarely infiltrate the adjacent brain. Although prolactinomas are usually microscopic, chromophobe adenomas typically grow large enough to exert pressure on surrounding structures (Fig. 19–4). Adenomas' upward pressure on the diaphragm sella causes bitemporal or generalized headache. Pressure on the optic chiasm, which is above the diaphragm, causes characteristic visual field cuts: bitemporal superior quadrantanopsia and then bitemporal hemianopsia (see Chapter 12).

In addition to headache, the earliest manifestations of pituitary adenomas are symptoms of hormone irregularities, such as infertility, amenorrhea, decreased libido, and galactorrhea. Eventually, pituitary hormone insufficiency results in a lack of energy, apathy, and listlessness. Patients may appear to be depressed, but their cognitive capacity is normal.

MRIs will reveal virtually all pituitary adenomas. In patients with prolactinomas and most chromophobe adenomas, the serum prolactin level is elevated. Visual field testing is helpful in detecting pituitary adenomas and following their course. Treatment varies with the exact tumor type, symptoms, and institutional expertise, but the usual options are radiation, transphenoidal microsurgery, and, with prolactin-secreting tumors, bromocriptine. Treatment

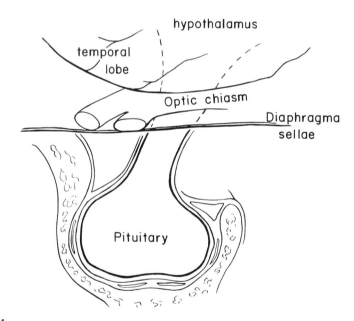

FIGURE 19–4

Pituitary adenomas grow laterally and inferiorly against the walls of the sella turcica and upward against the *diaphragm sella*. Large adenomas compress the optic chiasm, which causes a distinctive bitemporal hemianopsia or bitemporal superior quadrantanopsia (see Fig.12–9). Continuous pressure on the chiasm results in optic atrophy. Large pituitary tumors may first lead to pituitary insufficiency that may have an insidious onset.

Extraordinarily large pituitary tumors compress and damage the adjacent medial inferior surface of the temporal lobe. A craniotomy or radiotherapy directed at a pituitary tumor may also damage this area.

The suprasellar region of the brain, which is above the diaphragm sella, contains the hypothalamus. Lesions in this area, such as craniopharyngiomas, cause diabetes insipidus, as well as optic chiasm compression and pituitary insufficiency.

with radiation or craniotomy, which risks damaging the temporal lobes, can lead to memory impairment and partial complex seizures.

Less common pituitary growths secrete *growth hormone*, which can cause *acromegaly*, or *adrenocorticotropin hormone (ACTH)*, which can cause *Cushing's syndrome*. These growths are not really adenomas, but are mostly collections of hyperplastic cells. Their mass is insufficient to cause visual impairment or severe headache. Their hormones alter the patients' body habitus and reduce their energy. Various psychologic symptoms varying from depression to psychosis were attributed to acromegaly and Cushing's syndrome. However, these symptoms do not occur unless the conditions are advanced and characterized by a marked excess of hormones.

In contrast to these relatively benign pituitary lesions, the *craniopharyngioma*, a tumor that occurs in children as well as in adults, is frequently fatal or severely debilitating. This tumor is a calcified, cystic, congenital lesion derived from Rathke's pouch. Unlike pituitary adenomas, it grows within the hypothalamus, which is located above the diaphragm sella (Fig. 19–4). Since it disrupts endocrine function, affected children have retarded physical, sexual, and mental development; adults have symptoms of impaired libido, amenorrhea, and apathy; and children and adults develop diabetes insipidus. When craniopharyngiomas are large, they press downward on the optic chiasm. This pressure causes optic atrophy and visual field defects similar to those found with large pituitary adenomas. If the third ventricle is compressed, patients develop obstructive hydrocephalus, which causes papilledema with headache, nausea, and vomiting—the classic signs of increased intracranial pressure. Treatment begins with surgery to relieve the hydrocephalus by shunting and then proceeds to draining the cyst, or possibly removing the tumor.

An important non-neoplastic pituitary condition is *postpartum pituitary necrosis*, better known as *Sheehan's syndrome*. It is pituitary insufficiency that classically results from obstetric deliveries complicated by hypotension or another catastrophe. In overt cases, which are unmistakable, women who survive these complicated deliveries fail to lactate, remain hypotensive, lose weight, and have recession of their secondary sexual characteristics. Nevertheless, they do not report hot flashes or other signs of vasomotor instability. Many cases follow less dramatic obstetric problems, do not cause symptoms until several months to several years postpartum, and are responsible for less debilitating physical and mental problems. Affected women have scant menses, constant fatigue, and diminished libido. Similar symptoms may develop because of postpartum autoimmune hypothyroidism. Women with either condition are liable to be misdiagnosed as having psychogenic postpartum depression.

Acoustic Neuromas

The covering of the acoustic (eighth cranial) nerve sometimes proliferates to form a relatively benign tumor—the *acoustic neuroma*. (The term "acoustic neuroma" is a misnomer, however, because Schwann cells, not neurons, proliferate, and the growth develops in the vestibular, not acoustic, portion of the nerve.)

In any case, the tumor develops in the internal auditory canal and the cerebellopontine angle where it may compress adjacent structures, particularly the fifth (trigeminal) and seventh (facial) cranial nerves. Acoustic neuromas cause hearing impairment with speech discrimination being affected early.

Subsequent symptoms are tinnitus, imbalance, and vertigo and then, as the other cranial nerves are compressed, facial sensory loss and weakness.

Abnormalities of the acoustic neuromas can be detected by auditory tests and brainstem auditory evoked responses (see BAERs, Chapter 15). Acoustic neuromas, which usually develop unilaterally and spontaneously, can be visualized with an MRI. However, bilateral acoustic neuromas characteristically develop in young adults with neurofibromatosis-type 2 (NF2), which is an autosomal dominant disorder of chromosome 22 (see Chapter 13). Skilled neurosurgeons can now remove acoustic neuromas while carefully sparing the adjacent facial nerve and often a modicum of hearing.

Spine Metastases

Lung, breast, and other cancers often metastasize to the vertebrae, as well as the brain, where they can grow into the spinal epidural space (Fig. 19–5). These *epidural tumors* cause severe pain not only in the affected region (local pain) but also along the path of the affected nerve roots (radiating pain). For example, patients with thoracic spine metastases typically have interscapular spine pain that radiates around the chest in a bandlike pattern, and patients with lumbar spine metastases have lower back pain that radiates down the legs.

If the metastases continue to grow, they will compress the spinal cord. They will cause quadriplegia when the cervical spinal cord is compressed or paraplegia when the thoracic spinal cord is compressed (see Chapter 2). Spinal

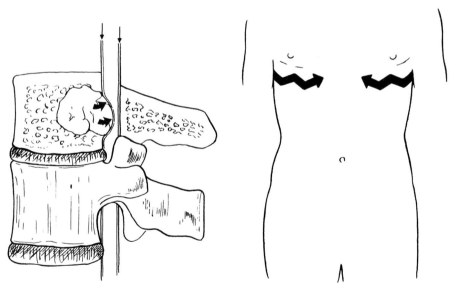

FIGURE 19–5

Left, Vertebral metastases typically grow posteriorly to encroach on the spinal *epidural space* (*thin arrows*), which contains the spinal cord and its nerve roots. This common situation, called an *epidural metastasis,* eventually causes spinal cord compression, which produces paraplegia or quadriplegia, loss of sensation (hypalgesia) below the level of the lesion, and fecal and urinary incontinence. *Right,* Patients have "local pain" from destruction of the vertebrae and a characteristic band-like "radiating pain," which follows the course of the nerves. The location of the pain, which is usually severe, and the level of the hypalgesia indicate the site of an epidural metastatic tumor (see Fig. 2–15).

cord compression generally causes loss of sensation and incontinence of urine and feces. Even with complete spinal cord compression, of course, mental functions are preserved.

In short, spinal cord compression by epidural tumors, a dreadful complication of cancer, causes pain, paraplegia or quadriplegia, and incontinence. Early diagnosis can prevent spinal cord compression, but once compression is complete, which might occur within 48 hours after the onset of weakness, the deficits are usually permanent. MRI of the spine can detect most metastases, but myelography is sometimes necessary. Therapy usually consists of steroids, radiation, and, sometimes, decompressive laminectomy.

Other Causes of Limb Weakness

Cancer-related muscle or peripheral nerve problems (myopathies or neuropathies) may cause weakness, which is the worst symptom of the illness. Patients are most often weak because of cachexia. They have muscle paresis and atrophy accompanied by systemic symptoms, such as anorexia, weight loss, and diffuse pain. Patients and clinicians alike recognize this situation and know that it reflects the extensive spread of cancer. Experienced physicians can acknowledge failure of their primary medical treatments, but can continue to provide realistic symptomatic treatment, including optimal nutrition.

Inflammatory conditions may affect the PNS as well as the CNS and produce weakness. Lung, breast, ovarian, gastric, and other solid tumors provoke *dermatomyositis*, which consists of diffuse, proximal muscle weakness, tenderness, and a heliotrope rash on the face and extensor skin surfaces.

A paraneoplastic syndrome involving the neuromuscular junction is the *Lambert-Eaton syndrome.* Unlike the symptoms of myasthenia gravis and botulism—two better-known neuromuscular junction disorders—the Lambert-Eaton syndrome causes proximal limb muscle weakness that is partially alleviated by repetitive actions. It does not cause the extraocular muscle palsy or dysarthria that characterizes myasthenia and botulism. (The Lambert-Eaton syndrome, botulism, and botulinum toxin, but not myasthenia, cause weakness by impairing the release of acetylcholine [ACh] from the presynaptic neuromuscular junction neuron. Myasthenia is also an inflammatory condition, but its weakness is caused by an abnormally rapid ACh inactivation at the postsynaptic site.)

Iatrogenic weakness from muscle or nerve impairment is common. Prolonged steroid use or the administration of diuretics without potassium supplements impairs muscle function and result in *steroid* and *hypokalemic myopathies*. A generalized impairment of nerves, *polyneuropathy* (see Chapter 5), may be caused by various chemotherapy agents, such as vincristine. Chemotherapy-induced polyneuropathy usually causes a sensory loss, as well as paresis. The paresis can be so sudden, profound, and extensive that it mimics a metastatic spinal cord compression; however, this neuropathy, as other neuropathies, is identifiable by its peripheral distal sensory loss and weakness, areflexia, and the absence of back pain. Most forms of chemotherapy-induced neuropathy improve over several months.

In contrast, injuries of individual peripheral nerves, *mononeuropathies*, cause paresis and sensory loss along the distribution of only one nerve, which is usually in the arm or leg (see Table 5–1). Most often the sequence begins with weight loss from anorexia and other factors leading to the loss of muscle bulk and subcutaneous fat. Then peripheral nerves, deprived of their protective cushion, are vulnerable to pressure even as little as the patient's own weight. The sciatic, peroneal, and radial nerves are most often injured when patients are bedridden, moved onto stretchers, or secured in wheelchairs. Sometimes these nerves are injured by misplaced injections or other accidents.

Probably the most painful cancer complication is tumor infiltration of a nerve plexus. When lung and breast cancers invade the brachial plexus or pelvic cancers invade the lumbosacral plexus, patients develop excruciating pain, as well as paresis of the limb. Since the nerves themselves are invaded, the pain is poorly responsive to routine treatments, such as radiotherapy and analgesics (see Chapter 14).

DISORDERS THAT MIMIC BRAIN TUMORS

CVAs, as well as tumors, occur predominantly in older people and cause mental impairments, physical deficits, and seizures. However, the course of CVAs and tumors is markedly different. Whereas CVAs usually occur acutely or occasionally develop over several days, often being felt when the patient awakens in the morning, brain tumors usually evolve over at least several weeks. Another difference is that even when patients develop extensive physical and intellectual deficits after a CVA, they usually remain alert and free of headaches. For example, a patient with a CVA may be fully alert despite having a homonymous hemianopsia, hemiparesis, and hemisensory loss. To produce a comparable extensive deficit, a tumor would have to extend through an entire cerebral hemisphere. It would then be so large that it would increase the intracranial pressure. Finally, whereas seizures from CVAs develop about 6 months after the CVA, they develop at the onset or early in the course of a tumor. Of course, CTs and MRIs usually can differentiate these conditions.

A *subdural hematoma* is another important, frequently occurring disorder that mimics tumors. Intracranial venous bleeding, usually initiated by head trauma, causes a hematoma in the potential space between the dura (the thick layer of the meninges) and the underlying brain (Figs. 19–1D and 20–11). Over a period of several weeks, the subdural hematoma, which may be either unilateral or bilateral, accumulates fluid and progressively enlarges. As it grows, the subdural hematoma compresses one or both cerebral hemispheres, causing generalized cerebral dysfunction (see Chapter 22).

Older people are especially prone to subdural hematomas because they have intracranial bleeding after minor or even no obvious head injury. Also, the bleeding continues unchecked after its onset because their frequently atrophied brains do not compress the bleeding veins.

Subdural hematomas typically cause headaches, personality changes, and cognitive impairments, but no lateralized signs. They may be easily evacuated through small "twist-drill" holes. When promptly treated, cerebral function can be restored. In other words, subdural hematomas are a relatively common and correctable form of dementia.

Common, nonmalignant cerebral mass lesions, which also begin with headaches, mental changes, lateralized signs, or seizures, are AVMs and brain abscesses. AVMs are congenital abnormalities in which large veins and arteries are directly joined without the normal intervening small vessels. They cause intraparenchymal hemorrhaging, as well as lateralized signs and seizures. Abscesses, which cause mass effect, follow intravenous drug abuse, dental procedures, sinusitis, bacterial endocarditis, and immunodeficiency. The infective organisms in most cases are bacteria, but in cases involving immunodeficiency, *toxoplasmosis* is usually responsible. Patients with *cysticercosis*, which is caused by a parasite that infects multiple regions of the brain, develop multiple focal neurologic deficits, seizures, and increased intracranial pressure. Since cysticercosis is endemic in Central and South America, *neurocysticercosis* can be anticipated in immigrants from these areas. *Tuberculosis* causes intracerebral masses, *tuberculomas*, particularly in patients with AIDS and residents of the Indian subcontinent. All these lesions can be detected by CT or MRI scans, even when they are not suggested by the clinical evaluation (see Fig. 20–20).

In contrast to malignant and nonmalignant mass lesions, *pseudotumor cerebri* is a metabolic disturbance characterized by excessive fluid accumulation in the brain parenchyma. As its name suggests, pseudotumor mimics real tumor because the fluid retention raises intracranial pressure and results in headaches and papilledema (see Chapter 9). Although its etiology is unknown, pseudotumor predominantly affects obese, young women who have menstrual irregularities. Thus, it may be seen as a complication of obesity.

In pseudotumor cerebri, the LP will disclose markedly elevated CSF pressure (300 to 600 mm H_2O) and no white cells. Since the differential diagnosis of pseudotumor is tumor, neurologists order CT or MRI scans. Those studies usually reveal cerebral swelling and compressed, small ventricles because of the brain swelling, but of course no mass lesions.

INDICATIONS FOR EVALUATION FOR BRAIN TUMORS

Brain tumors and related conditions should be considered without waiting for florid physical or mental deficits to appear. Physicians should not rely exclusively on the mental status examination to distinguish between psychogenic disorders and brain tumors. In addition, commonplace complaints of fatigue, weight loss, menstrual irregularity, or infertility might prompt evaluation for pituitary insufficiency or hypothyroidism.

Neurologists generally order a CT or MRI scan of the brain, admittedly quite liberally, for any patient who has intellectual decline; those over 50 years who develop substantial emotional changes; and most adults with headaches that are not attributable to migraines, cluster headaches, trigeminal neuralgia, or temporal arteritis (see Chapter 9). They often also suggest a scan and other tests (see Chapter 7) for patients who develop any new mental illness severe enough to warrant psychiatric hospitalization for the first time. In particular, they suggest a CT or MRI scan before depressed patients undergo ECT because a tumor or other mass lesion, in addition to possibly causing the depression, might either precipitate *status epilepticus* or cause transtentorial herniation. Finally, whenever the patient is worried about a brain tumor, no matter how groundlessly, a scan might be performed to settle the issue and permit appropriate therapy to begin.

REFERENCES

Barry M, Kaldjian LC: Neurocysticercosis. Sem Neurol *13*: 131–143, 1993
Black PM: Brain tumors. N Engl J Med *324*: 1471–1476, 1555–1564, 1991
Byrne TN: Spinal cord compression from epidural metastases. N Engl J Med *327*: 614–619, 1992
Clouston PD, DeAngelis LM, Posner JB: The spectrum of neurological disease in patients with systemic cancer. Ann Neurol *31*: 268–273, 1992

DeAngelis LM: Primary central nervous system lymphoma. Neurology *41*: 619–621, 1991

Duffner PK, Horowitz ME, Krischer JP, et al: Postoperative chemotherapy and delayed radiation in children less than three years of age with malignant brain tumors. N Engl J Med *328*: 1725–1731, 1993

Grunberg SM, Hesketh PJ: Control of chemotherapy-induced emesis. N Engl J Med *329*: 1790–1796, 1993

Newman NJ, Bell IR, McKee AC: Paraneoplastic limbic encephalitis: Neuropsychiatric presentation. Biol Psychiatry 27: 529–542, 1990

Pollack IF: Current concepts: Brain tumors in children. N Engl J Med *331*: 1500–1507, 1994

Scharf D: Neurocysticercosis: Two hundred thirty-eight cases from a California hospital. Arch Neurol *45*: 777–780, 1988

QUESTIONS and ANSWERS: CHAPTER 19

1. An 8-year-old boy, who had a 6-week history of progressively greater difficulty with athletic activities, develops a severe headache, papilledema, and ataxia. Of the following, which is the most likely illness?

a. Meningioma of the cerebellum
b. Glioblastoma of the cerebrum
c. Metastatic carcinoma
d. Astrocytoma of the cerebellum

> **answer:** d. Since he has ataxia as well as signs of increased intracranial pressure without lateralization, the lesion is probably in the cerebellum, causing obstructive hydrocephalus. In children, astrocytomas are a common variety of brain tumor. They typically develop in the cerebellum and are generally curable.

2. A 60-year-old man, who smoked two packs of cigarettes daily since age 20, develops partial complex seizures. He has headaches, a left superior quadrantanopia, and mild left hemiparesis. In addition, he has right-sided dysmetria and intention tremor. Of the following conditions, which is the most likely illness?

a. Subdural hematomas
b. Metastatic carcinoma in the right temporal lobe and right cerebellar hemisphere
c. Glioblastoma of the left temporal lobe
d. CVAs in the right temporal lobe and right cerebellar hemisphere

> **answer:** b. The patient has partial complex seizures, visual field loss, and hemiparesis from a right temporal lobe lesion. He also has right-sided coordination impairments from a right cerebellar lesion. These two lesions are probably manifestations of multiple metastatic tumors, but multiple embolic CVAs are possible. Strokes cause mild and transient headaches. Subdural hematomas rarely cause seizures or cerebellar dysfunction. Also, although subdural hematomas often occur over both cerebral hemispheres, they rarely occur in the posterior fossa. He is too old to have developed multiple sclerosis, and headaches are not a symptom of this illness.

3. A 60-year-old woman has apathy and an impaired ability to concentrate. Otherwise her history is unremarkable, and the neurologic examination is unrevealing. From a neurologic viewpoint, what is the next step in her evaluation?

a. CT or MRI scan
b. EEG
c. Neuropsychologic testing
d. Additional preliminary assessment

> **answer:** a or d. Patients who may have either psychologic or medical (including neurologic) illness should have a complete physical examination. They usually should have routine medical tests that include a CBC, routine chemistry tests, thyroid function, and serology studies. In any case, she probably needs a CT or MRI scan. As a screening test, a CT is sufficient because it would show a mass lesion large enough to cause these symptoms. An EEG may be helpful in diagnosing Creutzfeldt-Jakob disease. It may indicate a metabolic aberration, but the blood tests should detect most abnormalities. Of course, at the conclusion of the evaluation, the patient might be diagnosed as having pseudodementia.

4. A 50-year-old woman has an impaired ability to hear while listening with the telephone receiver next to her right ear. She also has tinnitus on the right and mild loss of auditory acuity on the right, but otherwise her neurologic examination is normal. Of the following, which is the most likely illness?

a. Left temporal lobe meningioma
b. Hysteria
c. Otitis media
d. Cerebellopontine angle tumor

> *answer:* d. Acoustic neuromas, the most common cerebellopontine angle tumor, typically cause speech discrimination impairment, tinnitus, and the gradual loss of auditory acuity. They do not cause vertigo because they develop slowly. Lesions of the cerebral hemispheres or the brainstem do not cause auditory disturbances. Acoustic neuromas are associated with neurofibromatosis type 2, but they are otherwise much less frequent than routine middle and inner ear disease.

5. A 55-year-old woman developed mild paresis of the left leg, which had hyperactive DTRs and a Babinski sign. She refused further evaluation until 11 months later, when she had a seizure that began with clonic movements of the left foot, then leg, and finally the arm. On examination, she has left hemiparesis, hyperactive DTRs, and a Babinski sign. Of the following, which is the most likely illness?

a. Right cerebral glioblastoma
b. Right cerebral meningioma
c. Left cerebral glioblastoma
d. Left cerebral meningioma

> *answer:* b. The evolution of a hemiparesis over a relatively long (11-month) time, especially when it is accompanied by a partial (motor) seizure, suggests a cerebral tumor. In view of the chronicity, a meningioma is more likely than a glioblastoma. Meningiomas are more common in women than men.

6. Which of the following are apt to cause headaches in the elderly?

a. Subdural hematomas
b. Open-angle glaucoma
c. Brain tumors
d. Pseudotumor cerebri
e. Temporal arteritis
f. Nitroglycerin and other vasodilator medications

> *answer:* a, c, e, f. Open-angle glaucoma (b) is not associated with headaches. Pseudotumor (d), although it causes headaches, occurs almost exclusively in young adults.

7. Brain tumor headaches often produce headaches that are worse in the early morning, waking patients from sleep. Which of the following headaches also begin in the early morning?

a. Muscle contraction, tension-type headache
b. Pseudotumor cerebri
c. Migraine
d. Trigeminal neuralgia
e. Postconcussive syndrome
f. Cluster headache
g. Sleep-apnea-induced headache

> *answer:* c, f, g. Migraine and cluster headaches characteristically develop during REM sleep, which occurs predominantly in the early morning. Hypoxia and carbon dioxide retention also cause headache.

8. An obese 22-year-old woman with moderately severe, generalized headaches has papilledema and paresis of abduction of her right eye, but no other neurologic abnormalities. Routine blood and chemistry tests are normal. A CT scan shows small ventricles, but no mass lesion. What would be the most appropriate next step?

a. An MRI to look for a brainstem glioma or cerebrovascular accident
b. EEG
c. Lumbar puncture to measure the pressure and withdraw CSF

> *answer:* c. The patient almost certainly has pseudotumor cerebri, which often causes a sixth cranial nerve palsy. The palsy results from increased intracranial pressure that stretches the nerve. In this setting, a sixth nerve palsy does not result from a localized mass and is called a "false localizing sign."
>
> Given the clinical situation, an MRI is unnecessary. Instead, an LP should be performed as soon as possible for diagnosis and therapy of pseudotumor cerebri

and to exclude chronic meningitis. In pseudotumor, the CSF pressure is usually above 300 mm, which is a marked elevation. Prolonged papilledema, for any reason, will lead to optic atrophy and then blindness. Pseudotumor is one of the rare exceptions when lumbar puncture is done in the presence of papilledema.

9. A 45-year-old policeman with various emotional difficulties has become obsessed with the thought that he has a brain tumor. Careful medical and neurologic examinations are normal. What would most neurologists do next?

a. Offer reassurance
b. Suggest psychotherapy
c. Give an antidepressant
d. Treat him for obsession
e. Take other steps

answer: e. Even though brain tumors are uncommon in middle-aged people, most neurologists would, of course, order a CT or MRI scan for several reasons. At the onset, about 50 per cent of the patients with tumors have no overt physical neurologic deficits. Other structural lesions, such as an AVM or subdural hematoma, could be responsible for the patient's symptoms. Furthermore, with a normal scan, a neurologist can give more secure reassurance, feel protected in the event of a medical-legal problem, and refer the patient to a psychiatrist who will feel more confident in accepting the patient.

10. A 60-year-old man with pulmonary carcinoma develops confusion and agitation. He refuses a full neurologic examination, but physicians find that he has no obvious hemiparesis or nuchal rigidity. A noncontrast head CT is normal. Which of the following are frequent causes of an alteration in mental state in such a patient?

a. Seizures
b. Pneumonia
c. Liver metastases with hepatic encephalopathy or slowed metabolism of medications
d. Increased intracranial pressure
e. Inappropriate ADH secretion
f. Hypercalcemia
g. Hyperkalemia

answer: a, b, c, d, e, f

11. Two months later, the man in the previous case undergoes a CT scan that reveals two ring-shaped lesions with surrounding lucency. The patient becomes combative during the evaluation. Which medication should be given?

a. A neuroleptic
b. An antidepressant
c. Steroids
d. Hypnotics

answer: a, c. A neuroleptic should be given at least until the patient's behavioral disturbances subside. Since steroids, such as dexamethasone, will reduce the edema and thus the volume of the lesion, they will bring about a rapid and dramatic, although short-lived, improvement. Some neurologists would also prophylactically give an anticonvulsant because cerebral metastases often cause seizures.

12. A 65-year-old woman with an onset of dementia over 9 months has no physical or neurologic abnormalities except for frontal release signs and hyperactive DTRs. A full laboratory and EEG evaluation reveals no specific abnormality. A CT scan shows atrophy and a small meningioma in the right parietal convexity. Which would be the most appropriate next step?

a. Have the tumor removed
b. Tentatively diagnose Alzheimer's disease and repeat the clinical evaluation and the CT scan in 6 to 12 months

answer: b. The meningioma is irrelevant to the dementia. These tumors grow so slowly that they can be followed with periodic scans. They should be removed, of course, if they are large enough to compress brain tissue or become symptomatic. An MRI scan might be more helpful in confirming that the lesion is a meningioma, but not whether the patient has Alzheimer's disease.

13. A 75-year-old man, who has had dementia for years, suddenly develops increased irritability and behavioral disturbances. His cognitive impairments are pronounced, but not much more than usual. He has no lateralized signs or indication of increased intracranial pressure. He is treated with a major tranquilizer. One week later, the patient became somnolent and had a seizure. He remains comatose with a left hemiparesis. No abnormalities are found on a general medical examination or routine laboratory tests, but a CT scan shows an extra-axial lucency with some dense regions and a shift of midline structures. Before any treatment can be instituted, the patient dies. An autopsy discloses cerebral atrophy and a large chronic subdural hematoma with recent hemorrhage. Which aspects of subdural hematomas does this case illustrate?

a. Subdural hematomas are apt to occur in the elderly, especially those with a history of dementia and cerebral atrophy, following little or no head trauma.
b. The location of subdural hematomas is outside or overlying the brain, i.e., extra-axial.
c. Unless they are large or rapidly expanding, subdural hematomas may not cause lateralized signs or give indications of increased intracranial pressure.
d. In chronic subdurals, CT scans portray blood as less radiodense than brain. With superimposed bleeding, densities appear within these lucent regions. In other words, chronic hematomas are black (radiolucent), and fresh ones are white (radiodense).

answer: a, b, c, d

14. Which structure is *not* located in the posterior fossa?

a. Sphenoid wing
b. Chemoreceptors for vomiting
c. Vertebrobasilar artery system
d. Cerebellum
e. Fourth ventricle

answer: a

15. Match the brain lesion (1−6) with the group at risk (a-j).

1. Chronic subdural hematoma
2. Cerebellar astrocytoma
3. Cerebral lymphomas
4. Cysticercosis
5. Tuberculosis
6. Acoustic neuromas

a. Drug addicts
b. Elderly individuals
c. Homosexuals
d. Children
e. Residents of Central America
f. Residents of India
g. Neurofibromatosis type 1
h. Neurofibromatosis type 2
i. Trisomy 21
j. AIDS patients

answer: 1-b; 2-d; 3-a, -c, -j; 4-e; 5-a, -c, -f, -j; 6-h

16. Which of the following is *not* usually indicative of a pituitary adenoma?

a. Increased serum prolactin level
b. Cognitive impairment
c. Galactorrhea
d. Bitemporal hemianopsia
e. Decreased libido
f. Menstrual irregularity
g. Headaches
h. Bitemporal superior quadrantanopia
i. Infertility

answer: b

17. Which of the following pituitary conditions is most likely to emerge in a 14-year-old child and delay growth, puberty, and social maturity?

a. Chromophobe adenoma
b. Prolactinoma
c. Cushing's syndrome
d. Craniopharyngioma

answer: d. Unlike other tumors that cause pituitary insufficiency, craniopharyngiomas are congenital lesions that emerge in children and adults. They are typically located in the hypothalamic region, are cystic, and contain calcium that can be seen on CT, MRI, and histologic studies. In children, craniopharyngiomas cause delayed puberty and poor school performance. When craniopharyngiomas are large, they cause the visual impairments characteristic of pituitary tumors, e.g., bitemporal hemianopsia or superior quadrantanopia and optic atrophy. They also cause diabetes insipidus because they grow into the hypothalamus, and obstructive hydrocephalus if they occlude outflow from the third ventricle.

18. Which of the following conditions are usually manifest by papilledema when they are first detected?

a. Chromophobe adenoma
b. Obstructive hydrocephalus
c. Normal-pressure hydrocephalus
d. Cerebellar astrocytoma
e. Cerebral astrocytoma

f. Pseudotumor cerebri
g. Cerebral glioblastoma
h. Optic glioma
i. Acoustic neuroma
j. Parasagittal meningioma

answer: b, d, f. Early in their course, tumors and other conditions that lead to obstructive hydrocephalus usually cause papilledema. In contrast, small or infiltrating tumors usually do not produce enough mass effect to cause papilledema. They cause symptoms referable to cerebral cortex damage, such as cognitive impairment, lateralized signs, and seizures. In other words, the physician should not exclude a tumor as a diagnostic consideration because a patient does not have papilledema.

19. A 65-year-old man with metastatic prostate carcinoma has been in agony from bone metastases. He is agitated, loud, and threatening in his demands for narcotics. He has become a major management problem, and his family is also becoming disruptive. What should be a psychiatry consultant's initial response to this situation after being assured that the patient has no cerebral metastases, hypercalcemia, or other metabolic aberrations?

a. Help the primary physician control the patient's pain with as much narcotics as he wants. Once the pain is controlled, the situation can be reassessed.
b. Stop all medications because they can be the cause of the behavioral disorder.
c. Use minor or major tranquilizers or antidepressants.
d. Before treating further, check with an MRI scan and a lumbar puncture for signs of cerebral metastases or opportunistic infections.

answer: a and possibly c. Metastases to the brain from prostatic cancer virtually never occur, but ones to bone are common—and they are agonizingly painful. Bone pain from metastatic prostate cancer is controlled with hormone manipulation, radiotherapy, and narcotic analgesics that are titrated to the patient's level of comfort. If the pain is poorly controlled, drug-seeking behavior is expectable. Long-acting narcotics, such as methadone, or narcotics given by patch or continuous intravenous infusion are quite effective. "Break-through pain" may be alleviated by "rescue doses" of parenteral narcotics, such as morphine. Narcotics, which act on the CNS, may be enhanced by steroids and nonsteroidal anti-inflammatory agents, which reduce inflammation of bone metastases. Judicious use of antidepressants and tranquilizers may provide additional analgesia, mood improvement, and restful sleep.

20. A 55-year-old man underwent a "total resection" of a right frontal astrocytoma. He was treated postoperatively with whole brain radiotherapy. Residual deficits include a mild left-sided hemiparesis and left homonymous hemianopsia.

Seven months later, he has emotional dulling, anorexia, anxiety, insomnia, marked cognitive impairments, and a tendency to cry. What are the likely neurologic causes of his apparent depression?

answer: He probably has recurrence of the tumor because astrocytomas, a common glial tumor, are infiltrating, and total removal is accomplished rarely. Total removal is possible only when a large section of brain can be sacrificed, as with tumors of the nondominant frontal lobe or sometimes the tip of the frontal, temporal, or occipital lobe.

The tumor has probably grown through the corpus callosum to invade the left frontal lobe. Bilateral frontal lobe involvement will cause depression, personality changes, and pseudobulbar palsy. Antidepressants might elevate the patient's mood, help his sleeplessness, and reduce the pathologic crying.

Another possibility is that the whole brain radiation has caused radiation necrosis. This complication of treatment, in which cerebral arteries become occluded, often causes cognitive and motor deficits. It typically begins between 6 and 18 months after the completion of radiotherapy.

Iatrogenic mental status changes should be considered in brain tumor patients who are routinely treated with anticonvulsants and steroids. Anticonvulsants can cause liver dysfunction, apathy, confusion, and sedation. Steroids can cause anxiety, insomnia, and, in high doses, marked mental aberrations, i.e., steroid psychosis.

21. Of the following lesions, which tend to be located extra-axially?

a. Butterfly gliomas
b. Astrocytomas
c. Meningiomas
d. Epidural hematomas
e. Subdural hematomas

answer: c, d, e

22. Which of the following is not a function of glial cells?

a. To provide structure for the spinal cord
b. To provide structure for the brain
c. To clear debris from infections and CVAs
d. To generate a myelin coat for CNS neurons
e. To generate a myelin coat for PNS neurons
f. To generate electrochemical potentials

answer: e, f

23. What do oligodendrocytes do?

a. Occasionally become oligodendrogliomas
b. Generate myelin for the CNS
c. Generate myelin for the PNS
d. Generate action potentials
e. Act as a glial cell

answer: a, b, e

24. How do brain tumors in children differ from ones in adults?

a. Childhood tumors are usually located in the cerebellum.
b. Childhood astrocytomas are usually relatively benign.
c. In children, tumors tend to present with signs of hydrocephalus.
d. Metastatic tumors in children are as common as primary brain tumors.
e. Meningiomas are relatively common in children.
f. Pituitary adenomas are relatively common in children.

answer: a, b, c

25. Match the condition that causes weakness (1–6) with the impairment of ACh transmission (a-d).

1. Myasthenia gravis
2. Lambert-Eaton syndrome
3. Botulism
4. Guillain-Barré syndrome
5. Botulinum toxin
6. Dermatomyositis
a. Impaired ACh release from the presynaptic neuromuscular neuron
b. Increased degradation or other increased inactivation at the postsynaptic neuron
c. Enhanced reuptake
d. None of the above

answer: 1-b, 2-a, 3-a, 4-d, 5-a, 6-d

26. Which statements are true regarding the chemoreceptor area of the brain?

a. It is located in the medulla.
b. Although stimulating the chemoreceptor area does not immediately produce vomiting, it initiates vomiting through the vomiting center.

    c.   It is located in the area postrema, which is unprotected by the blood-brain barrier.

    d.   The area is accessible to chemicals only during certain illnesses.

    answer: a, b, c

27.   Serum prolactin levels that are transiently elevated above the baseline are a useful diagnostic test for seizures. Which of the following conditions elevate the baseline serum prolactin level?

a.	Chromophobe adenoma	e.	Estrogens
b.	Prolactinoma	f.	Bromocriptine
c.	Phenothiazines	g.	Dopamine
d.	Butyrophenones		

    answer: a-e. Bromocriptine, dopamine, and L-dopa reduce prolactin secretion.

28.   What are complications of performing ECT on a patient with an undetected meningioma?

    a.   Skin necrosis

    b.   Status epilepticus

    c.   Transtentorial herniation

    d.   Exacerbating Parkinson's disease

    answer: b, c. ECT will alleviate, at least temporarily, the motor impairments of Parkinson's disease.

20 Lumbar Puncture, Computed Tomography, and Magnetic Resonance Imaging

LUMBAR PUNCTURE

Examination of a sample of cerebrospinal fluid (CSF), which is usually obtained by a lumbar puncture (LP), is most often required when patients have signs or symptoms of meningitis (headache, fever, and nuchal rigidity) or a subarachnoid hemorrhage (the sudden development of a severe headache, especially if described as the worst of the patient's life).

In evaluating patients with dementia, a lumbar puncture may be advisable. It is usually indicated for the diagnosis of relatively few conditions, which include hydrocephalus and infectious illnesses, such as acquired immunodeficiency syndrome (AIDS), neurosyphilis, Lyme disease, cryptococcal or tuberculous meningitis, and, in children, subacute sclerosing panencephalitis (SSPE). However, an LP is not indicated in patients suspected of having dementia attributable to Creutzfeldt-Jakob's disease, even though it is an infectious illness; Alzheimer's disease; multiple infarctions; Huntington's disease; and most other illnesses.

In several neurologic illnesses, the CSF can reveal a characteristic abnormality. For example, in Guillain-Barré syndrome (see Chapter 5), the CSF has a high protein concentration in contrast to only a slight increase in cell content. In multiple sclerosis (see Chapter 15), the CSF often contains oligoclonal bands and myelin basic protein. In SSPE, it contains antimeasles antibodies. Specific antigens may be detected in meningitis from many bacteria and fungi.

Diagnosing most other neurologic illnesses depends on abnormalities in the CSF color, white blood cell count, and concentration of protein and glucose —the *CSF profile*. With most infectious or inflammatory illnesses, but with the notable exception of Guillain-Barré syndrome, the CSF has an increase in the white blood cell count—a *CSF pleocytosis*—that is paralleled by a rise in protein concentration and a decrease in the glucose concentration. In bacterial meningitis, this trend is accentuated, and CSF pleocytosis is polymorphonuclear instead of lymphocytic. Unless antigen testing is immediately available, reliable identification of virus, fungus, and *Mycobacterium* often requires 1 to 3 weeks of culture. Therefore, the patient's initial diagnosis and first several days of treatment are usually based on the clinical evaluation and the CSF profile (Table 20–1).

In some circumstances, despite the potential value of the CSF examination, an LP is sometimes counterindicated. It should not be performed when patients have an extensive sacral decubitus ulcer because the LP needle may drive bacteria into the spinal canal. It should not be performed above the first lumbar vertebra, which is the lower boundary of the spinal cord, to prevent the spinal cord from being struck by the needle.

The most common counterindication to an LP is the presence of an intracranial mass lesion. This prohibition is based on the fear that an LP could suddenly reduce pressure in the spinal canal and lead to transtentorial herniation caused by the unopposed force of a cerebral mass (see Fig. 19–3). Moreover, CSF examination is not helpful in diagnosing most mass lesions—brain tumors, cerebrovascular accidents (CVAs), subdural hematomas, and toxoplasmosis abscesses—because their CSF profiles are not distinctive. Unless physicians suspect acute bacterial meningitis or subarachnoid hemorrhage, where rapid diagnosis is crucial, they usually do not perform an LP, or they postpone it until after an intracranial lesion has been excluded by computed tomography (CT) or magnetic resonance imaging (MRI).

COMPUTED TOMOGRAPHY

Computed tomography displays the brain, skull, other tissues, and various abnormalities in a black to white scale, with the normal brain being gray. Structures that are increasingly *more* radiodense than brain—tumors, blood,

TABLE 20–1. CEREBROSPINAL FLUID (CSF) PROFILES[a]

	Color	WBC/mm	Protein (mg/100 ml)	Glucose (mg/100 ml)	Miscellaneous
Normal	Clear	$0-4^b$	30–45	60–100	
Bacterial meningitis	*Turbid*	100–500	75–200	*0–40*	Gram stain may reveal organisms
Viral meningitis	*Turbid*	*50–100^b*	50–100	40–60	
TB and fungal meningitis[c]	*Turbid*	*100–500^b*	100–500	40–60	Cryptococcus antigen shoud be ordered
Neurosyphilis	Clear	$5-200^b$	45–100	40–80	VDRL positive[d]
Guillain-Barré syndrome	Clear	$5-20^b$	*80–200*	60–100	
Subarachnoid hemorrhage	*Bloody*	White and red cells in same proportion as in blood[e]	45–80	60–100	Supernatant usually xanthochromic

[a]Characteristic abnormalities in italics.
[b]Mostly lymphocytes.
[c]In carcinomatous meningitis, the CSF profile is similar to fungal meningitis, but malignant cells may be detected.
[d]About 40 per cent of neurosyphilis cases have a false-negative VDRL CSF test (see Chapter 7).
[e]1:1000.

bone, and calcifications—are increasingly closer to white. Structures that are increasingly *less* radiodense than the brain, particularly the ventricles, which are filled with CSF, are increasingly closer to black. Common lesions that are virtually black are cerebral infarctions, chronic subdural hematomas, cystic lesions, and the edema surrounding tumors.

When iodine-containing contrast solutions are administered, blood-filled structures become more radiodense and thus more white. This phenomenon, *contrast enhancement*, highlights vascular structures, such as arteriovenous malformations, glioblastomas, and the membranes of chronic subdural hematomas.

In several situations, CT should be avoided or modified. CT exposes the patient to a dose of ionizing radiation that is slightly greater than that of a conventional x-ray skull series. Even though that radiation dose is still relatively small and is confined to the head, ordering CT examinations should be considered carefully and should be avoided in pregnant women. Also, since the contrast solution can provoke a reaction in individuals who are allergic to iodine-containing substances, including shellfish, contrast solutions should be selectively administered. Hyperosmolar contrast solution administration should not be given to patients with diabetes, dehydration, or other hyperviscosity states because they might precipitate renal failure. However, hypoosmolar solutions, although expensive, can be used in these circumstances.

The warnings are trivial compared to the amazing benefit of CT and MRI scans. They are diagnostically indispensable, generally cost effective, and are far more reliable than the electroencephalogram (EEG), conventional x-ray skull series, or isotopic brain scan. They are routinely performed for numerous, common neurologic conditions, including dementia, delirium, aphasia, other neuropsychologic deficits, headaches in elderly individuals, and partial seizures (Figs. 20–1 to 20–12). On the other hand, these scans are not particularly indicated in sleep disturbances, absence (petit mal) seizures, cluster and migraine headaches, Parkinson's disease, tics, essential tremor, or diseases of the peripheral nervous system.

Although specific criteria are still not yet established for ordering CT or MRI scans for individuals who seem to have psychiatric illness, their use has become commonplace in the evaluation of patients who have developed a first episode of psychosis, atypical psychosis, depression after the age of 50 years, profound depression at any age, episodic behavioral disturbances, and in some cases of anorexia. These scans can exclude structural lesions that could conceivably account for those psychiatric symptoms; however, relationships remain problematic between psychiatric symptoms and cerebral atrophy, small cerebral lesions, and congenital abnormalities.

The most consistent correlation between CT and MRI abnormalities and psychiatric illness has been shown by several studies—about 20 per cent of chronic schizophrenic patients, compared to those with affective disorders and to control groups, have large CSF-filled lateral ventricles and a small brain volume. The hydrocephalus, also called the "increased ventricular-brain ratio," is most pronounced in the temporal horns of the lateral ventricles. The large lateral ventricles are usually accompanied by a large third ventricle and wide cerebral cortical sulci.

The abnormal ventricular enlargement occurs predominantly in schizophrenic patients with severe illness, a history of perinatal complications, preponderance of negative symptoms (in most studies), greater resistance to neuroleptics, more cognitive impairments, and worse outcomes. The enlargement

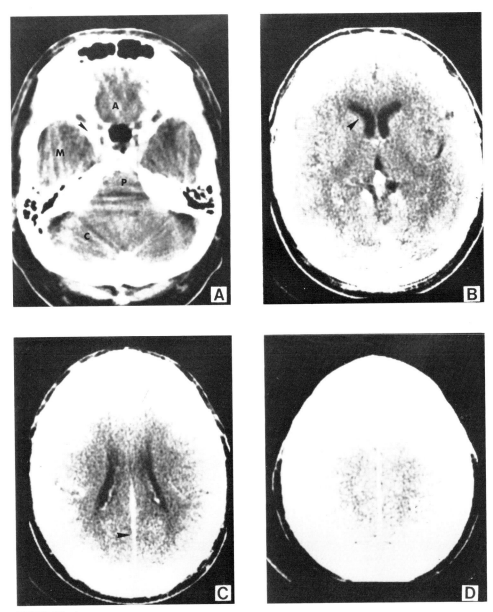

FIGURE 20-1

Four representative, progressively higher *transaxial* (*axial*) view CT scans of a normal brain. *A,*
The anterior fossae (*A*) contain the anterior frontal lobes and the olfactory nerves. Immediately
posterior is a circular black area, which represents the sella turcica. However, artifacts from
bone and relatively poor resolution prevent visualization of its pituitary gland. The middle fossae
(*M*) contain the anterior temporal lobes, which are situated behind the sphenoid wing (*arrowhead*). The posterior fossa contains the cerebellum (*C*) and the medulla and pons (*P*), which are
called the bulb. The black streaks that seem to cut across the posterior fossa are artifacts from
the skull. *B,* The anterior horns of the lateral ventricles are indented by the heads of the caudate
nuclei (*arrowhead*). A calcified pineal gland is the small white structure in the center. The third
ventricle is the small triangular black area anterior to the pineal gland. *C,* The lateral ventricles,
spread lengthwise in the hemispheres, are separated by the white, straight sagittal sinus
(*arrowhead*). *D,* The cerebral cortex is adjacent to the inner table of the skull. Since the normal
gyri are separated by thin sulci, individual gyri are not discernible.

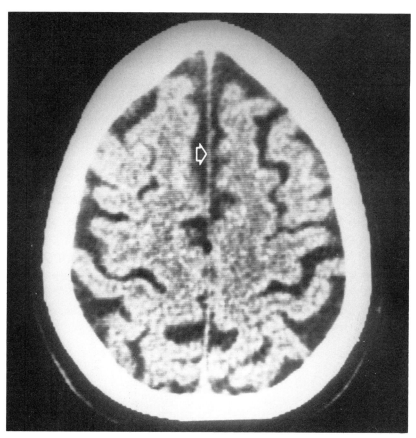

FIGURE 20-2

This CT scan shows cerebral atrophy (see Fig. 20-16 for MRI appearance of cerebral atrophy). The gyri are thin, and the sulci are wide. Because of the atrophy, the cerebral cortex is retracted from the inner table of the skull and from the sagittal sinus (*open arrow*)—in contrast to the normal situation (Fig. 20-1D) in which the gyri are indistinguishable, sulci are not discernible, and the cortex seems to blend into the skull. Cerebral atrophy, as pictured in this CT scan, is a normal concomitant of old age, and it is not necessarily associated with intellectual deterioration. However, it is closely associated with Alzheimer's disease, Down's syndrome (trisomy 21), AIDS dementia, alcoholism, cocaine abuse, degenerative neurologic illnesses, and treatment-resistant schizophrenia.

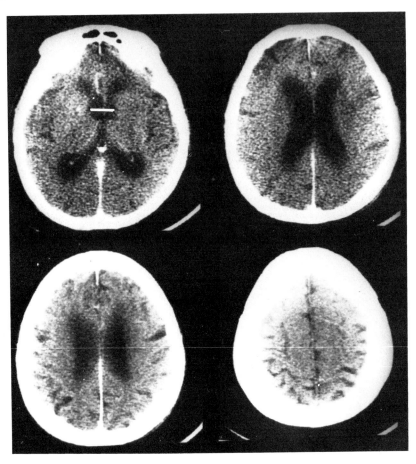

FIGURE 20–3

This CT scan illustrates that cerebral atrophy also leads to expansion of the lateral ventricles and widening of the third ventricle (*line*)—hydrocephalus ex vacuo or an increased ventricular-brain ratio.

is not attributable to age, neuroleptic use, or electroshock therapy. Although large ventricles mean worse schizophrenia, CT and MRI scans cannot be used to support the diagnosis.

Another difference in schizophrenia, according to some studies, is a lack of normal cerebral asymmetry, in which the cortex of the dominant (usually left) hemisphere is normally more convoluted than that of the nondominant (see Chapter 8). Finally, many of these studies reveal decreased volume of the amygdala and hippocampus (the temporal lobe components of the limbic system) in schizophrenic patients. Some children with autism have the loss of cerebral asymmetry, other dominant hemisphere abnormalities, and also relatively small cerebellar hemispheres; however, these cerebral abnormalities have been found inconsistently and were present mostly in children who also had mental retardation or congenital physical neurologic impairments.

MAGNETIC RESONANCE IMAGING

To perform an MRI, patients are placed in a strong magnet that forces protons' spin axis to be parallel with the magnetic field. Then radiofrequency (RF)

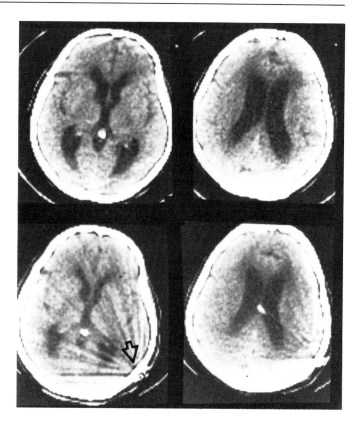

FIGURE 20–4

Top two scans, In normal-pressure hydrocephalus (NPH), CT scans show ventricular dilation, including widening of the ventricular horns of the lateral ventricles (see Fig. 20–15 for MRI of NPH), but little or no cerebral atrophy. *Bottom two scans,* After instillation of a shunt (*open arrow*), the size of the ventricles decreases. In this pair of scans, notice the linear artifacts emanating from the shunt. Unfortunately, the distinction between NPH and hydrocephalus ex vacuo, based exclusively on CT and MRI scans, is unreliable.

pulses are applied to orient the protons in the same direction. After the RF pulses, the protons resume their previous alignment ("relax") within the magnetic field and thereby emit energy. The energy (signal) is characteristic for the tissues and is detected readily. Changing relaxation times and other parameters highlight different features.

In the brain, the energy is emitted mostly from hydrogen nuclei (protons) in water-containing tissue. The 20 per cent greater water content of gray matter compared to white matter and the differences in water content between various tissues result in signals of different intensity. These signals eventually generate the MRI images (scans).

MRI scans offer extraordinary resolution and several other advantages over CT scans (Table 20–2). Although no physician should be a slave to photographs, the MRI permits extraordinarily accurate diagnoses. At the very least, it can offer assurance that structural lesions are not present. By simple manipulations in the software, rather than by having to contort the patient, the MRI machinery can generate images of the brain and its small components, including the acoustic and optic nerves, and display the images in the three major planes: transaxial (conventional top-down view), coronal (front-to-back view), and sagittal (side view). Another advantage of MRI is that since most of the skull is comprised of cortical bone, which contains no water, images of the brain are free of interference from the skull. Thus, MRI can generate detailed images of the cerebellum and other posterior fossa contents, pituitary gland, spinal cord, eyes, and other structures that are shielded from ionizing radiation by bony casings (Fig. 20–13). On the other hand, MRI poorly detects lesions with little or no water content, such as some meningiomas.

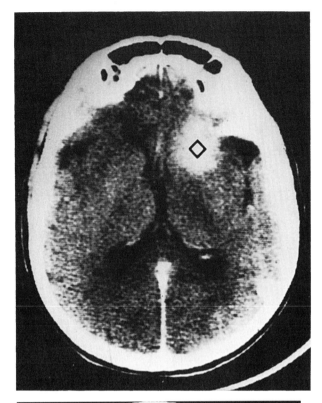

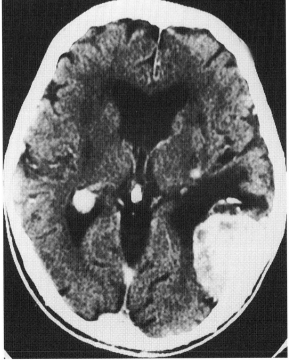

FIGURE 20–5

Top, This CT scan shows a radiodense lesion (*diamond*), typical of a meningioma, arising from the right sphenoid wing. These lesions can irritate the temporal lobe posteriorly, triggering partial complex seizures, or they can grow anteriorly and compress the frontal lobe and the olfactory (first cranial) nerve, i.e., causing the Foster-Kennedy syndrome (see Chapter 4). *Bottom*, This CT shows a large, radiodense meningioma that exerts relatively little mass effect. In contrast to glioblastomas (Fig. 20–6A), large infarctions (Fig. 20–8A), and subdural hematomas (Fig. 20–10), meningiomas develop slowly and thus may not produce symptoms until they are very large. In addition, small meningiomas, which are common, do not produce symptoms. Because they are composed of radiodense calcium and contain virtually no water, meningiomas are one of the few structural lesions that are more readily visualized on CT than MRI scans.

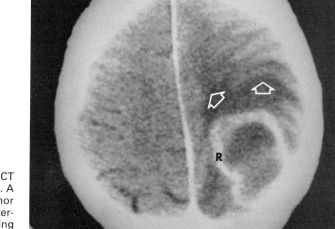

FIGURE 20-6

A, This contrast-enhanced CT scan illustrates a glioblastoma. A circular, dark region of the tumor is surrounded by the characteristic white, contrast-enhancing ring (*R*) and a large border of black brain edema (*open arrows*). The mass effect of the lesion compresses the adjacent brain and shifts midline structures, such as the sagittal sinus (see Fig. 20-19 for an MRI scan of a glioblastoma). *B,* This CT scan, which is also contrast enhanced, shows two metastatic tumors (*arrows*) in the right cerebral hemisphere. Each metastatic tumor is radiodense because of the contrast administration, relatively solid, and surrounded by edema. Distinguishing between a glioblastoma and a single metastatic lesion is often difficult.

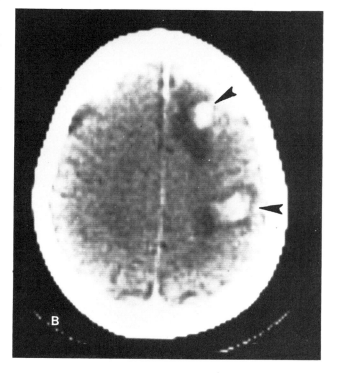

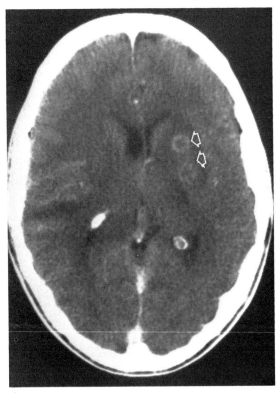

A

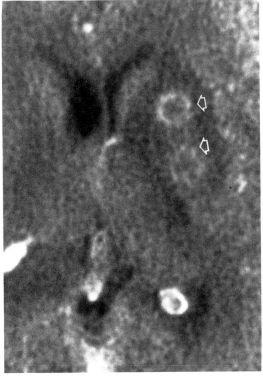

B

FIGURE 20–7

A contrast-enhanced CT (*A*) and an enlargement of a section (*B*) of two of numerous toxoplasmosis lesions (*open arrows*) in an AIDS patient. Both lesions are circular, white, and surrounded by dark areas that indicate cerebral edema. The adjacent anterior horn of the lateral ventricle is compressed, and the normally calcified choroid plexus, which is large, white, and circular, is pushed posteriorly—signs of swelling of the cerebral hemisphere (see Fig. 20–18 for toxoplasmosis detected by MRI).

FIGURE 20–8

A, CT and MRI machines typically display the brain with the sides reversed: With unilateral lesions, look for the "R" and "L" markings. This CT shows a right-sided, acute middle cerebral infarction. The area of infarction is darker (more hypodense) than the normal brain because it is no longer perfused with blood, which is relatively radiodense. In addition to its pie-shaped hypodensity, the infarction has a mass effect that compresses the adjacent lateral ventricle and shifts midline structures. *B,* The infarction is outlined. Its area includes the lateral portion of the right cerebral hemisphere, which contains the origin of the corticospinal tract for the left face and arm. The region medial and anterior to the infarction is supplied by the anterior cerebral artery, which gives rise to corticospinal tracts for the leg. The region posterior and medial, supplied by the posterior cerebral artery, contains the occipital lobe's visual cortex and the temporal lobe. *Illustration continued on following page.*

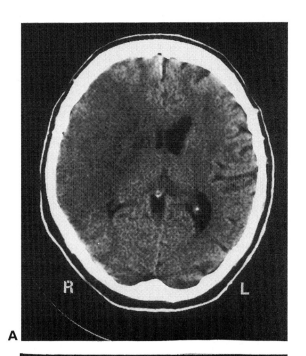

A

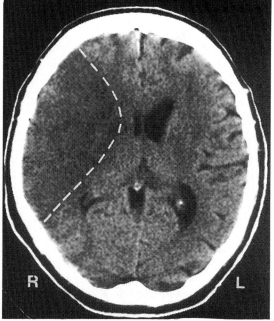

B

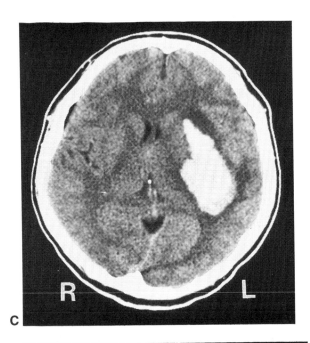

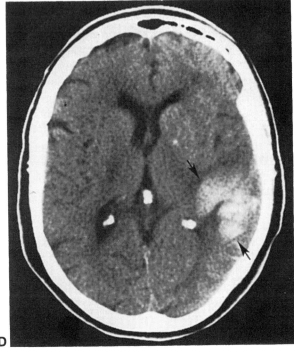

FIGURE 20-8

(*Continued*) *C*, This CT shows a cerebral hemorrhage that originated in the left thalamus and extended into the lateral ventricle. The blood, denser than the brain, is seen as a white plume. *D*, A parietal cerebral hemorrhage can be seen as a white globular area (*arrows*). It has a mass effect that obliterates the occipital horn of the ipsilateral lateral ventricle. The three small white areas are the normally calcified choroid plexus of the third and lateral ventricles.

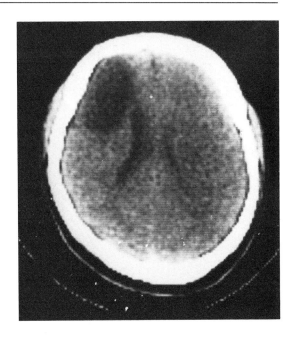

FIGURE 20-9

A frontal lobe porencephaly is a well-circumscribed oval lesion that, being less dense than brain, is radiolucent. It has the opposite effect of a mass lesion. Its absence of brain tissue leads to expansion of the adjacent lateral ventricle and the ipsilateral shift of midline structures. The porencephaly is a congenital cerebral injury that is often responsible for seizures, spastic contralateral hemiparesis, and mental retardation.

Although administration of contrast solutions is usually not necessary, newly available "paramagnetic" agents, such as gadopentetate (gadolinium), enhance intracranial abnormalities by altering the time that protons require to resume their natural alignment. Gadolinium does not cross the intact blood-brain barrier; however, it highlights lesions that disrupt the barrier, such as neoplasms, abscesses, and acute infarctions. Unlike CT contrast solutions, gadolinium almost never produces side effects.

In addition to detecting small intracranial and intraspinal structures, MRI can assist the diagnosis of illnesses in which the composition of the brain tissue is altered (Figs. 20-14 to 20-20). For example, MRI can reveal the characteristic white matter plaques of multiple sclerosis and the subtle white matter changes of progressive multifocal leukoencephalopathy (PML).

Also, with advanced equipment and software, MRI can generate images of the carotid and vertebral arteries (see Fig. 11-2). In many cases the images are so clear that they obviate the need for cerebral arteriography, which carries considerable risk and usually requires hospitalization.

However, MRI is no more effective than CT in diagnosing several major illnesses—Alzheimer's disease, AIDS-dementia complex, and psychiatric illnesses. In addition, compared to CT, MRI has some disadvantages (Table 20-3). The MRI procedure, which takes 30 to 40 minutes, requires that patients be placed entirely within the bore of the magnet, which is an awesome, long, and narrow tunnel with an opening that is just slightly wider than their body and a length of about 9 feet.

Even excluding individuals known to be claustrophobic, at least 10 per cent of patients, sometimes in a state of utter panic, will abort the procedure. Taking a minor tranquilizer helps most anxious patients undergo the MRI. Then wearing a sleep mask during the procedure might ameliorate fear. Heavy sedation is inadvisable because a patient's respiratory rate is difficult to monitor during the procedure.

A potentially life-threatening problem with MRI is that ferrous metals are attracted or adversely affected by the MRI magnet. Pacemakers, implanted

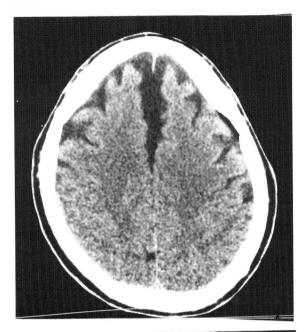

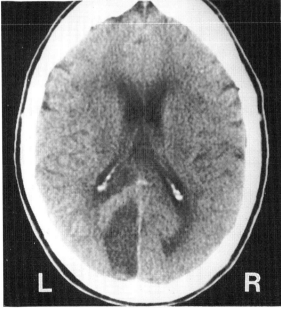

FIGURE 20–10

A, Limited atrophy has retracted the frontal lobes from each other, the falx, and the inner table of the skull. Other views reveal temporal lobe atrophy, but normal parietal lobes. The pattern of frontal and temporal lobe atrophy is indicative of Pick's disease and distinguishes it from Alzheimer's disease. *B,* A semicircular lucency in the left occipital lobe represents an infarction produced by a thrombosis of the left posterior cerebral artery. The infarction included the adjacent posterior corpus callosum (not pictured). This lesion produced alexia without agraphia (see Fig. 8–4).

hearing devices, intracranial aneurysm clips, and other implanted medical devices might be dislodged or ruined if the patient were exposed to the intense magnetic field of an MRI study.

POSITRON EMISSION TOMOGRAPHY

In contrast to CT and MRI, which can provide exquisitely detailed images of every nook and cranny of the CNS, *positron emission tomography (PET)*

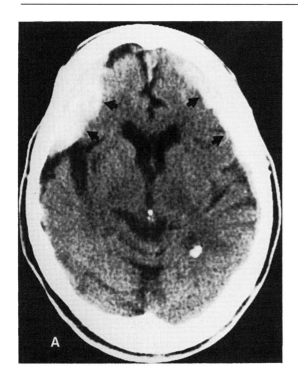

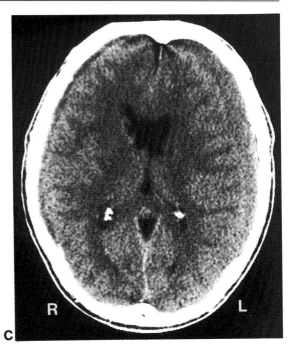

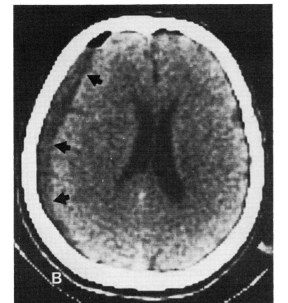

FIGURE 20–11

A, *Acute* subdural hematomas (*arrows*) contain fresh blood, which is radiodense compared to brain on CT scans. Large ones compress the underlying brain and cause headaches, stupor, and lateralized neurologic signs, such as hemiparesis. If these acute subdural hematomas are not removed by neurosurgery, they can cause transtentorial herniation (see Chapter 19). Although many subdural hematomas often result from overt head trauma that also leads to skull fractures, the trauma may have been hidden in cases of abuse or minimal in people with bleeding disorders or fragile vessels. B, *Chronic* subdural hematomas (*arrows*) contain aged, liquefied blood that is less radiodense than brain. They are black on a CT scan and are usually bordered by a radiodense, contrast-enhancing membrane. They compress the underlying brain, although to a lesser extent than with acute subdural hematomas. C, *Isodense* subdurals occur between the time that subdural hematomas are acute and chronic. Because their density is equal (isodense) to brain, they are almost indistinguishable from the underlying cerebral cortex. However, their presence is suggested by a unilateral "loss," by compression, of the gyri-sulci pattern and signs of a mass, such as shift of midline structures. In this CT scan, structures are shifted from the patient's left to right.

provides a rough map of the metabolic activity, chemistry, and physiology of the brain. The PET technique is based on positron-emitting radioisotopes, which must be produced in cyclotrons and incorporated into biologically active substrates. The compounds, which are inhaled or injected intravenously, release positrons as they are metabolized in the brain.

Most studies have measured cerebral metabolism of the radioisotope, fluorine-18 labeled fluorodeoxyglucose (FDG), which is absorbed into the brain

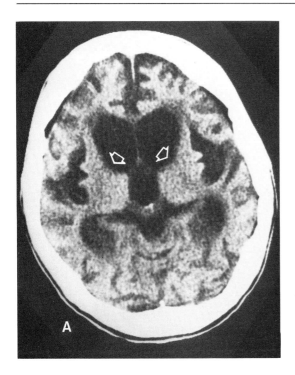

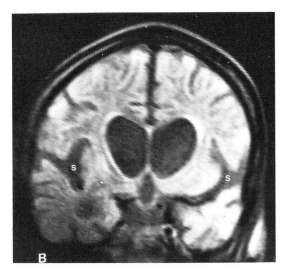

FIGURE 20–12

A, This CT scan shows the characteristic abnormality of Huntington's disease: The anterior horns of the lateral ventricles are convex because of atrophy of the caudate nuclei (*arrows*). Contrast that convex shape of the ventricles in Huntington's disease to the concave shape seen normally (see Fig. 20–1B) and in hydrocephalus ex vacuo (see Fig. 20–3). As in many other illnesses, Huntington's disease is associated with atrophy. The cortex is atrophied, sulci are copious, and ventricles are massively enlarged. *B,* This *coronal* view of the MRI scan of the same patient also shows the convex expansion of the ventricles, gigantic sulci, and sylvian fissures (*S*), as well as cerebral atrophy. Compare this scan to the coronal view of the normal brain (Fig. 20–13B). These changes, as dramatic as they may be, occur long after the disease can be diagnosed on clinical grounds. Positron emission tomography in Huntington's disease may show changes earlier than the CT or MRI scan.

and metabolized as though it were endogenous glucose. Positron emission from FDG reflects the rate of glucose metabolism. Other metabolic substrates are oxygen-15 labeled water, oxygen-15 labeled oxygen, and fluorine-18 labeled fluorodopa. All of them have a brief half-life. For example, oxygen-15 has a half-life of 2 minutes and fluorine-18, less than 2 hours.

PET has been used to analyze cerebral metabolism during normal activities, the administration of medications, and several illnesses. It has shown that, in partial complex epilepsy, the affected temporal lobe is generally hypoactive in the interictal period, but hyperactive during seizures. Deciding which temporal lobe is epileptogenic by this method, which is complementary to electroencephalography, is one step in determining whether a temporal lobectomy would benefit patients with intractable epilepsy (see Chapter 10).

TABLE 20–2. ADVANTAGES OF MRI OVER CT

Greater imaging ability
  MRI has greater resolution: can detect smaller objects
  Distinguishes white from gray matter
  Routinely displays images in three planes
Absence of interference from bone
  Can display posterior fossa structures, pituitary gland, optic nerves
  Can image the spinal cord
Does not utilize ionizing radiation
Can be applied to intra- and extracranial arteries
Can indicate certain conditions
  White matter plaques of multiple sclerosis and PML[a]
  Mesial temporal sclerosis, AVMs, and small gliomas[b]

[a]Progressive multifocal leukoencephalopathy, a complication of AIDS.
[b]Common findings in partial complex seizures.

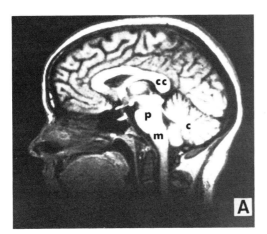

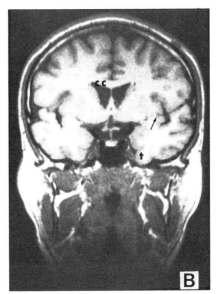

FIGURE 20–13

A, An MRI *sagittal* view of a normal brain reveals exquisitely detailed cerebral gyri and sulci, the corpus callosum (*cc*), and the three main structures of the posterior fossa, the pons (*p*), medulla (*m*), and cerebellum (*c*). In addition, the cervical-medullary junction and various non-neurologic soft tissue structures are apparent. *B,* The coronal view reveals the corpus callosum (*cc*), the "great commissure," bridging the cerebral hemispheres. The white matter of the corpus callosum and subcortical cerebral hemispheres is distinct from the ribbon of gray matter of the cerebral cortex. The anterior horns of the lateral ventricles, with their concave lateral borders, are beneath the corpus callosum and anterior and medial to the caudate nuclei and internal capsule (see Figs. 7–6 and 18–1A). The cerebral cortex around the left sylvian fissure (*arrow*), including the planum temporale, is usually more convoluted than that around the right, conferring greater cortical area for language function on the dominant hemisphere. The frontal lobe is above the sylvian fissure, and the temporal lobe is below. The medial-inferior surface of the temporal lobe (*t*), which is the origin of most partial complex seizures, is sequestered by the bulk of the temporal lobe above and the sphenoid wing anteriorly. It is far from the sites of conventional scalp EEG electrodes.

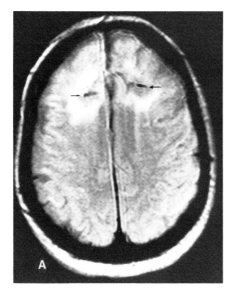
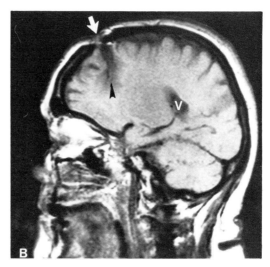

FIGURE 20–14

This MRI scan was performed on a patient who had undergone a frontal lobotomy. As in this case, the procedure did not involve removing the frontal lobes, but drilling a hole through the skull above each frontal lobe and passing a sharp instrument through the brain immediately anterior to the motor cortex. The surgeon would attempt to sever the white matter tracts that are connections to the anterior frontal lobe; however, the incision would usually only interrupt the superior connections. *A,* The axial view shows black horizontal slits, the incisions (*arrows*), which are surrounded by scar tissue. *B,* This sagittal view through the right cerebral hemisphere shows the skull defect (*white arrow*), where the incision starts, and the lowermost extent of the incision (*black arrow*), which is only about halfway down through the frontal lobe. The frontal lobe anterior to the incision is atrophied. A posterior portion of the lateral ventricle may be seen (*V*).

PET is especially helpful in studying early, presymptomatic stages of Parkinson's and Huntington's diseases. In those conditions, PET abnormalities develop before clinical signs or MRI abnormalities can be discerned. PET studies have followed basal ganglia changes in individuals exposed to MPTP before and after they developed in parkinsonism and in recipients of fetal cell transplantation (see Chapter 18).

In Alzheimer's disease, PET shows decreased cerebral metabolism, especially in the parietal and then frontal lobes' association areas. Multi-infarct

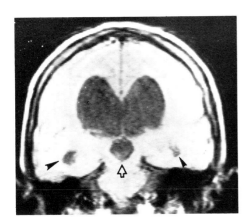

FIGURE 20–15

This MRI scan shows a coronal view of the brain of a patient with normal pressure hydrocephalus. It demonstrates the classic findings: in the absence of cerebral atrophy, dilation of the lateral ventricles, their temporal horns (*black arrows*), and the third ventricle (*open arrow*).

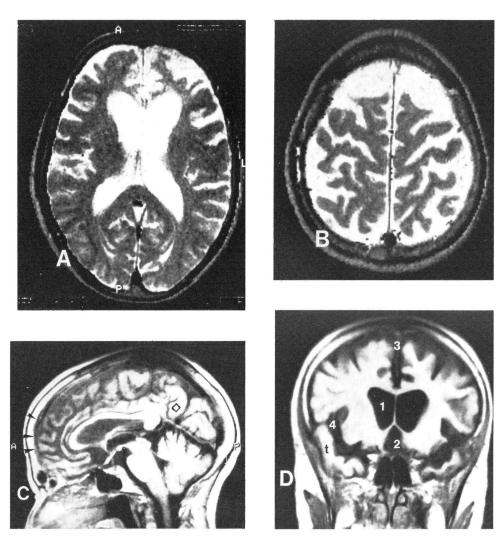

FIGURE 20–16

These MRI scans show four views of cerebral atrophy, which can be contrasted to the normal brain (see Fig. 20–13). MRI emphasizes cerebral atrophy because it does not detect the cortical bone of the skull, which contains virtually no water. The head is visualized because the scalp, blood, fat, and other soft tissue contain water. MRI provides exquisite detail, multiple views and little artifact, but no indication of the etiology of cerebral atrophy. *A,* In an axial view through the cerebral hemispheres, the CSF is white and fills the dilated lateral ventricles and sulci. Since the frontal lobe gyri are more atrophied than those of the other lobes, the CSF fills the frontal sulci and the anterior interhemispheric fissure. *B,* In a higher axial view, the surface of the brain has thin gyri and copious amounts of CSF in the sulci and over the cortex, occupying the void left by the atrophied brain. *C,* In a sagittal view, where the MRI is programmed not to detect a signal from CSF, it shows thin, ribbon-like frontal lobe gyri (*arrowheads*) and less atrophied parietal lobe gyri (*diamond*). The corpus callosum, pons, and cerebellum are easily visualized. The tentorium, which is seen as a straight line, lies above the cerebellum. *D,* In a coronal view through the frontal lobes, also where the CSF is not portrayed, the typical manifestations of cerebral atrophy include (1) dilated lateral ventricles, (2) an enlarged third ventricle, (3) enlargement of the anterior interhemispheric fissure because of separation of the medial surfaces of the frontal lobes, and (4) massively dilated Sylvian fissures with the atrophic temporal lobe (t) below and the atrophic frontal lobe above.

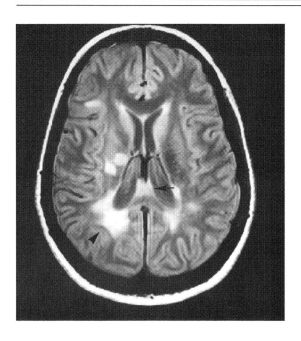

FIGURE 20–17

This MRI shows multiple cerebral plaques in a patient with multiple sclerosis. As is typical, the lesions are white and are clustered in the white matter deep in the cerebral hemispheres, particularly in the periventricular regions. A large plague is in the occipital lobe, posterior to the lateral ventricle (*arrowhead*). Others are adjacent to the ventricle in the middle and frontal lobe on the same side. One is in the posterior corpus callosum (*arrow*).

dementia, in contrast, produces multiple, random areas of decreased metabolism.

In schizophrenia, most studies show frontal lobe hypometabolism. In depression, although unipolar and bipolar varieties may differ, patients also have cerebral hypometabolism. As in MRI studies, PET studies of schizophrenia and depression cannot address the diagnosis of an individual patient, and in general, the results overlap those obtained from normal individuals and ones with other conditions. Ligands for dopamine, serotonin, GABA, and acetylcholine permit visualization of the distribution and activity of their receptors.

In its current form, PET will probably not attain widespread use. It is prohibitively expensive, and because of the radioisotopes rapid decay, the PET facility must be near a cyclotron.

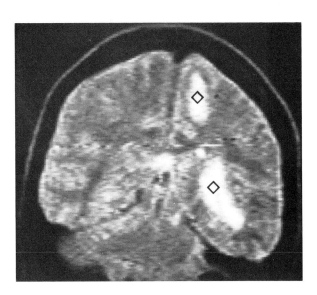

FIGURE 20–18

This MRI scan of a 21-year-old AIDS patient shows a coronal view of two toxoplasmosis lesions with surrounding edema (*diamonds*). Although MRI is more capable of detecting small and multiple toxoplasmosis lesions, CT is better able to portray their characteristic ring-like structure. Toxoplasmosis is the most common cause of mass lesions in young and middle-aged adults in North America.

FIGURE 20–19

Transaxial (*A*) and coronal (*B*) projections of an MRI scan show a large, lobulated hyperintense, right-sided, posterior parietal lesion. It has compressed the occipital horn of the lateral ventricle and shifted structures to the patient's left side. The coronal view reveals the cerebellum (*C*).

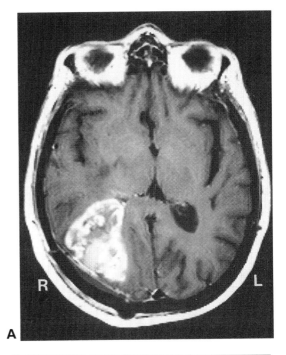

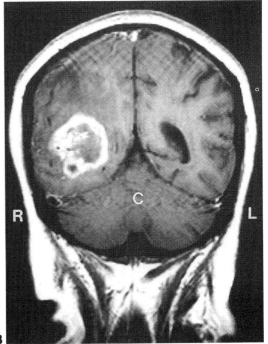

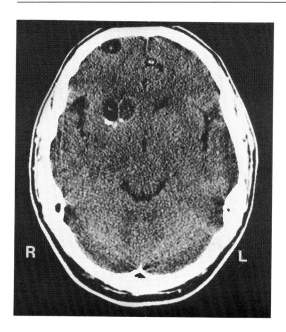

FIGURE 20-20

Cysticercosis, in contrast to most other cerebral mass lesions, causes multiple ring-like cysts, often with calcification, and little or no surrounding edema. However, they produce a substantial cumulative mass effect and irritate the cerebral cortex. This CT shows two "kissing" cysts compressing the right ventricle's anterior horn and another cyst in the right frontal cortex. Other CT slices showed numerous other cysts. Caused by the parasite, *Taenia solium*, cysticercosis is the most common cerebral mass lesion in South and Central America.

TABLE 20-3.   DISADVANTAGES OF MRI OVER CT

Cost is great, approximately three times greater than CT
Requires about 40 minutes, more than twice as long as CT
Being in the magnet often precipitates a claustrophobic reaction
Ferrous metal devices cannot be placed near the MRI magnet
    Patients cannot have a pacemaker, old intracranial aneurysm "clips," cochlear implants, or many other implanted ferrous metal devices
    Respirators and most other life-support machinery, unless specially designed, cannot be near the magnet
CT can detect acute hemorrhage—as occurs in acute intracranial hematomas and subarachnoid hemorrhage—rapidly and easily. Better than MRI as a screening procedure for head trauma and subarachnoid hemorrhage

SINGLE PHOTON EMISSION COMPUTED TOMOGRAPHY

A similar but less expensive technique is *single photon emission computed tomography (SPECT)*. This procedure uses readily available, stable substrates that do not require a cyclotron for preparation. Their relatively long life allows more detailed chemical studies. Moreover, unlike the radioisotopes in PET, those used in SPECT emit easily detectable gamma rays. However, the anatomic resolution with SPECT is even less than with PET.

SPECT can map cerebral blood flow and neurotransmitter receptors. It can thus indirectly show regional cerebral metabolic activity in cerebrovascular accidents, seizures, migraine, recurrent brain tumors, and Alzheimer's, Huntington's, and Parkinson's diseases.

REFERENCES

American College of Physicians: Magnetic resonance imaging of the brain and spine. Ann Intern Med *120*: 872–875, 1994
Andreasen NC (Ed): Brain Imaging: Applications in Psychiatry. Washington, DC: American Psychiatric Press, 1989

Carpenter WT, Buchanan RW: Schizophrenia. N Engl J Med *330*: 681–690, 1994

Cummings JL: The neuroanatomy of depression. J Clin Psychiatry *54*(Suppl): 14–20, 1993

Edelman RR, Warach S: Magnetic resonance imaging. N Engl J Med *328*: 708–716, 1993

Greenberg JO: Neuroimaging: A Companion to Adams and Victor's Principles of Neurology. Blue Ridge Summit, PA, McGraw-Hill, Inc, 1994

Masdeu JC, Brass LM, Holman L, et al: Brain single-photon emission computed tomography. Neurology *44*: 1970–1977, 1994

Therapeutics and Technology Assessment Subcommittee of the American Academy of Neurology: Assessment: Positron emission tomography. Neurology *41*: 163–167, 1991

Turner R: Magnetic resonance imaging of brain function. Ann Neurol *35*: 637–638, 1994

Weinberger DR: SPECT imaging in psychiatry: Introduction and overview. J Clin Psychiatry *54*(Suppl): 3–5, 1993

Author's Note: A Question and Answer section does not follow Chapter 20 because the information is included in other sections and in the End Question and Answer section.

21 Neurotransmitters and Drug Abuse

Previous chapters have referred to the neurotransmitters that underlie various neurologic conditions. This chapter presents this material from the neurotransmitters' perspective, recapitulating and expanding it. The chapter's latter half presents complementary information in discussion of the neurologic complications of drug abuse.

For the most well-recognized, clinically relevant neurotransmitters, this chapter describes their metabolism (synthesis, metabolism, and deactivation), anatomy (neurologic tracts), receptors, and neurologic conditions in which their activity is altered. With a few necessary exceptions, the chapter restricts the discussion to the neurotransmitters' role in the central nervous system (CNS) and to neurologic diseases. It includes discussions of the following neurotransmitters:

- monoamines: dopamine, norepinephrine, and serotonin
- acetylcholine
- GABA—an inhibitory amino acid
- glutamate and aspartate—excitatory amino acids
- neuropeptides
- nitric oxide

MONOAMINES

Dopamine

Metabolism

$$\text{Tyrosine} \xrightarrow{\text{tyrosine hydroxylase}} \text{DOPA} \xrightarrow{\text{DOPA decarboxylase}} \text{Dopamine}$$

The neurotransmitter dopamine is synthesized from tyrosine. In its synthesis, the rate-limiting step is the enzyme, *tyrosine hydroxylase*. Both endogenously produced DOPA and L-dopa, which is supplied as a medication for Parkinson's disease (see Fig. 18–3), undergo decarboxylation to form dopamine. The decarboxylation is purposefully blocked in non-CNS tissues by supplementing L-dopa with a dopa-decarboxylase inhibitor, *carbidopa* (as in Sinemet).

Dopamine's actions are terminated by several processes. It undergoes reuptake into the presynaptic neuron. It is also metabolized by a *monoamine oxidase* (*MAO*) or *catechol-O-methyltransferase* (*COMT*) enzymes.

The main metabolic product of dopamine is *homovanillic acid* (*HVA*). Its concentration in the cerebrospinal fluid (CSF) corresponds to dopamine activity in the brain.

Anatomy. Three long dopamine tracts have the greatest clinical significance. Most dopamine is synthesized in the *nigrostriatal tract*. As its name indicates, this tract projects from the substantia nigra, a pigmented nucleus, to the striatum. The *mesocortical* and *mesolimbic tracts* project from the midbrain (*meso*) to the frontal and other cortical areas and the limbic system. A short tract, the *tubero-infundibular tract*, connects the hypothalamic area with the pituitary gland.

Dopamine is also synthesized in the adrenal medulla and other organs outside the brain. Thus, adrenal cells have been transplanted into the brain in attempts to correct the dopamine deficiency in Parkinson's disease (see Chapter 18).

Receptors. At least five dopamine receptors—D_1 through D_5—have been described. D_1 and D_2 receptors are the most relevant to the extrapyramidal system. Both are located in the striatum (see Fig. 18–1), but D_1 receptors are also located in the cerebral cortex and limbic system. Although D_1 receptors are more plentiful, D_2 receptors seem to be the dopamine receptor involved when the typical antipsychotic medications induce parkinsonism (see Chapter 18). Clozapine, which does not induce parkinsonism, exerts little D_1 and D_2 receptor blocking effect. Stimulation of the D_1 and D_2 receptors has opposite effects on cyclic AMP production: D_1 receptors increase it and D_2 receptors decrease it.

Conditions Reflecting Changes in Dopamine Activity. Dopamine depletion in Parkinson's disease can be restored by administering the *dopamine precursor* L-dopa (see Fig. 18–3). L-Dopa is converted to dopamine as long as enough nigrostriatal (presynaptic) neurons remain intact. The activity of either naturally occurring or medically induced dopamine can be prolonged by inhibiting MAO with deprenyl (selegiline, Eldepryl). When presynaptic neurons have completely degenerated and can no longer convert dopa to dopamine, the postsynaptic effects can be duplicated by *dopamine agonists*, such as bromocriptine (Parlodel) and pergolide (Permax).

Neuroleptic-induced parkinsonism probably results from blockade of the D_2 receptors. Giving L-dopa when those receptors are blocked can stimulate frontal cortex and limbic system dopamine receptors and provoke mental aberrations.

In contrast to reduced dopamine activity, dopamine activity can be increased by several mechanisms: precipitating dopamine release from the presynaptic neuron, blocking its reuptake, or increasing the sensitivity of the postsynaptic receptors. Increased dopamine receptor sensitivity is postulated to underlie hyperkinetic disorders, such as tics, dystonia, chorea, and the oral-buccal-lingual variety of tardive dyskinesia. Cocaine and amphetamine increase dopamine activity, which also leads to hyperkinetic movement disorders accompanied by mental aberrations.

Through the tubero-infundibular tract, dopamine and dopamine agonists inhibit normal prolactin release from the pituitary gland. Thus, dopamine receptor blockers, especially the typical neuroleptics and risperidone—but not clozapine—provoke prolactin release from the pituitary and raise its serum concentration. Pituitary adenomas can either secrete prolactin or stimulate other cells to produce it. Prolactin production and the size of many adenomas can be reduced by bromocriptine. Also, generalized and partial complex seizures provoke a burst of prolactin detectable in the serum for about 20 minutes.

Norepinephrine

Metabolism.

Tyrosine $\xrightarrow{\text{tyrosine hydroxylase}}$ DOPA $\xrightarrow{\text{DOPA decarboxylase}}$ Dopamine $\xrightarrow{\text{dopamine}}$

$\xrightarrow{\text{β-hydroxylase}}$ Norepinephrine $\xrightarrow{\text{phenylethanolamine N-methyl-transferase}}$ Epinephrine

Dopamine is converted by *dopamine β-hydroxylase* to norepinephrine. Norepinephrine is converted into epinephrine almost exclusively in the adrenal gland. Dopamine, norepinephrine, and epinephrine are considered *catecholamines.*

In addition to the fact that norepinephrine retains dopamine's basic monoamine structure, the two neurotransmitters share many chemical characteristics. The rate-limiting enzyme in both of their syntheses is tyrosine hydroxylase. Their actions are both terminated primarily by reuptake. The remaining neurotransmitter is metabolized by the same enzymes: COMT and MAO.

Anatomy. The anatomy of norepinephrine and dopamine are considerably different. Unlike dopamine, norepinephrine is generated primarily in the *locus ceruleus*, which is located in the dorsal portion of the pons. Neurons from that nucleus, which is also pigmented, and from adjacent regions project to the cerebral cortex, limbic system, and the reticular activating system. Also unlike dopamine, norepinephrine tracts project down the spinal cord. In addition, norepinephrine serves as the transmitter in the sympathetic nervous system's postganglionic neurons.

Receptors. CNS receptors for norepinephrine are present in the cerebral cortex, brainstem, and spinal cord. Non-CNS, sympathetic nervous system receptors for epinephrine and norepinephrine produce clear-cut, virtually opposite effects. Moreover, various receptors have different agonists and antagonists (Table 21–1).

Conditions Reflecting Changes in Norepinephrine Activity. Norepinephrine depletion occurs in Parkinson's and Alzheimer's diseases, but its consequences are unknown. In Parkinson's disease, the locus ceruleus, as well as the substantia nigra, is depigmented.

Stimulation of β-2 adrenergic sites leads to tremor; bronchodilatation; and vasodilation of coronary, peripheral, and possibly meningeal arteries. Essential tremor's response to β-blockers suggests that it results from excessive β-adrenergic activity (see Chapter 18).

TABLE 21–1. PHARMACOLOGY OF EPINEPHRINE AND NOREPINEPHRINE RECEPTORS

Receptor	Effect of Stimulation	Agonists	Antagonists
α-1[a]	Vasoconstriction	Phenylephrine	Phenoxybenzamine, Phentolamine
α-2[b]	Vasodilation, hypotension	Clonidine	Yohimbine
β-1[a]	Cardiac stimulation	Dobutamine	Metoprolol
β-2[b]	Bronchodilation	Isoproterenol	Propranolol

[a]Postsynaptic.
[b]Presynaptic.

Serotonin

Metabolism.   Serotonin (5-hydroxytryptamine, 5-HT) is an *indolamine*. It is a monoamine, but not a catecholamine. Serotonin's synthesis parallels that of dopamine: hydroxylation then decarboxylation, with hydroxylation being the rate-limiting step. Likewise, its actions are terminated by reuptake and, to a lesser extent, by MAO metabolism. The primary metabolic product is 5-hydroxyindoleacetic acid (5-HIAA).

Tryptophan

Tryptophan hydroxylase →   ↓

5-hydroxytryptophan

Amino acid decarboxylase → ↓

Serotonin → 5-HIAA

Anatomy.   Serotonin-producing neurons are located predominantly in the *dorsal raphe nuclei*, which surround the aqueduct in the dorsal midbrain (see Fig. 18–2). These neurons project rostral (upward) to the cortex, limbic system, striatum, and cerebellum and caudal (downward) to the dorsal horn of the spinal cord. Within their rostral projections, serotonin neurons innervate intracranial blood vessels, particularly those around the trigeminal nerve. They are also involved with the brain's "vomiting center," which is in the medulla. Although the brain generates serotonin, platelets and other non-neurologic cells synthesize more than 98 per cent of the body's total serotonin.

Receptors.   At least three CNS serotonin receptors and several subtypes have been identified. They differ in their location, response to certain medications, and effect on second-messenger systems, such as adenyl cyclase. In most CNS systems, serotonin exerts an inhibitory influence.

Conditions Reflecting Changes in Serotonin Activity. Useful, effective medications, such as many antidepressants, enhance serotonin activity by blocking its reuptake. Likewise, pain-modulating systems enhance serotonin activity in the brain and spinal cord (see Chapter 14). Serotonin activity is normally absent during rapid eye movement (REM) sleep.

On the other hand, antagonizing serotonin is sometimes desirable. For example, migraines may be aborted or prevented by serotonin antagonists possibly because of their effect on trigeminal nerve and other intracranial blood vessel nerve endings (see Chapter 9). Blocking certain serotonin receptors has an antiemetic effect that is a useful adjunct to chemotherapy.

Serotonin levels are decreased in individuals with Parkinson's disease, perhaps more so if they are depressed, and those with Alzheimer's disease. Lysergic acid (LSD), which is a CNS serotonin agonist, produces a toxic psychosis characterized by hallucinations.

ACETYLCHOLINE (ACh)

Metabolism.   Acetylcholine (ACh) is formed by the combination of acetyl co-enzyme A and choline, with the rate-limiting factor being choline. The reaction depends on the enzyme *choline acetyltransferase (ChAT)*:

Acetyl CoA + Choline $\xrightarrow{\text{ChAT}}$ ACh

Unlike the monoamines, ACh does not undergo reuptake. Its action is terminated by *cholinesterase* metabolism. Similarly, its action may be prolonged by inhibiting cholinesterase with *anticholinesterases*. For example, edrophonium (Tensilon) and physostigmine prolong ACh activity by retarding its degradation (see Chapter 6 and Fig. 7–5).

Anatomy. ACh is an important neurotransmitter at the neuromuscular junction (see Fig. 6–1), in the autonomic nervous system, and throughout the CNS. In the CNS, most ACh neurons originate in the *nucleus basalis of Meynert* and adjacent nuclei in the *forebrain* (a rostral portion of the brainstem). These nuclei project cholinergic neurons to the limbic system and cerebral cortex.

Nerve growth factor (NGF) is a trophic factor, which is a molecule that promotes survival and helps maintain the health of groups of neurons. Administration of NGF may restore damaged cholinergic neurons.

Receptors. Two major types of ACh receptors have been described: *nicotinic* and *muscarinic*. Nicotinic receptors are excitatory and are blocked by curare. Neuromuscular junctions rely on nicotinic receptors. Muscarinic receptors are both excitatory and inhibitory and are blocked by atropine and scopolamine. The CNS has both types of receptors, but those in the cerebral cortex are predominantly muscarinic.

Conditions Reflecting Changes in ACh Activity. ACh activity may be altered at the neuromuscular junction by either pre- or postsynaptic influences. Both can lead to potentially fatal muscle paralysis. Botulism, whether received as a food poison or as medication for focal dystonia (see Chapter 18), and the Lambert-Eaton syndrome, a paraneoplastic disorder, impair ACh release from the presynaptic neuron. ACh receptors, which are on the postsynaptic (muscle) side of the neuromuscular junction, are blocked by poisons, such as curare, and by antibodies produced in myasthenia gravis (see Chapter 6). Anticholinesterases, such as edrophonium (Tensilon) and pyridostigmine (Mestinon), usually temporally increase ACh activity enough to overcome the weakness induced by receptor blockade in myasthenia gravis.

Reduced cerebral ACh concentrations, ChAT activity, and muscarinic receptors are well-established markers of Alzheimer's disease (see Chapter 7). Low ACh levels are also found in trisomy 21 and Parkinson's disease. A related observation is that scopolamine and other drugs, which block muscarinic ACh receptors, interfere with memory and learning—even in normal individuals. Similarly, directly anticholinergic medicines, such as some of those used for parkinsonism, and those with only anticholinergic side effects produce similar cognitive impairments.

To counteract the ACh deficiency in Alzheimer's disease, scientists have administered ACh precursors, such as choline and lecithin (phosphatidylcholine), but the dementia did not respond. A complementary strategy has been to administer long-acting anticholinesterases that cross the blood-brain barrier. Although physostigmine did not help, tacrine (Cognex) may provide some benefit (see Chapter 7).

GAMMA-AMINOBUTYRIC ACID—AN INHIBITORY AMINO ACID NEUROTRANSMITTER

Metabolism. Gamma-aminobutyric acid (GABA) and, to a lesser extent, glycine are the brain's major inhibitory neurotransmitters. GABA is formed from the decarboxylation of glutamate by the enzyme *glutamate decarboxylase (GAD)*. GABA is metabolized, in the Krebs cycle, to succinic semialdehyde.

$$\text{Glutamate} \xrightarrow{\text{GAD}} \text{GABA}$$

Anatomy. Reflecting the widespread role of inhibition, GABA is distributed throughout the entire CNS. Its highest concentrations are in the striatum, hypothalamus, spinal cord, and temporal lobe.

Receptors. Two GABA receptors, $GABA_A$ and $GABA_B$, are complex molecules. $GABA_A$, the more important, has binding sites for benzodiazepines, barbiturates, and convulsants as well as GABA. $GABA_A$-induced receptor activity is inhibitory because it opens chloride channels to hyperpolarize neurons. In other words, a GABA-induced intracellular movement of chloride (Cl^-) lowers (makes more negative) the normal resting potential, which is -70 mV.

Conditions Reflecting Changes in GABA Activity. In the opposite effect, viewed simplistically, a lack of GABA inhibitory effect leads to excessive neurologic activity, including chorea and seizures. In Huntington's disease, GAD and GABA concentrations in the basal ganglia are decreased, and CSF concentrations of GABA are decreased.

Pyridoxine (B_6) deficiency and INH overdose, which each decrease GABA concentration, lead to seizures. B_6 injections will abort such seizures. Along the same line, the anticonvulsant, valproate (Depakote), is effective, in part, because it increases GABA levels.

GLUTAMATE AND ASPARTATE—EXCITATORY AMINO ACID NEUROTRANSMITTERS

Metabolism. Glutamate and aspartate, both amino acids, are two of several excitatory neurotransmitters. The synthesis of these relatively simple molecules stems from several different pathways and is not dependent on particular enzymes. Their actions are terminated by reuptake and nonspecific metabolism.

Anatomy. Reflecting its role in cognition, motor function, and other fundamental activities, glutamate is the brain's principal excitatory neurotransmitter. Receptors for both amino acids are found throughout the CNS.

Receptors. The receptors are the well-described N-methyl-D-aspartate (*NMDA*) multimolecular complex and two others (AMPA and kainate). The NMDA receptor, which is modulated by the inhibitory neurotransmitter glycine, regulates the patency of a calcium channel.

Excessive NMDA activity floods the neuron with lethal concentrations of calcium (Ca^{++}) and sodium (Na^+). Through this process, called "excitotoxicity," glutamate-receptor interactions lead to neuron death.

Conditions Reflecting Changes in NMDA Activity. Illnesses have been more closely correlated with NMDA activity than with changes in amino acid concentrations. In contrast to its vital functions at normal levels of activity, excessive NMDA activity has been associated with epilepsy, stroke and other causes of cerebral ischemia, Parkinson's disease, and head trauma. Experimental studies show that NMDA blockade may protect neurons, i.e., provide a "neuroprotective" effect.

Deficient NMDA should also be deleterious. One example may be PCP (see below), which blocks the NMDA calcium channel.

NEUROPEPTIDES

Endorphins, enkephalins, and substance P, which are situated in the spinal cord and brain, primarily provide endogenous analgesia (see Chapter 14). Other neuropeptides are somatostatin, cholecystokinin, and vasoactive intestinal peptide (VIP). Substance P and, to a lesser degree, the other neuropeptides are depleted in Alzheimer's disease.

NITRIC OXIDE

Metabolism. Nitric oxide (NO), a newly recognized neurotransmitter, is synthesized in a complex reaction involving electron transfers:

$$\text{Arginine} + \text{Oxygen} \xrightarrow{\text{nitric oxide synthase}} \text{Nitric oxide} + \text{Citrulline}$$

Nitric oxide (NO) should not be confused with nitrous oxide (N_2O), which is an anesthetic gas ("laughing gas"). When inhaled daily as a form of drug abuse, N_2O results in peripheral neuropathy.

Anatomy. NO inhibits platelet aggregation, dilates blood vessels, and has diverse functions in the CNS. In particular, it is instrumental in regulating cerebral blood flow and generating penile erections.

Receptors. Bypassing specific membrane receptors, NO diffuses into cells and interacts directly with chemicals, such as enzymes and iron-sulfur complexes. In the CNS, depending on its chemical state, NO may mediate either glutamate-induced excitotoxicity or have a neuroprotective effect. Excessive glutamate-NMDA interactions, for example, lead to increased NO.

NEUROLOGIC COMPLICATIONS OF ILLICIT DRUGS

Standard statistics continue to reflect increased illicit drug use: increases in drug-related hospital admissions, deaths, motor vehicle accidents, and homicides. Novel discoveries also reflect widespread drug use. For example, cocaine is detectable on the surface of 75 per cent of paper money in Los Angeles.

In addition to the dangers of addiction and of procuring the drug by prostitution, violence, and other unsavory means, individuals using illicit drugs are exposing themselves to life-threatening complications. The most notorious complication is acquired immunodeficiency syndrome (AIDS; see Chapter 7). AIDS is not only a tremendous source of morbidity but it also leads directly to opportunistic infections, such as toxoplasmosis, and related infectious illnesses, such as syphilis and tuberculosis. Other frequently occurring, drug-related infectious illnesses are bacterial endocarditis, which causes cerebral infarctions (strokes) and mycotic aneurysms, and hepatitis B, which can cause hepatic encephalopathy (see Chapter 7). Several rare infectious complications of drug use—malaria, tetanus, and botulism—have distinct neurologic aspects.

Injections of illicit drugs also leads to several noninfectious complications. Intravenous injections may include particulate material, such as talc, that travels as an embolus to the brain, retinae, spinal cord, and other organs. Subcutaneous or intravenous injections can cause nerve injury, tissue fibrosis, or other soft tissue damage.

Cocaine

Pharmacology. Both cocaine and amphetamine are primarily CNS stimulants through their sympathomimetic qualities: They block the reuptake of norepinephrine, dopamine, and serotonin. One difference is that cocaine characteristically provokes massive discharges of dopamine from presynaptic storage vesicles. Another is that cocaine is a powerful local anesthetic.

Cocaine is usually smoked as *crack*, its alkaloid form, or inhaled through the nostrils as a powder. Its effects may be enhanced or confounded by mixing it with other illicit drugs, such as narcotics. Before being metabolized by plasma and liver cholinesterases, cocaine has a brief half-life of about 30 minutes to 1 hour. Its metabolic products may be detected in the urine for about 2 days.

Clinical Effects. The immediate effects of "standard" doses of cocaine may be a "rush," euphoria, and a sense of increased sexual, physical, and mental power. Concomitant sympathomimetic effects are hypertension and tachycardia. At higher doses, the sympathomimetic effects are magnified to dangerous proportions.

During an acute cocaine intoxication, patients typically become agitated, irrational, paranoid, delusional, and hallucinatory. Their being alert—even hypervigilant—is a prominent exception to the general rule that patients in delirium or a toxic-metabolic encephalopathy are lethargic or stuporous (see Chapter 7). However, with enough cocaine, patients become comatose.

The neurologic complications seem to stem from cocaine's sympathomimetic and dopaminergic effects. Cocaine-induced strokes and seizures are the most frequent, serious neurologic complications; however, those complications and others depend on the dose and route of administration, the co-administration of narcotics, and duration of use.

Most cocaine-induced strokes occur immediately or within 2 hours of drug exposure. Many are "bland," nonhemorrhagic cerebral infarctions, but characteristically they are cerebral hemorrhages related to hypertension and underlying aneurysms. Other causes of stroke-like brain damage in substance abusers are vasculitis, bacterial endocarditis, AIDS-related infections, emboli of particles, and head trauma. Cocaine users often suffer the cardiac counterpart of strokes—myocardial infarctions.

Cocaine-induced seizures likewise occur immediately or within 2 hours. They disproportionately follow first-time cocaine use and are often fatal. Most seizures are generalized and are not associated with abnormal CT scans or EEGs. Seizures that are focal or followed by hemiparesis may, of course, be a manifestation of an underlying stroke.

In contrast, seizures induced by alcohol, barbiturates, or benzodiazepines usually occur after withdrawal from high-dose and chronic use, but rarely with a severe overdose. Seizures related to those substances are more than a warning of casual or recreational use: They are a marker of dependency. In practical terms, the development of a seizure disorder in young adults should prompt an investigation for drug abuse.

Cocaine's other neurologic complications include movement disorders that are presumably related to excessive dopamine activity, such as tic-like facial movements, chorea, tremor, dystonia, and repetitive, purposeless behavior (stereotypies; see Chapter 18). Cocaine also seems to increase sensitivity to dystonic reactions from neuroleptics. Quite frequently, when cocaine induces chorea, patients cannot stand at attention and are said to have "crack dancing." Habitual cocaine use has been associated with cerebral atrophy.

Amphetamine

As commonly used, the term "amphetamine" refers to dextroamphetamine (Dexedrine), methamphetamine, methylphenidate (Ritalin), and several other related substances. Like cocaine, amphetamine is sympathomimetic and a dopamine reuptake blocker. It is usually taken orally, but sometimes intravenously ("speed"). Its half-life is about 8 hours, which is much longer than that of cocaine.

Standard doses of amphetamines produce excessive alertness, greater stamina, euphoria, and other effects of cocaine. Its chronic use causes anorexia with weight loss and decreased total sleep time, with a reduced percentage of sleep time spent in rapid eye movement (REM) sleep.

Acute amphetamine and cocaine intoxications produce virtually indistinguishable toxic psychoses. Other neurologic complications common to amphetamine and cocaine intoxication include hemorrhagic and bland strokes that, in some cases, may be related to vasculitis. Amphetamines also cause dyskinesias and stereotypies. However, seizures are relatively infrequent.

Opioids

Narcotics are now referred to as "opioids," which is actually a broader term applied to morphine, synthetic analgesics, heroin, other illicit drugs, and endorphins (see Chapter 14). Although opioids may affect dopamine and other neurotransmitters, their more important action is directly on several specific receptors in the brain and spinal cord.

Therapeutic opioid doses relieve pain and reduce anxiety. Higher doses, usually associated with abuse, lead to a rush of euphoria, a sense of well-being, and then sleepiness; however, they occasionally produce a paradoxical agitation. Opioids routinely lead to nausea and vomiting that presumably result from direct stimulation of the brain's "chemoreceptor trigger zone" (CTZ). The CTZ is in the medulla's *area postrema*, which is one of the few CNS regions unprotected by the blood-brain barrier.

Opioid overdose causes a characteristic triad of stupor or coma, "pin-point pupils" (miosis), and respiratory depression. The respiratory depression results from a slowed rate, rather than a reduced amplitude or depth. It may reflect an interaction of opioids with the brain's respiratory drive, which is centered in the medulla. Opioid overdose frequently results in neurogenic pulmonary edema. An overdose can also result in cerebral hypoxia with cerebral cortex and basal ganglia damage. These injuries cause cognitive impairment and stroke-like deficits.

Compared to the complications of amphetamines or cocaine, opioid-induced vascular occlusions and cerebral hemorrhages are infrequent. Except as a manifestation of overdose-induced hypoxia, seizures rarely complicate opioid use, addiction, or withdrawal. On the other hand, opioid overdoses are routinely complicated by compression of a major nerve or limb muscles (see Table 5–1).

Several unrelated facts are important. Physicians, dentists, nurses, and other health care workers are particularly at risk for surreptitious opioid abuse. Administration of a synthetic analogue of meperidine (Demerol), MPTP, routinely induces parkinsonism (see Chapter 18). Phenytoin (Dilantin) interferes with methadone and can precipitate opioid withdrawal symptoms. Likewise, administering opioid antagonists, such as naloxone, to counteract an overdose can precipitate withdrawal symptoms. Compared to morphine, heroin acts somewhat differently and, possibly because it more readily penetrates the blood-brain barrier faster, more rapidly, However, it holds no major, distinguishing advantage as a pain killer or treatment for cancer patients.

Phencyclidine (PCP)

Popular in America's drug culture of the late 1960s and early 1970s, phencyclidine (PCP) is simultaneously a central analgesic, depressant, and hallucinogen. As with cocaine, PCP blocks the reuptake of dopamine, serotonin, and norepinephrine. In a more important action, it interferes with the NMDA and other specific receptors. It is usually either swallowed or smoked with marijuana or tobacco.

In small doses, PCP causes signs similar to alcohol intoxication: euphoria, dysarthria, nystagmus, and ataxia. At higher doses, it causes disorganized thinking and hallucinations that progress to psychosis. Many of its mental effects mimic schizophrenia.

PCP users may have combinations of stereotypies, muscular rigidity, and a blank stare. They are often oblivious to pain. Overdoses can cause coma and seizures, but rarely strokes.

Marijuana

Marijuana (cannabis) is a cannabinoid that contains several psychoactive ingredients, with Δ9-THC being the most potent. Usually smoked, but sometimes swallowed, marijuana produces euphoria, alters perceptions, and impairs judgment. When acting as a sedative, marijuana reduces REM sleep.

In contrast to other illicit drugs, marijuana rarely causes neurologic injury. Initial reports of cerebral atrophy have been unconfirmed. Its chronic use has been associated only in anecdotal reports with cognitive impairment, strokes, and seizures. Also, marijuana possesses a mild anticonvulsant activity, reduces intraocular pressure, and suppresses chemotherapy-induced vomiting.

On the other hand, the strength of these benefits is overrated, and standard medicines are more effective. For example, dopamine blockers are very effective in reducing nausea and vomiting. Also, probably because of its psychologic effects, marijuana is involved in an inordinate number of highway fatalities. Very high doses can induce hallucinations and thought disorders. A related but important issue is that the herbicides sprayed on the plants in attempt to control their growth may be quite harmful when inhaled along with the marijuana smoke.

REFERENCES

Neurotransmitters

Abramowicz M (Ed): Yohimbine for male sexual dysfunction. Med Lett *36*: 115–116, 1994

Cooper JR, Bloom FE, Roth RH: The Biochemical Basis of Neuropharmacology, 6th ed. New York, Oxford University Press, 1991

Dawson TM, Dawson VL, Synder SH: A novel neuronal messenger molecule in brain: The free radical, nitric oxide. Ann Neurol *32*: 297–311, 1992

Greenamyre JT, Porter RHP: Anatomy and physiology of glutamate in the CNS. Neurology *44* (suppl): S7–S13, 1994

Lipton SA, Rosenberg PA: Excitatory amino acids as a final common pathway for neurologic disorders. N Engl J Med *330*: 613–622, 1994

Lowenstein CJ, Dinerman JL, Snyder SH: Nitric oxide: A physiologic messenger. Ann Intern Med *120*: 227–237, 1994

Perry EK: Neurotransmitters and disease of the brain. Br J Hospital Med *45*: 73–83, 1991

Drug Abuse

Burst JCM: Neurologic Aspects of Substance Abuse. Boston. Butterworth-Heinemann, 1993

Cardoso FE, Jankovic J: Cocaine-related movement disorders. Movement Disord *8*: 175–178, 1993

Daras M, Koppel BS, Atos-Radzion E: Cocaine-induced choreoathetoid movements ("crack dancing"). Neurology *44*: 751–752, 1994

Derlet RW, Rice P, Horowitz BZ, et al: Amphetamine toxicity: Experience with 127 cases. J Emerg Med *7*: 157–161, 1989

Foley KM: Opioids: Neurologic complications of drug and alcohol abuse. Neurol Clin *11*: 503–522, 1993

Holland RW, Marx JA, Earnest MP, et al: Grand mal seizures temporally related to cocaine use: Clinical and diagnostic features. Ann Emerg Med *21*: 772–776, 1992

Hollister LE: Health aspects of cannabis. Pharmacol Rev *38*: 1–20, 1986

Levine SR, Burst JCM, Futrell N, et al: A comparative study of the cerebrovascular complications of cocaine: Alkaloidal versus hydrochloride—a review. Neurology *41*: 1173–1177, 1991

McCarron MM, Schulze BW, Thompson GA, et al: Acute phencyclidine intoxication: Incidence of clinical findings in 1,000 cases. Ann Emerg Med *10*: 237–242, 1981

Pascual-Leone A, Dhuna A, Anderson DC: Cerebral atrophy in habitual cocaine abusers: A planimetric study. Neurology *41*: 34–38, 1991

Sanchez-Ramos JR: Psychostimulants: Neurologic complications of drug and alcohol abuse. Neurol Clin *11*: 535–553, 1993

Sloan MA, Kittner SJ, Rigamonti D, et al: Occurrence of stroke associated with use/abuse of drugs. Neurology *41*: 1358–1364, 1991

Spivey WH, Euerle B: Neurologic complications of cocaine abuse. Ann Emerg Med *19*: 1422–1428, 1990

QUESTIONS and ANSWERS: CHAPTER 21

1. Which features are characteristic of narcotic (n) or cocaine (c) administration?

a. Provokes dopamine discharge from presynaptic neurons
b. Agitation
c. Hypertension
d. Slowed respiratory rate
e. Stimulation of the area postrema
f. Miosis
g. Blockade of dopamine reuptake

answer: a-c, b-c, c-c, d-n, e-n, f-n, g-c

2. Which features are complications of narcotic (n) or cocaine (c) administration?

a. Cerebral hemorrhage
b. Cerebral anoxia
c. Seizures
d. Radial nerve palsy
e. Tics
f. Stereotypies
g. Psychotic thought
h. Pulmonary edema

answer: a-c, b-n, c-c, d-n, e-c, f-c, g-c, h-n

3. Which three causes of seizures are disproportionately more common in 15- to 50-year-old individuals than in older adults?

a. Marijuana use
b. Head trauma
c. Drug and alcohol abuse
d. Sleep deprivation
e. Narcolepsy
f. Brain tumors
g. Cerebrovascular accidents

answer: b, c, d

4. Which substance's active ingredient is Δ9-THC?

a. Cocaine
b. PCP
c. Amphetamine
d. Cannabis
e. Heroin

answer: d. Cannabis is marijuana.

5. What is the effect of amphetamine on sleep?

a. It increases the total sleep and increases the proportion of REM.
b. It increases the total sleep and decreases the proportion of REM.
c. It decreases the total sleep and increases the proportion of REM.
d. It decreases the total sleep and decreases the proportion of REM.

answer: d

6. A narcotic addict, who is being maintained on methadone, develops a seizure for which he is hospitalized and treated with an anticonvulsant. A psychiatry consultation is solicited when the patient becomes combative. The psychiatrist finds that the patient has piloerection, muscle cramps, nausea, and abdominal pain. Although a CT and EEG have not been performed, the preliminary laboratory results are normal. What should be the course of action?

a. Add a minor tranquilizer.
b. Add a major tranquilizer.
c. Increase the anticonvulsant.
d. Increase the methadone.
e. Demand a CT if not an MRI.
f. None of the above

answer: d. Narcotic addicts often undergo withdrawal when hospitalized. They may be given little or no methadone. Phenytoin (Dilantin) or other medications may interfere with methadone.

7. Which is probably the primary mechanism of action of cocaine?

a. It enhances dopamine activity.
b. It enhances serotonin metabolism.
c. It diverts serotonin innervation.
d. It leads to reduced GABA levels.

answer: a. Cocaine enhances dopamine activity by triggering its release from presynaptic nerve endings and simultaneously blocking its reuptake.

8. Which two signs are not manifestations of excessive sympathetic activity?

a. Tachycardia
b. Angina
c. Hypertension
d. Miosis
e. Abdominal cramps
f. Anxiety

answer: d, e

9. Which of the following is not a manifestation of amphetamine use?

a. Weight loss
b. Insomnia
c. Psychosis similar to cocaine-induced psychosis
d. Parkinsonism
e. Stereotypies

answer: d. Use of synthetic narcotics, particularly MPTP, has been complicated by parkinsonism. Many overweight people and students use amphetamines. Occasionally they develop addiction or complications.

10. A college student is brought to the Emergency Room in a coma. He has a weak and thready pulse, infrequent and shallow respirations, and miosis. He has pulmonary edema. Of the following, which should be the next procedure?

a. Inject naloxone.
b. Give thiamine.
c. Obtain a CT scan of the head.
e. Inject glucose.

answer: a. He has a narcotic overdose that typically causes coma, depressed respirations, and miosis. Pulmonary edema is a complication of a severe overdose. Naloxone is a narcotic antagonist; however, its half-life may be shorter than the duration of the narcotics (requiring further doses), and it may precipitate narcotic withdrawal.

11.   Which of the following are false regarding vomiting?

a.   It is typically induced by narcotics.
b.   Marijuana reduces nausea and vomiting induced by chemotherapy.
c.   The brain is well protected from vomiting-inducing substances.
d.   Lesions located in posterior fossa structures are more apt to induce vomiting than those in the other parts of the brain.

answer: c. Vomiting is induced by activation of the chemoreceptor trigger zone (CTZ), which is located in the area postrema of the medulla. This region is unprotected by the blood-brain barrier. Dopamine blockers as well as marijuana suppress nausea and vomiting.

12.   A 29-year-old man is revived from an opioid overdose, but he has paresis of his right wrist extensor muscles and impairment of his ability to make a fist. He is alert, has normal mental and language ability, no abnormalities in his legs, and no Babinski signs. Where is the most likely site of his injury?

a.   Left cerebral hemisphere
b.   Left internal capsule
c.   Near the spiral grove of the right humerus
d.   In or near the right wrist

answer: c. Most likely he has a "wrist drop" because he has compressed the right radial nerve as it winds around the humerus. He cannot make a fist because that action requires the wrist to be extended. The absence of aphasia and signs in the leg and upper arm indicate that the lesion is not likely to be in the CNS. Nerve compressions are a frequent complication of alcohol and drug overdose.

13.   Which is the metabolic product of dopamine that is measurable in the CSF?

a.   MAO
b.   HVA
c.   COMT
d.   VMA

answer: b

14.   Which is the rate-limiting enzyme in the synthesis of dopamine?

a.   DOPA decarboxylase
b.   Tyrosine hydroxylase
c.   MAO
d.   COMT
e.   Dopamine β-hydroxylase

answer: b

15.   Of the enzymes listed in the preceding question, which converts dopamine to norepinephrine?

answer: e

16.   Of the choices listed in the question 14, which is the rate-limiting enzyme in the synthesis of norepinephrine?

answer: b

17.   Which two are effects of stimulation of dopamine receptors?

a.   Stimulation of the D_1 receptor increases ATP to cyclic AMP production.
b.   Stimulation of the D_2 receptor decreases ATP to cyclic AMP production.
c.   Stimulation of the D_1 receptor decreases ATP to cyclic AMP production.
d.   Stimulation of the D_2 receptor increases ATP to cyclic AMP production.

answer: a, b. D_1 receptor activity increases ATP to cyclic AMP production through adenyl cyclase.

18.   Which dopamine tract is responsible for the elevated prolactin levels induced by many antipsychotic agents?

a.   Nigrostriatal
b.   Mesolimbic
c.   Tubero-infundibular
d.   None of the above

answer: c. The tubero-infundibular tract is the connection between the hypothalamus and the pituitary gland. Dopamine and dopamine agonists inhibit this tract and suppress prolactin release. Dopamine blockade provokes prolactin release, which is the basis of elevated serum prolactin levels produced by the use of typical neuroleptics.

19. Which is the primary site for conversion of norepinephrine to epinephrine?

a. Locus ceruleus
b. Stratum
c. Adrenal medulla
d. Nigrostriatal tact

answer: c

20. What is the major metabolic pathway for serotonin?

a. Metabolism by COMT to 5-hydroxyindoleacetic acid (5-HIAA)
b. Metabolism by MAO to 5-HIAA
c. Metabolism by decarboxylase to HVA (homovanillic acid)
d. Metabolism by HVA to 5-HIAA

answer: b. Although most serotonin undergoes reuptake, the remainder is subject to metabolism by MAO, which forms 5-HIAA.

21. Where is the main site of serotonin production?

a. Dorsal raphe nuclei
b. Regions adjacent to the aqueduct in the midbrain
c. Striatum
d. None of the above

answer: d. Almost all serotonin is produced in platelets and other non-neurologic cells. Within the brain, which generates less than 2 per cent of the total, serotonin-producing neurons are located predominantly in the *dorsal raphe nuclei*, which is adjacent to the aqueduct in the dorsal midbrain.

22. Which three regions describe primary site of norepinephrine production?

a. Locus ceruleus
b. A pigmented nucleus
c. The caudate nucleus
d. The dorsal portion of the pons
e. The hypothalamus
f. The striatum

answer: a, b, d

23. Which two statements are false regarding ACh receptors in the cerebral cortex?

a. They are predominantly muscarinic.
b. They are predominantly nicotinic.
c. Atropine blocks muscarinic receptors.
d. Scopolamine, which antagonizes muscarinic receptors, induces memory impairments that mimic Alzheimer's disease dementia.
e. Physostigmine penetrates the blood-brain barrier to block cholinergic receptors.
f. Botulinum toxin penetrates the blood-brain barrier to block cholinergic receptors and cause memory impairments.

answer: b, f. Cerebral cortex ACh receptors are predominantly muscarinic. Blocking CNS muscarinic receptors causes memory impairments, even in normal individuals. Botulinum toxin neither penetrates the blood-brain barrier nor causes memory impairments. However, it does impair release of ACh from the presynaptic neuron at the neuromuscular junction and thereby causes paresis and relief of focal dystonia.

24. In the reaction, acetyl CoA + choline to acetylcholine, which is the rate-limiting factor?

a. Choline acetyltransferase (ChAT)
b. Acetyl CoA
c. Choline
d. None of the above

answer: c

25. Which two comparisons of Lambert-Eaton syndrome and myasthenia gravis are valid?

a. Lambert-Eaton syndrome is a paraneoplastic syndrome, whereas myasthenia gravis is an autoimmune disorder.
b. Lambert-Eaton syndrome is associated with decreased ACh production, whereas myasthenia gravis is associated with excess ACh production.
c. Lambert-Eaton syndrome is characterized by impaired presynaptic ACh release, whereas myasthenia gravis is characterized by defective ACh receptor function.
d. Lambert-Eaton syndrome is alleviated by botulism, but myasthenia gravis is alleviated by anticholinesterases.

answer: a, c. Myasthenia gravis is alleviated by anticholinesterases.

26. When GABA interacts with postsynaptic GABA$_A$ receptors, which four events can be anticipated?

a. Sodium channels are opened.
b. Chloride channels are opened.
c. The electrolyte shift depolarizes the neuron.
d. The electrolyte shift hyperpolarizes the neuron.
e. The electrolyte shift in polarization leads to inhibition.
f. The electrolyte shift in polarization leads to excitation.
g. Glutamate provokes a similar response.
h. Glycine provokes a similar response.

answer: b, d, e, h. The GABA$_A$ receptor is a ubiquitous, multifaceted complex that is sensitive to benzodiazepines and barbiturates, as well as GABA. When stimulated, the GABA$_A$ receptor permits the influx of chloride. The electrolyte shift hyperpolarizes the neuron's membrane and inhibits depolarization. Glycine is a similar inhibitory amino acid neurotransmitter.

27. What is the approximate normal resting potential of neurons?

a. +100 mV
b. +70 mV
c. 0 mV
d. −70 mV
e. −100 mV

answer: d. When the resting potential is −100 mV, the neuron is hyperpolarized and thereby inhibited. When the potential is less negative than −70 mV, the neuron is excited.

28. Which two roles does glycine play?

a. Glycine is an inhibitory amino acid neurotransmitter.
b. Glycine modulates the NMDA receptor.
c. Glycine is the rate-limiting substrate in glutamate synthesis.
d. Glycine raises the resting potential, i.e., makes it less negative.

answer: a, b. Glycine is an inhibitory amino acid neurotransmitter that modulates the NMDA receptor. Inhibitory neurotransmitters generally make the resting potential more negative. Glutamate and aspartate can be synthesized through several pathways.

29. Which two roles does nitric oxide (NO) play?

a. It leads to cerebral vasodilation and may trigger penile erections.
b. Like aspirin (ASA), it promotes platelet aggregation.
c. Excessive NMDA activity leads to increased NO activity, which leads to neuron death.
d. When used excessively, NO causes a peripheral neuropathy.

answer: a, c. NO is a newly described neurotransmitter that bypasses secondary messengers to bind with enzymes and sulfur or iron-containing molecules. Both NO and ASA inhibit platelet aggregation. Nitrous oxide (N$_2$O) is a gas anesthetic that, when used daily, causes a peripheral neuropathy.

30.   Which CNS neurotransmitter is confined mostly or entirely to the brain?

a.   Dopamine   d.   Norepinephrine
b.   ACh   e.   Serotonin
c.   Glycine   f.   Glutamate

> ***answer:***   a. Dopamine is found in the adrenal medulla, but its primary tracts are confined to the brain. The other neurotransmitters are found in high concentrations in the spinal cord, as well as the brain.

31.   Which are two effects of glutamate-NMDA activity?

a.   Intracellular neuron calcium concentration increases.
b.   Inhibition occurs through hyperpolarization.
c.   Excitation occurs under normal circumstances.
d.   Excitotoxicity occurs under normal circumstances.
e.   Inhibition occurs under normal circumstances.

> ***answer:***   a, c. Glutamate, the principal CNS excitatory neurotransmitter, interacts with the NMDA and other receptors to open calcium channels. With excessive activity, the calcium influx raises intracellular concentrations that can be lethal to the cell or excitotoxic.

22 Head Trauma

MAJOR HEAD TRAUMA

In somewhat of an arbitrary separation, neurologists distinguish major from minor head trauma; major head trauma results in at least 1 hour of post-traumatic unconsciousness and then permanent residual neurologic deficits. Motor vehicle accidents (MVAs) are the most common cause of major head trauma in civilian life, particularly for 15- to 24-year-old men. Alcohol plays a role in innumerable, serious MVAs because it impairs drivers' judgment, coordination, and ability to stay awake. Work-related and athletic injuries and gunshot wounds (GSWs) are the other common causes of head trauma.

The type and forcefulness of head trauma determine the different pathologic patterns of *traumatic brain injury (TBI)*. As the head receives a blow, the underlying brain is injured (a *coup* injury). Then, as the brain is thrown against the opposite inner table of the skull, the opposite cerebral lobe is injured (a *contrecoup* injury). These reciprocal, *coup-contrecoup injuries* have their greatest impact on the temporal lobe and anterior-inferior surface of the frontal lobes because those lobes are pointed and they abut against sharp surfaces of the anterior and middle fossae (Fig. 22–1). In contrast, the occipital skull is relatively large, flat, and smooth. Thus, *coup-contrecoup injuries* rarely cause visual symptoms, but they frequently cause frontal and temporal lobe symptoms, such as memory impairment and personality changes.

Sometimes the pathologic pattern is not as obvious. In MVAs, for example, the force of the head striking a dashboard or windshield may lead to generalized shearing and stretching of axons (*diffuse axonal injury*) without gross changes.

Moderately severe, blunt trauma causes cerebral swelling, small hemorrhages, and ischemic areas, especially in the brainstem—all of which raise intracranial pressure. Such trauma can also produce hematomas within and over the surface of the brain, extensive brain damage, and, in the extreme, fatal herniation. In addition to all of those injuries, penetrating injuries deposit bone, shrapnel, and other foreign material in the brain. Any injury can leave an epileptogenic cerebral cortex scar.

Epidural hematomas, which typically stem from temporal bone fractures and concomitant middle meningeal artery lacerations, are large, rapidly expanding hematomas that develop between the inner table of the skull and the outer surface of the dura (Fig. 22–2). Their mass effect compresses the underlying brain and forces it through the tentorial notch, i.e, produces *transtentorial herniation.* Unless surgery can immediately arrest the bleeding and evacuate them, epidural hematomas are usually fatal.

Subdural hematomas are more common and are usually not fatal. They result from tearing of small or large veins and subsequent bleeding into the space between the undersurface of the dural and arachnoid matter, which is

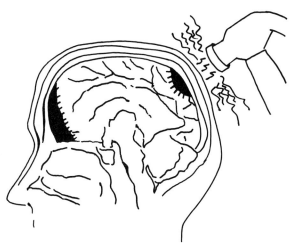

FIGURE 22–1

A *coup* refers to the brain injury immediately underlying a blow. In a *contrecoup* injury the opposite side of the brain is damaged though a rebound effect. In this drawing, a hammer blow to the back of the head typically inflicts a coup injury in the occipital region and, through contrecoup injury, a more extensive injury to the tips of the frontal and temporal lobes.

immediately over the brain. Minimal trauma can be a sufficient cause. In many cases, the trauma has been so mild and distant that it is forgotten. Since venous pressure is low, the rate of bleeding is slow. The blood exudes into the extensive subdural space until the pressure of the brain arrests the bleeding (see Fig. 20–11).

Chronic subdural hematomas are those hematomas that have spread diffusely in the subdural space and have persisted for weeks. They are typically responsible for the insidious onset of headaches, change in personality, and dementia, but curiously they cause minimal physical deficits (see Chapters 19 and 20). Psychiatrists are most likely to encounter patients with this variety of intracranial hematoma.

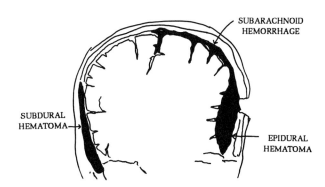

FIGURE 22–2

The inner table of the skull is lined by the dura matter. The potential space external to the dura is the *epidural* space. The space internal to it is the *subdural* space. Arterial bleeding, which generally results from blows forceful enough to cause skull fractures, usually causes *epidural hematomas*. Venous bleeding, which is usually slower and less forceful, typically produces *subdural hematomas*. Both hematomas cause potentially fatal mass effect with compression of the gyri and shift of midline structures.

The *arachnoid matter* closely covers the brain. The subarachnoid space, which is between the arachnoid and the underlying brain, normally contains cerebrospinal fluid (CSF). Trauma and ruptured aneurysms cause *subarachnoid hemorrhage*. With these hemorrhages, blood tracks through the subarachnoid spaces over the convexities, between the gyri, and sometimes into the interhemispheric fissure. Subarachnoid hemorrhages cause bloody or xanthochromic CSF. Meningitis, which is an infection predominantly in the subarachnoid space, causes purulent CSF.

People older than 65 years are especially prone to chronic subdural hematomas for several reasons. They have a tendency to fall and are often taking anticoagulants. More important, since the space between the inner table of the skull and the brain is enlarged because of cerebral atrophy, bleeding can be sizeable before the mechanical pressure of the brain compresses it. Other people susceptible to subdural hematomas are those with chronic renal failure, neoplasms, and bleeding disorders. A CT or MRI scan will diagnose chronic as well as acute subdural hematomas. Surgical evacuation is a relatively simple procedure that can reverse the dementia and other symptoms.

Coma

Survivors of major head trauma can remain in coma for days to weeks. The depth of coma is measured by the *Glasgow Coma Scale (GCS)*, which is an assessment of three readily apparent neurologic functions—eye opening, speaking, and moving (Table 22–1). Almost 90 per cent of patients with the worst (lowest) scores die during the first day. By the end of 3 weeks, comatose patients generally have either improved or succumbed.

When coma patients improve, their transition is frequently rocky. The TBI makes patients confused, disoriented, agitated, and combative. A psychiatrist called to assess these disturbances, which are often loosely termed *traumatic psychosis* or *delirium*, must maintain a global view and bear in mind neurologic problems in addition to those directly attributable to TBI. Head trauma patients, for example, may also be suffering from alcohol or drug intoxication or, after several days in the hospital, from withdrawal symptoms. Various agitated states can be produced by pain from diagnosed or undiagnosed extracranial injuries, adverse reactions to narcotics and other medications, and other medical complications, such as hypoxia, sepsis, and fat emboli. In addition, pre-existing dementia renders patients particularly susceptible to TBI.

TABLE 22–1. THE GLASGOW COMA SCALE (GCS)[a]

Category		Score
Eyes opening	Never	1
	To pain	2
	To verbal stimuli	3
	Spontaneously	4
Best verbal response	None	1
	Incomprehensible sounds	2
	Inappropriate words	3
	Disoriented and converses	4
	Oriented and converses	5
Best motor response	None	1
	Extension[b]	2
	Flexion[c]	3
	Flexion withdrawal	4
	Patient localizes pain	5
	Patient obeys	6
Total		3–15

[a]This standard scale indicates the level of consciousness, with the lowest scores indicating less neurologic function. Scores lower than 9 indicate coma. The GCS has great prognostic value.
[b]Decerebrate rigidity (see Fig. 19–3).
[c]Decorticate rigidity (see Fig. 11–5).

Focal Deficits

Focal neurologic deficits, such as hemiparesis, spasticity, and ataxia, are commonly occurring physical-neurologic consequences of TBI. They can be correlated with cerebral damage from lacerations, hematomas, and GSWs. Naturally, focal deficits are associated with focal seizures (see the section below on post-traumatic epilepsy). Recovery from neurologic deficits usually reaches a maximum within 6 months after the injury, but patients can further increase their mobility with physical and occupational therapy, braces and other devices, and modifications of their environment.

The cranial nerves may also be injured. They are vulnerable to lacerations, severing by skull fractures, or direct trauma to their sensory organs, such as the eye, ear, or nose. Cranial nerve injuries can cause functional impairment, sensory deprivation, disfigurement, and psychologic repercussions. In particular, the olfactory nerve fibers, on their way through the cribriform plate to the frontal lobes, are sometimes ripped. Whereas loss of the function of other cranial nerves is obvious, anosmia is often overshadowed by frontal lobe impairment.

Epilepsy

Cerebral scars and residual foreign bodies routinely evolve into epileptic foci. Post-traumatic epilepsy is one of the most troublesome and, with an incidence of 50 per cent, most commonly occurring complications of major head injury. The incidence is even greater when head trauma patients use alcohol.

Post-traumatic epilepsy takes the form of focal seizures, including partial complex seizures, that tend to undergo secondary generalization (see Chapter 10). The seizures themselves may be debilitating and lead to further head injury. Moreover, side effects of anticonvulsants may compound the neuropsychologic sequelae.

Neuropsychologic Impairments

In the worst case scenario, many months after sustaining extensive cerebral damage, patients remain with their eyes open, but—paradoxically—are capable of only rudimentary bodily functions. Always assuming a flexed, decorticate (fetal) posture, patients are devoid of communication, cognitive capacity, and purposeful activity. They are in a *persistent vegetative state* with no hope for a functional recovery (see Chapter 11).

Less devastated TBI survivors, such as Vietnam war veterans who sustained penetrating head wounds, have neuropsychologic impairments related to the size of the lesion and depth of coma as measured by low scores on the GCS. The lesion's location, in contrast, is a relatively poor predictor of neuropsychologic impairment, except for a vocabulary deficit induced by left temporal lobe injuries.

Recovery of motor and language skills usually reaches a maximum within 6 months after the injury, but intellectual recovery—to the extent that it occurs—may be delayed until 18 months. In general, older patients recover more slowly and less completely than younger ones.

Cognitive rehabilitation is a team approach that attempts to overcome intellectual deficits. It includes retraining and focusing attention on the task at hand. Although this discipline has its supporters, its benefit may stem entirely from classic rehabilitation approaches: social interaction with a peer group; identification and treatment of depression, anxiety, and insomnia; education; and physical, occupational, speech, and recreational therapy.

Memory impairment or *post-traumatic amnesia* is the most salient, specific neuropsychologic deficit. In addition to amnesia for the trauma and events immediately preceding it (retrograde amnesia), TBI interferes with learning or memorizing newly presented information (anterograde amnesia). The severity and duration of amnesia are directly proportional to low GCS scores.

Post-traumatic amnesia is often accompanied by another major handicap, *slowed information processing*. Other neuropsychologic sequelae—perseveration, inattention, cognitive inflexibility, and impaired problem solving—are additional, somewhat overlapping impairments.

Post-traumatic as well as congenital brain damage predisposes people to the *episodic dyscontrol syndrome*, dissociative states, impulsive behavior, and violence (see Chapter 9). TBI also makes people exquisitely sensitive to alcohol. In them, alcohol often precipitates violent outbursts even before they are overtly intoxicated. TBI-induced violence reportedly may be reduced by carbamazepine, propranolol, and lithium, as well as by major tranquilizers. Nevertheless, most individuals with brain damage are not violent. In fact, many are as docile as if they had undergone a frontal lobotomy.

Personality changes, such as being abrupt, suspicious, and argumentative, are commonplace. They presumably result from generalized cerebral or predominantly frontal and temporal lobe damage. *Post-traumatic depression* occurs in about 25 per cent of TBI patients. Although it is not related to the severity of the head trauma, post-traumatic depression is associated with damage to the left anterior cerebral hemisphere, drug and alcohol abuse, previous depression, and poor social functioning.

Although schizophrenia per se cannot be attributed to head trauma, after trauma some patients do develop schizophrenia-like symptoms. These symptoms, which are associated with left temporal lobe damage, include emotional lability, speech and language impairments, and thought disorders. They are accompanied by cognitive impairments.

Other Impairments

TBI has been alleged to be either a direct cause or at least a risk factor for Alzheimer's disease. The main evidence is taken from studies that found a statistical association between the two conditions, but most failed to establish a significant relationship. Other evidence is that severe head trauma causes a deposition in the brain of beta-A4 amyloid protein, which may be the nidus for amyloid plaques.

Despite commonly eliciting a history of preceding head trauma, the consensus among neurologists is that single head injuries do not cause Parkinson's disease (see Chapter 18). Similarly, when Parkinson's disease patients sustain head trauma, their Parkinson symptoms are only transiently exacerbated. Multiple injuries, however, can cause Parkinson-like problems (see the material below on dementia pugilistica). Isolated reports have also linked head trauma to dystonias, including spasmodic torticollis (see Chapter 18).

Child Abuse.   The "shaken baby syndrome" occurs in an infant who has sustained brain injury because violent shaking has thrown the brain within the skull. Although many infant victims probably also have sustained direct blows to the head, that component of the trauma is unnecessary. Without the blows, and in most cases even when they do occur, abused infants have neither external signs of trauma nor routine x-ray evidence of skull fractures. CT and MRI scans reveal blood—often of different ages—in the subdural, subarachnoid, or interhemispheric space. Funduscopic examination often shows retinal hemorrhages.

Overt cases of child abuse often include new and old fractures of the long bones, as well as skull, facial, and ocular trauma. Although young children may fall backward and injure their occiput, if they fall forward, they reflexively extend their arms and shield their face and eyes. In other words, facial, ocular, and anterior skull injuries are more suspicious than occipital injuries.

Dementia Pugilistica.   Dementia pugilistica, the "punch drunk syndrome," consists of progressive intellectual deterioration accompanied by dysarthria, stiffness and clumsiness from spasticity, and characteristic, Parkinson-like slow movements. These deficits end a boxing career. The disorder occurs most often in boxers who are lightweight, alcoholic, or have lost many fights, and it progresses after their retirement.

CT and MRI studies show white matter changes, focal contusions, and cerebral atrophy in proportion to the number of bouts. Autopsy studies demonstrate hydrocephalus and atrophy of the corpus callosum and cerebrum. As in Parkinson's disease, the substantia nigra is depigmented. Most important, histologic examination shows Alzheimer-like neurofibrillary tangles and, with special stains, plaques. The fact that boxing leads to dementia pugilistica, Alzheimer's-like histologic changes, and occasionally a fatal epidural or subdural hematoma has provoked demands for more stringent regulations—if not an outright ban of the sport.

MINOR HEAD TRAUMA

Concussions and *contusions*—minor injury head trauma—cause a loss or impairment of consciousness for less than 30 minutes and a GCS score no lower than 13. A concussion, a term with both physiologic and clinical aspects, is a blow, shaking, or jarring that results in an immediate although transient impairment in consciousness. In addition, victims typically have retrograde and anterograde amnesia. Studies have postulated shearing of neuron bundles, damage at gray and white matter boundaries, and production of intracellular vacuoles; however, pathologic studies have revealed no consistent abnormality.

A contusion, in contrast, consists of minute bleeding into the brain and overlying meninges that often causes scar formation, but the cerebral architecture is otherwise preserved. Compared to concussions, contusions cause more long-lasting loss of consciousness. As in *coup-contrecoup* injuries, contusion of the tips of the frontal and temporal lobes might explain personality changes and memory impairments. In any case, a seemingly invariable component of head trauma from MVAs is the wrenching or ripping of cervical muscles, ligaments, and nerve roots (see the section below on whiplash).

Most minor head injuries result from MVAs or occupational injuries. Athletic accidents and assaults are less common but important causes. Abuse of children, elderly, and spouses leads to both major and minor head injuries and all the sequelae.

Postconcussive Syndrome

The *postconcussive syndrome* includes a variety of symptoms persisting after either a contusion or concussion. It also occurs, along with more obvious problems, both in people who have sustained major head injury and those who have sustained only a trivial injury. Although components of the postconcussive syndrome may represent the *post-traumatic stress disorder syndrome*, the most frequent neurologic symptoms are a headache, neuropsychologic disturbances, and insomnia.

Even the neurologic aspects of the postconcussive syndrome are almost entirely subjective. Neuropsychologic testing may reveal certain patterns, but results are usually inconsistent. Neurologic examinations and CT or MRI scans are normal. Physiologic tests, which are exquisitely sensitive, such as EEGs, brainstem auditory evoked responses, electronystagmograms, and audiograms, are normal or show only minor, transient abnormalities.

Although the postconcussive syndrome's existence is accepted, patients' individual cases are regularly met with skepticism. They are disproportionately women; people with a history of learning disabilities, attention deficit disorders, or neuroses; and unskilled and semiskilled workers. Postconcussive syndrome rarely affects children, soldiers, athletes, or self-employed or professional people. The syndrome cannot be correlated with either the estimated force of impact or the usual neurologic parameters—GCS scores and duration of retrograde or anterograde amnesia. The symptoms typically are not corroborated by physical or laboratory abnormalities and are refractory to treatment.

The postconcussive syndrome sometimes has an extraordinarily long duration—seeming to take on a life of its own—with possibly 25 per cent of cases lasting longer than 3 years. The duration is longer in patients with certain premorbid intellectual and personality traits. The symptoms seem inextricably linked to monetary rewards, expectation of compensation, and unsettled litigation.

On the other hand, a great deal of data indicates that the postconcussive syndrome is primarily neurologic rather than psychogenic: The symptoms are similar from patient to patient, develop in some self-employed and highly motivated people including physicians, and do not prevent the majority of patients from returning to work. Neurologic symptoms are worse in patients with bodily injuries. Contrary to long-held opinion, symptoms are poorly correlated with outstanding litigation, and they often persist after legal claims are settled. Children and various stoics may rarely seem to develop the symptoms because they are unable to describe them, admit to pain, or have different manifestations. For example, rather than complaining of post-traumatic headaches, children may have somnolence and hyperactivity, and professionals may merely be more irritable.

Post-Traumatic Headache

The essential feature of the postconcussive syndrome is a dull, continuous headache in a generalized, diffuse, or band-like pattern. The headache is exacerbated by movement, bending, working, and alcohol. Post-traumatic headaches last longer than 1 year in 50 per cent and longer than 3 years in 25 per cent of patients. The headaches occur more frequently in mildly injured than in severely injured head trauma patients and in those with cervical spine degenerative changes. Of the various aspects of the postconcussive syndrome, headaches are most closely associated with memory and concentration impairments.

However, all headaches following trauma are not simply post-traumatic headaches. When headaches are hemicranial or throbbing, develop in a patient with a history of migraines, or are accompanied by autonomic nervous system dysfunction, they may be predominantly *post-traumatic migraines*, i.e., migraines triggered by the trauma (see Chapter 9). Other causes of headache are trauma to the muscles, ligaments, and cervical spine (see the section below on whiplash); temporomandibular joint; and supra-orbital nerve (neuralgia). Head trauma does not seem to provoke cluster headaches or trigeminal neuralgia. On the other hand, head trauma can cause chronic subdural hematomas that present with headaches and may not be apparent for weeks after the injury.

Neuropsychologic Disturbances

Symptoms include memory impairment especially for new information, slowed information processing, inattention or inability to concentrate, and difficulty completing complex mental tasks. Neuropsychologic tests show inconsistent impairments and lack of correlation with the severity of trauma. Cognitive function usually returns to the preinjury level in 1 to 3 months, even though the other symptoms persist—sometimes indefinitely.

Patients describe depression, anxiety, irritability, and moodiness, but rarely in so few words. They may also report decreased libido not just for sex, but for other previously enjoyable endeavors. These symptoms may be considered a post-traumatic stress disorder, rather than the result of physical neurologic damage.

In contrast, some patients may consciously or subconsciously minimize their impairments. They may not acknowledge amnesia, other cognitive deficits, or personality changes. Using poor judgment, they may undertake ambitious plans or attempt to fulfill major commitments.

Other Symptoms

Postconcussive syndrome patients often say that they have "dizziness." In most cases, their symptom is not authentic vertigo, but a nonspecific sensation with variable, idiosyncratic meanings that include lightheadedness, anxiety, and unsteadiness. This symptom is difficult to define and virtually impossible to treat. Occasionally, however, patients have sustained labyrinth damage from a temporal bone fracture, in which case they have nystagmus and ataxia, as well as unequivocal vertigo.

Another common symptom is hypersensitivity to light, sound, talking, and other stimuli. Patients seemingly cannot tolerate routine levels of conversation, reading, or socializing. The hypersensitivity is distracting, intensifies headaches, and contributes to inattention.

Insomnia likewise occurs frequently, and its underlying cause is not established. In some cases, headaches or other pain and lack of exertion may be responsible. Moreover, sedentary patients are liable to consume excessive coffee, narcotics and other medications, as well as alcohol. Of course, insomnia —as well as the other symptoms—is partially attributable to anxiety, depression, post-traumatic stress disorder, or a misperception of the time spent asleep (pseudo-insomnia; see Chapter 17).

Excessive daytime sleepiness (EDS), the opposite problem of insomnia, occurs frequently because of the poor night-time sleep and lack of daytime demands, as well as a direct effect of TBI. EDS also results from medications given to trauma patients, including narcotics, anticonvulsants, antidepressants, and minor tranquilizers.

Treatment

Neurologists attempt to educate the patient and family about the nature, extent, and course of the postconcussive syndrome. Many urge the patient to return to work, even with a reduced workload or on a part-time basis. Also, they encourage patients with neck and head pains to enter a physical therapy program.

For the headaches, neurologists prescribe mild, nonaddicting analgesics similar to those used for muscle contraction headaches. Sometimes, even with a minimal migraine component, antimigraine drugs are helpful (see Chapter 9). Neurologists also prescribe nonsteroidal anti-inflammatory drugs (NSAIDs).

Small doses of amitriptyline and related medications are useful for pain and insomnia. However, biofeedback has no demonstrable benefit, and cognitive retraining remains controversial. Psychotherapy and antidepressants in therapeutic doses may be indicated for anxiety, depression, and post-traumatic stress disorder.

Insomnia must be treated cautiously. Hypnotics can easily lead to EDS, mimic symptoms of TBI, and produce confusion and memory impairments. Alcohol must be forbidden because it may induce cognitive impairments, behavioral difficulties, insomnia and EDS, headaches, poor judgment, and fatigue.

WHIPLASH

Mechanism of Action

In rear-end MVAs, the head and neck of the driver and passengers are thrown backward by a sudden, unexpected, large force. Their neck is suddenly hyperextended because the anterior neck muscles are too weak and too slow to counteract the force. The hyperextension suddenly applies severe traction to the muscles and anterior spinal ligaments. It also compresses the posterior elements of the spine.

Immediately afterward, the head naturally rebounds suddenly forward and the neck is flexed. Sometimes the chin strikes the chest, or the forehead strikes the dashboard. Although the sequence may be reversed and occur in other injuries, this violent back-and-forth movement leads to a *flexion-extension* or *whiplash injury* (Fig. 22–3).

This injury can wrench, rip, tear, or compress—or merely strain—the neck's soft tissues: ligaments, tendons, and both the large trapezius and paraspinal muscles and the numerous, delicate, small muscles. Forceful, extreme movements also aggravate degenerative spine disease, such as cervical spondylosis (see Fig. 5–5). Cervical nerve roots may be transiently or permanently compressed by the vertebrae, soft tissues, or intervertebral disks.

Sometimes fragments of herniated intervertebral disks compress cervical nerve roots. When large fragments of the disk are herniated, the spinal cord

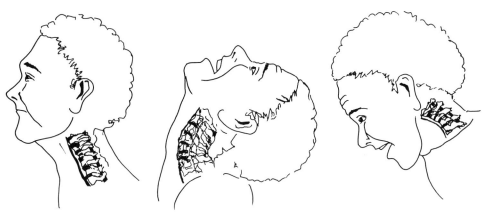

FIGURE 22–3

Flexion-extension or whiplash injuries can tear the longitudinal ligaments and other soft tissues, herniate intervertebral disks, and exacerbate cervical spondylosis (see Fig. 5–5). Most frequently, the forces that produce whiplash injuries are motor vehicle accidents in which the totally unsuspecting occupants of a car are struck from behind. With the impact from the rear, the head and neck are whipped backward. Then they snap forward, sometimes striking the head on the steering wheel, dashboard, or other firm surface.

may be compressed. In severe injuries, well beyond the severity of whiplash, cervical vertebrae may be fractured or dislocated and transect the spinal cord. In such injuries, bleeding can occur into the spinal cord.

Symptoms

Symptoms are greatest when the patient is an unprepared driver or passenger of the car that was struck from behind (i.e., "rear-ended") and when the head are neck are turned or flexed at the time of impact. Patients with whiplash injuries describe incapacitating neck pain that is increased by either moving or by holding still, as when reading or keyboarding. The pain radiates beyond their neck to their shoulders, arms, and thoracic region. With simultaneous head trauma and whiplash injuries, the symptoms seem to multiply.

When cervical intervertebral disks are herniated, patients typically have pain that radiates down the nerve roots (radicular pain), weakness, and loss of deep tendon reflexes in the arms. Herniated disks, as well as fractures and dislocations, are usually detectable with an MRI. Electromyograms (EMGs) are also helpful in establishing the nature, severity, and extent of the injury.

Whiplash injury typically prevents patients from working for 3 to 6 months. Outstanding litigation and pre-existing cervical spondylosis are each associated with more protracted disability. Some cases, even without head trauma, may be complicated by cognitive impairments, inattention, and headache. As in the postconcussive syndrome, the symptoms' duration does not correlate with the speed or severity of an MVA.

Treatment

The treatment of whiplash injury has not been subjected to rigorous examination, and it remains empiric and variable. Some patients respond to immobilization of their neck by rest, not working, and wearing a soft foam rubber cervical collar. Others respond to active therapy exercises and possibly traction. Most people report feeling better after massage, heat packs, and gentle manipulation; however, vigorous cervical manipulation, as occurs in chiropractic treatment, has led to injuries of the spinal cord and occlusion of the vertebral arteries.

Whiplash patients and most other adults would probably benefit from good "neck hygiene": not cradling the telephone in the neck, especially when typing; if the telephone is used a great deal, buying an expanded receiver or a headset; elevating the computer keyboard and monitor to avoid excessive neck flexion; using only one pillow; and curtailing tennis and other sports that strain the neck.

Useful medications include muscles relaxants, NSAIDs, non-narcotic analgesics, and, primarily for their analgesic and sedative effects, antidepressants. Migraine medications have also been reported to be helpful. With varying degrees of success, some physicians inject steroids and anesthetics into areas that incite the pain ("trigger point injections"), muscles with spasm, or cervical facet joints.

Settlement of lawsuits does not necessarily produce a cure. Although occupational, psychological, and legal issues must at least be acknowledged, the deleterious effects of litigation tend to be overestimated.

REFERENCES

DeGiorgio CM, Lew MF: Consciousness, coma, and the vegetative state: Physical basis and definitional character. Issues Law Med 6: 361–371, 1991
Ditunno JF, Formal CS: Chronic spinal cord injury. N Engl J Med 330: 550–556, 1994
Duhaime AC, Gennarelli TA, Thibault LE, et al: The shaken baby syndrome. A clinical, pathological, and biomechanical study. J Neurosurg 66: 409–415, 1987
Evans RW: Some observations on whiplash injuries. Neurol Clin 10: 975–977, 1992
Factor SA, Weiner WJ: Prior history of head trauma in Parkinson's disease. Movement Dis 6: 225–229, 1991
Fedoroff JP, Starkstein SE, Forrester AW, et al: Depression in patients with acute traumatic brain injury. Am J Psychiatry 149: 918–923, 1992
Grafman J, Jonas BS, Martin A, et al: Intellectual function following penetrating head injury in Vietnam veterans. Brain 111: 169–184, 1988
Jankovic J: Post-traumatic movement disorders: Central and peripheral mechanisms. Neurology 44: 2006–2014, 1994
Kelly JP, Nicholos JS, Filley CM, et al: Concussion in sports. Guidelines for the prevention of catastrophic outcome. JAMA 27: 2867–2869, 1991
Krauss JK, Mohadjer M, Braus DF, et al: Dystonia following head trauma: A report of nine patients and review of the literature. Movement Dis 7: 263–272, 1992
Lee MS, Rinne JO, Ceballos-Baumann A, et al: Dystonia after head trauma. Neurology 44: 1374–1378, 1994
Levin HS, Gary HE, Eisenberg HM, et al: Neurobehavioral outcome 1 year after severe head injury. J Neurosurg 73: 699–709, 1990
Mayou R, Brant B, Duthie R: Psychiatric consequences of road traffic accidents. Br Med J 307: 647–651, 1993
Pearce JM: Whiplash injury: A reappraisal. J Neurol Neurosurg Psychiatr 52: 1329–1331, 1989
Pearce JMS: Polemics of chronic whiplash injury (Editorial). Neurology 44: 1993–1197, 1994
Pincus JH: Neurologist's role in understanding violence. Arch Neurol 50: 867–868, 1993
Radanov BP, DiStefano G, Schnidrig A, et al: Cognitive functioning after common whiplash. Arch Neurol 50: 87–91, 1993
Radanov BP, Sturzenegger M, DiStefano G, et al: Factors influencing recovery from headache after common whiplash. Br Med J 307: 652–655, 1993
Roberts GW, Allsop D, Bruton C: The occult aftermath of boxing. J Neurol Neurosurg Psychiatr 53: 373–378, 1990
Schwab K, Grafman J, Salazar AM, et al: Residual impairments and work status 15 years after penetrating head injury: Report from the Vietnam Head Injury Study. Neurology 43: 95–103, 1993
Sturzenegger M, DiStefano G, Radanov BP, et al: Presenting symptoms and signs after whiplash injury: The influence of accident mechanisms. Neurology 44: 688–693, 1994

Teasdale G, Jennett B: Assessment of coma and impaired consciousness: A practical scale. Lancet *2*: 81–84, 1974

Volpe BT, McDowell FH: The efficacy of cognitive rehabilitation in patients with traumatic brain injury. Arch Neurol *47*: 220–222, 1990

White RJ, Likavec MJ: The diagnosis and initial management of head injury. N Engl J Med *327*: 1507–1511, 1992

Williams DB, Annegers JF, Kokman E, et al: Brain injury and neurologic sequelae: A cohort study of dementia, parkinsonism, and amyotrophic lateral sclerosis. Neurology *41*: 1554–1557, 1991

CHAPTER 22: QUESTIONS *and* ANSWERS

1. A 24-year-old man is brought to the Emergency Room after a MVA. He is stuporous with a Glasgow Coma Scale score (GCS) of 6. Skull x-rays show a fracture across the left temporal bone. On his way to a tertiary care hospital, he develops coma with decerebrate posturing and a left third cranial nerve palsy. What is the most likely cause of his deterioration?

a. A subdural hematoma
b. Alcohol intoxication
c. Laceration of the middle meningeal artery
d. None of the above

> *answer:* c. The young man has probably sustained a laceration of the middle meningeal artery by the temporal bone skull fracture. Bleeding from this artery has led to an epidural hematoma, which is a rapidly expanding, usually fatal, intracranial mass lesion. Low GCS scores are associated with fatal outcomes.

2. How do epidural hematomas differ from subdural hematomas?

a. Epidural hematomas originate from arterial bleeding, but subdural hematomas usually originate from venous bleeding.
b. Epidural hematomas are more likely to be fatal.
c. Epidural hematomas are more likely to be chronic.
d. Epidural hematomas are more likely to occur in the elderly.

> *answer:* a, b. Subdural hematomas originate in venous bleeding, which is under lower pressure. The bleeding is apt to stop spontaneously. Although the blood may be reabsorbed slowly, the mass effect may persist and increase over weeks.

3. Which is/are features of chronic subdural hematomas?

a. They appear in CT scans as curved, extra-axial lucencies (black regions).
b. They are a correctable cause of dementia.
c. They cause few physical deficits, such as hemiparesis, compared to nonspecific symptoms, such as headaches and personality changes.
d. The elderly are prone to subdural hematomas because they have cerebral atrophy and a tendency to fall.
e. Many chronic subdural hematomas are reabsorbed without the need for surgery.

> *answer:* All

4. Which condition is most likely to follow in a head trauma patient with a GCS score of 7?

a. Anterograde amnesia
b. Postconcussive syndrome
c. Whiplash injury
d. Seizures

> *answer:* a. Anterograde and retrograde amnesia are the most common residual effects of coma. Seizures are associated with coma, but the association is not as close. Postconcussive and whiplash injuries have relatively little association.

5. To which injury can the term *contrecoup* apply?

a. Temporal lobe, especially the temporal tip, injury after an occipital blow
b. Blindness after an occipital lobe blow
c. Diffuse axonal injury after localized head trauma
d. Neck pain after head injury

answer: a. Head trauma that damages the opposite side of the brain causes *contrecoup* injuries. These injuries can be envisioned as resulting from the brain "bouncing around the inside of the skull." They are most apparent in areas where the brain strikes rough or sharpened inner surfaces of the skull, such as in the middle fossa, which holds the temporal lobes. Temporal lobe injuries result in the characteristic post-traumatic memory impairments (amnesia).

6. Shrapnel and other foreign bodies that are retained in the brain are frequently uncorrectable sequelae of penetrating head injuries. What are their consequences?

a. They may act as a scar focus for seizures, i.e., post-traumatic epilepsy.
b. They are associated with general cognitive impairments depending on their position.
c. They may act as a nidus for a brain abscess.
d. They can cause a permanent state of coma.

answer: a, c. In general, post-traumatic cognitive impairments are related to the extent of the brain injury, not its location. Dominant temporal lobe lesions, however, are related to a post-traumatic aphasia or other language disorders. Traumatic brain-injured patients remain in coma for up to 3 weeks. If they do not succumb, their level of consciousness improves or changes to a persistent vegetative state.

7. Which cognitive function is most susceptible to head trauma?

a. Judgment
b. Language function
c. Memory
d. Constructional ability

answer: c

8. Of the following, which variety of seizure is the most common manifestation of post-traumatic epilepsy?

a. Psychogenic
b. Focal with secondary generalization
c. Petit mal
d. Primary generalized

answer: b. Since post-traumatic epilepsy results from cerebral cortex injury, focal (partial) seizures, including partial complex seizures, are common. Primary generalized seizures—petit mal (absences) and tonic-clonic—do not result from head trauma.

9. Which one of the following is not characteristics of dementia pugilistica?

a. It results from a single episode of brain injury.
b. Its manifestations mimic Parkinson's disease: tremors, rigidity, and depigmentation of the substantia nigra.
c. It causes cerebral plaques and tangles.
d. It occurs most frequently in lightweight boxers and alcoholics.
e. It results in atrophy of the corpus callosum and the cerebrum.

answer: a. Repeated head injury leads to dementia pugilistica.

10. Which are the two most reliable guidelines of the seriousness of a head injury?

a. GCS score
b. Duration of amnesia
c. Seizure on impact
d. Blood alcohol level

answer: a, b. The depth of coma is measured by the GCS. Both retrograde or anterograde amnesia correlate wi'h the seriousness of head injury.

11. Which two regions of the brain are most likely to be injured in a coup-contrecoup injury?

a. Frontal lobe
b. Parietal lobe
c. Occipital lobe
d. Temporal lobe
e. Cerebellum
f. Brainstem

answer: a, d. Reciprocal, coup-contrecoup injuries have their greatest impact on the temporal lobe and anterior-inferior surface of the frontal lobes because those lobes are pointed and they abut against sharp surfaces of the anterior and middle fossae.

12. Which combination of two injuries most suggests the "shaken baby syndrome"?

a. Retinal hemorrhages
b. Occipital skull fracture
c. Blood in the interhemispheric fissure

d. Nasal fracture
e. Wrist fracture

answer: a, c. Shaken babies succumb to raised intracranial pressure and intracranial bleeding without skull or long bone fractures. Most shaken babies do not have obvious soft tissue injuries.

Additional Review Questions

This group of questions is more than a quiz: It is a learning opportunity. To increase their value, most questions have more than one answer. Readers will, of course, benefit more by taking a self-quiz than by immediately reading the answer.

1. A 60-year-old man is brought for evaluation of dementia. On mental status testing he performs poorly on the questions that require memory. In contrast, he satisfactorily completes questions that require judgment, language skills, and abstract reasoning. He has a tendency to be verbally aggressive and excessively use profanities. He has a snout and bilateral palmar-omental reflexes. Of the following, which condition is most likely the cause of his mental status changes?

a. Alzheimer's disease
b. Tourette's syndrome
c. A nonspecific dementia
d. Multi-infarct dementia
e. None of the above

> *answer:* e. The patient has an amnestic syndrome, in which memory is impaired exclusively or to a much greater degree than other intellectual functions. In typical cases of Alzheimer's disease and multiple infarct dementia, memory is impaired less than or in proportion to other intellectual functions. Although Alzheimer's disease can produce an amnestic syndrome, this disorder is typical of Wernicke-Korsakoff syndrome, partial complex status epilepticus, temporal lobe injury, or *Herpes simplex* encephalitis. In some of these conditions, memory impairments are accompanied by features of the Klüver-Bucy syndrome. Frontal release signs, except perhaps for bilateral grasp reflexes, are not diagnostically helpful. Multi-infarct dementia produces physical impairments roughly in proportion to cognitive impairments.

2. A 22-year-old man with mental retardation and tonic-clonic seizures has about one seizure each week. Which of the following are likely causes of these seizures?

a. He does not comply with his anticonvulsants.
b. Psychogenic seizures are mixed with epileptic seizures.
c. He has narcolepsy.
d. He has Jakob-Creutzfeldt disease.
e. He has tuberous sclerosis.
f. He takes drugs, alcohol, or medications other than anticonvulsants.
g. The wrong anticonvulsant or the incorrect dose has been prescribed.

> *answer:* a, b, e, f, g. Routine evaluation will probably reveal the cause of the high frequency of his seizures. In cases that remain refractory, the definitive test is closed circuit television monitoring (CCTV) of behavior and the electroencephalogram (EEG), which can be combined with anticonvulsant blood level determinations and other measurements.

3. After a vigorous day of training, a 19-year-old Marine recruit suddenly develops a temperature of 103°F and stupor. He is brought to the Emergency Room where he is found to have nuchal rigidity. Which three therapies or diagnostic tests should be performed as soon as possible?

a. Intravenous anticonvulsants
b. Oral anticonvulsants
c. Thiamine (50 mg IV)
d. Lumbar puncture
e. Penicillin or penicillin in combination with chloramphenicol

> *answer:* a, d, e. Children and young adults brought together from different geographic locations occasionally develop outbreaks of meningitis. These small

epidemics typically occur in kindergartens and military recruit barracks. Most cases of acute bacterial meningitis are fatal unless treated promptly with intravenous antibiotics. In this setting, the stupor and nuchal rigidity indicate meningitis. A subarachnoid hemorrhage, which could be responsible, can be diagnosed by examination of the spinal fluid by the lumbar puncture.

4. A 30-year-old man has a long history of aggressive behavior and other antisocial activities. His EEG shows an isolated, phase-reversed spike focus intermittently over the left frontal lobe. Which single statement is valid?

a. In retrospect, the behavioral disturbances were the result of partial complex seizures.
b. The EEG has absolutely no bearing on the case.
c. Certain EEG abnormalities are characteristically found in antisocial people.
d. Both the EEG and the behavior may reflect cerebral damage.

answer: d. The EEG indicates the presence of a structural lesion in the left frontal lobe that could be a source of seizures. Lesions in the frontal lobe as well as those in the temporal lobe can cause the partial complex seizures. However, since there are no stereotyped behavioral disturbances and the EEG shows no paroxysmal activity, most neurologists would not make the diagnosis of seizures with the information at hand. Depending on the circumstances, further testing might be indicated in an attempt at diagnosing seizures.

5. An 8-year-old boy begins to have 10- to 20-second episodes of repetitive lip smacking, eyelid fluttering, and finger rubbing. During these episodes he is incoherent. Afterward he is confused and sleepy. What is the most likely diagnosis?

a. Absence (petit mal) seizures
b. Partial complex (psychomotor) seizures
c. Attention deficit disorder
d. Psychologic aberrations

answer: b. This child is having typical partial complex seizures: He has incoherence without loss of consciousness; stereotyped, simple, repetitive movements and sounds; and subsequent (postictal) confusion and somnolence. The distinction between absences and partial complex seizures in children is difficult but important.

6. During the course of evaluation for dementia, a 68-year-old patient's CT scan reveals a small, calcium-containing, dense lesion without surrounding edema that arises from the right parietal convexity. It does not compress the underlying brain. Which two symptoms might this lesion likely cause?

a. Dementia
b. Aphasia
c. Absence seizures
d. Partial seizures without secondary generalization
e. Partial seizures with secondary generalization

answer: d, e. The lesion is probably a small meningioma. Although a brain tumor, such meningiomas are common and usually innocuous. They might, however, cause seizures by irritating the underlying cortex. In this case, partial seizures arising from the parietal cortex might cause sensory symptoms on the left side of the body. Seizure activity might also undergo secondary generalization. Small meningiomas do not cause dementia. Especially in the elderly, they need not be removed.

7. Which one of the following patients is most likely to have a seizure?

a. A 65-year-old man with left Bell's palsy
b. A 70-year-old woman with a right third cranial nerve palsy and left hemiparesis
c. A 55-year-old woman with rapidly progressive paresis and sensory loss in her left arm and more so in her left leg, which has hyperactive DTRs and a Babinski sign
d. A 40-year-old man who, after an upper respiratory tract infection, develops ascending flaccid, areflexic weakness of both legs

answer: c. This patient has a lesion involving the right cerebral cortex that could cause seizures. She could have a parasagittal (parafalcine) meningioma, glioblastoma, or abscess. Patients are unlikely to have a seizure if they have lesions in noncerebral cortex locations, such as the left seventh cranial nerve (a), right midbrain (b), or peripheral nerves, such as the Guillain-Barré syndrome (d).

8. A 65-year-old man, who has nonfluent aphasia, understands and complies with most simple verbal requests. However, when asked to pretend to show how he would use a comb, he runs his hand and fingers through his hair. What is the name of this phenomenon?

a. Dementia
b. Ideational apraxia
c. Limb apraxia
d. Finger agnosia
e. Aphasia

answer: c. Because the patient employed his body part as the object (comb), he is said to have limb apraxia. Another classic example of limb apraxia would be if he had been asked to show how he would use a toothbrush, but he brushed his teeth with his finger. Unless he also suffered from dementia, the patient probably would have been successful if he had been handed either a comb or a toothbrush, in which case the actual object would have served as a cue. Likewise, he would have been able to mimic the examiner's actions.

In contrast, patients with ideational apraxia are unable to perform an abstract sequence of simple actions, such as pretending to address, stamp, and then mail an envelope. Ideational apraxia might also be overcome by using actual objects or having the patient mimic the examiner. Unlike limb apraxia, ideational apraxia is closely associated with dementia.

9. After partially successful resuscitation from a cardiac arrest, a 70-year-old man has apathy and psychomotor retardation. He says only a few simple words. However, he repeats many long, complex phrases, and he accompanies singers on the radio. He does not have a hemiparesis or homonymous hemianopsia. What is the nature of this patient's language impairment?

a. Nonfluent aphasia
b. Fluent aphasia
c. Frontal lobe dysfunction
d. Isolation (transcortical) aphasia

answer: d. Isolation (transcortical) aphasia results from isolation of the perisylvian language arc—Broca's area, the arcuate fasciculus, and Wernicke's area—from the remaining cerebral cortex. Most often, the nonlanguage cortex is destroyed by the anoxia. With the language arc remaining intact, patients are able to repeat words, phrases, and songs. However, since the language arc exists in isolation, patients are unable to integrate language with other intellectual functions. Although patients with language or other cognitive impairments may be difficult to examine, physicians should attempt to perform bedside testing for aphasia.

10–15. Below are six sketches of spinal cords stained such that normal myelin is stained black, gray areas are crosshatched, and demyelinated areas are white (unstained). Match the sketches with the descriptions of the clinical associations (a-f).

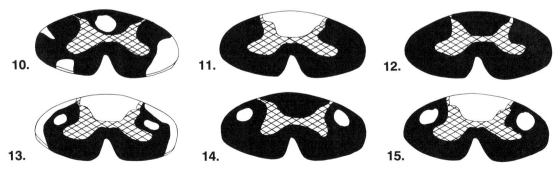

a. A 45-year-old man with progressively severe intellectual and personality impairment for 4 years has loss of vibration and position sensation, absent reflexes in the legs, and a floppy-foot gait. His pupils are miotic. They constrict to closely regarded objects but not to light.

b. A 65-year-old man, who had a complete gastrectomy 4 years ago, now has dementia, hyperactive DTRs, bilateral Babinski signs, and loss of vibration sensation in the legs.

c. A 70-year-old woman has weakness of the left leg, right arm, and neck muscles. She has atrophy of many limb muscles and fasciculations of the tongue and most of the atrophic muscles.

d. A 35-year-old man has optic neuritis, internuclear ophthalmoplegia, and gait impairment because of ataxia, weakness, and spasticity.

e. A 40-year-old woman and her sister have pes cavus, intention tremor of the limbs, and loss of position and vibration sensation.

f. A 70-year-old man who has schizophrenia sustains a frontal lobe gunshot wound. He takes phenytoin that leads to cerebellar dysfunction. He becomes so distraught that he becomes an alcoholic and suffers an episode of severe confusion, nystagmus, and bilateral abducens nerve palsy.

answers: 10–15.

10. *answer:* d. The spinal cord shows multiple areas (plaques) of demyelination (sclerosis). The patient has signs of optic nerve, brainstem, and spinal cord dysfunction. Both the clinical and pathologic information indicate multiple sclerosis.

11. *answer:* a. The spinal cord shows demyelination of the posterior columns. Loss of these tracts causes loss of position sensation, which makes patients walk with a high, uncertain, and awkward pattern, i.e., a steppage gait. This patient is described as having Argyll-Robertson pupils and mental abnormalities. This is a case of syphilis of the brain and spinal cord (tabes dorsalis).

12. *answer:* f. The spinal cord remains normal despite the cerebral injury, medication-induced cerebellar dysfunction, and Wernicke's encephalopathy.

13. *answer:* e. There is degeneration of the spinocerebellar, posterior column, and corticospinal tracts. Loss of the spinocerebellar and posterior column tracts, which indicates a spinocerebellar degenerative illness, such as Friedreich's ataxia, causes intention tremor, position and vibration sense loss, and a foot deformity (pes cavus).

14. *answer:* c. The spinal cord shows demyelination of the lateral corticospinal tracts and loss of the anterior horns, which contain the motor neurons. This is the picture of typical motor neuron disease, in which both the upper and lower motor neuron systems degenerate. The patient has the clinical features of amyotrophic lateral sclerosis (ALS), the most common form of motor neuron disease.

15. *answer:* b. The spinal cord shows demyelination of the posterior columns and the lateral corticospinal tracts. This pattern, combined system disease, is associated with B_{12} deficiency from pernicious anemia or surgical removal of the stomach because both conditions remove intrinsic factor. Combined system disease is associated with dementia, paraparesis, hyperactive DTRs, and position and vibration sense loss. These findings are similar to those of tabes dorsalis with dementia; however, while combined-system disease causes hyperactive DTRs and Babinski signs, tabes dorsalis causes hypoactive DTRs and Argyll-Robertson pupils, but neither paraparesis nor Babinski signs.

16–20. Match the visual field loss (16–20) associated with each condition (a-k).

a. Retinal injury, e.g., retinal detachment or embolus from carotid artery
b. Hysteria
c. Migraine with aura
d. Diabetes insipidus
e. Loss of libido
f. Optic atopy

g. Amaurosis fugax
h. Internal capsule infarction
i. Aphasia
j. Occipital infarction
k. Optic or retrobulbar neuritis

16. Left homonymous hemianopsia with macular sparing

answer: j

17. Fortification scotoma

answer: c

18. Central scotoma, lasting for 2 weeks

answer: k

19. Bitemporal hemianopsia

answer: d, e, f (all associated with pituitary tumors)

20. Unilateral superior quadrantanopia

answer: a

21. An 80-year-old man, who is being treated for depression, complains of right-sided frontal headaches. His vision in the right eye is impaired. Temporal arteries are prominent, but not especially tender. There is no papilledema, hemiparesis, or other neurologic sign. Which two conditions must be considered immediately?

a. Open-angle glaucoma
b. Metastases to the skull
c. Meningioma
d. Optic neuritis
e. Temporal arteritis
f. Narrow-angle glaucoma

answer: e, f. The diagnosis of temporal arteritis should be made rapidly. If untreated, this condition can cause blindness or cerebral infarction. The most commonly used diagnostic tests are the sedimentation rate and temporal artery biopsy. Likewise, untreated glaucoma (both narrow- and open-angle) can rapidly lead to blindness.

22–30. Match the ocular abnormality (22–30) with the most probable cause (a-k).

a. Neuromuscular junction impairment
b. Anticholinergic intoxication
c. Right pontine lesion
d. Left pontine lesion
e. Left midbrain lesion
f. Right midbrain lesion
g. Midline, dorsal brainstem lesion
h. Left lateral medullary lesion
i. Right lateral medullary lesion
j. Syphilis
k. Opioids

22. Right third cranial nerve paresis and left hemiparesis

answer: f

23. Left sixth cranial nerve paresis and right hemiparesis

answer: d

24. Right Horner's syndrome, right facial hypalgesia, right limb ataxia, and left limb and trunk hypalgesia

answer: i

25. Internuclear ophthalmoplegia

answer: g

26. Right sixth and seventh cranial nerve paresis and left hemiparesis

answer: c

27. Ophthalmoplegia with normally reactive pupils, ptosis, and facial diplegia

    answer: a (myasthenia gravis)

28. Small, irregular pupils that accommodate but do not react

    answer: j

29. Fever, agitated confusion, and dilated pupils

    answer: b (scopolamine intoxication)

30. Stupor, miosis, and pulmonary edema

    answer: k (heroin or methadone overdose)

31. Which of the following are found in Alzheimer's disease brains, but not in normal elderly brains?

a. Loss of weight
b. Increase in sulci width
c. Expansion of the lateral ventricles
d. Major loss of large cortical neurons
e. Marked reduction of choline acetyltransferase in the hippocampus
f. Mild memory impairment
g. Multiple neurofibrillary tangles
h. Similarity to brains of Down's syndrome patients and retired boxers
i. Presence of senile plaques

    answer: d, e, g, h. Cerebral atrophy (a, b, c) and plaques (i), neurofibrillary tangles, and granulovacuolar degeneration are found in normal brains. However, they are present in greater concentrations in Alzheimer's disease brains.

32. A 60-year-old gentleman with dementia has a gait abnormality in which he excessively raises his legs. He seems to be climbing as he walks. His pupils are small (miotic), poorly reactive, and irregular. What is the gait abnormality?

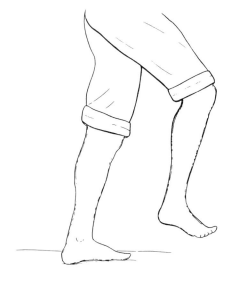

a. Gait apraxia
b. Congenital spastic paraparesis
c. Steppage gait from posterior spinal cord degeneration
d. Astasia abasia

answer: c. The patient has a steppage gait because he has lost position sense. He must raise his legs to avoid catching the tips of his toes when he walks or especially when he steps onto curbs. He has lost his position sense because he has tabes dorsalis and Argyll-Robertson pupils as a manifestation of tertiary syphilis. Loss of position sense from diabetic neuropathy or degenerative spinal cord diseases can also cause a steppage gait, but those diseases do not cause dementia.

33–35. Match the confabulation (33–35) with the lesion (a-c) that might produce it.

a. Nondominant parietal lobe infarction
b. Bilateral occipital lobe infarctions
c. Hemorrhage into the limbic system

33.   The patient, who is blind, "describes" clothing that an examiner is wearing. His pupils are round and reactive to light.

answer: b. In cortical blindness, some patients tend to confabulate (Anton's syndrome). Cortical blindness usually results from infarction or trauma of both occipital lobes. The pupils react normally because the optic and oculomotor nerves are unaffected.

34.   A man with recent onset of left hemiparesis claims that he cannot move his left arm and leg because he is too tired.

answer: a. Patients with hemiparesis from a nondominant hemisphere infarct often confabulate, deny, and use other defense mechanisms in ignoring their hemiparesis. Typically the right parietal lobe is the site of the lesion.

35.   An agitated, diaphoretic middle-aged man describes bizarre occurrences and experiences visual hallucinations. When asked to repeat six digits, he seems to select random numbers.

answer: c. Patients with alcohol withdrawal can have confabulations. They may occur alone or as part of delirium tremens. However, the frequency of confabulations in Wernicke-Korsakoff syndrome is usually overestimated. Petechiae in the mammillary bodies constitute hemorrhage into the limbic system.

36.   A 35-year-old man staggers into the Emergency Room. He is lethargic and disoriented. He has nystagmus, gait ataxia, and finger-to-nose dysmetria. Which illness is he most likely to have? What is the specific therapy?

a. Subdural hematoma   c. Wernicke-Korsakoff syndrome
b. Cerebral infarction   d. Psychogenic disturbance

answer: c. Thiamine 50 mg IV.

37.   An 11-year-old boy is admitted because of headache, nausea, and vomiting. He has had clumsiness for the 2 weeks before admission. He has papilledema, ataxia, bilateral hyperactive DTRs, and Babinski signs. Which is the most likely diagnosis?

a. Multiple sclerosis   c. Cerebellar tumor
b. Drug abuse   d. Spinocerebellar degeneration

answer: c. Cerebellar astrocytomas, which are relatively common in children, block the aqueduct of Sylvius, creating hydrocephalus (manifested by headaches, nausea, vomiting, and papilledema).

38.   Which of the following symptoms constitute the narcoleptic tetrad?

a. Inability to move on awakening (sleep paralysis)
b. Hunger or anorexia
c. Vivid dreams when falling asleep (hypnagogic hallucinations)
d. Excessive daytime sleepiness (narcolepsy)
e. Night terrors (pavor nocturnus)
f. Episodic loss of muscle tone (cataplexy)
g. HLA-DR2

answer: a, c, d, f. The human leukocyte antigen (HLA) DR2, which is located on chromosome 6, is a marker for the illness in more than 90 per cent of cases; however, it is not included in the clinical tetrad.

39. An adolescent with a chronic, psychiatric disorder begins to drink large quantities of water and other fluids. After 1 week, he develops a seizure. Which of the following conditions could be responsible?

a. The psychiatric condition
b. Diabetes insipidus
c. Diabetes mellitus
d. Parkinson's disease
e. Huntington's disease
f. Seizures
g. Steroid abuse

answer: a, b, c. Polydipsia usually leads to seizures because it causes hyponatremia, water intoxication, or another electrolyte imbalance.

40. In the previous question, assuming the patient did not have excessive salt intake, what might be the cause of the seizure?

a. A hypothalamic or pituitary tumor
b. Hyperglycemia-hyperosmolarity from diabetes mellitus
c. Hyponatremia (serum sodium of 120 or below) from compulsive water ingestion
d. All of the above

answer: d. The usual nonpsychiatric causes of this degree of polydipsia are excessive glucose serum concentration or, as a result of pituitary tumors, an absence of antidiuretic hormone.

41. A 29-year-old woman presents to a hospital with a 6-year history of progressively severe involuntary movements. Her limbs, trunk, and neck continuously move into grotesque postures. Her muscles are hypertrophied. In contrast, her cognitive function is normal. What are common causes of this condition?

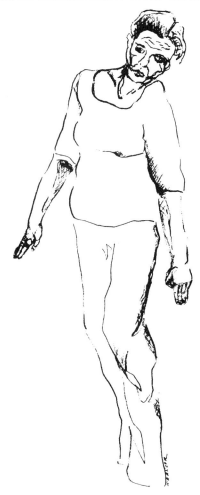

answer: This person has chronic dystonia. Its organic (nonpsychogenic) nature and chronicity are indicated by muscle hypertrophy and lack of bodily fat. In young adults, dystonia may be caused by Wilson's disease, Huntington's disease, neuroleptics (tardive dystonia), and dystonia musculorum deformans.

42. A 20-year-old sailor who has a history of glue sniffing develops paresthesias and mild weakness in his hands and toes. Of the following, which single portion of the nervous system has been damaged?

a. Spinal cord
b. Corpus callosum
c. Peripheral nerves

d. Spinal cord
e. Neuromuscular junction

answer: c. Major components of glue, which carries a great potential for abuse, include N-hexane and other volatile solvents. These substances are mostly lipophilic and are thus able to damage the lipid-rich myelin cover of peripheral nerves. Chronic exposure causes a peripheral neuropathy.

43. Three weeks after recovering from an apparently successful repair of an anterior communicating artery aneurysm, a patient is apathetic and almost mute, but not aphasic. A psychiatry consultation has been solicited. Which of the following is most likely to have complicated the aneurysm or surgery?

a. The spinal cord and brain have been damaged.
b. Depression has developed.
c. Both anterior cerebral arteries were occluded.
d. The patient developed normal-pressure hydrocephalus (NPH), i.e., dementia, gait apraxia, and incontinence.
e. Dementia has developed.
f. A major depression has developed.

answer: c. The anterior communicating arteries supply a large portion of the frontal lobes, including the medial surface of the motor cortex. Because this region controls the voluntary function of the legs and bladder, the patient should be tested for incontinence and paraparesis. Infarction of these arteries, from the aneurysm or surgery, creates marked personality impairments, as well as incontinence and paraparesis. NPH sometimes develops after subarachnoid hemorrhages, but NPH patients have gait apraxia, rather than paraparesis. Major depression after neurosurgery is rare.

44. Which three of the following conditions often lead to patient's sensing "putrid smells" that the physician cannot detect?

a. Seizures that originate in the uncus
b. Sinusitis
c. Migraines

d. Seizures that originate in the parietal lobe
e. Phenytoin
f. Dental infections

answer: a, b, f. Migraines, curiously, often include visual but rarely auditory or olfactory auras. Infections in the sinuses and mouth are the most common causes.

45. In which conditions might a lumbar puncture (spinal tap) be indicated?

a. Subdural hematoma
b. Brain abscess
c. Brain tumor
d. Unruptured arteriovenous malformation
e. Pseudotumor cerebri

f. Multiple sclerosis
g. Bacterial meningitis
h. Subacute sclerosing panencephalitis
i. Viral encephalitis
j. Sexual impairment

answer: e, f, g, h, i. Lumbar punctures should not be done when intracranial mass lesions are suspected because CSF analysis will not be helpful and the procedure might precipitate transtentorial herniation.

46. Which of the following are complications of alcoholism?

a. Mammillary body hemorrhage
b. Peripheral neuropathy

c. Neurofibrillary tangles
d. Central pontine myelinolysis
e. Corpus callosum degeneration (Marchiafava-Bignami syndrome)
f. Cerebellar degeneration
g. Granulovacuolar degeneration
h. Sclerotic plaques

answer: a, b, d, e, f

47. Which of the following illness(es) is (are) characterized by a normal mental state despite quadriparesis and respiratory distress?

a. Guillain-Barré syndrome
b. Locked-in syndrome
c. Persistent vegetative state
d. Porphyria

answer: a, b, d

48. An 11-year-old girl has developed twitchy, restless movements. She cannot protrude her tongue for 10 seconds. When her arms are extended, her fingers have individual flexion or extension movements. Except for irritability, her mental and emotional status is normal. Which tests would be most appropriate?

a. VDRL
b. Inquiries about oral contraceptives
c. Antistreptolysin O Titer (ALSO)
d. Pregnancy test
e. Lupus preparation

answer: b, c, d, e. Chorea in adolescents can be a manifestation of rheumatic fever (Sydenham's chorea), lupus, or pregnancy (chorea gravidarum) or a reaction to oral contraceptives.

49. Which procedures might be helpful in determining the dominant hemisphere?

a. Positron emission tomography (PET)
b. Computed tomography (CT)
c. EEG with sphenoidal electrodes
d. Magnetic resonance imaging (MRI)
e. Intracarotid sodium amobarbital injection
f. Wada test
g. Visual evoked responses (VER)
h. Brainstem auditory evoked responses (BAER)

answer: a, e, f. The Wada test is based on intracarotid amobarbital injections. Perfusion of the dominant hemisphere will induce aphasia.

50. When nonsteroidal anti-inflammatory agents are given for menstrual cramps, with which substance do they interfere?

a. Enkephalins
b. Endorphins
c. Prostaglandins
d. Serotonin
d. Dopamine

answer: c

51. Which two statements are true regarding the dorsal raphe nucleus?

a. It contains high concentrations of endorphins.
b. Stimulating it causes pain.
c. Stimulating it produces analgesia.
d. Stimulating it produces behavioral changes.
e. Its destructions causes analgesia.
f. It contains high serotonin concentrations.
g. Microinjections of procaine (Novocain) cause analgesia.
h. Microinjections of morphine cause analgesia.

answer: c, f

52. A 14-year-old boy is brought to the Emergency Room in a stupor. He is apneic, and his pupils are miotic. Which one of the following conditions is most likely to be the cause of this constellation of findings?

a. Brainstem stroke
b. Heroin overdose
c. Hypoglycemia

d. Postictal stupor
e. Psychogenic disturbance

answer: b. Heroin overdose typically causes stupor, miosis, and apnea. Brainstem strokes may cause this constellation; however, they rarely occur in this age group. The other conditions generally cause dilated pupils, but not apnea.

53–55. A 29-year-old woman has developed a tremor that is most pronounced when she writes, drinks coffee, and lights a cigarette.

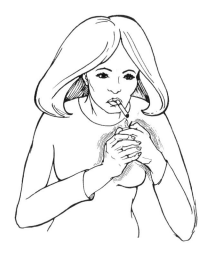

53. Which of the following conditions can lead to such a tremor?

a. Essential tremor
b. Wilson's disease
c. Anxiety
d. Huntington's chorea

e. Athetosis
f. Benign familial tremor
g. Dystonia

answer: a, b, c, f. Essential tremor and benign familial tremor are probably varieties of the same condition. Wilson's disease is a rare but important condition that might be considered in young adults who develop a tremor. Anxiety can produce a tremor that is indistinguishable from essential tremor. The two conditions may have a similar etiology and positive response to beta-adrenergic blockers.

54. Which tests should be performed to exclude Wilson's disease when only mild tremors are evident?

a. CT
b. EEG
c. Lumbar puncture

d. Serum ceruloplasmin
e. Serum copper concentration
f. Slit-lamp examination

answer: d, f

55. If the patient did have an essential tremor, which medications are often effective?

a. Anticholinergics
b. Dopamine agonists
c. Neuroleptics

d. Beta-adrenergic blockers
e. Antiviral agents
f. Alpha-adrenergic blockers

answer: d

56. How do neurotransmitters differ from endocrine hormones, such as T4?

a. They or their byproducts circulate in detectable quantities in the blood.
b. They are produced and stored at a site adjacent to the target organ.

c.   They or their byproducts are often present in detectable concentrations in the cerebrospinal fluid, but not in the blood.

d.   They are steroids.

answer: b, c

57.   Of the following, which single condition frequently increases REM latency?

a.   Depression
b.   Drug withdrawal
c.   Excessive alcohol use
d.   Narcolepsy

answer: c. The other conditions typically cause dreams to be present soon after sleep begins, i.e., a short REM latency.

58.   A 28-year-old woman complains of gait impairment. She has a history of vigorous exercise, taking large quantities of vitamins, and avoiding red meat. She consumes no alcohol. On examination, she has marked sensory loss and absent DTRs in all limbs, but her strength is normal. Which one of the following conditions is most likely to be responsible for her symptoms?

a.   Cervical spondylosis
b.   Myopathy
c.   Vitamin toxicity
d.   Iron-deficiency anemia

answer: c. Pyridoxine (vitamin B_6) in large daily doses creates a neuropathy that impairs sensation. The neuropathy is reversible after the vitamins are withdrawn. Iron deficiency does not create a neuropathy. However, thiamine and folate deficiency, often consequences of alcoholism, can produce a neuropathy.

59.   A 68-year-old house painter has weakness, atrophy, and areflexic DTRs in his arms. He has sensory loss in his right hand, brisk DTRs in his legs, and a right Babinski sign. Which one of the following features suggests that he has cervical spondylosis rather than amyotrophic lateral sclerosis (ALS)?

a.   Hand atrophy
b.   Hyperactive DTRs
c.   Sensory loss
d.   The Babinski sign

answer: c. House painting requires prolonged neck hyperextension, which leads to cervical spondylosis. Whatever its cause, cervical spondylosis leads to sensory and lower motor neuron loss in the arms and hands and upper motor neuron signs in the legs. Cervical spondylosis is a much more frequently occurring condition than ALS.

60.   Which is the most characteristic finding in standard intelligence tests in early dementia?

a.   Decreased performance, decreased verbal scales
b.   Decreased performance, relatively normal verbal scales
c.   Decreased verbal, relatively normal performance scales
d.   None of the above

answer: b

61.   What will standard intelligence tests show in patients with depression-induced cognitive changes?

a.   Decreased performance, decreased verbal scales
b.   Decreased performance, relatively normal verbal scales
c.   Decreased verbal, relatively normal performance scales
d.   None of the above

answer: a. Verbal and performance scales are usually both decreased. Performance scales might be lower than verbal scales because of psychomotor retardation, and they might fluctuate because of variable attention and mood.

62.   As people age, what is the most common EEG change?

a.   Loss of amplitude
b.   Slowing of the background activity
c.   Fragmentation of background
d.   Episodic beta activity

answer: b

63. In which two ways do hypnagogic hallucinations differ from partial complex seizures?

a. Hypnagogic hallucinations are associated with flaccid, areflexic musculature.
b. Hypnagogic hallucinations often have an auditory component.
c. Hypnagogic hallucinations are associated with EEG spikes.
d. Hypnagogic hallucinations have visual, auditory, and emotional aspects.
e. Hypnagogic hallucinations are varied.

answer: a, e

64. Which structure contains 80 per cent of the brain's dopamine content?

a. Third ventricle
b. Thalamus
c. Cerebral cortex
d. Corpus striatum

answer: d

65. Which condition is not associated with shortened REM latency?

a. Night terrors
b. Narcolepsy
c. Depression
d. Withdrawal from sedatives
e. Withdrawal from neuroleptics

answer: a. Night terrors, which occur in the early night, are not bad dreams and are not associated with REM sleep. In contrast, nightmares are bad dreams, which are associated with REM sleep.

66. One week after a right cerebral infarction, a 60-year-old man complains of pain, but he really describes an intense burning sensation in the left side of his face and arm. He has a marked sensory loss to all modalities in these regions and a mild left hemiparesis. What is the origin of the patient's symptom?

a. Parietal lobe injury
b. Brachial plexus injury
c. Lateral spinothalamic injury
d. Thalamic injury

answer: d. The patient really has *thalamic pain*, which is a distressing consequence of an infarction in the thalamus. This burning sensation is attributable to *deafferentation* or loss of sensory input to the brain. Similar unpleasant sensations result from phantom limbs and brachial plexus avulsions. Thalamic pain sometimes responds to anticonvulsants, but generally not to analgesics. Deafferentation pain should be distinguished from neuropathic pain in which pain results directly from nerve injury, such as postherpetic neuralgia.

67. Which two of the following tests rely on ionizing radiation?

a. CT
b. MRI
c. Isotopic brain scan
d. EEG
e. EMG
f. VER
g. BAER

answer: a, c

68. In patients with the human variety of the Klüver-Bucy syndrome, which symptom is least common?

a. Oral exploration
b. Amnesia
c. Uncontrollable sexual activity
d. Placid demeanor
e. Anger

answer: c. All these symptoms may be manifestations of the Klüver-Bucy syndrome in humans, as well as animals. Humans develop the Klüver-Bucy syndrome from Herpes encephalitis, contusion of the temporal lobes, or multiple strokes. Although they may have increased sexual activity, it is limited in humans to minor verbal and behavioral changes. Also unlike monkeys, humans do not have overt aggression, homosexual activity, or oral exploration. Moreover, their affect is usually bland, as with frontal lobe injury, but it may be punctuated by bursts of anger.

69. Medical treatments occasionally produce neurologic damage as a complication of an otherwise beneficial program. Which one of the following statements is false?

a. Human growth hormone injections given to correct short stature in children have caused Creutzfeldt-Jakob disease.
b. Smallpox vaccinations rarely cause an attack of disseminated CNS demyelination that mimics multiple sclerosis.
c. Measles vaccinations rarely cause subacute sclerosing panencephalitis (SSPE).
d. Artificial insemination with donor semen has induced acquired immunodeficiency syndrome (AIDS).

answer: c. Although elevated measles antibody titers are found in the CSF of SSPE patients (who are usually children), measles virus has not been proven to be the cause of this illness. In addition, similar abnormalities have been detected in patients with multiple sclerosis. Studies have shown that the incidence of SSPE has been markedly reduced after measles vaccination programs and that measles vaccinations have not caused SSPE.

The development of Creutzfeldt-Jakob disease in children given growth hormone extracted from human pituitary glands led to the use of growth hormone synthesis from genetically engineered bacteria. Creutzfeldt-Jakob disease has also been transferred by the use of depth EEG electrodes and corneal transplantation.

Smallpox vaccinations occasionally cause *postvaccinal demyelination*, a condition in which multiple areas of the CNS become demyelinated. The clinical and histologic features of postvaccinal demyelination mimic multiple sclerosis; however, attacks of postvaccinal demyelination are single events. This complication has been one of the major reasons that smallpox vaccinations are given sparingly.

AIDS transmission has been documented to have resulted from homosexual, heterosexual, and artificial semen transfer.

70. A 30-year-old woman has the sudden onset of "the worst headache of her life." She has nuchal rigidity, but no lateralized signs. A CT scan shows blood density material in the right Sylvian fissure. Of the following, which is the best diagnostic procedure to perform?

a. Lumbar puncture
b. EEG
c. Isotopic brain scan
d. Cerebral arteriography

answer: d. The patient probably has had a subarachnoid hemorrhage from a ruptured "berry" aneurysm. Cerebral arteriography would document the aneurysm, reveal its location and anatomy, and exclude the possibility of other sources of bleeding, such as a mycotic aneurysm or small arteriovenous malformation (AVM). If the resolution of MRI improves, the procedure may supplant arteriography. A lumbar puncture would probably be superfluous and possibly dangerous because it could lead to further rupture of the aneurysm. If a large hematoma were present, a lumbar puncture might lead to transtentorial herniation.

71. In Alzheimer's disease, which region has a pronounced neuron loss that results in an acetylcholine deficit?

a. Frontal lobe
b. Frontal and temporal lobe
c. Hippocampus
d. Nucleus basalis of Meynert

answer: d. Although the brain has a major loss of neurons in the hippocampus, the most striking loss occurs in the nucleus basalis of Meynert.

72. A 15-year-old waiter has episodes of feeling dizzy and dreamy that last 3 to 5 minutes. During them, he also has paresthesias in his fingertips and around his mouth. Sometimes his wrists bend and his fingers cramp together and his foot flexes. An EEG during an episode showed slowing of the background activity and bursts of high-voltage, smooth 3-Hz activity. Of the following conditions, which one is the most likely to be occurring?

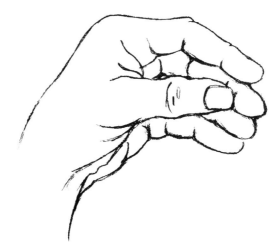

a. Partial complex seizures
b. Panic attacks
c. Petit mal (absence) seizures

d. Occupational cramps
e. None of the above

answer: e. He is probably having episodes of hyperventilation with carpopedal spasms and EEG slowing. These episodes might be a part of panic attacks, but they are not seizures. A clinical diagnosis of hyperventilation can be confirmed if patients reproduce their symptoms by hyperventilating for 2 to 4 minutes.

73. The patient in the preceding question is asked to hyperventilate. After 90 seconds, he becomes giddy and then irrational. What is the best way to abort the test?

answer: He probably has developed cerebral hypoxia because of a reduction in carbon dioxide tension in the blood, which reduces cerebral blood flow. He should be asked to breathe into a paper bag to increase his carbon dioxide blood tension.

74. A 32-year-old woman is referred to a psychiatrist for postpartum depression because, for the 5 months after a difficult delivery of her fifth child, she feels that she is "unable to cope" with the family. She describes not having enough energy to do her share of the housework or the inclination to resume her usual occupation (dentistry). She never resumed her menses or regained her libido. She has anorexia and mild weight loss. She has a mild continual headache, but no cognitive loss, visual changes, or other neurologic symptoms. Her obstetrician, internist, and a neurologic consultant all find no physical signs of illness. Nevertheless, which conditions may be responsible?

a. Multiple sclerosis (MS)
b. Lupus

c. Sheehan's syndrome
d. Pregnancy

answer: c. Postpartum pituitary necrosis (Sheehan's syndrome) is usually caused by deliveries complicated by hypotension. Its symptoms, which may not develop for several months to several years postpartum, include failure of lactation, scanty or no menses, sexual and generalized indifference, and being easily fatigued. Except for a subtle loss of secondary sexual characteristics, patients may have no physical abnormalities. Similar postpartum disturbances may be caused by autoimmune diseases and hyper- or hypothyroidism.

75. A 27-year-old man with a history of intractable seizures and violent behavior has had numerous EEGs that have shown only equivocal abnormalities. His serum phenytoin concentration has always been below the therapeutic range, despite a 500 mg/day prescription. He is suspected of abusing phenobarbital and other barbiturates, which he obtains on the basis of his diagnosis of epilepsy.

After seriously injuring a friend during a fistfight in a bar, his lawyer attributed the violence to the seizure disorder. As part of the medical-legal evaluation, an EEG was performed (see below). During the study, the patient became rigid and then had symmetric motor activity of all his limbs. Afterward, he remained unresponsive for several minutes and then became confused and amnestic. He was found to have had urinary incontinence. Evaluate the case in view of the history and the EEG.

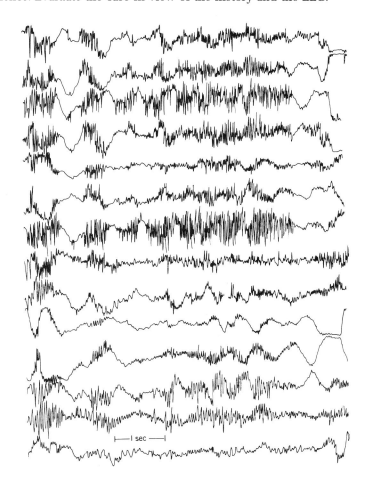

answer: The most prominent features of this EEG are bursts of high-voltage activity in the beginning and middle third of the sample. This activity is muscle artifact, which can be caused by either voluntary or involuntary muscle contraction. The diagnostic feature of this EEG is the alpha and beta activity. This normal activity, which occurs during a pause in the muscle artifact, can be seen above and below the 1-second marker. Muscle artifact cannot distinguish between epileptic and psychogenic seizures; however, normal (alpha) EEG activity in the midst of apparent generalized tonic-clonic movements clearly indicates that the activity is psychogenic.

Individuals with sociopathic behavior can convincingly mimic seizures. Alternatively, a patient with genuine seizures might let them become intractable by failing to take anticonvulsants. The most common explanation for a low-serum anticonvulsant level is neither impaired absorption nor rapid metabolism, but failure to take the prescribed dosage, i.e., noncompliance. Directed, purposeful violence (aggression) as a manifestation of a seizure is a rare phenomenon, if it exists at all. Moreover, aggression that occurs in bars is more likely to be the result of alcohol consumption than a seizure.

76. A 45-year-old woman has developed frequent blinking and involuntarily closure of her left eye (see below). The eyelid closure is forceful, lasts about 4 to 6 seconds, and is intensified by anxiety. She has no ocular abnormality, change in intellectual capacity, prior neurologic conditions, or medical illnesses. With which area is her problem associated?

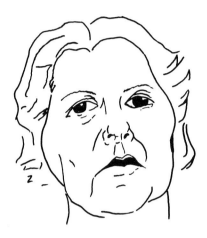 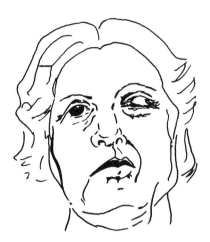

a.   Corpus striatum
b.   Lenticular nuclei
c.   Facial nerve at the cerebellopontine angle

d.   Autonomic nervous system
e.   Trigeminal nerve at the cerebellopontine angle
f.   Unknown regions

answer: c. The patient has hemifacial spasm, not blepharospasm. Note that, in addition to the closure of her left upper and lower eyelids, the muscles of the left side of her mouth contract, pull it laterally, and deepen the nasolabial fold. Hemifacial spasm, which develops in middle-aged and older individuals, is associated with an aberrant vessel compressing the facial nerve at its origin from the brainstem. Hemifacial spasm can be treated with botulinum toxin injections or neurosurgical decompression of the facial nerve as it exits from the brainstem at the cerebellopontine angle.

Although tics may involve one eye, they are momentary and affect only the eyes, singly or together. They usually do not affect the lower and upper face on the same side. Tardive dyskinesia may cause facial movements, but it does not cause such unilateral movements. Psychogenic movement disorders are rare, and their diagnosis requires intensive investigation.

77–78. A teenaged man and woman attempted suicide by sitting in a car with the engine running in a closed garage. They were discovered in a comatose state.

77. Three months later, the young man was alert, but bedridden, always in a flexed posture, mute, and unresponsive to stimulation. From which disorder did he suffer?

a.   Dementia
b.   Global aphasia
c.   Persistent vegetative state
d.   Depression

e.   Isolation aphasia
f.   Conduction aphasia
g.   None of the above

answer: c. He probably had generalized cerebral cortex destruction from carbon monoxide poisoning that resulted in dementia with a decorticate (fetal) posture, i.e., the persistent vegetative state.

78. Three months later, the young woman could be placed in a chair. Her eyes remained open. Although she did not follow verbal requests, initiate conversation, or respond purposefully, she would repeat incessantly whatever questions or phrases that she heard from visitors, television, and nearby casual conversations. Of the choices in Question 77, from which disorder did she suffer?

> *answer:* e. She sustained incomplete cortex damage that has resulted in isolation aphasia (also called "mixed transcortical aphasia"). Her injury spared the perisylvian language arc. The much larger surrounding watershed area of the cerebral cortex is more sensitive to carbon monoxide, hypoxia, and similar insults. She has lost all of her intellectual functions, except for her characteristic tendency—sometimes compulsion—to repeat (echolalia).

79. A 25-year-old man, who has been a drug abuser, while recovering from abdominal surgery, became agitated, severely anxious, irrational, and diaphoretic. When he had persistent postoperative pain, despite moderate doses of various narcotics, he was given pentazocine. A psychiatric consultation is requested. While a full investigation is being undertaken, which of the following medications would be most appropriate?

a. A major tranquilizer
b. Methadone
c. Alcohol
d. Phenobarbital
e. Steroids
f. Benadryl

> *answer:* b. Pentazocine (Talwin), butorphanol (Stadol), and other mixed narcotic agonist-antagonist preparations can precipitate withdrawal in narcotic addicts. (Being aware of their vulnerability, narcotic addicts often claim, with some justification, that they are allergic to these preparations.) Methadone or other narcotics will abort the withdrawal symptoms and provide analgesia.

80. A 28-year-old nurse, who has previously been well, is hospitalized for the sudden onset of generalized muscle weakness. An internist diagnoses hypokalemic myopathy. What are four causes of hypokalemic myopathy that develop in young and middle-aged adults?

a. Adrenal insufficiency
b. Pernicious anemia
c. Diuretic use or abuse
d. Vomiting
e. Diarrhea from laxative use or abuse
f. Steroid use
g. Excessive vitamin use

> *answer:* c, d, e, f. Hypokalemic myopathy in previously healthy young adults may be iatrogenic, a sign of underlying illness, or self-induced. Hypokalemia is especially likely to be self-induced by health care workers who surreptitiously take diuretics. Steroids may cause weakness by a direct muscle injury (steroid myopathy) or indirectly by depleting serum potassium (hypokalemic myopathy). Weakness is a paradoxical outcome when steroids are used by body builders.

81. Which two of the following statements concerning prions are true?

a. They contain RNA.
b. They contain reverse transcriptase.
c. They are infective agents.
d. They may be the cause of Creutzfeldt-Jakob disease.
e. They are identifiable in cerebral biopsy tissue of Alzheimer's disease patients.

> *answer:* c, d. Prions are protein-containing infective agents that contain neither DNA nor RNA. They are believed to cause Creutzfeldt-Jakob disease. Prions can be identified in cerebral biopsies of patients with Creutzfeldt-Jakob but not Alzheimer's disease. The human immunodeficiency virus (HIV) is an RNA virus that contains reverse transcriptase.

82–88. Match the clinical description of patients with mental status changes and the appropriate CT scan.

(*see illustrations on following pages*)

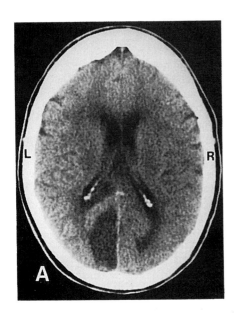

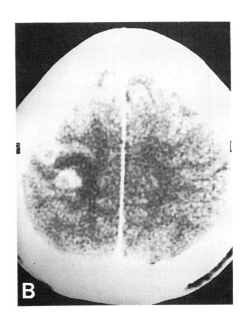

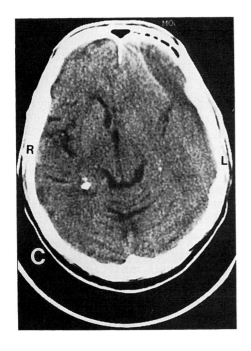

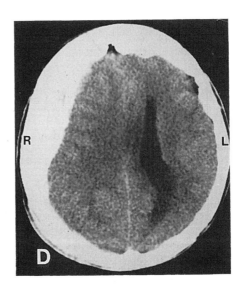

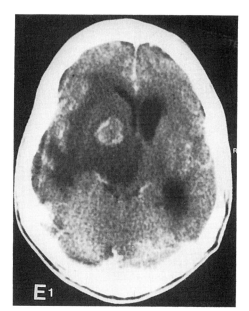

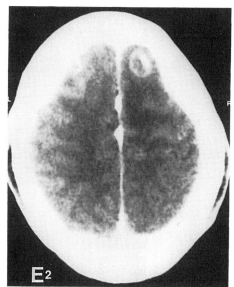

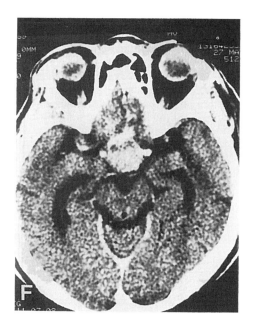

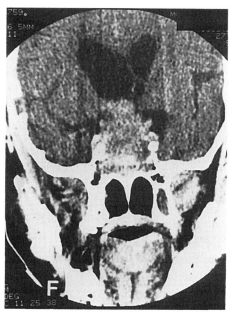

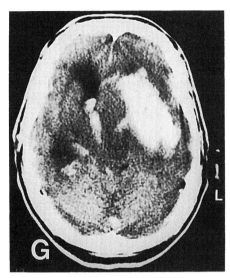

82. A 23-year-old woman, who had just delivered a baby boy 5 days before, had the sequential development of personality changes, agitation, garbled speech, seizures, and right hemiparesis. She had had an uneventful pregnancy. She did not use alcohol, tobacco, or drugs, but her boyfriend is a former drug addict.

answer: e. The two CT scans show two circular lesions that are each enhanced by contrast infusion. The use of contrast infusion can be surmised by the fact that the falx, a thick vascular structure, is white. The conventional representation consists of placing "L" or "R" notations on the appropriate side of the scan. A large lesion, surrounded by extensive edema, is deep in the left cerebral hemisphere (Scan E1). Another is in the right frontal lobe (E2). In the lower cut (E1), the anterior and occipital horns of the left lateral ventricle are compressed, and midline structures are shifted to the right. In the higher cut, a shift is not possible because the falx acts as a rigid barrier. The lesions, being multiple masses and enhanced by contrast, are indicative of toxoplasmosis, bacterial abscesses, and metastatic tumors. Given the history of the patient being the sexual partner of a drug addict, the most likely diagnosis is cerebral toxoplasmosis from AIDS.

83. A 45-year-old man was placed in restraints and given neuroleptics for agitated behavior. Later in the night, although the patient is stuporous, he screams about a headache. Examination reveals papilledema and a mild left hemiparesis that the patient, in his obtundation, seems to ignore.

answer: d. Before looking at the image of the brain, note that this CT follows the convention: The CT portrays the brain with the left and right sides reversed. It shows that a thick white border overlies the right side of the brain. In addition, the right lateral ventricle is obliterated by compression. Bone, fresh blood, and calcium are denser than brain tissue and therefore portrayed as white on a CT scan. The patient has an acute subdural hematoma compressing the right cerebral hemisphere.

84. A 65-year-old man complains that for several weeks he has had difficulty reading newspapers and books. Although his memory and other aspects of his general intellect are intact, he stumbles, almost incoherently, when reading. Nevertheless, he can repeat phrases, comprehend spoken statements, and even transcribe entire sentences.

answer: a. This CT scan shows a relatively large dark semicircular area, adjacent to the posterior falx, in the left occipital lobe. Its lucency and pattern indicate that it is an infarction of the posterior cerebral artery. The patient has the interesting and important neuropsychologic condition, *alexia without agraphia* or inability to read with preserved ability to write, which is a disconnection syndrome. Alexia without agraphia usually results from damage to the left occipital lobe and posterior corpus callosum.

85. An 80-year-old man has malaise, mild frontal headaches, and progressively severe cognitive impairments with prominent anomias. Otherwise, he has no abnormalities on neurologic or general medical examination. Routine laboratory tests, including a sedimentation rate, are normal.

> *answer:* c. This CT scan shows an abnormality overlying the left frontal lobe that has a white rim in its anterior portion. The mixed black and gray intensities indicate that its density is less than that of the brain. Cerebrospinal fluid, edema fluid, aged blood, and necrotic brain—all portrayed as black on the CT—are the most common hypodense tissues. The frontal horn of the left lateral ventricle is compressed, and the left frontal lobe is shifted slightly to the right. This CT scan indicates a chronic subdural hematoma. The symptoms of chronic subdural hematomas are usually a dull headache and cognitive impairments, including exacerbations of age-related language impairments, such as anomias. Although subdural hematomas are typically produced by trauma, the injury is often so trivial that patients often do not recall it. Since chronic subdural hematomas are slowly evolving, they do not cause papilledema or prominent lateralized signs. Subdural hematomas are a commonly occurring, correctable cause of dementia.

86. A 50-year-old man is unable to concentrate on his work, which consists of making architectural drawings. When he relates his history, he seems inattentive, but his cognitive capacity is grossly normal.

> *answer:* b. The CT scan shows a lesion, located in the posterior portion of the right cerebral hemisphere, that has a white center and fragments of a white ring surrounding it. The white falx indicates infusion of contrast material. The lesion is probably a tumor or other mass. Lesions in the nondominant parietal lobe, whatever their etiology, are associated with constructional apraxia, hemiinattention, anosognosia, and, according to some neurologists, impaired emotional communication. This patient's presenting symptom is probably a manifestation of constructional apraxia. Because symptoms of right hemisphere lesions are often accompanied by anosognosia, patients may ignore them or describe them only in imprecise terms.

87. A 38-year-old woman, who has been infertile, has the onset of headaches and bitemporal hemianopsia.

> *answer:* f. *Left,* This axial, contrast-enhanced CT scan reveals a circular radiodense lesion in the midline, just anterior to the midbrain. *Right,* In this coronal view, the lesion can be seen to be arising from the sella and growing into the hypothalamus. The lateral ventricles are pushed aside and dilated, which suggests that blockage of the third ventricle has caused hydrocephalus. The white, upside-down, wishbone-shaped structure in the posterior portion of the axial CT is the normal venous drainage. In adults, pituitary lesions are usually adenomas that cause endocrine disturbances, including elevated prolactin concentrations, headaches, and, when large, bitemporal hemianopsia. Craniopharyngiomas and meningiomas in that location are uncommon.

88. A 55-year-old hypertensive man has the sudden onset of a severe headache, aphasia, and right hemiparesis.

> *answer:* g. This CT reveals a large intracerebral hemorrhage with blood that has extended into the ventricle in the left side of the brain (the right side of the picture). Hypertensive cerebral hemorrhages, such as this one, usually occur in the putamen, thalamus, pons, or cerebellum.

89–90: A physician is called to see a colleague, who is known to be hypertensive and seriously depressed, because of severe headache, nausea, and vomiting. She finds that her colleague is stuporous and diaphoretic with nuchal rigidity and bilateral Babinski signs. His blood pressure is 210/130 mmHg. Bottles of chlorpromazine, isocarboxazid, propranolol, meperidine, and hydrochlorothiazide are in the medicine chest.

89. What are the two most likely diagnoses?

a. Medication interaction
b. Meningitis

c. Intracranial hemorrhage
d. None of the above

answer: a, c. The patient has classic signs of an intracranial hemorrhage: headache, stupor, nausea, vomiting, and nuchal rigidity. The origin could have been a hypertensive cerebral hemorrhage that was not prevented by the antihypertensive medications. Alternatively, the etiology could have been a drug-induced hemorrhage from the isocarboxazid (Marplan). That medication, like tranylcypromine (Parnate), phenelzine (Nardil), and others, is a monamine oxidase (MAO) inhibitor. MAO inhibitors cause acute, severe hypertension if certain foods, such as aged cheese, or medications are ingested. Sometimes depressed people purposely take prohibited foods in suicide attempts.

90. If the problem is caused by an MAO inhibitor, which of the following medications should be given?

a. Meperidine
b. Chlorpromazine
c. Propranolol

d. Hydrochlorothiazide
e. Phentolamine
f. Dibenzoxazepine

answer: e. The most specific treatment for a hypertensive reaction to an MAO inhibitor is the alpha-adrenergic blocking agent, phentolamine (Regitine), at a dose of 5 mg given slowly intravenously. Of the medications that are usually readily available, propranolol or chlorpromazine would be most helpful. Although the headache may be agonizingly severe, meperidine (Demerol) is contraindicated.

91. Which structure connects the hippocampus and the hypothalamus?

a. Corpus callosum
b. Cingulate gyrus

c. Fornix
d. None of the above

answer: c. The fornix connects the hippocampus with the mammillary bodies, which are an extension of the hypothalamus. The mammillary bodies communicate through the mammillothalamic tract with the anterior nucleus of the thalamus.

92. After extraction from a high-speed motor vehicle accident (MVA), the driver was stuporous and had facial contusions. After regaining consciousness, he was noted to have paresis of his right arm and leg, which also had decreased position sensation. The left arm and leg had decreased sensation to pinprick. He had a right-sided Babinski sign. The paresis persisted even though he fully regained consciousness and had no language, ocular, or visual impairment. Where would the lesion have to be located to explain the paresis?

a. Frontal lobe
b. Brainstem

c. Cervical spinal cord
d. Lumbar spinal cord

answer: c. He has a hemitransection of the cervical spinal cord. The cervical spinal cord is vulnerable because, when the forehead strikes the wheel or dashboard, the head and neck snap backward (hyperextension). Although it does not seem to be relevant in this case, drivers involved in a high-speed MVA, especially if they have behavioral abnormalities, should be evaluated for drug and alcohol use.

93. Which statement concerning the cerebellum is false?

a. Multiple sclerosis frequently involves the cerebellum.
b. Lesions in the cerebellum may cause scanning speech.
c. In adults, strokes and tumors involve the cerebellum less often than the cerebrum.
d. A lesion in a cerebellar hemisphere causes contralateral limb ataxia.

answer: d. A lesion in a cerebellar hemisphere causes *ipsilateral* limb ataxia. Reflecting that only about 10 per cent of the brain's blood supply perfuses the cerebellum, strokes and tumors involve the cerebellum in only about 10 per cent of cases.

94. Which sign is not found with the others?

a. Fasciculations
b. Spasticity

c. Babinski signs
d. Clonus

answer: a. Fasciculations are a manifestation of lower motor neuron injury. In contrast, spasticity, Babinski signs, and clonus are all manifestations of upper motor neuron injury.

95. In Parkinson's disease, which tract undergoes degeneration, and what is the function, origin, and destination of each tract?

a. Nigrostriatal
b. Geniculocalcarine

c. Spinothalamic
d. Corticospinal

answer: a. The nigrostriatal tract, which undergoes degeneration in Parkinson's disease, originates in the substantia nigra and terminates in the striatum. The geniculocalcarine tract conveys the visual pathways from the lateral geniculate bodies to the calcarine cortex of the occipital lobes. The spinothalamic tract conveys pain pathways from the dorsal horn of the spinal cord to the contralateral thalamus. (Crossing shortly after it originates, the spinothalamic tract ascends in the spinal cord contralateral to the side of its origin.) The corticospinal tract originates in the motor strips of the cerebrum and descends, after crossing in the medulla, in the spinal cord to the contralateral anterior horn cells of the spinal cord. It conveys voluntary motor system signals.

96. Of the following substances, which one is most likely to produce seizures during an acute intoxication?

a. Cocaine
b. Phencyclidine (PCP)
c. D9-TCH
d. Heroin

e. Valium
f. Amphetamine
g. Alcohol

answer: a. Cocaine, whether smoked, inhaled, injected, or swallowed, readily causes seizures. Almost one half of the cases of cocaine-induced seizures occur in first-time users. Phencyclidine (PCP) and amphetamine cause seizures much less frequently. Heroin and other narcotics usually do not cause seizures, except from hypoxia, massive overdose, or contaminants. Benzodiazepines and alcohol rarely cause seizures during an intoxication; however, withdrawal from these substances regularly produces seizures that are sometimes intractable, i.e., status epilepticus. The active agent in marijuana, D9-TCH, actually has a mild anticonvulsant effect.

97. Which two of the substances listed in Question 95 are associated with seizures after several days of abstinence?

answer: e, g

98. Which one of the substances listed in Question 95 is most likely to cause a stroke?

answer: a. Cocaine often causes cerebral hemorrhages and bland infarctions. All cocaine-induced strokes are likely to present with seizures. Amphetamine produces similar mental changes, but fewer strokes or seizures.

99. A 19-year-old college student was brought to the Emergency Room because of physical and mental agitation, vivid hallucinations, and combative behavior. Although she had often used marijuana, she had never previously developed such a reaction. She was hypertensive, oblivious to a laceration, and held her eyes wide open. She made repetitive, purposeless kissing movements. Which of the substances listed in Question 95 is probably responsible?

answer: b. Somebody probably laced her marijuana with phencyclidine (PCP).

100. Which are two effects of the normal GABA-induced influx of chloride ions?

a. Neurons are inhibited.
b. Neurons are excited.
c. The resting potential is made more negative.
d. The resting potential is made more positive.
e. NMDA receptors are activated.

answer: a, c. The normal resting potential is −70 mV. An influx of chloride ion (Cl^-), which makes the potential more negative, inhibits neuron activity.

101. In beginning to treat a depressed Parkinson's disease patient who is already being treated with L-dopa and selegiline, which medications are contraindicated?

a. Fluoxetine
b. Tricyclic antidepressants
c. MAO inhibitors
d. Amoxapine
e. All of the above

answer: e. None of these medications should be given in this situation. Amoxapine has dopamine-blocking activity that will exacerbate Parkinson's disease. Selegiline is a monoamine oxidase inhibitor that causes toxic reactions with fluoxetine and tricyclic antidepressants. Thus, in most cases, selegiline will have to be discontinued. Electroshock therapy is safe and effective in Parkinson's disease patients. Psychotherapy, support groups, and physical and occupational therapy may be helpful; however, Parkinson's disease depression almost always requires medications.

102. Insert the proper enzyme (a-d) into the synthetic steps for epinephrine synthesis.

Tyrosine $\xrightarrow{1}$ DOPA $\xrightarrow{2}$ Dopamine $\xrightarrow{3}$ Norepinephrine $\xrightarrow{4}$ Epinephrine

a. DOPA decarboxylase
b. Phenylethanolamine N-methyl-transferase
c. Dopamine β-hydroxylase
d. Tyrosine hydroxylase

answer:

Tyrosine $\xrightarrow{\text{tyrosine hydroxylase}}$ DOPA $\xrightarrow{\text{DOPA decarboxylase}}$ Dopamine $\xrightarrow{\text{dopamine β-hydroxylase}}$

Norepinephrine $\xrightarrow{\text{phenylethanolamine N-methyl-transferase}}$ Epinephrine

103. Which is the rate-limiting enzyme?

answer: Tyrosine hydroxylase

104. A 23-year-old man who has been an intravenous drug abuser and has been prescribed neuroleptics develops spasmodic contractions of his left arm where he has a deep skin infection. He is fully alert, and his neurologic examination is otherwise normal. What conditions may be responsible?

answer: Although several conditions might be present—neuroleptic-induced dystonia, a bacterial abscess, and, unlikely, a partial seizure—localized tetanus must be considered. The localized form of tetanus occurs in individuals, especially drug addicts, who have partial immunity. The generalized form of tetanus, which develops in individuals who were not immunized, causes the muscles of the entire body to have contractions and the jaw to close forcefully (trismus).

105. Which mental aberration is least frequently a component of Alzheimer's disease?

a. Delusions
b. Suicide ideation
c. Hallucinations
d. Anxiety

answer: b. With the onset of dementia, Alzheimer's disease patients typically develop anxiety. Delusions and hallucinations are manifestations of moderate-to-severe dementia. Remarkably few Alzheimer's disease patients have suicidal ideation.

106. Which of the following conditions is (are) associated with spasticity?

a. Multiple sclerosis that effects only the spinal cord
b. Parkinson's disease
c. Cerebellar degeneration
d. Poliomyelitis
e. HTLV-1 myelitis
f. Myotonic dystrophy
g. Neuroleptic-induced parkinsonism
h. Middle cerebral artery occlusion

answer: a, e, h. Spasticity is increased muscle tone resulting in an increased resistance to stretching. It is a sign of injury to the upper motor neurons of the corticospinal tract, which can occur in the cerebrum, brainstem, or spinal cord. Spasticity is characteristic of multiple sclerosis affecting the brain or the spinal cord, HTLV-1 myelitis (spinal cord infection), and cerebrovascular accidents. However, muscle rigidity, which is an inflexibility of muscle, is characteristic of basal ganglia disorders, such as naturally occurring or neuroleptic-induced parkinsonism. Cerebellar degeneration leads to muscle hypotonicity. Poliomyelitis is an infection of the lower motor neurons that leads to flaccidity. Myotonic dystrophy induces the myotonia, which is delayed muscle relaxation after a contraction or after percussion.

107. In the preceding question, which of the choices are associated with clonus?

answer: a, e, h. Clonus, like spasticity, is a manifestation of injury to the upper motor neurons of the corticospinal tract.

108. Which of the following structures is the beginning of the lower motor neuron?

a. Spinal cord
b. Cauda equina
c. Anterior horn cells of the spinal cord
d. Neuromuscular junction
e. Corticospinal tract

answer: c. The corticospinal tract, which contains the upper motor neurons, terminates on the anterior horn cells of the spinal cord to synapse with the lower motor neuron.

109. Onto which of the following structures do the corticobulbar fibers terminate?

a. Anterior horns cells of the spinal cord
b. Cranial nerve nuclei I to XII
c. Certain cranial nerve nuclei
d. Sympathetic nervous system pathways

answer: c. The corticobulbar tract, which is analogous to the corticospinal tract, conveys motor information to the motor nuclei of the brainstem. It contains upper motor neurons and innervates nuclei of cranial nerves that have motor function, but not those that are sensory, such as the olfactory, optic, and acoustic nerves.

110. Microscopic examination of brains with Alzheimer's disease will almost always reveal all except which of the following structures?

a. Neurofibrillary tangles
b. Senile plaques
c. Loss of neurons
d. Prions
e. Lewy bodies

answer: d, e. Prions are found in Creutzfeldt-Jakob's disease. Lewy bodies are found in Parkinson's and diffuse Lewy body diseases.

111. In which illnesses are prions and Lewy bodies found?

answer: Prions, protein-containing infectious agents that have no nucleic acid, are found in Creutzfeldt-Jacob disease. Lewy bodies, intracytoplasmic eosinophilic inclusions, are characteristically found in Parkinson's disease in the substantia nigra. They are also found in the cerebral cortex in a variant of the disease, Lewy body disease, which occurs in about 20 per cent of Alzheimer's patients.

112. Which structure forms the roof of lateral ventricles? ... the fourth ventricle?

a. Caudate nuclei
b. Corpus callosum
c. Pons

d. Medulla
e. Cerebellum

> *answer:* b and e. The corpus callosum forms the roof of the lateral ventricles, and the cerebellum forms the roof of the fourth ventricle.

113. Match the cranial nerve nuclei with their location.

1. Oculomotor
2. Trochlear
3. Abducens
4. Trigeminal motor
5. Vagus motor
6. Hypoglossal
7. Locus ceruleus
8. Substantia nigra
9. Red nucleus
10. Facial nerve

a. Midbrain
b. Pons
c. Medulla
d. Cerebral hemisphere
e. Cerebellum

> *answer:* 1-a, 2-a, 3-b, 4-b, 5-c, 6-c, 7-b, 8-a, 9-a, 10-b

114. This is a sketch of a high cervical level of the spinal cord with a myelin stain of a veteran who had a gunshot wound that transected the thoracic spinal cord 10 years before death. Identify the demyelinated tracts.

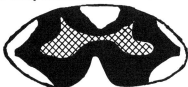

> *answer:* The salient feature is that certain ascending tracts, which are sensory, are unstained and presumably demyelinated because of the spinal cord injury. The spinothalamic tract, which is antero-lateral and peripheral, and the spino-cerebellar tract, which is posterior-lateral and also peripheral, are both mostly unstained. In addition, the medial portion of the posterior column, the fasciculus gracilis, is unstained, but the lateral segment, f. cuneatus, is stained. The difference occurs because the f. gracilis originates in the legs and thus is interrupted and unstained in this case, whereas the f. cuneatus is undamaged and normally stained.

115. Which is the most common cause of dementia in people older than 65 years?

a. Multiple infarctions
b. AIDS

c. Alzheimer's disease
d. None of the above

> *answer:* c. The most common causes of dementia in that age group are Alzheimer's disease, multiple infarcts, and then their combination.

116. A patient who has sustained a left cerebral embolus has left-right confusion, finger agnosia, and agraphia. Which other neuropsychologic abnormality is expectable?

a. Alexia
b. Dementia

c. Acalculia
d. Amnesia

> *answer:* c. Gerstmann's syndrome, which is usually caused by a dominant parietal lobe lesion, consists of left-right confusion, finger agnosia, agraphia, and acalculia; however, all four components are rarely present, and each may be incomplete, e.g., dysgraphia and dyscalculia.

117. In the limbic system, which tract conveys impulses between the hippocampus and the mammillary bodies?

a. Mammillothalamic tract
b. Cingulate gyrus

c. Fornix
d. None of the above

answer: c. The sequence in the limbic system is hippocampus and adjacent amygdala; fornix; mammillary bodies; mammillothalamic tract; anterior nucleus of the thalamus; cingulate gyrus.

118. Which chromosome contains the gene for β-amyloid?

a. 4
b. 14

c. 21
d. X

answer: c. Chromosome 21 contains the gene for β-amyloid and is triplicated in most cases of Down's syndrome (trisomy 21).

119. At birth, a male infant is found to have a delicate sac-like protrusion in the small of his back, at the base of the spine. His legs have flaccid, areflexic paraplegia, and urine dribbles continually from his penis, which never has erections. What condition is present?

a. Cerebral diplegia
b. Meningomyelocele
c. Dandy-Walker syndrome

d. Arnold-Chiari malformation
e. Spina bifida

answer: b. Most likely the baby has a meningomyelocele. This congenital abnormality consists of a deformed spinal cord or cauda equina protruding through an incompletely closed spinal canal. It causes paraplegia with bladder, bowel, and sexual dysfunction. Meningomyeloceles have been attributed to maternal exposure to environmental toxins, such as potato blight, and medications, including (in rare instances) valproic acid and carbamazepine. The abnormality, which may be detected in utero, might be prevented with folic acid and other vitamins during pregnancy.

120. Which of the following clinical features distinguish amyotrophic lateral sclerosis (ALS) from cervical spondylosis?

a. Weakness of the arms
b. Atrophy of the arms
c. Hyperactive DTRs in the legs

d. Fasciculations in the tongue
e. Sensory loss in the fingers and hands

answer: d, e. Sensory loss in the fingers and hands would be present in cervical spondylosis, but not in ALS. Fasciculations are found in both conditions, whereas tongue fasciculations are found only in ALS.

121. Which of the following are features of ataxia-telangiectasia?

a. Deficiency in IgA and IgE
b. Autosomal dominant inheritance
c. Onset of ataxia in childhood

d. Dilated vessels on the conjunctiva
e. Death from sinus or respiratory infection

answer: a, c, d, e. Ataxia-telangiectasia is a neurocutaneous disorder that is inherited in a recessive pattern. In this disorder, children have telangiectasia of conjunctival blood vessels, ataxia, and potentially fatal IgA and IgE deficiencies. They may also have cognitive impairment.

122. Which is the definitive test for Alzheimer's disease?

a. WAIS-R and other neuropsychologic tests
b. MRI
c. PET

d. EEG
e. Scopolamine administration
f. None of the above

answer: f. No clinical test is definitive.

123. Which of the following areas of the brain is most vulnerable to chronic alcoholism?

a. Cerebellar hemispheres
b. Optic nerves

c. Cerebellar vermis
d. Corpus callosum

answer: c. Although each of these areas may be damaged, cerebellar vermis atrophy is a frequently occurring and highly reliable sign of chronic alcoholism. Cerebellar vermis atrophy causes the gait ataxia.

124. A 66-year-old hypertensive businesswoman had the sudden painless onset of left-sided hemiparesis. She remains fully alert, comfortable, oriented, and with good memory and judgment. In addition, she has right-sided ptosis, the right pupil is dilated, and the right eye is laterally deviated. Which of the following events probably developed?

a. Periaqueductal petechial hemorrhages
b. Subdural hematoma with herniation

c. Midbrain arterial thrombosis
d. Cerebral hemorrhage

answer: c. A midbrain arterial thrombosis would damage the third cranial nerve and the adjacent corticospinal tract (Weber's syndrome). Since midbrain, pons, and medulla lesions are distant from the cerebrum, cognitive functions are almost always preserved. In contrast, periaqueductal petechial hemorrhages are indicative of Wernicke's encephalopathy, a condition in which patients have memory impairments, nystagmus, and ataxia, as well as oculomotor paresis. Subdural hematoma with herniation causes brainstem compression that leads to stupor if not coma and to decerebrate posturing. A cerebral hemorrhage could cause a third cranial nerve palsy only by its mass effect herniating downward to compress the nerve and necessarily the brainstem. Moreover, a cerebral hemorrhage would usually cause stupor, confusion, and headache.

125. What is the most caudal extent of the central nervous system (CNS)?

a. Foramen magnum
b. Occipital-cervical junction
c. Thoraco-lumbar junction

d. Sacrum
e. Neuromuscular junction

answer: c. The CNS terminates at the junction of vertebrae T12–L1. At this point, the spinal cord terminates by dividing into the cauda equina.

126. Which of the following EEG patterns indicates that a patient might have epilepsy?

a. Theta waves
b. Sharp waves
c. K complexes

d. Spindles
e. Vertex sharp waves
f. Spikes-and-wave complexes

answer: f. Spikes-and-wave complexes at 3 Hz are indicative of petit mal (absence) epilepsy. Theta waves, which are merely slow waves, are found when people are sleepy, in normal people older than 65 years, in metabolic disturbances, and as a sign of a structural lesion. Sharp waves, which are often occasionally found in normal people, may signify an underlying structural lesion. K complexes, spindles, and vertex sharp waves are all EEG patterns found in normal sleep.

127. Which condition will be detected or excluded most reliably by a routine EEG?

a. Partial complex seizures
b. Persistent vegetative state
c. Metabolic encephalopathy

d. Anterior cerebral infarction
e. Cerebellar hematoma

answer: c. The EEG is very sensitive to the diffuse changes induced by metabolic aberrations, as occurs in hepatic encephalopathy and drug use. Partial complex seizures may simply not be captured by a routine EEG, and interictal patterns are inconsistent. The persistent vegetative state, although leading to EEG slowing and disorganization, is not associated with a particular pattern. Structural lesions cannot be identified or excluded reliably by an EEG.

128. Which of the following are more characteristic of sleep terrors than nightmares?

a. Occur in deep NREM sleep
b. Are actually frightening dreams
c. Are associated with sleepwalking
d. Follow a partial awakening
e. Have contents that are often recalled on awakening

f.   Are accompanied by sweating and tachycardia
g.   Are associated with epileptiform EEG activity

> ***answer:***   a, c, d, f. Sleep terrors are a variety of parasomnia, but nightmares are dreams with a frightening content. Although seizures occasionally develop during sleep and sometimes exclusively, the clinical features of sleep terrors are virtually diagnostic.

129.   Which of the following is/are said to have led to people developing tics?

a.   Methylphenidate   c.   Encephalitis
b.   Anticholinergics   d.   Seizures

> ***answer:***   a, c. Although reports have described tics developing in children treated with methylphenidate (Ritalin) and other stimulants for attention deficit hyperactivity disorder, the number of cases is minute, and a causal relationship remains unproven. In contrast, tics as well as Parkinson's disease have routinely followed encephalitis.

130.   On several occasions, a 21-year-old college student has been unable to rise from bed upon awakening in the morning. He becomes terrified, and twice he found himself having visual hallucinations. He is otherwise in good mental and physical health. Which of the following conditions is the most likely cause of these symptoms?

a.   Incipient psychosis
b.   A paroxysm of spikes and waves from the mesial temporal cortex
c.   An intrusion or persistence of REM sleep into wakefulness
d.   Cerebral artery vasospasm

> ***answer:***   c. He is probably having sleep paralysis and sleep hallucinations. Although other aspects of narcolepsy should be sought, sleep deprivation and alcohol abuse should be considered.

131.   A psychiatric consultation is requested for a 30-year-old woman who is agitated and confused. Before reaching a conclusion about diagnosis or treatment, the psychiatrist finds that the patient has no lateralized signs or indications of increased intracranial pressure. Although the blood glucose is normal and no illicit drugs were detected, the serum sodium concentration is 122 mEq/L and the BUN is 9. Which of one of the conditions might explain the electrolyte disturbance?

a.   Postpartum pituitary necrosis   c.   Dehydration
b.   Diabetes insipidus   d.   Water intoxication

> ***answer:***   d. Of the choices, the patient most likely has water intoxication and mild cerebral edema. The electrolytes are diluted. Water intoxication can result from psychogenic disturbances, e.g., compulsive water drinking. It can also result from overhydration by intravenous fluids, especially in the presence of renal disease. The same electrolyte pattern can result from inappropriate antidiuretic hormone (ADH) secretion, which can result from neurologic injuries, cancer, and various medicines, including carbamazepine, amitriptyline, and thioridazine.
>
> In contrast, postpartum pituitary necrosis, diabetes insipidus, and dehydration cause an elevation in BUN. Postpartum pituitary necrosis and diabetes insipidus would lead to a loss of sodium, whereas dehydration would lead to retention of sodium.

132.   Six weeks after a cardiac arrest with asystole, a 48-year-old man opens his eyes and may establish eye contact briefly. He appears to have sleep-wake cycles. However, he is mute and unresponsive to verbal and gestured communication. Although he breathes normally, he has flexion of his limbs, cannot eat or swallow food that is placed in his mouth, and is incontinent of urine. An electroencephalogram (EEG) shows slow, low-voltage disorganized activity. What is his mental status, cognitive capacity, and prognosis?

> ***answer:***   He is in a persistent vegetative state. He has no cognitive capacity. His prognosis for a functional recovery is less than one in a thousand. A living will is applicable, and withdrawal of mechanical supports, which are necessary in the majority of cases, may be appropriate.

133. Six months after a cerebrovascular accident in which his basilar artery was occluded, a 75-year-old retired merchant seaman remains quadriplegic, mute, unable to follow verbal or gestured requests, and unable to breathe, eat, or swallow. However, through eyelid blinks, he can communicate using Morse code, which he had used in the Navy. An EEG often shows 10-Hz activity over the occipital area. What condition is present, and what is his cognitive capacity? How does he compare to the prior patient?

> *answer:* In contrast to the prior case, this man has intact cognitive capacity. He has the locked-in syndrome, in which the base of the pons and medulla are damaged, injuring breathing and swallowing brainstem centers and cutting off communication between the brain and the spinal cord.

134. Match the cell type (a-f) with its function (1–6).

a.	Microglia	1. Form the myelin in the central nervous system
b.	Astrocytes	2. Serve a chemical and physical supportive role for neurons
c.	Oligodendrocytes	
d.	Schwann cells	3. Act as phagocytes
e.	Ependymal cells	4. Form the myelin in the peripheral nervous system
f.	Neurons	5. Line the ventricles
		6. Basic element of the nervous system

> *answer:* a-3, b-2, c-1, d-4, e-5, f-6

135. Which test (a-d) will be most able to identify the conditions (1–10):

a. Positron emission tomography (PET)
b. Magnetic resonance imaging (MRI)
c. Computed tomography (CT)
d. Electroencephalograph (EEG)

1. Cerebral multiple sclerosis plaques
2. Cerebral calcifications
3. Mesial temporal sclerosis
4. Earliest basal ganglia changes in Parkinson's disease
5. Hepatic encephalopathy
6. Pituitary adenoma
7. Small cerebral metastases
8. An infarction that causes a third cranial nerve palsy with a contralateral hemiparesis
9. Impaired frontal lobe glucose metabolism in Alzheimer's disease
10. Skull fracture

> *answer:* a-4, -9; b-1, -3, -6, -7, -8; c-2, -10; d-5

136. Which of the following is the most common cause of coma in the United States?

a.	Cerebral hemorrhage	d.	Drug overdose
b.	Subarachnoid hemorrhage	e.	Subdural hematoma
c.	Seizures		

> *answer:* d. Drug overdose, not cerebral mass lesions, is the most common cause of coma in the United States. Head trauma, unlike the causes listed above, is rarely a diagnostic problem.

137. Which of the following neurologic infections is caused by a spirochete? Which is the most common? Which is the most common sporadic (nonendemic) illness?

a.	AIDS encephalitis	c.	Herpes simplex encephalitis
b.	Meningococcal meningitis	d.	Lyme disease

> *answer:* d, a, c. Lyme disease, which is a spirochete *Borrelia burgdorferi* infection, can cause a meningitis, encephalitis, facial nerve injury (which mimics Bell's palsy), or a polyneuropathy. AIDS encephalitis, a retrovirus (HIV-1) infec-

tion, is the most common of the neurologic infections. *Herpes simplex* is the most common form of sporadic encephalitis.

138. Which finding is not characteristic of Parkinson's disease?

a. Lewy bodies
b. Dementia in advanced cases
c. Impairment of postural reflexes
d. Kayser-Fleischer corneal rings

answer: d. Kayser-Fleischer rings, which reflect copper deposition in the cornea, are a finding in Wilson's disease when it affects the CNS.

139. In which way does Huntington's disease differ from Wilson's disease ?

a. Huntington's disease is a genetic illness.
b. Huntington's disease can become apparent in teenagers.
c. Huntington's disease can cause dementia in teenagers.
d. In Huntington's disease, the dementia cannot be reversed.

answer: d. Huntington's disease is an autosomal dominant illness, whereas Wilson's disease is an autosomal recessive illness. Both illnesses can become apparent in teenagers in whom Huntington's disease typically causes rigidity or chorea, whereas Wilson's disease causes tremor, rigidity, or dystonia. Haloperidol suppresses chorea in Huntington's disease and also in other hyperkinetic movement disorders, such as Sydenham's chorea and hemiballismus; however, there is no cure for either the chorea or dementia. In Wilson's disease, penicillamine or other copper-chelating agents may correct the dementia and involuntary movements.

140. Which of the following headaches occur predominantly in the morning?

a. Muscle contraction headaches
b. Sleep apnea
c. Brain tumors at their onset
d. Chronic obstructive lung disease
e. Subarachnoid hemorrhage
f. Trigeminal neuralgia

answer: b, c, d. Pulmonary dysfunction increases carbon dioxide blood levels, which lead to vasodilation.

141. Insert the proper substrates (a-e) into the synthesis and metabolism of dopamine.

$$1 \xrightarrow{\text{tyrosine hydroxylase}} 2 \xrightarrow{\text{DOPA decarboxylase}} 3 \xrightarrow{\text{dopamine } \beta\text{-hydroxylase}} 4$$

$$\xrightarrow{\text{phenylethanolamine N-methyl-transferase}} 5$$

a. Dopamine
b. Epinephrine
c. DOPA
d. Norepinephrine
e. Tyrosine

answer:

$$\text{Tyrosine} \xrightarrow{\text{tyrosine hydroxylase}} \text{DOPA} \xrightarrow{\text{DOPA decarboxylase}} \text{Dopamine} \xrightarrow{\text{dopamine } \beta\text{-hydroxylase}}$$

$$\text{Norepinephrine} \xrightarrow{\text{phenylethanolamine N-methyl-transferase}} \text{Epinephrine}$$

142. Which tract conveys information between the mammillary bodies and the thalamus?

answer: The mammillothalamic tract connects the mammillary bodies with the anterior nucleus of the thalamus.

143. Complete the indolamine pathway

$$\text{Tryptophan} \xrightarrow{\text{tryptophan hydroxylase}} \text{5-???} \xrightarrow{\text{amino acid decarboxylase}} \text{5-??} \rightarrow \text{5-???}$$

answer:

$$\text{Tryptophan} \xrightarrow{\text{tryptophan hydroxylase}} \text{5-hydroxytryptophan} \xrightarrow{\text{amino acid decarboxylase}}$$

5-hydroxytryptamine (serotonin) → 5-HIAA

144. A 70-year-old man, who sustained a right cerebrovascular accident with left hemiplegia, was examined by a neurologist. As the neurologist was washing his hands at a bedside sink, the patient asked the physician, "Doc! Did you forget your arm?" What disturbance probably gave rise to this question?

a. Inappropriate humor
b. Dementia
c. Anosognosia
d. A psychogenic disturbance

answer: c. Patients with nondominant hemisphere lesions, unable to comprehend their left hemiplegia, often disown their body parts and assign them to others.

145. Match the disorder that might follow a cerebrovascular accident in a 70-year-old person in the absence of paresis, sensory loss, and dementia with the appropriate terminology.

a. Inability to put on a shirt
b. Inability to assemble a simple kitchen device from directions
c. Use of paraphasias
d. Inability to read
e. Inability to sleep because of interruption in breathing
f. Inability to walk heel-to-toe (tandem gait)
1. Alexia
2. Dressing apraxia
3. Ideomotor apraxia
4. Aphasia, fluent
5. Ataxia
6. Sleep apnea

answer: a-2, b-3, c-4, d-1, e-6, f-5

146. During which period of gestation is the neural tube formed?

a. First trimester
b. Second trimester
c. Third trimester
d. Variable time
e. At the moment of conception

answer: a. During the third and fourth weeks of gestation, the dorsal ectoderm invaginates to form a closed, midline neural tube that eventually gives rise to the spinal cord and other elements of the CNS. This is a delicate maneuver that is susceptible to disruption by medications, including anticonvulsants, and toxins. Improper neural tube formation leads to neural tube defects, such as the Arnold-Chiari malformation, spina bifida, and meningomyelocele.

147. Although most hyperkinetic movement disorders cannot be treated, the movements might be suppressed. Which of the following medication would be most effective as a temporary measure?

a. Pergolide
b. L-dopa
c. Deprenyl (selegiline)
d. Bromocriptine
e. Haloperidol

answer: e. As a temporizing measure, which may be appropriate in Sydenham's chorea, Huntington's disease, hemiballismus, and rare cases of buccolingual dyskinesia, dopamine-blocking neuroleptics are appropriate to suppress the movements. Since sedation and sleep reduce or abolish the involuntary movement disorders, a sedating neuroleptic is often preferable.

148. Which characteristic distinguishes dementia from toxic-metabolic encephalopathy?

a. Permanence
b. Development only in adults
c. Development only in individuals with normal intelligence
d. Inattention
e. Being alert
f. Disorientation

answer: e. Both dementia and toxic-metabolic encephalopathy can be reversed (depending on the etiology). Both develop in children, young adults, and individuals who have been mentally retarded. They share many clinical features, including inattention and disorientation. In contrast, patients with toxic-metabolic encephalopathy are characteristically lethargic or stuporous, but sometimes are overly vigilant, whereas those with dementia must be fully alert. A potentially confusing situation arises when patients with dementia develop a toxic-metabolic encephalopathy. They are much more susceptible to delirium and stupor than previously normal individuals.

149.   With which condition is long-standing methysergide (Sansert) treatment associated?

a.	Retroperitoneal fibrosis	c.	Neural tube closure defects
b.	Liver function abnormalities	d.	Insomnia

answer: a

150.   A 19-year-old female college student who seemed to have developed a chronic, noninfectious hepatitis the preceding year begins to have a subtle decline in her grades, dysarthria, tremor, and depression. Except for abnormal liver function tests, routine laboratory testing and also CT, MRI, CSF, and EEG reveal no abnormalities. Which test should be ordered next?

a.	HIV	d.	Antistreptolysin O titer
b.	HTLV-1	e.	Serum ceruloplasmin
c.	Mononucleosis spot test	f.	Lupus evaluation

answer: e. This patient has hepatic dysfunction, cognitive impairment, depression, tremor, and dysarthria. The patient may have Wilson's disease (hepatolenticular degeneration), in which case the sooner the diagnosis is made and the sooner treatment is instituted, the better the prognosis is for reversal of the deficits. A low serum concentration of ceruloplasmin, the copper-carrying serum protein, is indicative of Wilson's disease. This illness, which is transmitted as an autosomal recessive condition, may affect only the liver, but when it has neurologic complications, a Kayser-Fleischer ring may be found on a slit-lamp examination of the cornea. Other causes of hepatic dysfunction and mental changes include mononucleosis, alcoholism, and other substance abuse. Multiple sclerosis is unlikely given the progressive course, early onset of cognitive impairment, and normal MRI.

151.   Match the spinal cord tract with its function.

a. Pyramidal
b. Spinothalamic
c. Fasciculus gracilis
d. Spinocerebellar
1. Provides cerebellar input for coordination
2. Descends to innervate the anterior horn cells
3. Transmits pain sensation
4. Transmits position sense from the upper extremities
5. Transmits position sense from the lower extremities

answer: a-2, b-3, c-5, d-1

152.   Which characteristics indicate that facial weakness is more likely due to a seventh cranial nerve lesion than a cerebral lesion?

a. Only flattening of the nasolabial fold
b. Loss or alteration of taste sensation
c. Inability to close the eyelid muscles and to smile on the same side of the face
d. Hyperacusis or tinnitus ipsilateral to the facial weakness
e. Aphasia
f. A recent tick bite
g. Pain in the mastoid area before the facial weakness

answer: b, c, d, f, g. Weakness of upper as well as lower facial muscles and the disruption of hearing and taste sensations characterize a seventh cranial nerve injury.

153. A 35-year-old woman who has difficulty describing her symptoms seems to have, several times yearly, a several-hour episode of monocular visual obscurations followed by a throbbing, generalized headache. A general medical and neurologic evaluation and CTs with and without contrast infusion are normal. Which of the following conditions is most likely?

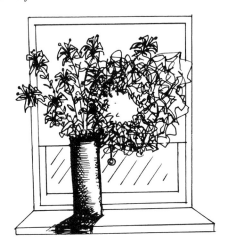

a. Migraine without aura (common migraine)
b. Transient ischemic attacks (TIA) from basilar artery stenosis
c. Migraine with aura (classic migraine)
d. Transient ischemic attacks (TIA) from carotid artery stenosis
e. An arteriovenous malformation (AVM)
f. Multiple sclerosis
g. Tension headaches

answer: c. Transient monocular visual disturbances that result from TIAs of the carotid artery (amaurosis fugax) usually last for less than 20 minutes, are unaccompanied by headache, and either resolve or culminate in a cerebrovascular accident after a few episodes. Basilar artery TIAs may cause bilateral visual changes accompanied by vertigo and ataxia, but usually not headaches or numerous recurrences. Multiple sclerosis may cause episodes of unilateral visual loss and pain in or around the eye (optic neuritis), but the symptoms have a duration of several days to weeks and usually are accompanied by other neurologic deficits. AVMs may cause repeated bouts of an homonymous hemianopsia and headache, but they are almost always evident on CT scans with contrast. Migraine with aura (classic migraine), but not migraine without aura (common migraines), by definition, includes visual auras. Often patients have mild forms of migraine with aura that are unrecognized because they do not describe dramatic visual hallucinations or have prostrating headaches accompanied by nausea and vomiting. Tension headaches are frequently episodic, discrete, or associated with monocular visual symptoms.

154. Which are common side effects of dopamine precursor or agonist treatment for Parkinson's disease?

a. Dyskinesias
b. Vivid dreams
c. Neuroleptic malignant syndrome

d. Seizures
e. Elevated serum prolactin concentration

answer: a, b. Neuroleptic malignant syndrome has occurred in rare cases after the abrupt withdrawal of such medications. They do not cause seizures, but do suppress serum prolactin concentrations.

155. A teenage boy and a female friend attempted suicide by running his car in the closed garage. The friend never recovered consciousness and during the next month developed a persistent vegetative state. The boy had only mild cognitive impairments during the 2 weeks after the incident, but then he developed confusion and excitement accompanied by spasticity, rigidity, and tremors. Of the following, which most likely caused his apparent relapse?

a. Reaction to neuroleptic medications
b. A delayed psychologic reaction
c. Postanoxic encephalopathy
d. Neuroleptic malignant syndrome

answer: c. Although a biphasic course is uncommon and not peculiar to carbon monoxide, both victims had typical consequences of carbon monoxide poisoning. The second phase of cerebral damage from anoxia, postanoxic encephalopathy, is poorly understood except that it results from necrosis of the globus pallidus (a major section of the lenticular nuclei), hippocampus, and cerebral white matter. Postanoxic encephalopathy is characterized by mental aberrations, rigidity and tremors from basal ganglia, and spasticity from upper motor neuron damage. It may be mistaken for neuroleptic-induced parkinsonism in a psychotic patient.

156. Which varieties of tremor may be suppressed with β-blocker medication?

a. Essential
b. Performance anxiety
c. Resting
d. Lithium-induced
e. Benign
f. Cerebellar
g. Hyperthyroid
h. End-point

answer: a, b, d, e, g. β-blockers suppress the tremor associated with excessive autonomic nervous system activity that may result from anxiety, medications, or genetic factors. The tremor in as many as 10 per cent of Parkinson's disease patients responds somewhat to β-blockers.

157. Match the lesion (a–f) with the movement disorder (1–6).

a. Atrophy of the caudate nuclei heads
b. Lewy bodies
c. Depigmentation of the substantia nigra
d. Infarction of the contralateral subthalamic nucleus
e. Compression of the seventh cranial nerve by an aberrant vessel
f. Depigmentation of the locus ceruleus
1. Parkinson's disease
2. Huntington's disease
3. Dystonia musculorum deformans
4. Hemifacial spasm
5. Meige's syndrome
6. Hemiballismus

answer: a-2, b-1, c-1, d-6, e-4, f-1

158. Several days after an automobile accident in which he sustained a whiplash injury, a 16-year-old boy begins to notice progressively worsening neck pain and weakness in his fingers. He has loss of pin sensation in a shawl pattern over his shoulders and upper arms and in his hands and fingers, but intact joint position and vibration sensation. Deep tendon reflexes in his arms are diminished, but those in his legs are brisk. Plantar reflexes are equivocal. Which of the following processes may be developing?

a. Worsening of the whiplash symptoms
b. Development of a herniated cervical intervertebral disk
c. Bleeding into the center of the spinal cord
d. Emergence of poststress symptoms

answer: c. Hematomyelia, bleeding into the center of the spinal cord, which usually occurs in the cervical portion of the spinal cord, may follow neck injuries from motor vehicle, trampoline, horseback riding, or diving accidents. Hematomyelia forms a lesion similar to a syringomyelia (syrinx), in which the crossing fibers of the lateral spinothalamic tract are stretched and the anterior horn cells are compressed—impairing pin and temperature sensation and also lower motor neuron function in the arms. In addition, the corticospinal tracts are mildly compressed, causing long tract motor signs in the legs. The congenital, nontraumatic variety of this disorder, syringomyelia, develops more insidiously, but the findings are the same.

159. Four months after delivering a healthy child, a 29-year-old woman complains of constant fatigue and bitemporal headaches. She has remained amenorrheic and has galactorrhea. What is the most likely cause of her chronic fatigue?

a. Chronic Epstein-Barr virus (EBV) infection	e. Myasthenia gravis
	f. Medication side effect
b. Lyme disease	g. Drug or alcohol abuse
c. Secondary adrenal insufficiency	h. Infectious mononucleosis
d. Excessive daytime sleepiness	

answer: c. All of the conditions are purportedly a cause of the so-called chronic fatigue syndrome. One condition—postpartum fatigue, headaches, amenorrhea, and galactorrhea—is associated with pituitary adenomas (Chiari-Frommel syndrome). Another cause of excessive postpartum fatigue is pituitary infarction after a delivery complicated by profound hypotension (Sheehan's syndrome). In both cases, pituitary damage leads to (secondary) adrenal insufficiency.

160. In the preceding question, which visual field abnormality is associated with her condition?

a. Homonymous hemianopsia
b. Bitemporal hemianopsia or superior quadrantanopia
c. Binasal hemianopsia or superior quadrantanopia
d. None of the above

answer: b. Bitemporal hemianopsia or superior quadrantanopia is associated with pituitary lesions that compress the overlying optic chiasm. However, with small lesions, especially infarctions, no visual field impairments may be present.

161. In normal-pressure hydrocephalus, (1) which feature is the most reliable in establishing its presence, (2) which feature responds most reliably to shunting, and (3) which of the following features is not part of the syndrome?

a. Headache	c. Urinary incontinence
b. Gait apraxia	d. Dementia

answer: 1-b, 2-b, 3-a

162. A 40-year-old man was struck on the back of his head with a baseball bat. He sustained a compound skull fracture and was rendered comatose for 2 days. When he became conversant, he confabulated about whomever visited him and often mistook people. He seemed to have marked visual impairment but he denied it, his pupils were round and reactive, funduscopy revealed no abnormalities, and extraocular movements were normal. What is the nature of his visual impairment?

a. Retinal detachments	d. Cortical blindness
b. Ocular trauma	e. Anosognosia
c. Ocular blindness	

answer: d. He has sustained cortical blindness because of trauma to the visual cortex in the occipital lobes. In cortical blindness, the eyes, optic nerves, and oculomotor nerves—which form the light reflex arc—are spared. His denial of blindness and tendency to confabulate about questions that depend on sight—Anton's syndrome—is a variety of anosognosia that usually follows sudden loss of vision. Anton's syndrome may result from occlusion of both posterior cerebral arteries, usually from an embolus that lodges at the tip of the basilar artery, leading to infarction of both occipital lobes.

163. Match the system with the associated group of nuclei.

a. Cholinergic
b. Serotonergic
c. Noradrenergic (norepinephrine-containing)
d. Dopaminergic

1. Nucleus basalis of Meynert
2. Dorsal raphe nucleus
3. Locus ceruleus
4. Mesolimbic and mesocortical tracts

answer: a-1, b-2, c-3, d-4

164. What is the cardinal feature of conduction aphasia?

a. Patients cannot name objects.
b. Patients cannot follow simple requests.
c. Patients cannot repeat.
d. Patients have diffuse cognitive impairment.

answer: c. In conduction aphasia, a lesion, which interrupts the perisylvian language arc, severs the connection between Wernicke's and Broca's areas. Thus, patients cannot repeat what they hear.

165. Which of the following conditions is not a disconnection syndrome?

a. Alexia without agraphia
b. Conduction aphasia
c. Split-brain syndrome
d. Gerstmann's syndrome
e. Ideomotor apraxia

answer: d. All conditions except Gerstmann's syndrome are disconnection syndromes. Another distinction is that all of the conditions, except for the split-brain syndrome, usually result from dominant hemisphere lesions.

166. Which part of the body is most commonly involved in tardive akathisia?

a. Head
b. Arms
c. Legs
d. Trunk

answer: c. In tardive akathisia, the legs are involved most frequently and most severely, but the trunk, head, neck, and arms may also be involved. When akathisia is extensive it mimics chorea.

167. Which are the two most common movements in tardive akathisia?

a. Walking or marching in place
b. Tremor of legs
c. Crossing or rapidly adducting and abducting the legs
d. Periodic flexion at the hip and ankle, especially when asleep

answer: a, c.

168. What treatable neurologic illness, which might be confused with tardive dystonia, often develops in young adults and causes mental aberrations, dystonia, or both?

a. Athetosis
b. Cerebral palsy
c. Wilson's disease
d. SSPE

answer: c. The diagnostic tests would be determination of the serum ceruloplasmin and a slit-lamp examination of the eye. In Wilson's disease, the serum ceruloplasmin is low or absent, and if the disease affects the brain, an ophthalmologist can usually detect Kayser-Fleischer rings in the cornea on a slit-lamp examination.

169. A 68-year-old waitress develops tremor at rest, rigidity, and bradykinesia. Otherwise her neurologic examination reveals no abnormalities. What is the best initial treatment of her condition?

a. Providing the missing enzyme
b. Giving the deficient neurotransmitter
c. Transplanting cells that synthesize the deficient neurotransmitter
d. Providing precursors that cross the blood-brain barrier for the deficient neurotransmitter

answer: d. She probably has Parkinson's disease. Repleting dopamine would correct her symptoms and also provide a therapeutic trial. Although dopamine is the deficient neurotransmitter, orally administered dopamine does not penetrate the blood-brain barrier. L-Dopa, its precursor, crosses the blood-brain barrier and, by the action of dopa-decarboxylase, is metabolized to the active neurotransmitter, dopamine. Transplanting cells and ablative neurosurgical procedures have not been perfected and are not indicated in the initial stages of the illness.

170. Match the condition (a-e) with the most common cause (1–6).

a. Athetosis
b. Huntington's disease
c. Wilson's disease
d. Sydenham's chorea
e. Hemiballismus
1. Infarction of a portion of the brainstem
2. Autosomal dominant inheritance
3. Autosomal recessive inheritance
4. Effect of a viral infection
5. Effect of a bacterial infection
6. Prematurity, low birth weight, hyperbilirubinemia, or other perinatal injury

answer: a-6 (athetotic cerebral palsy), b-2, c-3, d-5 (streptococcal infections associated with rheumatic fever), e-1 (infarctions in the subthalamic corpus of Luysii)

171. A 58-year-old soldier sustained a gunshot wound of the thoracic spine. He had paresis of the right leg and sensory loss to pinprick of the left leg and left lower trunk below the umbilicus. After the wound healed, which took 3 weeks, he was transferred for rehabilitation. Which two of the following problems would impair his walking?

a. Hypoactive left deep tendon reflexes
b. Spasticity of the right leg
c. Bilateral Babinski signs
d. Position sense loss of the right leg

answer: b, d. The soldier has the Brown-Séquard syndrome caused by a lateral transection of the spinal cord at the T10 level. Spasticity, a manifestation of upper motor neuron impairment that is usually accompanied by paresis, impairs function. Sometimes spasticity is a greater problem than paresis. Position sense loss on the same leg, which would be accompanied by pain and temperature loss on the opposite leg, is another major problem that would impair walking.

172. What is the lowermost level of the body to which upper motor neurons descend?

a. Foramen magnum
b. Medulla
c. Beginning of the spinal cord
d. First lumbar vertebrae (L1)

answer: d. The spinal cord contains upper motor neurons, which are carried in the corticospinal tract. Since it terminates at L1 by giving rise to peripheral nerve roots of the cauda equina, that level is the lowermost extent of upper motor neurons and the central nervous system.

173. Which one of the following structures is not part of the central nervous system?

a. Cerebellum
b. Basal ganglia
c. Optic nerves
d. Sciatic nerves

answer: d. The sciatic nerve and other peripheral nerves are formed from motor neurons in the anterior horn cells of the spinal cord. The optic nerves are an extension of the brain and are covered with myelin made from oligodendroglia. The optic nerves are affected by illnesses, such as multiple sclerosis, that involve injury of the central nervous system.

174. Of the following, which is the most significant risk factor for cerebrovascular accidents?

a. Birth control pills
b. Race
c. Hypertension
d. Obesity

answer: c. Of the numerous risk factors for cerebrovascular accidents, hypertension and advanced age are the two greatest. Many risk factors, such as obesity, diabetes, and hypertension, are so closely associated with each other that their independent influence is difficult to assess.

175. A 50-year-old person complains of diplopia on looking to the left. The right pupil is poorly reactive to light and larger than the left. There is right-sided ptosis. Which injury is most likely to have occurred?

a. Left sixth cranial nerve palsy
b. Right third cranial nerve palsy
c. Right transtentorial herniation
d. Left third cranial nerve palsy
e. Left transtentorial herniation

answer: b. Although diplopia on left lateral gaze might be attributable to either a left sixth or right third cranial nerve palsy, in this case the other signs of a third cranial nerve palsy indicate that the right third cranial nerve is responsible. Patients with herniation are stuporous or comatose: they are not alert enough to complain of anything, except perhaps headache.

176. With which other finding is tremor on intention most closely associated?

a. Dysdiadochokinesia (impaired rapid alternating movements)
b. Rigidity
c. Bradykinesia
d. Ataxia of gait
e. Tremor at rest

answer: a. Tremor on intention and other limb coordination problems, such as dysdiadochokinesia, are associated with cerebellar hemisphere injury. Tremor at rest is a manifestation of Parkinson's disease. Ataxia of gait is related to injury of the midline cerebellum (vermis) or the entire cerebellum.

177. Which features are common to partial complex and petit mal (absence) seizures?

a. 3-Hz spike-and-wave EEG activity
b. Auras
c. Automatisms
d. Postictal confusion

answer: c. Both conditions may induce repetitive, purposeless activities, such as lip smacking movements. Thus, on clinical grounds alone, partial complex and absences may be confused.

178. Which of the following medications does not lower the seizure threshold?

a. Maprotiline (Ludiomil)
b. Diazepam (Valium)
c. Clomipramine (Anafranil)
d. Chlorpromazine (Thorazine)

answer: b

179. Which single problem is not a side effect of anticonvulsants?

a. Allergic reactions
b. Liver or bone marrow toxicity
c. Gastrointestinal disturbances
d. Teratogenicity
e. Potentiating oral contraceptives

answer: e. Phenytoin and possibly carbamazepine can interfere with oral contraceptives.

180. Videotaped monitoring of seizure patients is useful in determining which of the following?

a. The variety or frequency of the seizures
b. The presence of psychogenic seizures
c. The site of the origin of seizures
d. Correlation of seizures with anticonvulsant blood levels
e. All of the above

answer: e

181. The presence of Todd's hemiparesis after a generalized tonic-clonic seizure indicates that the patient probably has which of the following type of epilepsy?

a. Absence
b. Partial with secondary generalization

c. Primary generalized tonic-clonic epilepsy
d. Partial elementary

answer: b. Hemiparesis for as long as 24 hours after a seizure (Todd's paresis) suggests a cortical origin and temporary dysfunction of the adjacent motor area. Todd's paresis is often found with seizures induced by cerebrovascular accidents or tumors.

182. Which of the following medications inhibits HIV-reverse transcriptase?

a. Trimethoprim-sulfamethoxazole (Bactrim, Septra, and others)
b. Pyrimethamine (Daraprim)
c. Ganciclovir (Cytovene)

d. Zidovudine (Retrovir)
e. Pentamidine

answer: d. Previously known as AZT and often given when HIV infection is first detected, zidovudine has increased median survival after diagnosis. Side effects include myopathy, headache, fatigue, malaise, and confusion. Trimethoprim-sulfamethoxazole and pentamidine are each effective for *Pneumocystis carinii* pneumonia (PCP). Pyrimethamine (Daraprim) is the treatment of choice for cerebral toxoplasmosis. Ganciclovir (Cytovene) is useful for cytomegalovirus (CMV) infections, especially CMV retinitis and colitis.

183. Which of the following infections is not a common complication of AIDS?

a. Pneumococcal meningitis
b. Mycobacterium tuberculosis
c. Mycobacterium avian complex

d. Syphilis
e. Mucosal candidiasis (oral thrush)

answer: a. Cellular immunity is impaired in AIDS.

184. Which of the following areas of the brain is most susceptible to anoxia?

a. Medulla
b. Wernicke's area

c. Globus pallidus
d. Hippocampus

answer: d. Although the hippocampus is exquisitely sensitive to anoxia, the entire cerebral cortex is sensitive. The globus pallidus is damaged not only with anoxia but also with carbon monoxide poisoning.

185. Which feature(s) characterize partial complex seizures compared to petit mal absences?

a. Impaired consciousness
b. Fluttering eyelids
c. Symptoms that might constitute an aura
d. Childhood onset in many cases
e. Duration of 5 seconds in many cases
f. Tendency toward retrograde amnesia, personality change, or sleep after the seizure

answer: c, f. Unlike absences, partial complex seizures originate in the cerebral cortex, often begin with certain recognizable symptoms that warn the patient of an impending event (the aura), and are associated with impaired consciousness, rather than the loss of consciousness. The aura is actually part of the seizure. Lack of retro- or anterograde amnesia or other lingering symptoms is characteristic of absences. Partial complex seizures often begin in childhood or teenaged years, but absences begin almost exclusively in childhood. Both varieties may have durations of only a few seconds, but partial complex seizures are longer and are further protracted by postictal symptoms. They routinely last for 30 seconds or longer and are followed by somnolence, confusion, and amnesia.

186. Which of the following are found in Alzheimer's disease?

a. Neuron loss in nucleus basalis of Meynert

b. Amyloid surrounded by abnormal neurites

c. Paired helical filaments within neurons

d. Loss of synapses

e. Lewy bodies in the cortex

f. All of the above

answer: f. Amyloid, surrounded by abnormal neurites, plaques, and paired helical filaments, and neurofibrillary tangles are characteristic of Alzheimer's disease. However, they are also found in the normal brains of elderly people and also those with Down's syndrome and dementia pugilistica. Lewy bodies, which are characteristic of Parkinson's disease, are found in the cerebral cortex in about 20 per cent of Alzheimer's brains.

187. When botulinum toxin treatment is administered for focal dystonias, such as spasmodic torticollis, what is its mechanism of action?

a. Like curare, botulinum blocks acetylcholine neuromuscular receptors.

b. Botulinum impairs acetylcholine neuromuscular presynaptic release.

c. Botulinum depletes dopamine.

d. Like Mestinon, botulinum enhances acetylcholine activity.

e. Like nerve gas, botulinum creates a depolarization of the postsynaptic acetylcholine receptor site.

f. Acetylcholine strength is increased because its reuptake is blocked by botulinum.

answer: b. Botulinum inhibits dystonic muscle contractions by impairing acetylcholine release from the presynaptic neuron at the neuromuscular junction. This process also induces some weakness, but usually much less than the reduction in dystonia. Curare and many nerve gases block the acetylcholine neuromuscular receptors, and in this way they can induce lethal paralysis. Whereas the activity of dopamine and many other neurotransmitters is partly terminated by reuptake, acetylcholine activity is terminated entirely by cholinesterase enzyme metabolism.

188. Match the area of the nervous system (a-i) with its location (1–4).

a. Anterior horn cells

b. Corpus callosum

c. Locus ceruleus

d. Bulb

e. Vermis

f. Cranial nerve nuclei for swallowing

g. Origin of phrenic nerve

h. Heschl's gyrus

i. Hippocampus

1. Cerebrum

2. Cerebellum

3. Brainstem

4. Spinal cord

answer: a-4, b-1, c-3, d-3, e-2, f-3, g-4, h-1, i-1

189. Match the brainstem region (a-l) with its location (1–5).

a. Cranial nerve nucleus that innervates the jaw muscles

b. Cranial nerves that move eyes medial

c. Trochlear nerve

d. Cranial nerves that move eye laterally

e. Beginning of the nigrostriatal tract

f. Cranial nerves that innervate the tongue muscles

g. Cranial nerves that govern speech and swallowing

h. Thalamus

i. Hypothalamus

j. Locus ceruleus

k. Crossing of the pyramids

l. Cranial nerve that innervates the upper and lower face muscles

1. Diencephalon
2. Midbrain
3. Pons
4. Medulla
5. None of the above

   answer: a-3, b-2, c-2, d-3, e-2, f-4, g-4, h-1, i-1, j-3, k-4, l-3

190. Which statements concerning syphilis or neurosyphilis are true?

a. In an appropriate clinical setting, a positive CSF-VDRL test confirms the diagnosis of neurosyphilis.
b. A dramatic increase in the incidence of syphilis has occurred and has been attributed to the AIDS epidemic.
c. A negative CSF-VDRL test is strong evidence against a diagnosis of neurosyphilis.
d. A positive serum VDRL or RPR at a dilution of 1:2 is strong evidence of syphilis.

   answer: a, b. A large proportion of patients with neurosyphilis—40 per cent in one study—have a negative CSF-VDRL. One the other hand, a positive CSF-VDRL is very strong evidence that a patient has neurosyphilis. False-positive serum results, which are generally 1:4 or less, are attributable to other infection, rheumatologic diseases, drug addiction, and changes in serum proteins found with old age. False-negative serum results may be found when the disease is "burnt out," the infectious activity is low, or in rare cases when the antibody concentration is so great that a visible reaction is prevented, which is called prozone inhibition.

191. Match the skin lesions (a-k) with its associated neurologic disorders (1–11).

a. Adenoma sebaceum
b. Kaposi's sarcoma
c. Vaginal chancre
d. Congenital facial angioma in the distribution of the first division trigeminal nerve
e. Acute eruption of vesicales in the distribution of the first division trigeminal nerve
f. Café-au-lait spots
g. Protuberance of skin and soft tissue at the base of the spine
h. Erythema migrans
i. Anesthetic, depigmented patches on the coolest regions of the face and body
j. Dermatitis, diarrhea, and dementia
k. White lines across the nails (Mees' lines)

1. Possible later development of *Treponema* in the CNS
2. Round growths in the brain that cause dementia and seizures
3. Intracerebral angioma that causes seizures, but usually not bleeding
4. Development of encephalitis and cerebral lymphoma
5. Neurofibromas
6. Lancinating pain in the distribution of the skin lesion
7. Impotence
8. Pellagra
9. Lyme disease
10. Leprosy
11. Arsenic poisoning

   answer: a-2, b-4, c-1, d-3, e-6, f-5, g-7, h-9, i-10, j-8, k-11

192. In the limbic system, in which area of the brain do direct thalamic projections terminate?

a. Frontal lobe
b. Mammillary bodies
c. Temporal lobe
d. Cingulate gyrus
e. Amygdala

   answer: a

193. From which cell are congenital illnesses that result from mitochondria defects derived?

a. The egg and the sperm in equal proportion
b. The egg exclusively
c. The sperm exclusively
d. The amniotic fluid

answer: b. All the mitochondria in the embryo derive from the egg. Mitochondria in the sperm are contained in the tail, which drops off as the head penetrates the egg.

194. Match the neurotransmitter (a-d) with the area of the brain in which it is formed (1–4).

a. Norepinephrine
b. Dopamine
c. Serotonin
d. Acetylcholine

1. Nucleus basalis of Meynert, which is inferior to the globus pallidus in the basal forebrain
2. Raphe nucleus, which runs diffusely in the brainstem
3. Substantia nigra, in the midbrain
4. Locus ceruleus, which is in the pons

answer: a-4, b-3, c-2, d-1

195. Which of the following are associated with meningomyeloceles?

a. Mental retardation
b. Hydrocephalus
c. Neurofibromatosis
d. Intravenous drug abuse

answer: a, b. Meningomyeloceles, which are lower neural tube closure defects, are associated with abnormalities of the upper end of the neural tube, including hydrocephalus and mental retardation.

196. About 10 days after beginning treatment with phenytoin, a 10-year-old child develops blister-like lesions on the skin, eyes, mouth, and other mucous surfaces. Which condition is most likely?

a. Meningococcal meningitis
b. Child abuse
c. Allergy
d. Seizure associated trauma

answer: c. The child has developed the Stevens-Johnson syndrome, which is a rare but severe life-threatening allergic reaction. Its danger lies in its predilection to involve mucous surfaces, including the intestine, and also in permitting infections to enter through interruption of the skin.

197. Which anticonvulsant has a chemical structure that most closely resembles a tricyclic antidepressant?

a. Phenytoin
b. Phenobarbital
c. Carbamazepine
d. Valproic acid

answer: c. Carbamazepine closely resembles imipramine.

198. Which is the best study in attempting to locate mesial temporal sclerosis?

a. CT
b. MRI
c. EEG
d. Routine x-rays

answer: b. MRI provides better resolution than CT. Also, with the MRI, the skull does not create artifacts that obscure structures virtually surrounded by the skull.

199. After a small cerebrovascular accident in the right cerebral hemisphere, a patient is found by the hospital staff to be belligerent and inattentive. To a psychiatry consultant, the patient is hostile, but is generally oriented and able to converse and recall a series of six numbers. The patient permitted only a brief examination, during which the psychiatrist found no hemiparesis, asterixis, or ataxia. Which physical abnormalities might be the cause of the mental aberrations?

> ***answer:*** Further evaluation of the patient's cognitive function must be undertaken to determine if the problem has been an underlying dementia that became overt because of the stroke. In other words, the patient could have developed a mild but devastating global cognitive stroke-induced impairment, i.e., multi-infarct dementia. On the other hand, the patient might have a limited, specific neuropsychologic disorder—anosognosia—as the result of a nondominant hemisphere infarction. Lesions that cause anosognosia may be overlooked because they do not necessarily cause hemiparesis, although they usually cause cortical hemisensory deficits. Another common cause of confusion that presents as disruptive behavior is a toxic or metabolic encephalopathy that led to delirium. Although physicians generally approach patients as though they all speak English, are not deaf or blind, are not aphasic, and are physically comfortable (or at least not in pain), these assumptions may have to be reconsidered when patients seem to be uncooperative.

200. After a flurry of generalized, tonic-clonic seizures, a 24-year-old man with epilepsy is found by the hospital staff to be amnestic, belligerent, and inattentive. To a psychiatry consultant, the patient is hostile, generally disoriented, and unable to converse or to recall a series of six numbers. What might be the cause of the mental aberrations?

> ***answer:*** Patients are often confused and amnestic during the postictal period, as though they had undergone electroshock treatment. Although the seizures themselves may be responsible, other factors that may occur during the seizures are important. Anticonvulsants, which are generally given intravenously and in high doses, may cause an encephalopathy. Head trauma and metabolic derangements may have occurred. Of course, whatever had caused the seizures may be causing the subsequent mental aberrations, e.g., a brain tumor that expanded, a degenerative neurologic condition, and drug or alcohol withdrawal.

201. Which one of the following is inconsistent with a diagnosis of Alzheimer's disease?

a. Aphasia
b. Apraxia
c. Amnesia
d. Apathy
e. Altered level of consciousness

> ***answer:*** e. Patients with Alzheimer's disease are alert unless another condition, such as a toxic-metabolic encephalopathy, has supervened. Of the other conditions that often accompany or are manifestations of the dementia, aphasia is most likely to confuse the diagnosis. Word-finding difficulty, which may result in an anomic aphasia, is characteristic of Alzheimer's disease; however, more extensive language difficulties may complicate testing, overshadow other cognitive impairments, and more often result from discrete cerebral lesions, such as cerebrovascular accidents.

202. For which conditions are psychostimulants approved by the Food and Drug Administration?

a. Attention deficit disorder
b. Parkinson's disease
c. Huntington's disease
d. Narcolepsy
e. Obesity
f. Petit mal epilepsy

> ***answer:*** a, d, e

203. Of the following, which is the most common form of inherited mental retardation?

a. Alzheimer's disease
b. Rett syndrome
c. Trisomy 18
d. Fragile X syndrome
e. Turner's syndrome

> ***answer:*** d. Of the choices, the fragile X syndrome is the most common cause of inherited mental retardation. It sometimes has features of autism. The fragile

X syndrome causes retardation in one boy in 1000 to 1500. These boys tend to have a long, thin face, large ears, and large testes. In one girl in 2000 to 2500, the fragile X syndrome causes retardation that is milder. The condition has no specific clinical features, but may now be diagnosed by DNA analysis.

204. Why is carbidopa administered along with L-dopa in the treatment of Parkinson's disease?

a. It is a decarboxylase inhibitor that retards the metabolism of all dopa.
b. It maximizes the nigrostriatal L-dopa concentration.
c. It is a monoamine oxidase inhibitor.
d. It is a dopa agonist.

answer: b. Carbidopa is a decarboxylase inhibitor that is administered in fixed combinations with L-dopa (Sinemet). It does not cross the blood-brain barrier, but it retards the metabolism of systemic L-dopa. Using less L-dopa minimizes systemic side effects.

205. In the preceding question, which of the neurotransmitters are not significantly altered in Alzheimer's disease?

answer: a, d

206. Match the treatment of Parkinson's disease (a-d) with its mechanism of action (1-4).

a. Pergolide
b. L-dopa
c. Deprenyl (selegiline)
d. Bromocriptine

1. A dopamine precursor
2. A dopamine agonist
3. A monoamine oxidase A inhibitor
4. A monoamine oxidase B inhibitor

answer: a-2, b-1, c-4, d-2

207. With which condition(s) is violent (directed, aggressive) behavior associated?

a. Epilepsy, all forms
b. Partial complex seizures
c. Episodic dyscontrol syndrome
d. Mental retardation
e. Males with the genotype XYY

answer: c

208. A 68-year-old man, who had been in good health, experienced a 20-minute episode of aphasia and right hemiparesis 2 days before an evaluation. He has a bruit over the right carotid artery, but otherwise he has normal general and neurologic examinations. An EEG, MRI of the head, and routine tests are normal. An angiogram discloses 50 per cent stenosis of the left common carotid artery at its bifurcation. Which is the best course of treatment?

a. Investigate the right carotid artery.
b. Suggest a daily aspirin.
c. Refer him for left carotid surgery.
d. Continue to follow him, but add no treatment.

answer: b. Recent, large studies indicate that in patients who have had a TIA (symptomatic patients), carotid endarterectomy was preferable to aspirin in reducing strokes when carotid stenosis was at least 70 per cent. Although carotid bruits often are detectable over a nonstenotic carotid artery, they should not necessarily be taken as a sign of underlying carotid stenosis. Carotid bruits may be due to blood turbulence from minor atherosclerotic changes or greater blood flow through a normal artery because its counterpart is stenotic.

209. In Alzheimer's disease, with which pathologic feature is dementia most closely associated?

a. Cerebral atrophy
b. Senile plaques
c. Neurofibrillary tangles
d. Pick bodies

answer: c. Although the initial studies indicated that plaques were the abnormality most closely associated with dementia, recent work indicates that the tangles are more closely associated. Cerebral atrophy is an age-related change.

210. Which is the most commonly occurring brainstem infarction?

a. Midbrain infarction
b. Pontine infarction
c. Lateral medullary syndrome
d. Medial medullary syndrome

answer: c

211. Which of the following conditions does a positive response to the Tensilon (edrophonium) test indicate?

a. Muscular dystrophy
b. Myasthenia gravis
c. Myotonic dystrophy
d. None of the above

answer: b. Tensilon (edrophonium) is a cholinesterase inhibitor that prolongs the effectiveness of acetylcholine at the neuromuscular junction. This test temporarily reverses ocular and facial weakness in an individual with untreated myasthenia gravis.

212. Which of the following neurotransmitters project from the brainstem to the spinal cord?

a. Norepinephrine
b. Dopamine
c. Serotonin

answer: a, c. Projections of norepinephrine and serotonin are probably crucial in analgesia. Dopamine tracts may be extensive, but they are confined to the brain.

213. Which of the following neurotransmitters is not a catecholamine?

a. Norepinephrine
b. Dopamine
c. Serotonin
d. Epinephrine

answer: c. Serotonin is an indole, which is a five-member ring containing nitrogen joined to a benzene (six-member) ring. Catecholamines have a benzene ring with two hydroxyl groups and one amine group.

214. Which of the prior neurotransmitters is not derived from tyrosine?

answer: c. Serotonin is derived from tryptophan. The others are derived from tyrosine.

215. Which features of Alzheimer's disease are also present in Parkinson's disease with dementia?

a. Senile plaques, abundant neurofibrillary tangles, and loss of neurons
b. Depletion of cholinergic neurons in the nucleus basalis
c. Decreased choline acetyltransferase (ChAT)
d. Improvement with L-dopa replacement
e. Lewy bodies in the cerebral cortex, as well as the basal ganglia

answer: a, b, c. The histology and biochemistry of Alzheimer's disease and Parkinson's disease with dementia are similar. Although Lewy bodies are not found in Alzheimer's disease, they are found in the cerebral cortex of diffuse Lewy body disease and Parkinson's disease with dementia. The dementia of neither condition improves with L-dopa.

216. Where does the corticospinal tract cross as it descends?

a. Internal capsule
b. Base of the pons
c. Pyramids
d. Anterior horn cells

answer: c. The crossing of the corticospinal tracts in the pyramids gives rise to their alternative name, pyramidal tracts.

217. In right-handed individuals, which artery supplies Broca's area and the adjacent corticospinal tract?

a. Anterior cerebral
b. Middle cerebral
c. Posterior cerebral
d. Basilar

answer: b. The left middle cerebral artery supplies these areas and also the underlying internal capsule. The handedness of patients should be ascertained.

218. Which group of illnesses are *all* suggested by the presence of spasticity, hyperactive deep tendon reflexes, and Babinski signs?

a. Poliomyelitis, cerebrovascular accidents, spinal cord trauma
b. Bell's palsy, cerebrovascular accidents, psychogenic disturbances
c. Spinal cord trauma, cerebrovascular accidents, congenital cerebral injuries
d. Brainstem infarction, cerebellar infarction, spinal cord infarction
e. Parkinson's disease, dystonia musculorum deformans, cerebellar infarction

answer: c. These signs indicate upper motor neuron injury, which would be found in central nervous system diseases that injure the corticospinal (pyramidal) tract. They would not be found in disease of the (1) peripheral nerves, (2) cranial nerves outside the brainstem (Bell's palsy), (3) cerebellum, or (4) extrapyramidal system (Parkinson's disease and dystonia musculorum deformans).

219. Patients with which group of illnesses usually have muscles that are paretic, atrophic, and areflexic?

a. Poliomyelitis, diabetic peripheral neuropathy, traumatic brachial plexus injury
b. Amyotrophic lateral sclerosis, brainstem infarction, psychogenic disturbance
c. Spinal cord trauma, cerebrovascular accidents, congenital cerebral injuries
d. Brainstem infarction, cerebellar infarction, spinal cord infarction
e. Parkinson's disease, cerebrovascular accidents, cerebellar infarction
f. Guillain Barré syndrome, multiple sclerosis, and uremic neuropathy

answer: a. These signs indicate lower motor neuron injury, which includes diseases of the anterior horn cell (polio), peripheral nerves, and their plexuses.

220. A 73-year-old woman has had the sudden onset of the following signs: right-sided limb ataxia, dysarthria, lack of facial sensation on the right face and left side of the body, and a right-sided Horner's syndrome. To which side will the palate deviate when she attempts to say "ah."

a. Right   c. Both
b. Left   d. Neither

answer: b. She has a right-sided lateral medullary syndrome. The lesion encompasses the right nucleus ambiguus, which leads to paresis of the right palate. Right-sided paresis causes the palate to deviate to the left when the palatal muscles contract.

221. Bat wing is to a butterfly as which of the following?

a. Peripheral neuropathy is to multiple sclerosis.
b. A glioma is to Huntington's disease.
c. Myelopathy is to myopathy.
d. Huntington's disease is to a glioma.

answer: d. Bat wing ventricles, which result from atrophy of the caudate nuclei, are characteristic of Huntington's disease. Gliomas often seem to develop in the corpus callosum and spread bilaterally and symmetrically into the cerebral hemispheres, giving the appearance of a butterfly, i.e., butterfly glioma.

222. Of the following, which two tests provide the most reliable confirmation of the clinical diagnosis of MS (multiple sclerosis) when it is in a quiescent state?

a. MRI of the head   d. CSF studies for myelin basic
b. VERs   protein
c. CSF studies for oligoclonal bands   e. CT of the head

answer: a and c. The MRI shows plaques, which may be enhanced after gadolinium infusion, as hyperintense white patches. Oligoclonal bands in the CSF are also a reliable marker. However, the multiplicity of tests indicates that no one test is definitive. Most may be abnormal in non-MS demyelinating conditions, chronic CNS infections, and inflammatory diseases. Although large doses of contrast and delayed studies increase the sensitivity of CT, it is still insensitive to cerebral lesions and unable to detect lesions in the optic nerves and the spinal cord. CSF myelin basic protein concentrations may be elevated in an acute attack of MS, but other inflammatory conditions and infectious illnesses may also produce an increased concentration. When MS is quiescent, the concentration of this substance is usually normal.

223. Which of the following descriptions best characterize the MRI changes of MS?

a.   Multiple, white areas scattered in the cerebrum
b.   Conversion of the cerebral hemisphere white matter to gray
c.   Loss of the myelin signal throughout the corpus callosum
d.   Periventricular, high-intensity abnormalities

answer: d. The MRI shows white, hyperintense lesions characteristically in the periventricular region. It may also reveal lesions in the optic nerve or spinal cord. Bright, small, or punctate intracerebral lesions may result from cerebro-vascular disease. Since their etiology is not established, they are called "unidentified bright objects" or "UBOs."

224. When is MS most likely to be exacerbated?

a.   During pregnancy
b.   During times of stress
c.   In adolescence
d.   After trauma
e.   For the first 3 postpartum months

answer: e. Although pregnancy is associated with some protection, the first 3 postpartum months are associated with MS exacerbations. The other factors are unproven precipitants of MS exacerbations.

225. When contemplating having a second child, a young mother who had developed MS during the postpartum period of her first delivery inquires about the effect of a second or third pregnancy on her MS. What is the current thinking?

a.   Deliveries are almost always more complicated when the mother has MS.
b.   MS worsens in a stepwise pattern with each succeeding pregnancy.
c.   The number of pregnancies has little or no effect on the ultimate outcome of MS.
d.   Her offspring, compared to the general population, will have an increased risk of developing MS.
e.   Fetal malformations are more common than in the general population.

answer: c and d

226. Which MS features are associated with cognitive impairment?

a.   Paraparesis and blindness
b.   Chronicity of the illness
c.   Enlarged cerebral ventricles
d.   Corpus callosum atrophy
e.   Number and size of cerebral plaques
f.   Decreased glucose metabolism on positron emission tomography

answer: All

227. After being comatose for 2 weeks after an attempted strangulation, a 35-year-old woman babbles incoherently. She seems to repeat conversations that take place around her. Although weak, she can eat, sit, and watch television. Although she does not seem to see the television, she repeats the dialogue. She does not respond to visual stimulation. Her pupils are equal and reactive to light. Which is the best description of her condition?

a.   Coma
b.   Psychosis
c.   Vegetative state
d.   Locked-in syndrome

e.   Isolation aphasia, probable dementia, and cortical blindness from watershed infarctions
f.   None of the above

answer: e. She has isolation aphasia because of her ability only to repeat. She also has cortical blindness because she cannot see, but her pupil function is spared. She is not comatose because she has interaction with her environment and verbal and motor activity. In the vegetative state and the locked-in syndrome, patients cannot vocalize, eat, or sit.

228.   Which of the following are characteristics of the N-methyl-D-aspartate receptor?

a.   It is usually called the NMDA receptor.
b.   It regulates calcium channels.
c.   Excitatory neurotransmitters, such as glutamate, bind onto this receptor.
d.   Overstimulation of the receptor leads to cell death by calcium flooding.
e.   The NMDA receptor has been suggested to be cytotoxic in cerebrovascular accidents, epilepsy, and Huntington's disease.

answer: All

229.   Which of the following is (are) not characteristics of the carpal tunnel syndrome?

a.   Compression of the median nerve at the wrist
b.   Tinel's sign
c.   Caused by repetitive stress injury
d.   Results in pain and weakness of the forearm extensor and supinator muscles
e.   Typically worse at night

answer: d. Tennis elbow is pain and weakness of the forearm extensor and supinator muscles from bursitis, muscle swelling, or entrapment of branches of the radial nerve. The most common cause is occupational injury, not tennis.

230.   What is the pattern of innervation of the fecal and urinary sphincters?

a.   An internal sphincter is innervated by the peripheral nervous system, and an external sphincter is innervated by the autonomic nervous system.
b.   An internal sphincter is innervated by the autonomic nervous system, and an external sphincter is innervated by the peripheral nervous system.
c.   An internal sphincter is innervated by the central nervous system, and an external sphincter is innervated by the autonomic nervous system.
d.   An internal sphincter is innervated by the peripheral nervous system, and an external sphincter is innervated by the central nervous system.

answer: b. In both cases, the autonomic nervous system and the internal sphincter are more powerful, but damage to the peripheral nervous system and the external sphincter, which can result from alcoholism, diabetes, and trauma, can cause incontinence.

231.   A 49-year-old man in the Emergency Room, being treated for alcohol withdrawal seizures, became progressively more stuporous. Which conditions might be considered?

a.   Hypoglycemia
b.   Anticonvulsant intoxication
c.   Bleeding from the small intracranial veins
d.   Alcoholic stupor
e.   All of the above

answer: a, b, c. Chronic alcoholism leads to cirrhosis that depletes stored glycogen. Unless glucose is supplied continuously, patients may develop hypoglycemia that causes seizures, as well as stupor. Inadvertent excessive treatment with anticonvulsants is relatively common, especially if a cirrhotic liver cannot metabolize medications. Bleeding from small veins, which characteristically leads to a subdural hematoma, is common is alcoholics because they have head trauma and an impaired coagulation ability.

232. Through which structure is CSF normally absorbed?

a. Spinal cord
b. Inner surface of the lateral ventricles
c. Choroid plexus
d. Arachnoid membrane
e. Cerebral hemisphere tissue

> *answer:* d. CSF is normally formed in the choroid plexus and absorbed through the arachnoid membrane of the meninges, predominantly at the base of the brain. When the arachnoid membrane is inflamed by infection (as in meningitis) or blood (a subarachnoid hemorrhage), CSF absorption is impaired, and communicating or normal-pressure hydrocephalus may develop. In those conditions, CSF may be absorbed through the ventricles.

233. A 75-year-old woman, after a vigorous hair washing at her local beauty parlor, develops vertigo, nausea, and diplopia. She has marked ataxia when she begins to walk. A CT scan shows no abnormalities. What is the most likely cause of her disturbance?

a. Cerebral infarction
b. A small brainstem infarction
c. A chemical in the hair wash
d. Labyrinthitis

> *answer:* b. She probably has had hyperextension (excessive backward bending) of her neck that crimped her vertebral arteries and precipitated a small infarction in the vertebrobasilar distribution. People who have osteophytes that press against the vertebral arteries as they pass upward through the cervical spine are apt to have interrupted vertebral blood flow if the neck is bent backward. Brainstem infarctions usually cannot be detected by CT scans because of artifact generated by the surrounding skull.

234. A 35-year-old psychiatrist in her last trimester of pregnancy has painful tingling in most of her hands and all her fingers. She also finds that small objects seem to drop from her fingers. The symptoms are worse in the late afternoon and early morning hours. She has no objective abnormalities. Percussion of the wrist re-creates the paresthesias. What is the cause of her problem?

a. Entrapment of a nerve in each wrist
b. Peripheral neuropathy
c. Cervical spondylosis
d. Guillain-Barré syndrome
e. Lyme disease

> *answer:* a. She has bilateral carpal tunnel syndrome, i.e., median nerve compression or entrapment at the wrist. The usual distribution of the median nerve is the palmar surface of the thumb, adjacent two fingers, and the lateral portion of the palm, but many people with carpal tunnel syndrome have sensory disturbances that do not strictly conform to the textbook's map. Paresthesias in the median nerve distribution produced by tapping the flexor surface of the wrist—Tinel's sign—are virtually pathognomonic. This disorder usually results from fluid accumulation in the carpal tunnel, as occurs during pregnancy, before menses, and after trauma to the wrist, including "repetitive stress injuries," e.g., keyboarding, wrist exercising, and sometimes excessive driving. Nerve conduction velocity studies that demonstrate slowing across the flexor surface of the wrist confirm the diagnosis. Her carpal tunnel syndrome will probably resolve after delivery. Most patients respond to wrist splints, diuretics, or change in activities. Sometimes treatment requires steroid injections into the carpal tunnel or surgery.

235. A 19-year-old student at a small New England college develops ascending, flaccid, and areflexic weakness of her legs, trunk, then arms. When she develops ocular, facial, and pharyngeal weakness, she is intubated for ventilator support. During periods of agitation, she was found to be hypoxic. Which of the following conditions is the most likely cause?

a. Multiple sclerosis
b. Conversion disorder
c. Poliomyelitis
d. Guillain-Barré syndrome
e. Herniated cervical intervertebral disk

> *answer:* d. She most likely has Guillain-Barré syndrome or acute inflammatory demyelinating polyradiculoneuropathy (AIDP) because of the extensive lower

motor neuron pattern. Poliomyelitis is asymmetric and does not involve ocular motility. Many infectious illnesses—mononucleosis, Lyme disease, AIDS, Hepatitis—can produce a Guillain-Barré syndrome, but no particular agent is identified in most cases. The mental changes result from hypoxia rather than direct cerebral involvement.

236. Which of the following statements about myelin are true?

a. CNS and PNS myelin are produced by the same cells.
b. Oligodendrocytes are to Schwann cells as the CNS is to the PNS.
c. They insulate electrochemical transmissions.
d. They are affected by the same illnesses.
e. The optic nerves are covered by CNS myelin.

answer: b, c, e

237. Which conditions might an HIV infection produce?

a. Dementia
b. Myelopathy
c. Guillain-Barré syndrome
d. Myopathy

answer: All

238. A 30-year-old homeless, epileptic, intravenous drug abuser becomes psychotic and is treated with parenteral dopamine-blocking neuroleptic medications. Thirty minutes later, although alert, he develops involuntary facial muscle contractions. What are the possible causes of these conditions?

answer: Multiple causes exist. The most likely would be a dystonic reaction to the antipsychotic medications and focal seizures. Less commonly occurring causes would be tetanus, rabies, and strychnine poisoning.

239. How does neuroleptic malignant syndrome differ from neuroleptic-induced parkinsonism?

a. Fever
b. Muscle rigidity
c. Brain damage
d. Markedly elevated CPK
e. Tachycardia
f. Familial tendency

answer: a, c, d, e. An elevated CPK is found in parkinsonism because of patients' immobility. Fever, tachycardia, and other autonomic disorders are attributable to the neuroleptic malignant syndrome. Malignant hyperthermia, which is also characterized by fever, rigidity, and rhabdomyolysis, has a familial tendency. In many cases it has a genetic basis.

240. Which of the following statements are true regarding acetylcholine?

a. It is a neurotransmitter at the neuromuscular junction.
b. It is a neurotransmitter in the CNS.
c. Like GABA, acetylcholine is an inhibitory neurotransmitter.
d. Like dopamine, acetylcholine is deactivated more by metabolism than by reuptake.

answer: a, b

241. Which condition is characterized by absence of dystrophin on a muscle biopsy?

a. Myotonic dystrophy
b. Becker's dystrophy
c. Duchenne's dystrophy
d. Diabetic neuropathy

answer: c. Absence of dystrophin, the muscle cell membrane protein, is virtually diagnostic of Duchenne's dystrophy. In Becker's dystrophy, the relatively benign variant of Duchenne's dystrophy, dystrophin is reduced or abnormal. In the dystrophin test, muscle biopsies are tested for dystrophin to distinguish among these conditions and exclude others that might mimic them.

242. Against which single site are antibodies directed in myasthenia gravis?

a. AChE receptors
b. All ACh receptors
c. ACh quanta
d. ACh receptors only at the neuromuscular junction

answer: d

243. Which are characteristics of myotonic but not Duchenne's dystrophy?

a. Presence of dystrophin on muscle biopsy
b. Cataracts
c. Baldness
d. Cardiac conduction abnormalities
e. Reduced or absent fertility
f. Autosomal inheritance
g. Dementia
h. Distal muscle weakness
i. Pseudohypertrophy
j. Genetic anticipation

answer: a, b-f, h, j

244. Which two conditions are associated with episodic quadriparesis?

a. Low potassium (hypokalemia)
b. REM activity
c. Hyponatremia
d. Cocaine

answer: a, b. Hypokalemic periodic paralysis, cataplexy, and REM periods during normal sleep cause episodic areflexic quadriparesis. When quadriparetic, patients are alert, except during sleep, and can breathe without assistance. Hyponatremia, when severe, causes stupor and seizures, but not quadriparesis.

245. Regarding mitochondrial (mtDNA), which statement(s) is (are) true?

a. Ragged red fibers are virtually pathognomonic of an mtDNA abnormality.
b. An individual's mtDNA is inherited exclusively from the mother.
c. mtDNA is not inherited in the chromosomes.
d. mtDNA abnormalities are not inherited in a classic, Mendelian pattern.
e. Abnormalities often produce combinations of myopathies, lactic acidosis, and progressively severe encephalopathies.
f. All of the above

answer: f

246. Which of the following is true regarding dystrophin?

a. Dystrophin is located in the muscle cell's surface membrane.
b. Dystrophin is absent in Duchenne's dystrophy.
c. Dystrophin is absent in myotonic dystrophy.
d. Dystrophin absence is a reliable marker of Duchenne's dystrophy that can be detected with a commercially available test.
e. Dystrophin is abnormal in Becker's dystrophy, which results from the same gene as Duchenne's dystrophy.
f. Dystrophin is abnormal in myotonic dystrophy, which results from the same gene as Duchenne's dystrophy.

answer: a, b, d, e

247. Which are genetic characteristics of myotonic dystrophy?

a. Females as well as males are likely to develop the illness.
b. Mitochondrial DNA might be affected.
c. In successive generations, the disease appears at a younger age because of a phenomenon called anticipation.
d. In successive generations, the disease is more severe because of anticipation.
e. Like other dominantly inherited nervous system disorders—Huntington's disease, dystonia musculorum deformans, tuberous sclerosis, and neurofibromatosis—myotonic dystrophy is not associated with storage of a particular metabolic product.

answer: a, c, d, e

248–252. What is the mechanism of action of the following poisons?

a. Blocks the release of the inhibitory neurotransmitter, glycine
b. Poisons the respiratory energy pathway
c. Interferes with the oxygen-carrying capacity of hemoglobin
d. Inactivates acetylcholinesterase (AChE), which causes excessive ACh activity
e. Blocks the release of acetylcholine from the presynaptic membrane of the neuromuscular junction
f. Blocks the release of acetylcholine from the presynaptic membranes in the brainstem

248. Poison gases

answer: d

249. Tetanus

answer: a

250. Botulism

answer: e

251. Cyanide

answer: b

252. Carbon monoxide

answer: c

253–258. Match the life-style (252–257) with its consequences (a-e).

a. Myositis
b. Eosinophilia-myalgia syndrome
c. Upper and lower facial nerve paresis
d. Hypertrophied muscles, excessive facial hair, amenorrhea
e. Peripheral neuropathy

253. Steroid injections for body building

answer: d

254. Deer hunting in Connecticut

answer: c or e, a. Tics in Connecticut are vectors for Lyme disease. Undercooked venison may contain *Trichinella.*

255. Using tryptophan-containing products as a hypnotic

answer: b. Tryptophan has been contaminated by substances that cause eosinophilia and myalgia.

256. Alcoholism

answer: e. Alcoholism, probably through the associated nutritional deficiency, causes peripheral neuropathy.

257. *Trichinella*

answer: a. *Trichinella* causes trichinosis.

258. Excessive pyridoxine consumption

answer: e. Taking excessive vitamin B_6 causes a peripheral neuropathy.

259. Which three are features of Huntington's disease dementia?

a. It correlates with caudate atrophy on the CT.
b. Neuropsychologic tests can usually detect it in presymptomatic carriers.

c.   It is responsible for impetuous actions.

d.   Chorea develops in proximity to the dementia.

   answer: a, c, d

260.   A 25-year-old right-handed patient underwent a commissurotomy for intractable seizures. It was successful, but he complained of not being able to express himself fully. What are possible explanations?

a.   Aphasia is a complication of the procedure.

b.   Commissurotomy patients lose cognitive function.

c.   Emotions generated in the left hemisphere are not as readily verbalized as those in the right hemisphere.

d.   Emotions generated in the right hemisphere are not as readily verbalized as those generated in the left hemisphere.

   answer: d

261–266.   With which conditions (a-h) are the various forms of apraxia (260–265) associated?

a.   Aphasia

b.   Hemi-inattention

c.   Dementia

d.   Dysarthria

e.   Incontinence

f.   Left homonymous hemianopsia

g.   Right homonymous hemianopsia

h.   Aprosody

261.   Gait

   answer: c, e

262.   Constructional

   answer: b, f, h

263.   Ideational

   answer: c

264.   Limb

   answer: a, g

265.   Buccofacial

   answer: a, d, g

266.   Ideomotor

   answer: a, g

267.   Which forms of communication are based, like speech and hearing, in the dominant hemisphere perisylvian language arc?

a.   Reading and writing

b.   Melody for most people

c.   American Sign Language

d.   Cursing

e.   Prosody

f.   Body language

   answer: a, c

268.   Which of the following is a disconnection syndrome?

a.   Nonfluent aphasia

b.   Conduction aphasia

c.   Fluent aphasia

d.   Isolation aphasia

e.   Dementia

f.   Global aphasia

   answer: b. Disconnection syndromes generally refer to neuropsychologic disorders in which connections between the primary neuropsychologic centers are severed, but the centers themselves are intact and capable of functioning. Conduction aphasia consists of the separation of Wernicke's and Broca's areas. Other disconnection syndromes are the split-brain syndrome and alexia without agraphia.

269. Which of the following arteries supply the cerebral cortex in which Broca's area is located?

a. Anterior cerebral artery
b. Middle cerebral artery
c. Posterior cerebral artery
d. Internal carotid artery system

answer: b, d

270. What is the common neurologic term for the zone of cerebral cortex between branches of the major cerebral arteries?

a. Watershed area (borderzone)
b. Limbic system
c. Cornea
d. Arcuate fasciculus

answer: a

271. What condition is caused by hypoperfusion of the watershed area?

a. Alexia without agraphia
b. Fluent aphasia
c. Hemiparesis
d. Isolation aphasia

answer: d. The perisylvian language arc is well perfused by relatively large branches of the middle cerebral artery. The more distal cortical regions, the watershed areas, have a tenuous blood supply from distal branches of the anterior, middle, and posterior cerebral arteries. With hypotension, the watershed areas often receive insufficient blood supply and develop ischemia; however, the language arc generally continues to receive an adequate supply. When the perisylvian language arc survives, but the outlying cortex is damaged, language function is isolated. It will be devoid of cognitive input, and the patient will be able only to perform repetition.

272. Which cerebral artery is the primary supply of the cerebral cortex motor center for the contralateral leg?

a. Anterior cerebral artery
b. Middle cerebral artery
c. Posterior cerebral artery

answer: a

273. After a CVA in which the main symptom was left-sided sensory loss, a patient's left hand had involuntary or unconscious movements. The patient alternated between being distraught, oblivious to the hand's movements, and ascribing the hand to his roommate. Which conditions are potential explanations?

a. Hemiballismus
b. Alien hand syndrome
c. Dementia
d. Aphasia
e. Anosognosia

answer: b, possibly a. The alien hand syndrome, which may follow a nondominant parietal lobe syndrome, is the misperception that the hand acts independently or under another person's control. Although he may have anosognosia, the unique features are that the hand acts independently and that the patient assigns control to another individual.

274. Which of the following apraxias is most closely associated with dementia and incontinence?

a. Ideational
b. Dressing
c. Ideomotor
d. Buccofacial
e. Oral
f. Gait

answer: f. In normal-pressure hydrocephalus, patients have gait apraxia, urinary incontinence, and dementia. The apraxia is the most characteristic feature and the most responsive to treatment—insertion of a ventriculoperitoneal shunt.

275. A 40-year-old woman, who had had migraine headaches as a teenager and tension headaches afterward, has evolved a pattern of dull, symmetric, nonthrobbing headaches that are present continuously every day. She has come to rely on prescription medications, but not narcotics. However, when the headaches flareup, which is about once a month, she visits an Emergency Room where physicians give her narcotic injections. Further evaluation reveals no underlying neurologic or serious psychiatric disorder. How should this problem be classified?

a. Chronic daily headaches
b. Tension headaches
c. Status migrainosus
d. Obsessive-compulsive disorder

answer: a. This woman has a distinct entity, chronic daily headache (CDH), that typically evolves from migraine and superimposed tension headaches. Its key feature is usually abuse or at least daily use of analgesic or vasoconstrictor medications. Occasionally patients are addicted to narcotics, sedatives, or anxiolytics. Of course, in some patients, depression leads to CDH, but in others, depression results from it. Patients with CDH take medication to avoid "rebound" headaches and withdrawal symptoms. CHD is a major diagnostic problem because patients request treatment for headaches, but the symptom is medication induced.

276. Patients often perceive migraine pain in or behind their eye (i.e., in the periorbital or retro-orbital location), even though the abnormality is in the meninges or extracranial vessels. What accounts for this discrepancy?

answer: The trigeminal nerve innervates the meninges, as well as the eye and its orbit. The brain itself probably has no pain receptors. Thus, neurosurgeons can operate on the brain without using anesthesia, and the patient can remain awake during certain neurosurgical procedures. In migraines and cluster headaches, pain is referred to the eye, which is supplied by the first division of the trigeminal nerve.

277. Serotonin has been implicated as a cause of migraine. Which two statements are true regarding the role of serotonin in migraine?

a. Effective abortive medications, such as sumatriptan, dihydroergotamine, and ergotamine, act on serotonin receptors.
b. Aspirin interferes with serotonin.
c. Serum 5HT concentration falls at the onset of a migraine.
d. Effective abortive medications lead to nausea.

answer: a, c

278. In which of the following conditions might the standard medication regimen produce an adverse reaction if monoamine oxidase inhibitor (MAOI) antidepressants are added?

a. Parkinson's disease
b. Seizures
c. Chronic pain
d. Depression
e. All of the above

answer: e. L-Dopa and selegiline, which is a MAOI, are common medications for Parkinson's disease. Patients with seizures may be taking carbamazepine as an anticonvulsant. Patients with chronic pain may be taking meperidine, possibly surreptitiously. Some patients with depression are under treatment with tricyclic antidepressants. When patients are taking any of these medications, MAOIs are absolutely or relatively contraindicated because the combination may cause a hypertensive crisis.

279. Which two of the following statements are true regarding saccades?

a. Their speed is about 30°/sec.
b. Their speed is rapid and can reach 700°/sec.
c. They are governed by supranuclear centers.
d. Abnormalities in saccades characterize the onset of Alzheimer's disease.

answer: b, c. Saccades, the high-velocity conjugate gaze movements, are generated by cerebral conjugate gaze centers. Abnormal saccades are one of the first findings in Huntington's disease and are also found in schizophrenia.

280. Which of the three following statements are true regarding pursuit eye movements?

a. They are the smooth, steady tracking movements used to follow moving objects.
b. They are found only in humans.
c. They are governed by supranuclear centers.
d. They are abnormal in many patients with schizophrenia.

> *answer:* a, c, d. Pursuits, the relatively slow, smooth conjugate gaze movements, are generated mostly by the pontine conjugate gaze centers. They are abnormal in schizophrenia and, to a lesser extent, in affective disorders. Both saccades and pursuit ocular movements are abnormal in a variety of neurologic illnesses.

281. In which three conditions might the combination of unilateral miosis, ptosis, and anhidrosis be found?

a. Pancoast tumors
b. Cluster headache
c. Migraine with aura
d. Lateral medullary syndrome
e. Midbrain infarction

> *answer:* a, b, d. Horner's syndrome includes ptosis, miosis (small pupil), and anhidrosis (lack of sweating). It results from injury to the sympathetic supply of the face and eye. Migraines and midbrain infarctions may impair parasympathetic innervation and cause dilation of the pupil. Parasympathetic innervation of the pupil is carried along with the third cranial nerve, which originates in the midbrain.

282. To which four vision-impairing conditions are the elderly particularly susceptible?

a. Cataracts
b. Glaucoma
c. Strabismus
d. Amblyopia ex anopia
e. Macular degeneration
f. Temporal arteritis
g. Psychogenic visual loss

> *answer:* a, b, e, f. Strabismus is congenital extraocular muscle weakness. If uncorrected, the affected eye will become blind from disuse, i.e, amblyopia ex anopia.

283. Why do psychotropic medications usually cause blurred vision?

a. They cause glaucoma.
b. They cause cataracts.
c. Their anticholinergic properties cause paresis of accommodation.
d. Their cholinergic properties stimulate accommodation.
e. Their anticholinergic properties cause paresis of the light reflex.

> *answer:* c. Psychotropic medications rarely precipitate glaucoma or cause cataracts, but about 5 per cent of patients have blurred vision because anticholinergic effects impair accommodation.

284. A 14-year-old boy with pronounced mental retardation with repetitive, stereotyped movements has a large forehead, large lobulated ears, and macro-orchidism. He has a sister who reportedly is physically normal, but is slow in school. The mother, who is 43 years old, is planning on remarrying and conceiving. Which of the following statements is true?

a. The boy probably has the fragile X chromosome.
b. Since her son's condition is rare, the mother's next pregnancy has no more significant risk than for other women of her age.
c. The sister probably is, as the mother says, merely a mediocre student and does not need to be evaluated further.
d. Since she is 43 years old, further evaluation is indicated for future pregnancies.

answer: a, d. The boy has the fragile X syndrome, which is an inherited disorder transmitted via a faulty X chromosome. It is the most frequent cause of inherited mental retardation and is responsible for about 15 per cent of cases of mental retardation. As if the disorder were transmitted as an incompletely recessive sex-linked trait, fragile X occurs in a modified form—mild mental retardation—in girls.

This mother must be concerned. As she is 43 years old, she might have a child with Down's syndrome (trisomy 21). Down's syndrome is not considered inherited "on a technicality": an affected child did not receive the condition from an affected parent. Down's syndrome causes mental retardation and, in the fifth and sixth decades, an Alzheimer-like dementia. The mother must also be concerned because the fragile X syndrome is inherited, and future conceptions are in danger of this disease as well as Down's syndrome. A different father will not reduce her risk because the mother is the carrier of the defective gene.

As a general rule, when genetic conditions cause mental retardation, they are apparent early and are accompanied by physical abnormalities.

The younger sister must also be evaluated. She could have a modified form of the fragile X syndrome and thus herself be a carrier. In any case, she ought to be evaluated for her poor school performance.

Another general rule is that pregnant women over 40 years old should have amniocentesis to detect Down's syndrome, fragile X, and numerous other conditions. Also, more extensive screening is indicated because she has one child with mental retardation.

285. A 17-year-old boy has numerous light-brown, flat "birthmarks" that are each larger than 3 cm by 1 cm and axillary "freckles." He inquires about some nodules that have been developing on his arms and face. Which statements concerning these new lesions are true?

a. They represent Recklinghausen's disease or neurofibromatosis.
b. They are closely associated with bilateral acoustic neuromas.
c. His siblings and parents ought to be examined because one of them is likely to have the same condition.
d. They are adenoma sebaceum, which is the cutaneous manifestation of tuberous sclerosis.

answer: a, c. He has Recklinghausen's disease or neurofibromatosis type 1 (NF1), which is a common inherited neurocutaneous disturbance characterized by a triad of six or more café-au-lait spots and nodules on peripheral nerves that become apparent in adults (neurofibromas). Patients tend to develop meningiomas. About 50 per cent of NF1 patients acquire the disorder through inheritance. The other 50 per cent apparently acquire it by mutation.

In contrast, a different disorder, previously also called Recklinghausen's disease and now called neurofibromatosis type 2 (NF2), causes bilateral acoustic neuromas and sometimes several café-au-lait spots. These disorders are transmitted on different autosomal chromosomes: NF1 is transmitted on chromosome 17 and NF2 on 22.

Tuberous sclerosis is a completely different inherited neurocutaneous disorder. It consists of a combination of nodules on the malar surface of the face and tubers in the brain that cause seizures and mental deterioration. Depending on the family, tuberous sclerosis is transmitted on chromosome 9 or 11. Tuberous sclerosis and NF1 offer the clinician an excellent opportunity to make a diagnosis by inspection.

286. A 4-year-old girl's parents notice that she has begun to lose her beautiful voice and charming conversational ability. Moreover, she has developed a habit, they feel, of playing repetitively with her hands. She seems to be washing them or clapping for hours at a time. The physician fails to keep her attention. Although he finds the child's eyes to be blue, her hair blond, and her head circumference relatively smaller compared to her height and age than he previously recorded, he diagnoses autism and refers her to a psychiatrist. Which disorder may be misdiagnosed, in this setting, as autism?

a. Down's syndrome
b. PKU deficiency
c. Mental retardation
d. Rett syndrome
e. Nonspecific mental retardation

> *answer:* d. The child probably has Rett syndrome. This condition is diagnosed on clinical criteria: young girls with acquired microcephaly who lose their verbal abilities and begin to perform repetitive, purposeless hand movements (stereotypies). It is a cause of autistic behavior. Its manifestations are often present, in retrospect, by age 2 years; however, the diagnosis is usually not made until age 5 years.

287. Which of the following statements are true regarding REM (rapid eye movement) latency?

a. REM latency is normally 90 to 120 minutes.
b. REM latency can be determined by a polysomnogram (PSG), but the standard test is the multiple sleep latency test (MSLT), which is performed during the day.
c. REM periods with latencies shorter than 5 to 10 minutes are often considered to be sleep-onset REM periods (SOREMPs).
d. REM latency is dependent on sleep latency.
e. Sleep latency is dependent on REM latency.
f. Alcohol-induced sleep is associated with SOREMPs.
g. Restless leg syndrome is associated with SOREMPs.
h. Alcohol and hypnotic withdrawal is associated with SOREMPs.
i. Depression is associated with SOREMPs.
j. Narcolepsy is associated with SOREMPs.
k. Sleep apnea is associated with SOREMPs.
l. Sleep deprivation is associated with SOREMPs.

> *answer:* a, b, c, h, i, j, k, l

288. A 17-year-old high school student begins to fall asleep in class. Despite being warned to get more sleep at night, she continues to fall asleep not only in class but also during more stimulating times, such as watching football games. A complete evaluation shows that she is otherwise in good health. After being assured that she does, in fact, get at least 6 hours of sleep a night, what should be the physician's next steps?

a. Delaying the sleep phase
b. Additional blood tests
c. PSG (polysomnography) and MSLT (multiple sleep latency test)
d. EEG

> *answer:* b, c. Teenagers vary between being excessively sleepy and never being ready to go to bed. Although they often normally have excessive daytime sleepiness (EDS), sleeping in class and during exciting events is abnormal. If the patient does seem to sleep 6 to 8 hours at night, physicians should then consider common causes of EDS in teenagers: depression, medical illness, and drug and alcohol use. Then narcolepsy and sleep apnea should be considered. Blood tests should be done for medical illnesses, such as mononucleosis, evidence of drug and alcohol use, and HLA typing. Narcolepsy is closely associated with HLA-DR2. The PSG and particularly the MSLT will reveal SOREMPs in narcolepsy. The EEG is not suitable for detecting the onset of sleep or the presence of REM.
>
> Narcolepsy is often overlooked in teenagers despite its onset before age 25 in 90 per cent of cases. Only after several years do patients with narcolepsy develop the dramatic cataplexy. Overall, only 10 per cent of patients with narcolepsy have the narcolepsy-cataplexy tetrad: narcolepsy, cataplexy, sleep paralysis, and sleep hallucinations.
>
> Delayed sleep phase syndrome, which does cause EDS and can occur in teenagers, is associated with a full, restful 6 to 8 hours of sleep, but at the "wrong" time. Patients remain awake until late at night and, if possible, sleep late into the next day. Since this teenager had at least 6 hours of sleep, she should have been rested.

289. A 77-year-old man developed EDS at age 75 years. He takes no medications, does not use alcohol, and is in good health. During the night, his wife reports, he has violent movements of his whole body. She does not know if he has restful sleep, but her sleep is restless. Which one of the following should be the next step?

a. Delaying the sleep phase
b. Additional blood tests
c. PSG
d. EMG
e. MSLT

answer: c. People with potentially injurious movements during sleep should be tested with a PSG. An MSLT is unnecessary because narcolepsy is unlikely in view of the lack of daytime naps. Several disorders cause nocturnal movements in 77-year-old individuals: periodic limb movements, restless leg syndrome, sleep apnea, seizures, and REM sleep disorder. All of these conditions interrupt sleep—the bed partner's, as well as the patient's—and lead to EDS.

290. Which three effects can be attributed to benzodiazepines?

a. Increase in total sleep time of 10 per cent
b. Increase in total sleep time of 33 per cent
c. Increase in total sleep time of 67 per cent or more
d. Reduced sleep fragmentation
e. Increase in slow-wave NREM sleep
f. Hip fractures from an increased tendency to fall
g. Weight gain
h. Lowered seizure threshold
i. Anterograde amnesia

answer: a, d, f, i

291. From which structures do subdural hematomas arise?

a. Lacerated middle meningeal arteries
b. Ripped bridging veins
c. Lacerated great vein of Galen
d. Aneurysms of the middle or anterior cerebral arteries

answer: b. Meningeal arterial bleeding leads to epidural hematomas. Aneurysms lead to bleeding that is predominantly subarachnoid. Venous bleeding, which is often so slow that it may be called oozing, leads to subdural hematomas.

292. Which three of the following are closely associated with spastic cerebral palsy?

a. Necrotic areas in the white matter around the ventricles, *periventricular leukomalacia*
b. Kernicterus
c. Detection by neonatal ultrasound examination
d. Foreshortened, spastic limbs
e. Thalidomide

answer: a, c, d. Kernicterus is associated with basal ganglia bilirubin staining. Thalidomide causes congenital limb deformity (phocomelia).

293. Which one of the following is most closely associated with neonatal periventricular leukomalacia?

a. Athetosis
b. Spastic cerebral palsy, all varieties
c. Spastic diplegia
d. Multiple sclerosis

answer: c. Neonatal periventricular white matter necrosis leads to spastic diplegia. Multiple sclerosis and sometimes multiple infarct dementia cause periventricular white matter changes, but these are conditions that affect adults.

294. One hour after a grilled tuna fish dinner in a fancy Chicago restaurant, a 29-year-old previous healthy physician feels "very sick" and has profound nausea and vomiting. She has beet-red skin and hypotension, but a temperature of only 100°F. The episode begins to subside after 2 hours. In addition to general supportive measures, which of the following is the best treatment?

a. Antibiotics
b. Antidiarrhea medication
c. Antihistamines
d. Antiparasitic medications

answer: c. Even when eaten raw, tuna fish and most other deep water fish are usually safe. However, if these fish are not refrigerated, bacteria in their gut and gills may proliferate and produce histidine. The histidine, which resists cooking, is transformed into histamine in the human intestine. As in this case, victims develop *histamine poisoning* that responds to antihistamine injections. In other circumstances, people who eat any fish, especially freshwater fish, can become infested with parasites, but routine cooking usually eliminates that threat. Uncooked shellfish harbor hepatitis virus. Barracuda and grouper fish are often contaminated with toxins that are heat sensitive. Antidiarrheal medications are not effective and counteract the body's natural protective reaction to expel toxins.

295. Which one of the following is incorrect regarding the Glasgow Coma Scale (GCS)?

a. It measures only three clinical parameters: eye opening, verbal response, and motor response.
b. A high score indicates a greater depth of coma.
c. GCS scores can be correlated with post-traumatic amnesia.
d. GCS scores cannot be correlated with post-traumatic headaches.

answer: b. GCS scores range from 3 to 15. Patients with low scores are less responsive, have deeper coma, are more likely to succumb, and have longer post-traumatic amnesia. However, GCS scores cannot be correlated with post-traumatic headaches or whiplash injury.

296. Which one of the following statements is false regarding the relationship of alcohol to head trauma?

a. Alcohol is a frequent contributory factor in motor vehicle, diving, and other accidents that result in head trauma.
b. Alcohol withdrawal may complicate recovery from post-traumatic coma.
c. Alcohol use in patients surviving major head trauma increases the incidence of seizures.
d. Although all the above are true, alcohol is a good sedative and minor tranquilizer in patients who have survived minor head trauma.
e. Patients with head trauma who use alcohol are particularly susceptible to violence, as in the episodic dyscontrol syndrome.

answer: d. Alcohol is neither a good sedative nor minor tranquilizer in patients who have survived minor head trauma. It induces insomnia and excessive daytime sleepiness. Excessive use, which occurs in many head trauma patients, impairs memory and judgment. Post-traumatic insomnia and anxiety may require specific medications, possibly antidepressants, and, for a stress disorder, psychotherapy. Patients with prolonged anxiety and insomnia should be investigated for cognitive impairments.

297. When confronted with patients who have sustained multiple trauma, attention is often exclusively directed at head injuries. During examinations and transportation, an unstable cervical spine can lead to spinal cord injury. Which of the following are complications of cervical spine injury?

a. Respiratory failure
b. Quadriplegia or paraplegia
c. Herniated intervertebral disks
d. Urinary retention
e. All of the above

answer: e. Acute cervical spinal cord injury is sometimes overshadowed by head injury. Facial and scalp lacerations, which bleed profusely, are compelling and distracting. Manipulation of the head and neck can be disastrous. Combined head and neck injuries occur in motor vehicle accidents in which the face or forehead strikes the windshield and the neck snaps backward. This type of injury also occurs in diving accidents in which people strike their head in a shallow pool and compress their cervical spine.

298. A 22-year-old Marine, who survived a penetrating frontal lobe shrapnel injury, has episodes of violent, aggressive, destructive behavior. These episodes occur when he drinks only one or two beers and are precipitated by little provocation. A careful neurologic examination reveals hyper-reflexia on the left side and a Babinski sign on the right. His MRI scan shows bilateral frontal lucencies. An EEG shows intermittent sharp waves that are phased reversed in the left temporal lobe and intermittent slowing when he is drowsy. Which one of the following should a consultant psychiatrist first recommend?

a. Further neurologic evaluation
b. Psychotherapy
c. Use of an anticonvulsant
d. Use of a minor or major tranquilizer
e. None of the above

> **answer:** a. The patient probably has episodic dyscontrol syndrome, which is violent behavior—often with aggression (directed violence)—that typically follows congenital or acquired head trauma. Patients often have abnormal reflexes. Although their EEGs have minor, nonspecific abnormalities and anticonvulsants may ameliorate the outbursts, the disorder is not epilepsy. In this case, the sharp waves on the EEG might indicate seizures apart from the violence. He should undergo EEG-TV monitoring that would determine if he has seizures, but the episodes of violence are probably not ictal events.

299. A 68-year-old woman loses her accuracy in her relatively complicated assembly-line job. She is brought by her family for evaluation for depression and dementia. Soon after the interview begins, she becomes upset and attempts to put on her robe. However, she becomes confused and frustrated. She tries to put both hands through the left sleeve. Then she puts the robe on backward. Finally, she is perplexed as to how to extricate herself. Which process is she displaying?

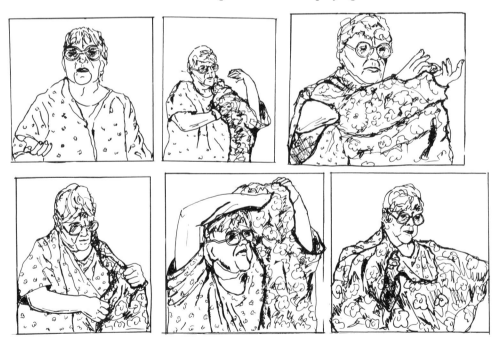

a. Dementia
b. Apraxia
c. Dressing apraxia
d. Left-right confusion
e. Neglect
f. Anosognosia
g. Inattention

> **answer:** c. Dressing apraxia is an uncommon, dramatic manifestation of non-dominant hemisphere injury, such as a tumor (as in this case), with the parietal lobe being the primary site of involvement. Dressing apraxia is an inability to

clothe oneself caused by a combination of visual-spatial impairment, somatotopagnosia, and motor apraxia. Like other apraxias, dressing apraxia is more than inattention, visual loss, or lack of sensation on one side of the body. Patients with dressing apraxia are befuddled or stymied when attempting to put on a coat, shirt, or hospital robe. Unlike patients with anosognosia, those with dressing apraxia are aware of their problem and are frustrated.

Examiners, wishing to demonstrate the phenomenon, will ask the patient to dress in a hospital robe with one sleeve turned inside-out. Even when warned about the sleeve's being reversed, patients will be unable to dress. Not appreciating the problem or being unable to solve it, they tend to change the normal sleeve into an abnormal sleeve, reverse any of their corrections, put both arms through the same sleeve, or drastically misalign the two sides. (The MRI scan of the patient is reproduced in Figure 20–19.)

300.   Which of the following tumors originate from glial cells?

a.   Astrocytomas
b.   Glioblastoma multiforme
c.   Oligodendrogliomas
d.   Lymphomas
e.   Meningiomas

answer: a, b, c

301.   A 31-year-old right-handed waiter has had partial complex seizures since he was 16 years old. His seizures have been refractory to anticonvulsants, except in intoxicating doses. CCTV documented that his seizures originate in a right-sided temporal lobe focus. MRI showed atrophy of the right hippocampus. PET could not be performed. Which of the following is probably the best therapy?

a.   Partial or complete right temporal lobectomy
b.   A commissurotomy
c.   Adding an antidepressant
d.   None of the above

answer: a. Surgery that removes an epileptic focus has been a major medical advance that, in skilled hands, benefits about 75 per cent of selected epilepsy patients. PET scans are unnecessary. Preoperative Wada tests are, however, often used to determine if the proposed surgery will lead to aphasia. A commissurotomy has limited usefulness: blocking the spread to seizures through the corpus callosum.

302.   Which statements are true regarding EEG changes that follow ECT?

a.   Unilateral ECT is associated with predominantly unilateral beta activity.
b.   Bilateral ECT induces generalized theta and delta activity.
c.   Greater post-ECT slowing is associated with greater antidepressant effect.
d.   Greater post-ECT slowing is associated with greater amnesia.

answer: b, c, d. Unilateral ECT is associated with unilateral EEG slowing (theta and delta activity).

303.   What structure lies immediately medial and anterior to the mesial surface of the temporal lobe?

a.   The temporal bone
b.   The eye
c.   The sphenoid wing
d.   The petrous pyramid
e.   The nasopharynx

answer: c. The mesial surface of the temporal lobe is immediately adjacent to the sphenoid wing. Insertion of nasopharyngeal EEG electrodes places them as close as possible to the mesial surface of the temporal lobe. Scalp EEG electrodes, which are placed over the temporal bones, are lateral to the temporal lobe's lateral surface.

304. In which lobe of the cerebrum (a-e) are the following structures (1–8) located?

1. Amygdala
2. Angular gyrus
3. Nucleus basalis of Meynert
4. Olfactory nerves
5. Broca's area
6. Medial longitudinal fasciculus
7. Uncus
8. Thalamus

a. Frontal lobe
b. Parietal lobe
c. Occipital lobe
d. Temporal lobe
e. Deep in the cerebrum
f. Cerebellum
g. In the dorsal, medial aspect of the pons and midbrain

answer: 1-d, 2-b, 3-e, 4-a, 5-a, 6-g, 7-d, 8-e (diencephalon)

305. Which structure is immediately medial and superior to the hypothalamus?

a. Thalamus
b. Corpus of Luysii

c. Corpus callosum
d. Third ventricle

answer: d

306. A 10-year-old boy has had three seizures during the previous 4 years. All have occurred during sleep at night and have consisted of facial paresthesias, abnormal sensations in his right arm, and speech arrest. His neurologic examination, routine laboratory testing, and an MRI are all normal. An EEG performed during sleep shows centrotemporal spikes. Which two of the following statements regarding the boy are true?

a. He has rolandic epilepsy.
b. He has a sleep disorder, not a seizure disorder.
c. As an adult, he is likely to develop epilepsy.
d. This condition will almost certainly disappear by the time he is 21 tears old.

answer: a, d. He has rolandic epilepsy, which is an inherited seizure disorder peculiar to children that is readily responsive to anticonvulsants.

307. In which conditions do examination of brains usually reveal intracytoplasmic eosinophilic inclusion bodies?

a. Patients with rigidity, tremor, and bradykinesia
b. Former boxers with dysarthria, cognitive changes, and rigidity
c. Elderly patients who develop dementia accompanied by mild extrapyramidal signs
d. Schizophrenic patients who have medication-induced parkinsonism

answer: a, c. Lewy bodies are routinely found in the brains of patients with Parkinson's disease or diffuse Lewy body disease.

308. Which conditions are associated with an increased incidence of suicide?

a. Huntington's disease
b. Absence (petit mal) seizures
c. Partial complex seizures
d. Cerebellar lesions
e. Spinal cord lesions

f. Multiple sclerosis
g. Guillain-Barré syndrome
h. AIDS dementia
i. Cerebral palsy

answer: a, c, e, f, h. In most of these illnesses, dementia causes impetuous behavior and lack of judgment. Spinal cord lesions, which usually result from gunshot wounds, motor vehicle accidents, or athletic injuries in young men, are associated with despondency that leads to suicide.

309. Which three statements are true regarding the relationship of interictal violence to epilepsy?

a. Violent behavior is no more prevalent among patients with partial complex seizures than other seizures.
b. The consensus among neurologists is that epilepsy does not cause crime, but that epilepsy, head trauma, and other brain injuries lead to conditions, such as poor impulse control and lower socioeconomic status, that predispose people to crime.
c. Interictal violence often stems from schizophrenia or mental retardation.

d. Interictal violence is associated with childhood-onset seizures.

e. Interictal violence can be reduced with benzodiazepines.

answer: a, b, c

310. In which patients might brain biopsies reveal intracytoplasmic eosinophilic inclusion bodies?

a. A 78-year-old person, who had encephalitis as a young adult, with tremor, rigidity, and bradykinesia

b. A 70-year-old person who presents with 6 months of dementia, rigidity, and bradykinesia

c. A 40-year-old retired boxer with slurred speech, festinating gait, mild dementia, and resting tremor

d. A 30-year-old former intravenous drug abuser with tremor, rigidity, and bradykinesia

answer: a, b. Intracytoplasmic eosinophilic inclusion bodies—Lewy bodies— are found in the substantia nigra in Parkinson's disease, especially if in the postencephalitic variety (a). They are also found in diffuse Lewy body disease, which causes dementia and mild parkinsonism (b). However, Lewy bodies are not found in dementia pugilistica (c) or MPTP-induced parkinsonism (d).

311. Called to evaluate a 63-year-old man who demands to be released from the oncology service of a general hospital, a psychiatrist finds the patient to be relatively calm, oriented, and aware that he has "a melanoma that will be fatal in the near future." Physical examination and laboratory tests reveal no major abnormalities; however, the patient seems to fall to his left and be inattentive to friends and family who stand on his left side. Before making a determination about whether the patient is competent, which of the following tests should the psychiatrist request?

a. Serum calcium determination
b. EEG
c. Mini-Mental Status Examination
d. CT or MRI of the brain
e. Liver function tests

answer: d. Melanomas tends to spread widely by blood-borne dissemination. Although the patient seems to be making a rational decision, an element of anosognosia might be present in view of his left-sided inattention and motor difficulties. A CT or MRI would be the best test to detect a metastasis in the nondominant parietal lobe. Of course, the psychiatrist would have to judge whether an element of anosognosia rendered the patient incompetent.

312. Which is the single most commonly occurring risk factor for falls in the elderly?

a. Transient ischemic attacks
b. Use of sedatives or hypnotics
c. Cardiac arrhythmias
d. Neurologic disease

answer: b

313. A psychiatrist is called because a patient has developed agitated, belligerent behavior. He is a 25-year-old methadone-maintenance patient hospitalized after his first seizure. A previous CT showed a small, ring-enhancing lesion in the right frontal lobe. He had started taking phenytoin and anti-toxoplasmosis medications. Methadone was continued. Of the following, which is the most likely cause of his behavior?

a. Cerebral toxoplasmosis
b. AIDS dementia
c. Phenytoin-enhanced hepatic metabolism
d. Anti-toxoplasmosis medications

answer: c. Phenytoin induces hepatic enzymes that metabolize other medications. Instituting phenytoin in methadone patients can thus precipitate narcotic withdrawal. Individuals in methadone-maintenance programs are often HIV positive because of prior or concomitant intravenous drug abuse. Many have AIDS. This patient may have cerebral toxoplasmosis, but a small lesion in the right frontal lobe is not likely to be the cause of his behavioral disturbances.

314.   Which three are characteristics of neurosyphilis in AIDS patients?

a.   Neurosyphilis is likely to be accompanied by ocular involvement.
b.   The diagnosis may be obscured by negative serologic tests.
c.   Treatment with penicillin may be deleterious.
d.   Neurosyphilis occurs rarely in AIDS patients.
e.   The usual doses of penicillin may be inadequate.

answer: a, b, e

315.   Which two are the greatest risk factors for dementia in AIDS patients?

a.   The CD4 count below 1,000 cells/cu mm
b.   Being HIV positive
c.   Anemia
d.   Depression
e.   Weight loss

answer: c, e. Dementia is usually a relatively late manifestation of AIDS. It occurs when immunodeficiency is pronounced and anemia and systemic symptoms have developed. A low CD4 count is an early manifestation of AIDS and long precedes dementia in almost all cases. Only profound CD4 depletion, such as less than 50 cells/cu mm, is a risk factor for AIDS dementia.

316.   Although the distinction's value has been questioned, many neurologist continue to divide dementia into cortical and subcortical varieties. Which of the following illnesses are considered examples of cortical (c) or subcortical (sc) dementia?

a.   AIDS dementia
b.   Alzheimer's disease
c.   Huntington's disease
d.   Normal-pressure hydrocephalus
e.   Parkinson's disease
f.   Pick's disease

answer: a-sc, b-c, c-sc, d-sc, e-sc, f-c. The distinction is arbitrary because several of these illnesses have overlapping features. The dementia in both AIDS and Huntington's disease, for example, has cortical as well as subcortical features.

317.   Which one of the following statements concerning hallucinations in Alzheimer's disease is false?

a.   Hallucinations are mostly visual, but are sometimes auditory or olfactory.
b.   They are associated with a rapid decline in cognitive function.
c.   They have little prognostic value.
d.   They are associated with clearly abnormal EEGs.

answer: c. They are clearly indicative of a poor prognosis.

318.   If a man is 45 years old, in which decade of life is he?

a.   Third
b.   Fourth
c.   Fifth
d.   Sixth

answer: c. This nomenclature is often a source of confusion.

319.   Which statement most closely describes the gate control theory?

a.   Descending pathways inhibit pain.
b.   Endogenous opioids suppress pain.
c.   Activity of large-diameter, heavily myelinated fibers inhibit pain transmission by small, sparsely myelinated fibers.
d.   Pain transmission is carefully regulated by a balance of substance P and serotonin.

answer: c

320.   Which of the following statements are true regarding the periaqueductal gray matter?

a.   Stimulation of the periaqueductal gray matter produces analgesia by liberating endogenous opioids.

b.   Hemorrhage into the periaqueductal gray matter is associated with thiamine deficiency.

c.   The periaqueductal gray matter surrounds the aqueduct of Sylvius, which is the passage for CSF between the third and fourth ventricles.

d.   The periaqueductal gray matter is in the midbrain.

e.   All of the above

answer: e

321.   Which are characteristics of enkephalins?

a.   They are peptides.

b.   They are neurotransmitters.

c.   Naloxone inhibits enkephalins.

d.   Serotonin inhibits enkephalins.

answer: a, b, c

322.   Which of the following substances serves as the neurotransmitter for pain?

a.   Enkephalins

b.   Serotonin

c.   Substance P

d.   Endogenous opioids

answer: c

323.   Nonsteroidal anti-inflammatory drugs (NSAIDs) can be as potent analgesics as opioids. In which other ways are they similar to opioids?

a.   They are addictive.

b.   They produce greater analgesia with increasingly higher doses.

c.   They promote tolerance to the analgesia.

d.   They cause gastrointestinal bleeding.

e.   None of the above

answer: e. Unlike opioids, NSAIDs are not addictive and do not cause tolerance to themselves. Also, at a certain dose, their analgesic effect reaches a maximum, ceiling effect. Increased doses do not produce additional analgesia. Moreover, additional medication will expose patients to side effects, particularly gastrointestinal bleeding.

324.   What is the primary mechanism of action of NSAIDs?

a.   They inhibit prostaglandin synthesis.

b.   They enhance serotonin activity.

c.   They enhance opioid activity.

d.   They cause opioid-like psychological side effects.

answer: a

325.   Which of the following two features are included in a syndrome that mimics autism in 3- to 6-year-old girls?

a.   Stereotypical hand-wringing movements

b.   Acquired microcephaly

c.   Low-set, large ears

d.   Large testicles

e.   Simian palm crease

answer: a, b. Rett syndrome, which has prominent autistic features, is characterized by repetitive hand movements and acquired microcephaly in young girls. Boys with mental retardation from the fragile X syndrome have large, low-set ears and large testicles. The simian palm crease is a characteristic of trisomy 21.

326.   A first-grade boy runs with his left hand fisted. When asked to walk on the sides of his feet, the left thumb tends to flex toward the palm, as though he were starting to make a fist. Which three other stigmata of neurologic injury can be expected?

a.   Hyperactive DTRs in the left arm

b.   Mental retardation

c.   Clumsy movements with the left arm

d.   Posturing of the arm

e.   Hypoactive DTRs in the left arm

f.   Athetosis

answer: a, c, d. He is displaying a "cortical thumb." This sign usually indicates congenital corticospinal tract injury that, in turn, would be accompanied by hyperactive DTRs and clumsiness. A unilateral cortical thumb and other soft signs are indicative of (contralateral) congenital cerebral injury; however, when they occur bilaterally, they have less significance. After strokes or traumatic brain injury, adults may develop a cortical thumb.

327.   Which are four advantages of nonsteroidal anti-inflammatory drugs (NSAIDs) over opioids?

a.   NSAIDs do not create tolerance.
b.   Additional NSAIDs produce greater analgesia, i.e., they have no ceiling.
c.   Patients develop no withdrawal symptoms when NSAIDs are stopped.
d.   NSAIDs can be as effective as opioids.
e.   NSAIDs have virtually no psychological side effects.
f.   NSAIDs produce gastric irritation much less frequently than opioids.

answer: a, c, d, e

328.   Where do peripheral nerves carrying pain sensation synapse with ascending spinal cord tracts?

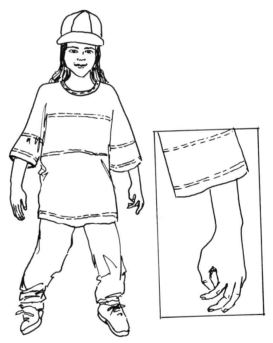

a.   Sympathetic nervous system
b.   In the spinal cord
c.   Lateral spinothalamic tract
d.   Substantia gelatinosa

answer: b, d. PNS fibers enter the spinal cord and synapse with the lateral spinothalamic tract in the substantia gelatinosa. The spinothalamic tract crosses the spinal cord and ascends to the thalamus where it undergoes another synapse.

329.   Which two of the following painful conditions are considered examples of neuropathic pain?

a.   Reflex sympathetic dystrophy
b.   Brain tumors
c.   Postherpetic neuralgia
d.   Trigeminal neuralgia
e.   Thalamic infarction

answer: c, d. When nerves are injured directly, such as in postherpetic neuralgia, the pain is called *neuropathic*. This type of pain is severe, but partially responsive to anticonvulsants.

330. Which four statements are true concerning reflex sympathetic dystrophy?

a. The disorder is mediated, at least in part, by the sympathetic nervous system.
b. Dry, shiny, and scaly skin is a characteristic.
c. Because the pain is increased by touch, patients protect their affected limb.
d. Sympathetic blockage will provide temporary relief in most cases.
e. The pain is confined to the injured nerves' dermatomes.
f. Anticonvulsants provide a cure and diagnostic confirmation.

> *answer:* a, b, c, d

331. Why is succinylcholine used in conjunction with electroshock therapy?

a. It makes the brain more susceptible to the beneficial effects of ECT because it lowers the seizure threshold.
b. It relaxes muscles by binding to the neuromuscular junction ACh receptors.
c. It reduces subsequent amnesia.
d. It is given to enhance ECT effect, but its usefulness has never been established.
e. It reduces oral secretions that the patient could aspirate.
f. It interferes with cerebral ACh and induces amnesia for the event.

> *answer:* b. Succinylcholine blocks the neuromuscular junction and prevents ECT-induced seizures from causing massive muscle contractions. These seizures can cause fractures and other bodily injuries. Succinylcholine does not cross the blood-brain barrier and thus would not influence the seizure threshold or memory pathways. Atropine is administered to reduce secretions.

332. An AIDS patient has the slow development of dementia, aphasia, left hemiparesis, and pseudobulbar palsy. A noncontrast CT scan of the head and CSF analysis reveal no abnormalities. Which one of the following is the most likely diagnosis?

a. Toxoplasmosis
b. Lymphoma
c. Cysticercosis
d. Progressive multifocal leukoencephalopathy (PML)
e. Multiple sclerosis (MS)

> *answer:* d. The patient's signs—pseudobulbar palsy, aphasia, and left hemiparesis—indicate multiple lesions. Toxoplasmosis, cerebral lymphoma, and progressive multifocal leukoencephalopathy (PML) are complications of AIDS, but PML is a relatively late developing complication. Toxoplasmosis, cysticercosis, PML, and MS cause multiple lesions. CT scans will reveal most cases of toxoplasmosis, lymphoma, and cysticercosis; however, MRI scans are usually required to demonstrate the demyelination induced by PML and MS.

333. Which condition is not associated with cerebral atrophy?

a. Dementia pugilistica
b. AIDS dementia
c. Down's syndrome
d. Schizophrenia
e. Subacute sclerosing panencephalitis (SSPE)

> *answer:* e. Although schizophrenia is not uniformly associated with cerebral atrophy, about 20 per cent of patients with poor response to treatment and other indicators of a poor prognosis have cerebral atrophy.

334. Which are three features of Pick's disease that are not found in Alzheimer's disease?

a. Dementia
b. Familial tendency
c. Oral exploration
d. Argentophilic inclusions
e. Age-proportional incidence
f. Neuron depletion in the nucleus basalis of Meynert
g. CAT depletion in the cerebral cortex
h. CT showing selective frontal pole atrophy

answer: c, d, h. Except for elements of the Klüver-Bucy syndrome and preserved spatial orientation in Pick's disease, the clinical features of Pick's and Alzheimer's diseases are virtually indistinguishable. Moreover, both have a familial tendency (although it is more pronounced in Pick's), produce neuron depletion in the nucleus basalis of Meynert, and deplete CAT in the cerebral cortex. By way of contrast, the incidence of Alzheimer's increases in proportion to age, but the incidence in Pick's disease peaks in late middle age. Whereas the CT scan in Pick's disease shows frontal or temporal lobe atrophy, in most cases of Alzheimer's disease it shows generalized atrophy. Also, Pick's disease is associated with diagnostic silver staining (argentophilic) inclusions in the neurons.

335. Which one of the following MRI abnormalities is most closely associated with chronic schizophrenia that has been resistant to treatment?

a. Cerebellar atrophy
b. Corpus callosum atrophy
c. Symmetry of the planum temporale
d. Enlargement of the lateral ventricles

answer: d. Schizophrenic patients with chronic, progressive illness that is resistant to treatment have large lateral ventricles accompanied by a large third ventricle and cerebral cortical atrophy. In addition, their amygdala and hippocampus are decreased in volume, and the planum temporale is unlikely to have normal symmetry.

336. Which two of the following are advantages of MRI over PET imaging of the brain in patients suspected of having Parkinson's or Huntington's disease?

a. Greater spatial resolution
b. Ability to see metabolic changes before clinical signs
c. Ability to see metabolic changes before anatomic changes
d. Less cost

answer: a, d. In Parkinson's and Huntington's diseases, PET scans, although expensive and anatomically crude, show metabolic abnormalities before clinical signs or anatomic changes are apparent.

337. Which one of the following results from sequential mental status tests indicates Alzheimer's disease?

a. A precipitous decline in the first 6 months
b. A decline over 6 months and then a plateau for 2 years
c. A borderline score in a well-educated individual
d. An uneven decline, including some plateaus, over 2 years

answer: d. A precipitous decline suggests a rapidly progressive illness, such as Creutzfeldt-Jakob's disease, AIDS, or a glioblastoma. A plateau of 2 years or more is unusual for Alzheimer's disease. A borderline score in well-educated individuals is a common diagnostic dilemma. They might not have been so bright in the first place; they could have developed other problems, such as alcoholism; or they could have depression (pseudodementia), rather than dementia. An uneven decline, including some plateaus, is typical of Alzheimer's disease.

338. Match the view (a-c) with its common description (1–3).

a. Transaxial
b. Coronal
c. Sagittal
1. Front-to-back or head-on
2. Top-down view
3. Side view

answer: a-2, b-1, c-3

339. Numerous soldiers were exposed to Agent Orange during the war in South Vietnam. Which of the following neurologic problems have been found, in scientific reviews, to have been attributed to Agent Orange exposure?

a. Brain tumors
b. Peripheral neuropathy
c. Cognitive impairment
d. Neuropsychologic deficits
e. None of the above

answer: e. No evidence has correlated Agent Orange exposure to any neurologic problem. Intense exposure to hydrocarbon solvents, such as toluene and hexane, can cause combinations of pyramidal and cerebellar damage, peripheral neuropathy, and cognitive changes.

340. In which two regions of the brain are pathologic changes most pronounced in Alzheimer's disease?

a. Primary motor cortex
b. Occipital cortex
c. Association areas, such as the parietal-temporal junction
d. Olfactory lobe
e. Limbic system, especially the hippocampus

answer: c, e. These regions are especially atrophic and contain high concentrations of plaques and tangles.

341. Which of the following medications elevate the serum prolactin concentration?

a. Thorazine
b. Bromocriptine
c. Haloperidol
d. Clozapine
e. Pergolide
f. L-dopa
g. Resperidone

answer: a, c, g. Dopamine normally inhibits the release of prolactin. Dopamine agonists also inhibit its release. Thus, dopamine-blocking neuroleptics trigger prolactin release and produce elevated serum concentrations. Prolactin concentration is also elevated for about 20 minutes after most generalized and partial complex seizures. Prolactinomas, a common pituitary adenoma, secrete prolactin. Bromocriptine can inhibit prolactinomas and obviate surgery.

342. Which two of the following nuclei constitute the corpus striatum?

a. Caudate
b. Putamen
c. Globus pallidus
d. Subthalamic
e. Substantia nigra

answer: a, b

343. In hepatolenticular degeneration, to which two structures does "lenticular" refer?

a. Caudate
b. Putamen
c. Globus pallidus
d. Subthalamic
e. Substantia nigra
f. Corticospinal tract
g. Thalamus
h. The liver
i. The cornea

answer: b, c. Being adjacent and forming a pie-shaped or lens-like structure, the putamen and globus pallidus form the lenticular nuclei. These basal ganglia structures are usually damaged, along with the liver, in hepatolenticular degeneration (Wilson's disease). The cornea, which develops Kayser-Fleischer rings, kidneys, and other organs may also be damaged.

344. Which two of the following are common manifestations of basal ganglia damage?

a. Paresis
b. Spasticity
c. Akinesia
d. Impairment of postural reflexes
e. Essential tremor
f. Seizures

answer: c, d. Basal ganglia damage causes many involuntary movements, but not essential tremor, tics, or focal dystonias. Paradoxically, it causes slowed or absent voluntary movements. Basal ganglia damage also changes muscle tone, most often inducing rigidity. It leads to the loss of postural reflexes.

345. Match the speech pattern (a-c) with the disorder (1–3).

a. Strained and strangled
b. Hypophonic and monotonous
c. Scanning

1. MS affecting the cerebellum
2. Parkinson's disease
3. Spasmodic dysphonia

answer: a-3, b-2, c-1

346. Which one of the following is not characteristic of apolipoprotein E (Apo-E)?

a. Apo-E is cholesterol-carrying protein, produced in the liver and brain.
b. Apo-E binds amyloid.
c. Apo-E is encoded on chromosome 19 in three isoforms: Apo-E2, Apo-E3, and Apo-E4.
d. Apo-E is a risk factor for cerebrovascular accidents (strokes).

answer: d. Being homozygote for an Apo-E allele, Apo-E4, increases the risk of Alzheimer's disease several fold.

347. Which structures are depigmented in Parkinson's disease?

a. Substantia nigra
b. Locus ceruleus
c. Dorsal motor nuclei

d. Anterior thalamic nuclei
e. Lewy bodies

answer: a, b, c

348. A 72-year-old man is brought by his family for the evaluation of dementia that developed along with mild rigidity and bradykinesia during the past several months. If he were to undergo an autopsy immediately, what might the brain show?

a. Plaques and tangles in the hippocampus
b. Lewy bodies in the cerebral cortex
c. Lewy bodies in the substantia nigra
d. Atrophy of the head of the caudate

answer: b. He probably has diffuse Lewy body disease. Lewy bodies in the substantia nigra are characteristic of Parkinson's disease, which does not cause dementia at its onset. Alzheimer's disease causes plaques and tangles in the cerebral cortex and especially the hippocampus, but it usually does not present with either pyramidal or extrapyramidal signs. Huntington's disease characteristically causes atrophy of the head of the caudate nuclei.

349. In the treatment of Parkinson's disease, with which dopamine receptors do dopamine agonists stimulate?

a. D_1
b. D_2

c. Both
d. Neither

answer: b. All commercially available dopamine agonists stimulate D_2. They may stimulate or inhibit D_1.

350. In a pallidotomy for treatment of Parkinson's disease, in which structure is the lesion placed?

a. The putamen
b. The basal ganglia medial to the putamen
c. The corpus striatum

d. The substantia nigra
e. The thalamus

answer: b. The globus pallidus is medial to the putamen. Lesions placed in the globus pallidus markedly reduce rigidity and bradykinesia in the contralateral limbs. Lesions placed in the thalamus reduce tremor, but have much less effect on the more incapacitating symptoms.

351. A 50-year-old draftsman complains that his hand forms a painful cramp several minutes after he starts to work. Early in his career, he would develop similar cramps only after many hours of nonstop work. Which condition forces his hand into his position?

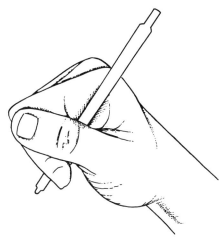

a. Psychogenic disturbance
b. Age-related disturbance
c. Motor neuron disease
d. Focal dystonia
e. Exercised-induced cramp

answer: d. He has developed writer's cramp, which is an occupational cramp. These disorders are focal dystonias, not psychologic reactions. After several decades, musicians, writers, draftsmen, and other workers who use their hand in a repetitive fashion sometimes develop focal dystonias related to their work. His writer's cramp might respond to botulinum toxin injections carefully placed into the muscles that go into spasm.

352. A 60-year-old man has been developing involuntary contractions of all the facial muscles. The contractions, which began around the eyes, are bilateral, symmetric, and accumulate to have a duration of several seconds. He remains conscious during the episodes. Jaw, tongue, and ocular muscles are unaffected. Which type of illness most likely underlies the involuntary movement?

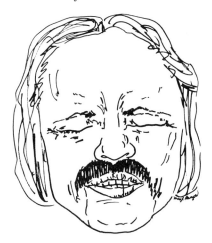

a. Seizure disorder
b. Iatrogenic illness
c. Cranial dystonia
d. Psychogenic condition

answer: c. He has Meige's syndrome, which is a cranial dystonia that is more extensive than blepharospasm. Most individuals with cranial dystonias have no history of psychiatric illness or exposure to neuroleptics. When tardive dyskinesia involves facial muscles, it usually involves the tongue and jaw muscles.

Meige's syndrome and blepharospasm respond to botulinum injections, but the tongue cannot be injected easily because if it were weakened, it might fall back and occlude the airway.

353.   Which three illnesses result from trinucleotide repeats?

a. Huntington's disease
b. Wernicke-Korsakoff
c. Wilson's disease
d. Dystonia

e. Fragile X syndrome
f.   Duchenne's muscular dystrophy
g. Myotonic dystrophy

answer: a, e, g. Excessive repeats of three nucleotide bases in the DNA create those illnesses. Moreover, the instability of trinucleotide repeats causes these illnesses to appear in younger family members in successive generations. The appearance in younger generations is called anticipation.

354.   In which three ways does the DNA in the juvenile and adult varieties of Huntington's disease differ?

a. Unlike the DNA in the adult variety, the DNA in the juvenile variety typically has more than 60 trinucleotide repeats.
b. The juvenile variety has a greater tendency toward anticipation in successive generations.
c. The juvenile variety usually results from the father's unstable, abnormal DNA.
d. The juvenile variety tends to cause rigidity, rather than chorea.
e. The juvenile variety affects girls more often than boys.

answer: a, c, d

355.   Which nuclei are most atrophied in Huntington's disease?

a. Lenticular nuclei
b. Corpus striatum

c. Subthalamic nuclei
d. Mammillary bodies

answer: b. Atrophy of the head of the caudate nuclei is characteristic of Huntington's disease.

356.   A 33-year-old person with AIDS develops vision impairment, confusion, and word-finding difficulties. His MRI is shown below. Which process is causing his symptoms?

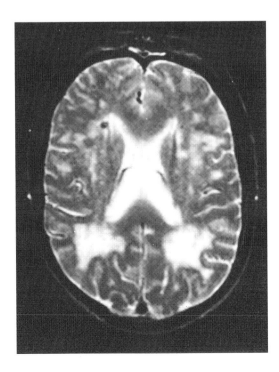

a. HIV encephalitis
b. Multiple sclerosis (MS)
c. Toxoplasmosis
d. Progressive multifocal leukoencephalopathy (PML)
e. Lymphoma

answer: d. The MRI shows two large, hyperintense lesions in the white matter of the occipital lobes. Similar, scattered lesions are located in the dominant hemisphere (on the right side of the MRI). The occipital lesions have caused the visual difficulties. The dominant hemisphere lesions have caused the language problems.

HIV encephalitis does not cause discrete lesions. Like PML, MS can cause white matter lesions. However, this case is unlikely to be MS: MS is rare in AIDS patients, such lesions would have to be a manifestation of long-standing MS, and the lesions would surround the ventricles, i.e., be periventricular. Toxoplasmosis, a common complication of AIDS, causes circular lesions that are not restricted to the white matter. Cerebral lymphomas in AIDS patients are more commonly singular than multifocal.

357. A 60-year-old man, who had been in excellent health, develops apathy, inattention, and a flattened affect during a 3-week vacation. His MRI scan is shown. Which is the most likely diagnosis?

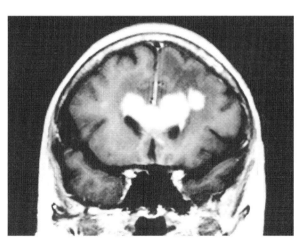 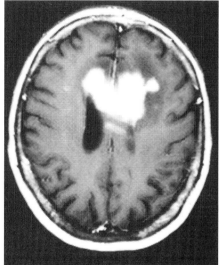

a. A frontal lobe glioblastoma
b. Multiple sclerosis (MS)
c. Lymphoma
d. Progressive multifocal leukoencephalopathy (PML)

answer: a. The MRI (on the *left*, the coronal view, and the *right*, axial view), shows a hyperintense lesion in both frontal lobes, spreading through the corpus callosum. There is relatively little mass effect or surrounding edema. This pattern, sometime referred to as a "butterfly," is indicative of glioblastomas.

His symptoms are manifestations of a frontal lobe lesion. His age at the onset of the illness and lack of risk factors virtually exclude MS, lymphoma, and PML. In contrast, glioblastomas are relatively common in this age group. Metastatic carcinoma is a possibility, but metastases are usually multiple, surrounded by edema, and do not spread through the corpus callosum.

358. With which neurotransmitter alteration is Huntington's disease most closely associated?

a. Increased GABA
b. Decreased GABA
c. Decreased NMDA
d. Increased ACh
e. Decreased ACh

answer: b. GABA is markedly decreased. ACh is also decreased, but less severely than GABA. The NMDA receptor has increased activity in Huntington's disease.

359. Which two illnesses are associated with genetic anticipation?

a. Muscular dystrophy
b. Myotonic dystrophy
c. Dystonia musculorum deformans
d. Huntington's disease

answer: b, d. The tendency of individuals in successive generations to show signs of the illness at a younger age, termed *anticipation*, is attributable to the instability of abnormal DNA.

360. Which of the following findings indicate a nonaccidental head injury in an infant?

a. Retinal hemorrhages
b. Discrepancy between history and contusions
c. CT or MRI showing cerebral atrophy
d. CT or MRI showing dural hemorrhages of varying ages
e. Absence of the corpus callosum

answer: a, b, c, d. Blood of varying ages in the face, retinae, subdural spaces, and brain of an infant indicates nonaccidental trauma, i.e., the shaken baby syndrome. Absence of the corpus callosum is a congenital defect.

361. Which three of the following involuntary movements are typically preceded by an urge to move?

a. Essential tremor
b. Tics
c. Stereotypies
d. Akathisia
e. Chorea
f. Restless leg syndrome

answer: b, d, f

362. Which two conditions typically produce brief, random, involuntary movements, accompanied by motor impersistence, that develop over several days in a 10-year-old child?

a. Tourette's syndrome
b. Lyme disease
c. Mononucleosis
d. Sydenham's chorea
e. Neuroleptic-induced dystonia
f. Withdrawal-emergent dyskinesia

answer: d, f. The child has chorea, which indicates Sydenham's chorea or withdrawal-emergent dyskinesia. Tourette's syndrome evolves slowly and produces stereotyped tics. Neuroleptic-induced dystonia produces backward extension of the head and neck (retrocollis) and is rare in children. Lyme disease and mononucleosis, which both occur in children, do not regularly produce chorea.

363. Which of the following children is most apt to have a mitochondria disorder?

a. A 10-year-old boy who develops dystonia of one foot that begins to spread to the ipsilateral hand
b. An 8-year-old boy who has had a head toss intermittently for 2 years and then develops an intermittent cough for which there is no pulmonary explanation
c. A 6-year-old girl who develops polyuria and polydipsia
d. An 11-year-old autistic girl
e. A 9-year-old boy with mild mental retardation
f. A 9-year-old boy who is short and mildly mentally retarded and has repeated hospitalizations for lactic acidosis

answer: f. The lactic acidosis indicates a systemic metabolic impairment. Curiously, it occurs on an intermittent basis.

364. In which three ways does palatal myoclonus differ from classic movement disorders?

a. Palatal myoclonus results from an injury in the inferior olivary nucleus, rather than the basal ganglia.

b. It persists during sleep, stupor, and coma.
c. It is regularly associated with dementia.
d. It often results from an infarction of the medulla.

answer: a, b, d. The inferior olivary nuclei are located in the medulla. Injuries specifically affecting that region of the brain do not cause dementia.

365. To which mechanism is clozapine's freedom from extrapyramidal side effects attributable?

a. D_1 dopamine receptor blockade
b. D_2 dopamine receptor blockade
c. ACh receptor blockade
d. NMDA receptor blockade
e. GABA receptor stimulation
f. GABA receptor blockade
g. D_4 dopamine receptor blockade

answer: b. Clozapine has little affinity for caudate D_2 dopamine and GABA receptors, but a relatively high affinity for muscarinic ACh receptors and possibly D_4 dopamine receptors.

366. An 18-year-old suburban high-school student, with newly developing social and academic difficulties, begins to have rapid, involuntary facial movements and a continual cough. The neurologist finds an otherwise normal neurologic examination including cognitive function, MRI, EEG, and blood tests to a determination of HIV, serum ceruloplasmin, Lyme titer, and syphilis tests. She concludes that the patient has no primary neurologic illness and refers him for a psychiatry consultation. During the course of a psychiatric evaluation, which other testing should be performed as soon as possible?

a. A complete family history
b. IQ and other academic-psychologic testing
c. Therapeutic trial of haloperidol
d. Testing for multiple sclerosis (MS)
e. Other testing

answer: a, b, e. The neurologist is "half-right." The development of tics occurs before age 13 years in 90 per cent of patients. Therefore, development of tics— vocal or respiratory as well as motor—in a teenager should prompt evaluation for use of cocaine and other stimulants. MS does not usually cause movement disorders because it is a white matter disease: The basal ganglia are gray matter. Huntington's disease and Sydenham's chorea would be very unlikely in this situation.

367. Which two features are present in the involuntary neck movements of tardive dystonia, but are absent in idiopathic spasmodic torticollis?

a. Response to botulinum injections
b. Movements being predominantly retrocollis
c. Hypertrophy of the neck muscles
d. Accompanying oral-buccal-lingual movements

answer: b, d. Both varieties of involuntary neck movements respond to botulinum toxin, but neither responds consistently to anticholinergic or other oral medications. Tardive dystonia is apt to be accompanied by other tardive dyskinesias.

368. Which of the following substances has an unpaired electron?

a. Monoamines
b. Free radicals
c. Dopamine
d. Choline acetyl transferase (ChAT)

answer: b. Free radicals are unstable atoms or molecules because they contain a single, unpaired electron. They seize electrons from adjacent atoms or molecules, which oxidize them. Methylphenylpyridinium (MPP^+), which is the metabolic product of MPTP, is the best-known example of a free radical.

369. Which of the following does not occur during sleep?

a. Periodic leg movements
b. Restless leg syndrome
c. Parkinson's disease tremor
d. Tics

e. Palatal myoclonus
f. Generalized seizures
g. Partial seizures
h. Migraines

> *answer:* c

370. A 19-year-old student developed progressively severe intellectual impairments over 1 year. Examination reveals a resting tremor, dysarthria, and rigidity. The cornea has a brown-green discoloration in its periphery. Liver function tests are abnormal. Which of the following is most likely to be found on further evaluation?

a. Trinucleotide repeats
b. Atrophy of the caudate nucleus
c. History of drug abuse
d. Decreased concentration of the serum protein that transports copper

> *answer:* d. He has Wilson's disease. His serum would contain insufficient ceruloplasmin, the copper-carrying protein. Trinucleotide repeats and atrophy of the caudate nucleus indicate Huntington's disease. Although not the case in this patient, drug abuse should be considered in progressive impairments in teenagers and young adults.

371. A 35-year-old alcoholic man with mild, chronic cirrhosis is brought to the Emergency Room because of agitation and belligerent behavior. Examination reveals disorientation, slurred speech, and asterixis. He has no nystagmus, extraocular paresis, pupillary abnormality, or lateralized signs. Laboratory data include the following: mildly abnormal liver function tests, 26% hematocrit, and blood in the stool. Which condition is the most likely cause of his behavioral disturbances and confusion?

a. Wernicke's encephalopathy
b. Alcohol-induced hypoglycemia
c. Hepatic encephalopathy

d. Subdural hematoma
e. Delirium tremens (DTs)

> *answer:* c. Hepatic encephalopathy from gastrointestinal bleeding is the most likely cause. People with cirrhosis or other causes of hepatic insufficiency will develop encephalopathy when gastrointestinal bleeding results from esophageal varices or gastric ulceration. Sometimes encephalopathy will follow a high-protein meal. In both cases, the protein breaks down in the intestine to form ammonia or other toxins. Mental changes and asterixis often occur, as in this case, before liver function tests become markedly abnormal. Medications for mental aberrations that require hepatic metabolism should be avoided or used sparingly.
>
> Wernicke's encephalopathy, alcohol-induced hypoglycemia, and subdural hematomas should be considered in alcoholics with mental changes. Even without particular indications of these diagnoses, treatment might include intravenous thiamine and, after blood tests are drawn, intravenous glucose.

APPENDIX 1
Patient and Family Support Groups

The following organizations provide patients and their families with educational, legal, medical, emotional, personal, or other assistance. However, people should be cautioned that, because sometimes these groups disproportionately represent incapacitated patients, a personal visit may be discouraging.

Acquired immune deficiency syndrome (AIDS)

Gay Men's Health Crisis
129 West 20th Street, New York, NY 10011
(212) 807-6664
FAX (212) 337-3656

Alzheimer's disease

Alzheimer's Disease and Related Disorders Association
919 North Michigan Avenue, Suite 1000, Chicago, IL 60611-1676
(312) 335-5720
(800) 272-3900
FAX (312) 335-1110

Amyotrophic lateral sclerosis (ALS)

The Amyotrophic Lateral Sclerosis Association
21021 Ventura Boulevard, #321, Woodland Hills, CA 91364
(818) 340-7500

Aphasia and related disorders

American Speech-Language-Hearing Association
10801 Rockville Pike, Rockville, Maryland 20852
(301) 897-5700
FAX (301) 571-0457

National Aphasia Association
P.O. Box 1887, Murray Hill Station, New York, NY 10156-0611
(212) 340-6025
(800) 922-4622

Blindness

American Foundation for the Blind
15 West 16th Street, New York, NY 10011
(212) 620-2000
FAX (212) 727-7418

Blepharospasm

Benign Essential Blepharospasm Research Foundation
P.O. Box 12468, Beaumont, TX 77726-2468
(409) 832-0788

Brain tumors

American Brain Tumor Association
2720 River Road, Suite 146, Des Plaines, IL 60018
(708) 827-9910
(800) 886-2282
FAX (708) 827-9918

American Cancer Society
19 West 56th Street, New York, NY 10019
(212) 586-8700
FAX (212) 237-3852

National Brain Tumor Foundation
785 Market Street, Suite 1600, San Francisco, CA 94103
(800) 934-CURE
FAX (415) 284-0209

Cerebral palsy

United Cerebral Palsy Foundation
330 West 34th Street, 13th Floor, New York, NY 10001
(212) 947-5770

Dystonia

Dystonia Medical Research Foundation
One East Wacker Drive, Suite 2900
Chicago, IL 60601-2001
(312) 755-0198
FAX (312) 321-5710

Dystonia Medical Research Foundation
777 Hornby Street, Suite 1800, Vancouver, B.C. V6Z 2K3
(604) 661-4886

Epilepsy

Epilepsy Foundation of America
4351 Garden City Drive, Landover, MD 20785
(301) 459-3700
FAX (301) 577-4951

Guillain-Barré syndrome

Guillain-Barré Syndrome Support Group
P.O. Box 262, Wynnewood, PA 19096
(215) 649-7837

Head injury

National Head Injury Foundation
1776 Massachusetts Avenue NW, #100, Washington, DC 20036
(202) 296-6443
(800) 444-6443
FAX (202) 296-8850

Huntington's disease

Huntington's Disease Association
140 West 22nd Street, 6th Floor, New York, NY 10011-2420
(212) 242-1968
FAX (212) 243-2443

Migraine and headache

American Association for the Study of Headache
875 Kings Highway, Suite 200, Woodbury, NJ 08096
(609) 845-0322

The National Headache Foundation
5252 North Western Avenue, Chicago, IL 60625
(312) 878-7715
FAX (312) 907-6278

Multiple sclerosis

National Multiple Sclerosis Association of America (MSAA)
601 White Horse Pike, Oaklyn, NJ 08107
(800) 833-4MSA
FAX (609) 858-8882

National Multiple Sclerosis Society
30 West 26th Street, New York, NY 10010-2094
(212) 463-7787
FAX (212) 989-4362

Muscular dystrophy and related disorders

Muscular Dystrophy Association of America
810 Seventh Avenue, New York, NY 10019
(212) 689-9040

Muscular Dystrophy Association
3300 East Sunrise Drive, Tucson, AZ 85718
(602) 529-2000
FAX (602) 529-5300

Myasthenia gravis

Myasthenia Gravis Foundation
61 Gramercy Park North, Room 605, New York, NY 10010
(212) 533-7005

The Myasthenia Gravis Foundation of America—National Office
222 South Riverside Plaza, Suite 1540, Chicago, IL 60606
(312) 258-0522
(800) 541-5454
FAX (312) 258-0461

Neurofibromatosis

The National Neurofibromatosis Foundation
95 Pine Street, 16th Floor, New York, NY, 10005
(212) 344-6633
FAX (212) 747-0004

Pain

American Chronic Pain Association
P.O. Box 850, Rocklin, CA 95677
(916) 632-0922
FAX (916) 632-3208

International Association for the Study of Pain
909 N.E. 43rd Street, Suite 306, Seattle, WA 98105-602
(206) 547-6409
FAX (206) 547-1703

Parkinson's disease

National Parkinson Foundation
1501 NW 9th Avenue / Bob Hope Road, Miami, FL 33136
(800) 327-4545
(800) 433-7022 (Florida)
FAX (305) 548-4403

Parkinson's Disease Foundation
710 West 168th Street, New York, NY 10032
(212) 923-4700

United Parkinson's Foundation
833 West Washington Boulevard, Chicago, IL 60607
(312) 733-1893

Paraplegia

See *Spinal cord injury*

Postpolio syndrome

International Polio Network
5100 Oakland Avenue #206, St. Louis, MO 63110
(314) 534-0475
FAX (314) 534-5070

Rett syndrome

International Rett Syndrome Association
9121 Piscataway Road, Clinton MD 20735
(800) 818-RETT

Sleep disorders

American Sleep Disorders Association
1610 14th Street NW, Suite 300, Rochester, MN 55901
(507) 287-6006
FAX (507) 287-6008

Spasmodic dysphonia

National Spasmodic Dysphonia Association
P.O. Box 203, Atwood, CA 92601-0203
(800) 714-6732

Our Voice
799 Broadway, Suite 640, New York, NY 10003
(212) 929-4299

Spasmodic torticollis

National Spasmodic Torticollis Association
P.O. Box 476, Elm Grove, WI 58122
(800) HURTFUL

Spinal cord injury

American Paralysis Association
500 Morris Avenue, Springfield, NJ 07081
(800) 526-3456

Paralyzed Veterans of America
801 18th Street NW, Washington, DC 20006
(202) 872-1300

Stroke

American Heart Association
7272 Greenville Avenue, Dallas, TX 75231
(214) 373-6300

National Stroke Association
8948 East Orchard Road, Suite 1000, Englewood, CO 80111-5015
(303) 762-9922
(800) STROKES
FAX (303) 771-1886

Tourette syndrome

Tourette Syndrome Association
42-40 Bell Boulevard, Bayside, NY 11361-2861
(718) 224-2999
(800) 237-0717
FAX (718) 279-9596

Tuberous sclerosis

National Tuberous Sclerosis Association
8000 Corporate Drive, Suite 120, Landover, MD 20785
(301) 459-0394
(800) 225-6872
FAX (301) 459-0394

Tremor

International Tremor Foundation
833 West Washington Boulevard, Chicago, IL 60607
(312) 733-1893

Wilson's disease

National Center for the Study of Wilson's Disease
432 West 58th Street, Suite 614, New York, NY 10019
(212) 523-8717
FAX (212) 523-8708

APPENDIX 2
Expenses of Medical and Diagnostic Procedures

The approximate cost of various medical and diagnostic procedures in New York City in 1995 are given below.

Procedure	Cost (dollars)
Annual cost of azidothymidine (AZT) treatment for AIDS	10,000
Computed tomography (CT) of head	350
CT of head with contrast	375
CT of spine	450
DNA test for	
Fragile X	250
Huntington's disease	250
Myotonic dystrophy	250
Dystrophin Western blot (for Duchenne's muscular dystrophy)	750
Electroencephalogram (EEG)	240
With video-telemetry	500
Electromyography (EMG)	250–500
Evoked response testing	300–500
Lumbar puncture (spinal tap)	500
Magnetic resonance imaging (MRI) of head	1000
MRI of head with gadolinium	1200
Nerve conduction velocity (NCV), per nerve	50
Typical cost for a study	500
Nocturnal penile tumescence (NPT) studies	1000
Nursing home care, annual	62,000
Penile prostheses and other treatment for erectile dysfunction	
Implants	
Inflatable	4000
Semirigid	4000
Injections of vasoactive medications, per erection	8
Vacuum devices	400
Polysomnography (PSG) sleep studies	2000
Positron emission tomography (PET)	1500
Single-photon emission computed tomography (SPECT)	600
Syphilis tests	
Fluorescent treponemal antibody absorption (FTA-ABS)	35
Rapid plasma reagin (RPR)	11
Treponema microhemagglutination assay (MHA-TP)	35
Venereal Disease Research Laboratory (VDRL)	18

APPENDIX 3
Chromosomes and the Diseases They Transmit

Chromosome Number	Disease
4	Huntington's disease
5	Tay-Sachs disease
	Infantile and juvenile spinal muscular atrophy
6	Narcolepsy
9	Dystonia musculorum deformans
	Tuberous sclerosis
	Friedreich's ataxia
10	Metachromatic leukodystrophy
11	Acute intermittent porphyria
	Ataxia telangiectasia
12	Phenylketonuria
	Tuberous sclerosis
13	Wilson's disease
14	Porphyria variegata
	Alzheimer's disease, early onset
15	Tay-Sachs disease, GM2 gangliosidosis
	Dyslexia
16	Tuberous sclerosis
17	Charcot-Marie-Tooth
	Neurofibromatosis-1, peripheral, von Recklinghausen
18	Tourette's syndrome
19	Myotonic dystrophy
	Alzheimer's disease, familial, late onset
	Malignant hyperthermia (ryanodine receptor)
20	Creutzfeldt-Jakob, familial prion disease (Gerstmann-Scheinker-Strauss)
21	Alzheimer's disease, early onset familial
	Amyotrophic lateral sclerosis (ALS), familial
	Progressive myoclonic epilepsy
22	Neurofibromatosis-2, familial acoustic neuroma
	Metachromatic leukodystrophy
X	Mental retardation, nonspecific
	Duchenne's muscular dystrophy
	Lesch-Nyhan syndrome
	Becker's muscular dystrophy
	Fragile X, mental retardation
	Adrenoleukodystrophy
	Spastic paraplegia

DISEASES TRANSMITTED BY MITOCHONDRIA

Kearns-Sayre syndrome
Progressive external ophthalmoplegia
MERRF (myoclonic epilepsy, ragged red fibers)
MELAS (mitochondrial encephalomyopathy, lactic acidosis, stroke)
Cytochrome c oxidase deficiency
Leigh's syndrome

DISEASES TRANSMITTED BY CHROMOSOMES (NUMBER) OR MITOCHONDRIA (*)

Acute intermittent porphyria (11)
Adrenoleukodystrophy (X)
Alzheimer's disease, early onset familial (21)
Alzheimer's disease, late onset familial (14, 19)
Amyotrophic lateral sclerosis (ALS), familial (21)
Ataxia telangiectasia (11)
Becker's muscular dystrophy (X)
Charcot-Marie-Tooth (17)
Creutzfeldt-Jakob, familial prion disease (20)
   (Gerstmann-Scheinker-Strauss)
Cytochrome c oxidase deficiency*
Duchenne's muscular dystrophy (X)
Dyslexia (15)
Dystonia musculorum deformans (9)
Fragile X, mental retardation (X)
Friedreich's ataxia (9)
Huntington's disease (4)
Kearns-Sayre syndrome*
Leigh's syndrome*
Lesch-Nyhan syndrome (X)
Malignant hyperthermia (ryanodine receptor) (19)
MELAS (mitochondrial encephalomyopathy, lactic acidosis, stroke)*
Mental retardation, nonspecific (X)
MERRF (myoclonic epilepsy, ragged red fibers)*
Metachromatic leukodystrophy (10)
Myotonic muscular dystrophy (19)
Narcolepsy (6)
Neurofibromatosis-1, peripheral, von Recklinghausen (17)
Neurofibromatosis-2, acoustic neuroma (22)
Phenylketonuria (12)
Porphyria variegata (14)
Progressive external ophthalmoplegia*
Progressive myoclonic epilepsy (21)
Spastic paraplegia (X)
Spinal muscular atrophy (5)
Tay-Sachs disease (5)
Tay-Sachs disease, GM2 gangliosidosis (15)
Tourette's syndrome (18)
Tuberous sclerosis (9, 16)*
Wilson's disease (13)

*Some uncertainties or discrepancies are attributable to different families transmitting on different chromosomes.

REFERENCES

Rowland LP: The first decade of molecular genetics in neurology. Ann Neurol *32*: 207–214, 1992
Martin JB: Molecular genetics in neurology. Ann Neurol *34*: 757–773, 1993
Rosenberg RN: A neurological gene map. Arch Neurol *50*: 1269–71, 1993

INDEX

Note: Page numbers in *italics* indicate figures; page numbers followed by t indicate tables.

ISBN 0-7216-5829-6

90038